HINNENTHAL

Emerging Strategies for the Treatment of Neuropathic Pain

Mission Statement of IASP Press®

The International Association for the Study of Pain (IASP) is a nonprofit, interdisciplinary organization devoted to understanding the mechanisms of pain and improving the care of patients with pain through research, education, and communication. The organization includes scientists and health care professionals dedicated to these goals. The IASP sponsors scientific meetings and publishes newsletters, technical bulletins, the journal *Pain,* and books.

The goal of IASP Press is to provide the IASP membership with timely, high-quality, attractive, low-cost publications relevant to the problem of pain. These publications are also intended to appeal to a wider audience of scientists and clinicians interested in the problem of pain.

Emerging Strategies for the Treatment of Neuropathic Pain

Editors

James N. Campbell, MD

Department of Neurosurgery, The Johns Hopkins University School of Medicine, Baltimore, Maryland, USA

Allan I. Basbaum, PhD

Department of Anatomy, W.M. Keck Foundation Center for Integrative Neuroscience, School of Medicine, University of California, San Francisco, California, USA

André Dray, PhD

AstraZeneca Research and Development Montreal, Montreal, Quebec, Canada

Ronald Dubner, DDS, PhD

Department of Oral and Craniofacial Biomedical Sciences, Dental School, University of Maryland, Baltimore, Maryland, USA

Robert H. Dworkin, PhD

Anesthesiology Clinical Research Center, Department of Anesthesiology, School of Medicine, University of Rochester, Rochester, New York, USA

Christine N. Sang, MD, MPH

Translational Pain Research, Department of Anesthesiology, Pain, and Perioperative Medicine, Brigham and Women's Hospital, School of Medicine, Harvard University, Boston, Massachusetts, USA

IASP PRESS® • **SEATTLE**

Library of Congress Cataloging-in-Publication Data

Emerging strategies for the treatment of neuropathic pain / editor, James N. Campbell ... [et al.].
   p. ; cm.
 Includes bibliographical references and index.
 ISBN 0-931092-61-2 (alk. paper)
  1. Pain--Chemotherapy--Congresses. 2. Neuralgia--Chemotherapy--Congresses. 3. Central pain--Chemotherapy--Congresses. I. Campbell, James N., 1948- II. International Association for the Study of Pain.
 [DNLM: 1. Pain--therapy--Congresses. 2. Nervous System Diseases--therapy--Congresses. WL 704 E53 2006]
 RB127.E52 2006
 616'.0472--dc22

2005055225

Published by:

IASP Press
International Association for the Study of Pain
111 Queen Anne Ave N, Suite 501
Seattle, WA 98109-4955, USA
Fax: 206-283-9403
www.iasp-pain.org
www.painbooks.org

Printed in the United States of America

Contents

Contributing Authors

Ralf Baron, Dr med *Department of Neurological Pain Research and Therapy, Christian-Albrechts University, Kiel, Germany*

Allan I. Basbaum, PhD *Department of Anatomy, W.M. Keck Foundation Center for Integrative Neuroscience, San Francisco, California, USA*

M. Catherine Bushnell, PhD *McGill Centre for Research on Pain, Montreal, Quebec, Canada*

Beata Buzas, PhD *Pain and Neurosensory Mechanisms Branch, National Institute of Dental and Craniofacial Research, National Institutes of Health, Department of Health and Human Services, Bethesda, Maryland, USA*

James N. Campbell, MD *Department of Neurosurgery, The Johns Hopkins University School of Medicine, Baltimore, Maryland, USA*

Sandra R. Chaplan, MD *Johnson & Johnson Pharmaceutical R&D, San Diego, California, USA*

Iain Chessell, PhD *Neurology CEDD, GlaxoSmithKline, Harlow, United Kingdom*

Michael J. Detke, MD, PhD *Lilly Research Laboratories, Eli Lilly and Company, Indianapolis, Indiana; Indiana University School of Medicine, Indianapolis, Indiana; McLean Hospital and Harvard Medical School, Belmont, Massachusetts, USA*

Marshall Devor, PhD *Department of Cell and Animal Biology, Institute of Life Sciences and Center for Research on Pain, Hebrew University of Jerusalem, Jerusalem, Israel*

André Dray, PhD *AstraZeneca Research and Development Montreal, Montreal, Quebec, Canada*

Ronald Dubner, DDS, PhD *Department of Biomedical Sciences, University of Maryland Dental School, Baltimore, Maryland, USA*

Robert H. Dworkin, PhD *Department of Anesthesiology, University of Rochester School of Medicine and Dentistry, Rochester, New York, USA*

James C. Eisenach, MS, MD *Department of Anesthesia, Wake Forest University School of Medicine, Winston Salem, North Carolina, USA*

M. Dolores Ferrer-Garcia, MD, PhD *Department of Anesthesiology, IMAS Hospitals, Barcelona, Spain*

Robert W. Gereau IV, PhD *Washington University Pain Center, Departments of Anesthesiology and Anatomy and Neurobiology, Washington University School of Medicine, St. Louis, Missouri, USA*

John W. Griffin, MD *Department of Neurology, Johns Hopkins University School of Medicine, Baltimore, Maryland, USA*

Michael S. Gold, PhD *Department of Biomedical Sciences, Dental School; Program in Neuroscience; and Department of Anatomy and Neurobiology, Medical School, University of Maryland, Baltimore, Maryland, USA*

Donna L. Hammond, PhD *Department of Anesthesia, The University of Iowa, Iowa City, Iowa, USA*

Ahmet Höke, MD, PhD, FRCP *Department of Neurology, Johns Hopkins Hospital, Baltimore, Maryland, USA*

Smriti Iyengar, PhD *Neuroscience Research, Lilly Research Laboratories, Eli Lilly and Company, Indianapolis, Indiana, USA*

Fredrik Kamme, PhD *Johnson & Johnson Pharmaceutical R&D, LLC, San Diego, California, USA*

Stefanie A. Kane, PhD *Pain Research Department, Merck & Co. Inc., West Point, Pennsylvania, USA*

Martin Koltzenburg, Dr med *Institute of Child Health, University College London, London, United Kingdom*

Jean Claude Louis, MD, PhD *AMGEN, Thousand Oaks, California, USA*

Katalin Lukacs, MD, PhD *School of Medicine, Chelsea and Westminster Hospital, London, United Kingdom*

Donald C. Manning, MD, PhD *Celgene Corporation, Summit, New Jersey, USA*

Patrick W. Mantyh, PhD *NeuroSystems Laboratory, University of Minnesota, Minneapolis, Minnesota, USA*

Mitchell B. Max, MD *Pain and Neurosensory Mechanisms Branch, National Institute of Dental and Craniofacial Research, National Institutes of Health, Department of Health and Human Services, Bethesda, Maryland, USA*

Michael Merzenich, PhD *Department of Otolaryngology, University of California San Francisco, San Francisco, California, USA*

Richard A. Meyer, MS *Departments of Neurosurgery and Biomedical Engineering and Applied Physics Laboratory, Johns Hopkins University, Baltimore, Maryland, USA*

Randall W. Moreadith, MD, PhD *Renovis, Inc., South San Francisco, California, USA*

Istvan Nagy, MD, PhD *Department of Anaesthesiology and Intensive Care, Imperial College London; School of Medicine, Chelsea and Westminster Hospital, London, United Kingdom*

Michael H. Ossipov, PhD *Health Sciences Center, University of Arizona, Tucson, Arizona, USA*

Karin L. Petersen, MD *UCSF Pain Clinical Research, San Francisco, California, USA*

Frank Porreca, PhD *Department of Pharmacology, Health Sciences Center, University of Arizona, Tucson, Arizona, USA*

Donald D. Price, PhD *Departments of Oral and Maxillofacial Surgery, University of Florida College of Dentistry, Gainesville, Florida, USA*

Matthias Ringkamp, MD *Department of Neurosurgery, The Johns Hopkins University School of Medicine, Baltimore, Maryland, USA*

Michael W. Salter, MD, PhD *The Hospital for Sick Children, Toronto, Ontario, Canada*

Christine N. Sang, MD, MPH *Translational Pain Research, Brigham and Women's Hospital, School of Medicine, Harvard University, Boston, Massachusetts, USA*

Peter Santha, MD, PhD *Department of Physiology, University of Szeged, Szeged, Hungary*

William K. Schmidt, PhD *Renovis, Inc., South San Francisco, California, USA*

Toni Shippenberg, PhD *Integrative Neuroscience Section, National Institute of Drug Abuse, National Institutes of Health, Bethesda, Maryland, USA*

Roland Staud, MD *McKnight Brain Institute, Gainesville, Florida, USA*

Rolf-Detlef Treede, Dr med *Institute of Physiology and Pathophysiology, Johannes Gutenberg-University, Mainz, Germany*

Laszlo Urban, MD, PhD *Preclinical Compound Profiling, Lead Discovery Center, Discovery Technologies, Novartis Institutes for BioMedical Research, Inc., Cambridge, Massachusetts, USA*

Charles J. Vierck, PhD *Department of Neuroscience and McKnight Brain Institute, University of Florida College of Medicine, Gainesville, Florida, USA*

Joachim F. Wernicke, MD *Lilly Research Laboratories, Eli Lilly and Company, Indianapolis, Indiana, USA*

William D. Willis, Jr., MD, PhD *Department of Neuroscience and Cell Biology, University of Texas Medical Branch, Galveston, Texas, USA*

Jon-Kar Zubieta, MD, PhD *Mental Health Research Institute, University of Michigan, Ann Arbor, Michigan, USA*

Acknowledgments

The editors gratefully acknowledge unrestricted educational grants from each of the following organizations that made possible the conference and this publication:

Abbott Laboratories
Adolor Corporation
AlgoRx Pharmaceuticals, Inc.
Amgen
AstraZeneca Pharmaceuticals LP
Celgene Corporation
GlaxoSmithKline Inc.
Johnson & Johnson/Ortho McNeil Pharmaceutical, Inc.
Eli Lilly and Company
Merck & Co., Inc.
Novartis Pharmaceuticals Corporation
Pfizer, Inc.
Renovis, Inc.

Preface

On April 13, 2005, we began a five-day meeting in Scottsdale, Arizona, with the express purpose of furthering the development of new ways to treat the problem of neuropathic pain and to produce this book. This book provides the background for our deliberations and also summarizes the discussions themselves. This intensive effort involved 40 participants from academia and the pharmaceutical industry, all regarded internationally as leading experts in the field.

Pain is a major health care problem for which current treatments are often inadequate. The tangible costs economically are in the many tens of billions of dollars, and the costs in terms of human suffering, while difficult to measure in dollars, are known only too well to practitioners who seek to help these patients. Demographics indicate that with the aging population these problems will only grow. Moreover, we see setbacks. One innovation of the past decade was the introduction of selective COX-2 inhibitors. Now use of this therapy has been sharply curtailed because of the emerging evidence for cardiovascular risks.

The problem of neuropathic pain has always intrigued scientists and clinicians, but only in recent years has this particular form of pain been appreciated for its overall magnitude as a clinical problem. Gabapentin deserves much of the credit. Although developed to treat epilepsy, gabapentin was soon shown by clinicians to help many patients with neuropathic pain. Peak annual sales of the drug for pain have exceeded a billion dollars. This staggering growth in sales reveals the true magnitude of the problem of neuropathic pain.

The pharmaceutical industry has made definite strides in bringing new therapies to bear on the problem of neuropathic pain, but to the suffering patient this progress must seem glacially slow. In an age of medical miracles, why should people still suffer from severe chronic pain? Many would say that the best therapy for serious pain remains one of the oldest treatments— morphine. However, opioid therapy remains entangled in the morass of the pervasive problem of drug abuse. Policy makers strive for a balance between patient access to legitimate care and the fight against addiction. One might think that by now we would have found a way to deliver opioids in a way that obviates the abuse problem, but we have not. Of course, for all drug treatments we strive to maximize benefit and minimize adverse effects. For new and old therapies, this ratio is often unfavorable. For too many patients, the current choice is between barely tolerable side effects versus pain relief, if indeed pain relief is to be had at all.

There is hope, however, and this book, the outcome of a novel think-tank conference among industry leaders and researchers from the academic sector, addresses this hope. There has been a rapid acceleration in the discovery of new molecular targets, and opportunities are abundant. The choices for industry in terms of selecting these targets for drug development are, however, formidable.

Costs for drug development are daunting, particularly when it comes to clinical trials. We need to pick targets accurately and have methods that will establish clinical "proof of concept" as expeditiously as possible. We still see a mismatch between animal model outcomes and limitations of clinical information and modeling. New therapeutic concepts have progressed slowly because of weaknesses in translational methods that bridge animal and human pain research.

By way of a seed grant from Novartis Pharmaceuticals, we convened a series of strategy meetings to determine how to confront these issues. Many traditional conferences offer conventional lectures, with only minutes left for discussion. These meetings are important and useful, but they do not offer the opportunity to delve in depth into the many issues that bar progress. Our approach was to put the lectures into written materials that could be digested before the meeting and use the meeting time to create, critique, and debate how best to develop new treatments for neuropathic pain. This effort had, in our opinion, to be a marriage of academia and industry. We needed to keep the group small. And we wanted an end product. Much of the book was written before the meeting. Nearly all of these chapters were then re-written post-meeting. Finally, four of the chapters, which summarize the deliberations of the different groups that met in discussion, were written during the meeting. The contents of these rapporteurs' reports were discussed on the final day of the meeting, revised after the meeting, and included in the book along with the chapters that were written in advance of the meeting.

This meeting was modeled after the well-known Dahlem workshops held in Berlin. In most meetings, many participants come and go, but not in this Dahlem-styled meeting. Cell-phones, e-mail, and much of the rest of the world were shut out over the course of four and a half days. Meetings started early and went into the evening. There were four main groups. The groups met by themselves initially, but then met with each of the other groups, pursuing an agenda that was established on the first day. Rapporteurs, with the help of their colleagues, kept careful notes of the proceedings. Smaller groups engaged in intense writing sessions just before all four groups met together for a final summation.

The topics for each group were chosen with great care and reflected themes for drug development.

PERIPHERAL NERVOUS SYSTEM TARGETS

Many neuropathic pain conditions stem from a lesion that affects primary afferent nociceptive fibers. Thus it is appealing to develop strategies of treatment that specifically focus on this group of patients. The concept that abnormal activity in nociceptive afferents triggers and maintains neuropathic pain remains a heuristic model. Nociceptive afferents express receptors, surface molecules, and channels and use a variety of biochemical processes that distinguish them from other sensory neurons, and from other cells in general. Attacking these targets provides promise, but the utility of targeting individual molecules is unclear. Nerve injury leads to events that promote nerve regeneration, some of which may be maladaptive, contributing to the phenotype of the neuropathic pain condition. In addition, some of the molecules and cellular processes concerned with regeneration may lead to abnormal discharges in nociceptive afferents.

CENTRAL NERVOUS SYSTEM TARGETS

Therapies directed at the CNS provide further opportunities for pain treatment. The CNS is important because maladaptive plasticity of function at several levels of the neuraxis almost certainly contributes to the development and persistence of neuropathic pain. Neurotransmitter modulators hold the promise of beneficially affecting nociceptive processing. Neuronal interactions with glial and other support cells may promote lasting pain. Attacking these interactions may be beneficial. Changes in neural processing brought about by neural injury may also lead to persistent pain. Clearly, injury to the spinal cord and brain, through trauma, vascular disease, and other pathological processes may lead to pain problems with very limited therapeutic options. The dorsal horn has been extensively studied, and many new directions for pain treatment should emerge from this knowledge. However, we ignore the rest of the CNS at our peril. How can drug development aimed at other central targets proceed in a practical way?

DISEASE-SPECIFIC TARGETS

Certain diseases are notorious for producing neuropathic pain. Postherpetic neuralgia, diabetic neuropathy, compression neuropathies, and trigeminal neuralgia are but a few examples. The extent to which the pain in these diseases represents distinctive nervous system pathophysiology must be determined. It is entirely possible that advances in treatment for neuropathic pain must await the development of specific disease therapies. For example, the effects of a simple axotomy have often been used as a model for neuropathic pain. In actuality, traumatic axotomy in humans accounts for a small percentage of the cases of neuropathic pain. Understanding how diabetes affects nociceptive neurons may lead to therapies that address this underlying pathophysiology.

How can molecules be screened better in early-stage clinical trials to determine the likelihood of correcting the effects on nociceptive processing? Will it be possible in the future to develop a signature of different diseases based on biomarkers, psychophysics, brain imaging, and genomic approaches?

DEVELOPMENT OF MEASUREMENT TOOLS AND APPLICATIONS OF NEW TECHNOLOGIES

Success will also involve the development of novel technologies. Among the approaches to be considered are downregulation of pronociceptive molecules, which might be achieved, for example, by delivery of RNAi by intrathecal injection. By contrast, viral delivery techniques may open doors to altering gene expression in dorsal root ganglion cells, for example, by upregulating expression of "pain" inhibitory molecules and receptors. Molecular "neurosurgery" may be accomplished with toxins, such as saporin-tagged ligands or antibodies that allow selective destruction of pain-signaling cells. The introduction of midline myelotomy to treat visceral pain and motor cortex stimulation to treat atypical facial and post-stroke pain suggests that ablative and stimulation strategies have yet to be fully exploited.

A second charge for this group was to consider how improvements in measurement might facilitate drug development and treatment. At present, simple withdrawal measurements dominate animal psychophysical techniques. Advances in imaging, development of biological markers, and advances in psychophysical techniques should improve our chances to learn more about mechanisms and treatment.

Finally, there are generic issues that crosscut all these considerations. What is neuropathic pain, and how do mechanisms of neuropathic pain differ from those that lead to persistent pain that is not neuropathic? What are the models that should be used in drug development? What proof-of-concept models can be used in phase I/II human trials that will expedite better decision making about whether to pursue phase II/III testing? Success in finding new therapies depends on finding capital-efficient techniques to order to make the cost manageable.

THE END PRODUCT

We intend for this book to represent not only the state of the art, but also a blueprint for what is to come. Neuropathic pain is a daunting and important problem. We need new approaches, new understandings of mechanisms, and finally new treatments. We will have achieved our goal if a reader coming into the field uses this book to frame the specific aims and the background and significance of a new NIH research proposal. Did we achieve our goal? We shall see.

It is hard to represent the intensity and intellectual vigor that permeated this meeting in a book. It is also hard to write by committee. On the other hand, it is a thing of beauty to watch colleagues working together in small groups, debating the course of our young field.

This is our best shot for the moment. Clearly there is momentum, but many challenges and opportunities await us. The editors recognize the great effort put forward by the attendees from both academia and the pharmaceutical industry. To them we offer our heartfelt thanks for an unforgettable meeting and, we hope, an unforgettable book. We also thank the talented staff of IASP Press, who worked faithfully to make this book a reality. This book and the meeting would simply not have happened except for the masterful stewardship of Paul Lambiase. We all owe him heartfelt gratitude. This meeting was financed entirely by the pharmaceutical industry. The grants were made without strings attached. The sponsors have the vision that the community of science is the engine of new ideas. Finally, we extend our thoughts to the many patients who suffer the ravages of neurological diseases that lead to pain and suffering. We dedicate this book to them.

JAMES N. CAMPBELL, MD
ALLAN I. BASBAUM, PhD
ANDRÉ DRAY, PhD
RONALD DUBNER, DDS, PhD
ROBERT H. DWORKIN, PhD
CHRISTINE N. SANG, MD, MPH

Part I

Peripheral Nervous System Targets

Emerging Strategies for the Treatment of Neuropathic Pain, edited by James N. Campbell, Allan I. Basbaum, André Dray, Ronald Dubner, Robert H. Dworkin, and Christine N. Sang, IASP Press, Seattle, © 2006.

1

Peripheral Nervous System Targets: Rapporteur Report

Michael S. Gold,[a] Iain Chessell,[b] Marshall Devor,[c] Andy Dray,[d] Robert W. Gereau IV,[e] Stefanie A. Kane,[f] Martin Koltzenburg,[g] Jean Claude Louis,[h] Matthias Ringkamp,[i] and Rolf-Detlef Treede[j]

[a]Department of Biomedical Sciences, Dental School; Program in Neuroscience; and Department of Anatomy and Neurobiology, Medical School, University of Maryland, Baltimore, Maryland, USA; [b]Neurology CEDD, GlaxoSmithkline, Harlow, United Kingdom; [c]Department of Cell and Animal Biology, Institute of Life Sciences and Center for Research on Pain, Hebrew University of Jerusalem, Jerusalem, Israel; [d]AstraZeneca Research & Development Montreal, Montreal, Quebec, Canada; [e]Washington University Pain Center, Departments of Anesthesiology and Anatomy and Neurobiology, Washington University School of Medicine, St. Louis, Missouri, USA; [f]Pain Research Department, Merck & Co, Inc., West Point, Pennsylvania, USA; [g]Institute of Child Health, University College London, London, United Kingdom; [h]AMGEN, Thousand Oaks, California, USA; [i]Department of Neurosurgery, Johns Hopkins University, Baltimore, Maryland, USA; [j]Institute of Physiology and Pathophysiology, Johannes Gutenberg-University, Mainz, Germany

Depending on the site of damage to the somatosensory system, neuropathic pain syndromes may be classified as peripheral or central. Because the underlying lesions and diseases differ, peripheral and central syndromes have distinct diagnoses, necessitating a differential clinical approach. As to mechanisms, those of central pain appear to reside entirely within the central nociceptive system, whereas peripheral neuropathic pain involves both peripheral and central neural mechanisms.

Potential peripheral nervous system (PNS) targets for the treatment of neuropathic pain can be evaluated within the following framework, which is summarized in Fig. 1. (1) Sensory transduction processes underlying the conversion of energy from the environment (thermal, mechanical, or chemical)

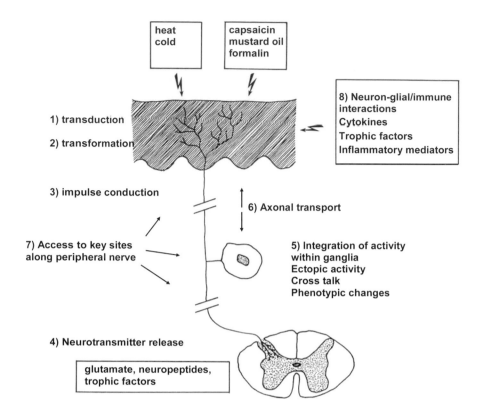

Fig. 1. The primary sensory neuron. Primary nociceptive afferents terminate as free nerve endings of Aδ or C fibers in the skin and other tissues. Their principal sensory functions consist of (1) transduction of external or internal chemical or physical stimuli into generator potentials, (2) transformation of generator potentials into trains of action potentials, (3) action potential propagation toward the central nervous system, and (4) presynaptic release of neurotransmitters and neuromodulators. The sensory neuron cell body (5) appears to be a site critical for the integration of neural activity in nociceptive afferents under normal conditions and may become a site of aberrant activity under pathological conditions. Axonal transport (6) of proteins in both anterograde and retrograde directions appears be critical for maintaining afferent phenotype under normal conditions, and for initiating changes in phenotype under pathological conditions. Axonal transport may also be a mechanism of shuttling critical mediators such as cytokines from the periphery to central targets. Blood- and tissue-nerve barriers (7) limit drug access to potential therapeutic targets in peripheral nerves. However, both the cell body and peripheral terminals are relatively accessible under normal conditions, and their accessibility may increase at critical points following nerve injury. Neuroimmune interactions have been depicted in the peripheral tissue, where they play an important role in inflammatory pain. In neuropathic pain, neuron-glial and neuroimmune interactions (8) may occur along the entire length of the primary sensory neuron. These nerve fibers are axons of neurons situated in the dorsal root ganglion or trigeminal ganglion.

into a change in membrane potential (generator potential). (2) Transformation of generator potentials into trains of action potentials. (3) Action potential propagation. (4) Neurotransmitter release. (5) Integration of activity within the dorsal root ganglion (i.e., the impact of action potential invasion on transcription and translation, cross-excitation, and ectopic action potential generation). (6) Axonal transport and trophic signaling. (7) Access to the systemic and local chemical milieu through the blood-nerve barrier or tissue-nerve barrier. (8) Neuron-glial interaction and neuroimmune interaction.

The first two processes usually occur at the peripheral terminals within the innervated target tissue. Following nerve injury, they may also occur at other sites ("ectopic activity"). One possible site of ectopic action potential generation is the soma within sensory ganglia (i.e., the dorsal root and trigeminal ganglia), which may also be a site for the integration of sensory signals under both physiological and pathophysiological conditions. Action potential propagation is an important common pathway for information transmission to the central nervous system (CNS), but it is not the only pathway. Axonal transport and trophic signaling also appear to be critical for maintenance of target connection, which in turn determines the stable phenotype of both sensory neurons and their spinal targets of innervation. Neurotransmitter release, occurring within the CNS, is clearly critical for the transmission of sensory information and is usually considered in the context of central neural mechanisms of neuropathic pain. Given that the same cellular mechanisms that mediate transmitter release may also operate in other parts of the primary nociceptive neuron (i.e., in peripheral terminals and within the sensory ganglia), these mechanisms should also be considered as potential targets for peripheral analgesia. Because the peripheral parts of the primary nociceptive neuron are situated outside the blood-brain barrier, these sites may be more accessible for drug intervention. However, drug penetration through the blood-nerve barrier or tissue-nerve barrier also needs to be considered. Finally, neurons can interact with glial cells and, in the case of neural damage, also with immune cells.

This chapter is based on the consensus of its authors, who were all participants of a group focused on PNS targets at a colloquium on neuropathic pain. It has been organized into sections that reflect the discussions of key issues. Each section is followed by consensus statements as well as research questions.

CONCEPTUAL FRAMEWORK AND TERMINOLOGY

Key terminology related to neuropathic pain is defined in this section. We discuss the prioritization of neuropathic pain mechanisms into four hierarchical levels and consider the general concept of what insight may be expected from models of neuropathic pain.

ALLODYNIA VERSUS HYPERALGESIA

In the current IASP taxonomy (Merskey and Bogduk 1994), allodynia and hyperalgesia, cardinal features of neuropathic pain, are defined as follows: *Allodynia:* pain induced by stimuli that are not normally painful. *Hyperalgesia:* increased pain to a stimulus that is normally painful. Taken literally, these definitions would mean that any reduction in pain threshold is termed "allodynia," whereas increased pain in response to suprathreshold stimuli is termed "hyperalgesia" (Cervero and Laird 1996). Because the neural mechanisms of sensitization (both peripheral and central) typically cause a leftward shift in the stimulus-response function, which encompasses both reduced thresholds and increased suprathreshold responses, allodynia and hyperalgesia might co-exist in most cases. The overuse of the term "allodynia" in animal behavioral studies is largely due to the use of withdrawal threshold measures without any suprathreshold tests. In most cases, this "allodynia" bears no resemblance to the clinical phenomenon (Treede et al. 2004). The clinical characteristics of the phenomenon for which IASP commissioned the new word "allodynia" (Merskey et al. 1979; Koltzenburg et al. 1992) consist of pain elicited by gentle, often moving, tactile stimuli. This phenomenon is appropriately called "dynamic mechanical allodynia." For other types of increased pain sensitivity (e.g., to heat), the terms *hyperalgesia* and *allodynia* are used inconsistently. We recommend that use of these terms should be clarified by IASP's Task Force on Taxonomy.

Terms referring to pain perception should not be used to describe reflexes in animals, while terms for nociceptive behavior observed in sensitized states would be better termed "reflex correlate of" or "behavioral correlate of" dynamic mechanical allodynia. "Mechanical hypersensitivity" may be appropriate to describe the decrease in mechanical threshold to von Frey hairs in models of neuropathic pain.

HIERARCHICAL LEVELS OF MECHANISM

A hierarchical structure should be considered for the systematic evaluation of neuropathic pain (Table I). At the top of this hierarchy is the clinical presentation encompassing the pain "phenotype," which may include features such as ongoing pain, dynamic mechanical allodynia, and sensory loss. The second level of evaluation encompasses disease processes that can be used to explain pain phenotypes. Processes include ongoing neuronal activity,

Table I
Hierarchical levels of analysis of neuropathic pain mechanisms

Clinical presentation	Sensory loss, ongoing pain, hyperalgesia, allodynia
Processes	Degeneration, regeneration, ectopic activity, central sensitization
Cellular mechanisms	Wallerian degeneration, increased excitability, long-term potentiation
Molecular mechanisms	Channel phosphorylation, channel upregulation

ectopic firing, central sensitization, and nerve degeneration. Cellular mechanisms, such as protein trafficking, constitute a third level of evaluation that can be used to explain processes underlying pain phenotypes. Finally, a fourth level of evaluation consists of molecular mechanisms, such as changes in gene expression patterns. Inherent in this hierarchical approach is the acknowledgment that not all neuropathic pain is the same, with variability in the presentation, incidence, severity, and co-expression of specific phenotypes. However, this approach allows the prioritization of potential targets at each level and permits a focus on the higher priorities.

NEUROPATHIC PAIN MODELS

In the effort to gain a mechanistic understanding of neuropathic pain, the appropriate choice of models is critical. By definition, a model can represent some, but not all, aspects of clinical reality. Therefore, it is essential to specify which aspects are being modeled: clinical signs and symptoms, processes of disease progression, processes of symptom generation, cellular mechanisms, and/or molecular mechanisms.

CONSENSUS

1) "Dynamic mechanical allodynia" is the appropriate term with which to describe pain elicited by moving gentle tactile stimuli. For other positive sensory signs, the terms "allodynia," "hyperalgesia," and "hyperpathia" have been used inconsistently. We need a consistent nomenclature for positive sensory signs.

2) The term "mechanisms" can have different meanings. We propose that the problem of neuropathic pain should be addressed at four hierarchical levels of evaluation: clinical presentation, disease processes, cellular mechanisms, and molecular mechanisms.

3) Models reflect only part of reality. Researchers should state whether their chosen model represents a disease process, a cellular or molecular mechanism, or symptoms.

HOW DOES DIVERSITY IN CLINICAL PRESENTATION
INFLUENCE THE IDENTIFICATION OF PERIPHERAL TARGETS?

Peripheral targets in neuropathic pain can be separated into (1) targets that can be utilized for the development of novel therapeutic strategies, even if they are not directly implicated in the neuropathic process; and (2) targets that are thought to be involved in the generation and maintenance of neuropathic pain.

While it would be desirable to target those processes that are a primary source of neuropathic pain, there is currently no evidence to suggest that such drugs would have greater clinical utility than agents that provide symptomatic pain relief alone. For example, opioids are often effective for pain relief in neuropathy, even though opioid mechanisms are not implicated in the genesis of the pain (Dworkin et al. 2003).

The cardinal symptoms and signs of neuropathic pain can be grouped into ongoing pain, positive sensory signs (an increase in evoked pain, i.e., allodynia and hyperalgesia), and negative sensory signs (a decrease in evoked pain, i.e., sensory loss). Mechanisms underlying these components may be distinct. Knowledge about the neurobiological mechanisms underpinning these clinical phenomena will be an important step toward target selection.

Ongoing pain has distinct qualities. The most commonly described spontaneous symptoms are deep aching in the extremities and a superficial burning, stinging, or prickling pain. Verbal descriptors from the McGill Pain Questionnaire that are used more frequently by patients with neuropathic pain than by those with non-neuropathic pain include "electric shocks," "burning," "tingling," "itching," and "prickling," whereas descriptions such as "dull," "heavy," and "tiring" are more often reported by patients with non-neuropathic pains (Boureau et al. 1990; Bouhassira et al. 2004). Patients also report paroxysmal, shock-like lancinating pains, sometimes radiating through an entire limb. However, none of the terms used for characterizing neuropathic pain symptoms are pathognomonic, and careful neurological work-up is required. One of the primary aims of the clinician should be to provide disease-modifying therapy (which might also result in resolution of pain) in addition to offering symptomatic therapy.

Evoked pains, also described as positive sensory signs, include several forms of mechanical hypersensitivity, notably dynamic mechanical allodynia or punctate hyperalgesia, the Tinel sign, and several types of thermal hypersensitivity, including hyperalgesia to cold and heat. Trigger points are particularly striking in some disorders such as trigeminal neuralgia, but they are absent in others such as painful diabetic polyneuropathy. Symptoms and signs can be similar across neuropathic pain conditions such as painful polyneuropathy and postherpetic neuralgia, but there can also be substantial differences between these conditions and others such as trench foot neuropathy or complex regional pain syndrome (see Table II) (Scadding and Koltzenburg 2005). However, the diagnosis of neuropathic pain is often not possible on the basis of the patient's description of symptoms in the absence of confirmatory clinical examination and tests. Patients who were referred to a tertiary neurological center with the "suspected" diagnosis presented more often with superficial ongoing pain and brush-evoked pain. Cold or pinprick hyperalgesias were more frequently found in patients with definitive and probable neuropathic pain than in patients with "unlikely" neuropathic pain (Rasmussen et al. 2004).

The expression of pain associated with nerve injury is variable. The prevalence of phantom limb pain is 35–80% (Nikolajsen and Jensen 2001), whereas that of neuropathic pain in diabetic polyneuropathy is on the order of 10–20% (Daousi et al. 2004). There is also variability in the expression of negative sensory signs. Fiber loss is clearly an important factor in the development of peripheral neuropathic pain. However, current evidence does not show that the degree of fiber loss is correlated with the development of pain. Indeed, it has been difficult to assess small-fiber loss, and a more systematic analysis of this issue is necessary (Cruccu et al. 2004). Importantly, pain is found in neuropathy with small-fiber involvement with or without large-fiber involvement (Scadding and Koltzenburg 2005), although most of the clinical studies have investigated cutaneous painful symptoms. Symptoms arising from deep somatic domains are not well characterized, although animal studies indicate that there may be profound abnormalities of sensory neurons innervating skeletal muscle (Michaelis et al. 2000). Damage to visceral nerves could also be a source of neuropathic pain, but this possibility remains unproven.

Variability in the expression of neuropathic pain after nerve injury remains a hurdle in the mechanistic understanding of neuropathic pain. More than 80% of Sprague Dawley rats will develop mechanical hypersensitivity following traumatic nerve injury such as spinal nerve ligation (SNL), while in the clinical situation far fewer patients develop pain following a distinct peripheral nerve disease. However, the incidence of clinical pain following peripheral nerve trauma is not well documented. There may be a difference in incidence between traumatic injury (the most prevalent animal model) and metabolic or infectious peripheral nerve disease (the most common human painful neuropathies). Genetic factors could also contribute to pain susceptibility. For example, the Holtzman strain of rats fails to develop neuropathic pain behavior following traumatic nerve injury. Genetic variability may be critical in humans (Valder et al. 2003), and this is an important issue for future research.

Table II
Symptoms and signs of neuropathic pain

	Peripheral Neuropathic Pain	Postherpetic Neuralgia	Trench Foot	Complex Regional Pain Syndrome	Capsaicin
Ongoing pain	100%	100%	None	100%	83%
Brush-evoked pain	36%	60%	None	60%	68%
Pinprick hyperalgesia	38%	37%	None	Present	83%
Static hyperalgesia	35%	52%	None	Present	80%
Joint hyperalgesia	None	None	None	90%	None
Heat hyperalgesia	29%	29%	5%	30%	90%
Cold hyperalgesia	46%	21%	50%	30%	None
Edema	Low	Low	Early	50%	None
Trophic changes	Present	Scars	Low	90%	None
Sympathetically maintained pain	Low	Low	Low	90% (early)	Low

Source: Data are from published and unpublished sources: Liu et al. (1998); Pappagallo et al.; Peters and Nurmikko (for a group of patients with mixed peripheral neuropathic pain), Jørum (for trench foot) and Wasner et al. (for complex regional pain syndrome).

*In other data sets, the incidence of cold hyperalgesia is lower than mechanical allodynia and pinprick hyperalgesia.

CONSENSUS

1) There is an astounding variability in clinical manifestations in patients with a seemingly identical underlying lesion or disease.

2) Ongoing neuropathic pain can have at least two different qualities (burning or shock-like) and temporal characteristics (continuous or paroxysmal).

3) Ongoing neuropathic pain can be found with sensory loss, with or without positive sensory signs.

4) Generally, among the positive sensory signs, there is a rank order of frequency and clinical relevance of stimulus modalities: mechanical > cold > heat.

RESEARCH QUESTIONS

1) Is there any evidence that a drug or drug class has a specific action on one pain quality (e.g., carbamazepine for paroxysmal pain)?

2) How are pain qualities encoded in the peripheral and central nociceptive system?

3) Is peripheral neuropathic pain restricted to cutaneous nerves? How about muscle or visceral nerves?

UNDERLYING MECHANISMS: PROCESS LEVEL

It is generally accepted that neuropathic pain is due to aberrant or inappropriate activity in both the peripheral and central nervous systems. Activity in the PNS plays two important roles. One is the mediation of ongoing pain, because the PNS provides the primary afferent signal perceived as pain by a conscious brain. The second is the initiation or maintenance of an increase in excitability within the CNS, a process referred to as "central sensitization." Signals perceived as pain normally arise from the peripheral terminals of nociceptive afferents (Fig. 1), although it is now clear that following nerve injury, action potentials can be generated outside the normal site of transformation ("ectopically"), i.e., along the peripheral nerve, in the dorsal root ganglion (DRG), or in the dorsal root itself (see the chapter by Devor, this volume). Pain sensation might arise entirely through signaling in the CNS ("central pain") as a result of CNS injury. However, in the absence of convincing examples, it remains to be determined whether such "pain centralization" occurs following peripheral nerve injury.

WHICH AFFERENTS ARE RESPONSIBLE?

Dynamic mechanical allodynia is abolished with selective A-fiber block (Campbell et al. 1988; Torebjork et al. 1992; Magerl et al. 2001), and C fibers do not appear to be capable of acquiring such exquisite mechanical sensitivity, even after nerve injury (Ørstavik et al. 2003; Tsuboi et al. 2004; Shim et al. 2005). Therefore, large, myelinated, low-threshold mechano sensitive (LTM) afferents must mediate this positive sensory sign. Sensitization of central "pain-processing" neurons (i.e., central sensitization) is an accepted mechanism that accounts for the ability of LTM afferents to signal pain. Whether or not ongoing pain requires central sensitization depends on whether that pain reflects activity in the PNS. If the latter is true, the requirement of central sensitization would also depend on whether ongoing pain reflects activity in non-nociceptive afferents that require changes in the central nervous system to mediate the change in perceptual quality associated with ongoing activity, activity in nociceptive afferents, or activity in non-nociceptive afferents that have undergone a phenotypic switch and now signal pain. What is clear, however, is that under experimental conditions in healthy humans and animals, activation of C fibers, probably mechanically insensitive C fibers, is necessary for the initiation and maintenance of central sensitization, at least in the short time frames that have been studied (Schmelz et al. 2000; Magerl et al. 2001). Input from LTM afferents is not normally sufficient to produce central sensitization.

A ROLE FOR INJURED Aβ FIBERS?

Data from animal models of neuropathic pain suggest that activity in myelinated Aβ LTMs may induce signs of central sensitization under pathological conditions. Following chronic constriction injury of the sciatic nerve, spontaneous ectopic activity is observed within 3 days after injury, about the time that mechanical hypersensitivity appears. This activity predominantly occurs in injured Aβ afferents (Kajander and Bennett 1992). Similarly, ectopic spontaneous activity is generated in injured myelinated Aβ afferents within 24 hours following SNL, again corresponding to the time of onset of mechanical hypersensitivity (Liu et al. 2000). Obvious spontaneous activity is absent in injured unmyelinated afferents (Liu et al. 1999, 2000). However, the methods used in these studies would not have revealed the extremely low firing rates reported to occur in uninjured unmyelinated afferents (Wu et al. 2001). Therefore, it is not known whether ectopic activity in unmyelinated afferents at the time of onset of tactile allodynia is a special property of adjacent uninjured C fibers, or whether it also occurs in injured C fibers.

At later times after nerve injury, ectopic spontaneous activity in severed unmyelinated afferents may become prominent, often more prominent than ectopic activity in A fibers.

Additional support for a causal role for injured Aβ fibers in neuropathic pain comes from the observation that lidocaine injection into the nucleus gracilis reverses the behavioral signs of mechanical hypersensitivity observed in the SNL model (Sun et al. 2001). However, these interesting findings are paradoxical for two reasons. First, in humans with neuropathic pain, dorsal column stimulation produces pain relief, and second, the nucleus gracilis is thought to be a relay station for mainly non-nociceptive input.

Under conditions of nociceptive (non-neuropathic) pain, Aβ LTM afferents produce neither pain sensations nor signs of central sensitization. This situation may change, however, following nerve injury. For example, myelinated afferents begin to synthesize neurotransmitters such as substance P and neuropeptide Y that normally are expressed only in nociceptive afferents (Noguchi et al. 1995). These transmitters may both activate nociceptive circuitry in the spinal cord and trigger central sensitization. Such "phenotypic switching" could indeed give non-nociceptive myelinated afferents access to nociceptive circuitry and enable activity in Aβ fibers to drive central sensitization. In the SNL model, mechanical hypersensitivity and nerve-injury-induced morphological changes develop within 24 hours, but it is unclear whether phenotypic switching contributes to mechanical hypersensitivity within this time frame.

THE "PROBLEM" WITH DORSAL RHIZOTOMY

Dorsal rhizotomy has been used as a means of identifying the afferent population "responsible" for the manifestation of neuropathic pain behavior. Unfortunately, results from these experiments have been contradictory. On the one hand, there is evidence that dorsal rhizotomy is able to both reverse and prevent the development of neuropathic pain behavior associated with SNL (Sukhotinsky et al. 2004). On the other hand, conflicting evidence shows that such an intervention fails to influence the development of neuropathic pain behavior (Li et al. 2000). A further complication is evidence that dorsal, and even ventral, rhizotomy produces mechanical hypersensitivity in animals (Sheth et al. 2002). In humans, however, dorsal rhizotomy appears to always eliminate pain of peripheral origin. Although, this clinical impression has not been verified in a formal clinical trial, and "deafferentation pain" may emerge weeks or months after the rhizotomy.

A ROLE FOR "UNINJURED" C FIBERS?

Recent evidence demonstrates that uninjured, unmyelinated afferents in the L4 spinal nerve develop spontaneous activity following L5 SNL (Wu et al. 2001). The significance of this finding is controversial, since the observed spontaneous activity is low, and we do not know whether such activity, even in a large percentage of uninjured, unmyelinated afferents, is able to produce central sensitization. However, low-frequency electrical stimulation of C fibers produces signs of secondary hyperalgesia in humans (Koppert et al. 2001; Klein et al. 2004). Recent evidence from microneurographic experiments in patients suffering from erythromelalgia suggests that unmyelinated, mechanoinsensitive afferents (MIAs) become spontaneously active in this painful neuropathic condition (Ørstavik et al. 2003). Indeed, activation of MIAs must be critical for the induction of capsaicin-induced secondary hyperalgesia (i.e., central sensitization), given that only this class of afferents is adequately activated by intradermal capsaicin injection (Schmelz et al. 2000). Whether MIAs also show spontaneous activity in other neuropathic pain syndromes is currently unknown.

The role of C-fiber activity in neuropathic pain has been called into question by the lack of effect of systemic capsaicin or resiniferatoxin (RTX) on SNL-induced mechanical hypersensitivity. For example, neonatal treatment with capsaicin does not prevent mechanical hypersensitivity following SNL (J.M. Chung, personal communication). Furthermore, systemic RTX treatment does not reverse SNL-induced mechanical hypersensitivity (Ossipov et al. 1999). However these data should be interpreted with caution. Such treatment also produces central effects (as indicated by loss or impairment of thermal regulation) that could result in the reorganization of sensory pathways. Moreover, systemic RTX treatment in adult animals does not ablate DRG neurons (Szallasi and Blumberg 1992).

In summary, the currently available data from animal models do not conclusively define the role of different classes of afferents in central sensitization. While ectopic neuronal activity in injured fibers and its modulation by different drugs have been studied in the laboratory, the clinical pharmacology of ectopic activity needs further advancement. The mechanisms underlying the development of spontaneous activity in uninjured afferents are also unknown. Observations in a human surrogate model of secondary hyperalgesia suggest that central sensitization is induced by C-fiber input and does not outlast a peripheral driving input by more than a day. The resulting allodynia is mediated by increased central responsiveness to peripheral input from Aβ-fiber LTMs (Magerl et al. 2001). The extent to which the experimental findings can be transferred to clinical neuropathic pain is still limited. Some clinical studies suggest that even long-standing central sensitization can reverse quickly when the peripheral maintaining input is removed (Gracely et al. 1992). However, we need more studies using diagnostic peripheral nerve blocks in patients suffering from neuropathic pain.

NEURAL-IMMUNE INTERACTIONS

It has long been appreciated that Schwann cell–axonal interactions are critical for maintenance of axonal function and that changes in this interaction are part of the response to peripheral nerve injury. Schwann cells appear to express nerve growth factor (NGF) (Rush 1984), and following nerve injury they demonstrate a rapid and dramatic increase in NGF receptors (Taniuchi et al. 1988). This increase in NGF receptors appears to be associated with a more generalized change in Schwann cell properties (Popovic et al. 1996), including initiation of mitosis and a structural reorganization of Remak bundles (Murinson et al. 2005). Evidence also suggests increased connectivity among satellite cells within sensory ganglia following nerve injury (Cherkas et al. 2004). The relative contribution of all these changes to neuropathic pain, however, has yet to be clearly demonstrated.

Considerable evidence now supports the conclusion that nerve-injury-induced changes in glial cells within the spinal cord contribute to behavior associated with nerve injury. However, this area requires additional research, given our incomplete understanding of the mechanisms by which glial and in particular, Schwann cell activation enhances neuronal transmission of nociceptive information (Watkins and Maier 2003). Activation of these cells is likely to cause the release of substances that act directly on neurons involved in pain transmission through several mechanisms including direct excitation, sensitization, potentiation of action potentials, the sensitization of neuronal receptors such as the purinergic $P2X_3$ receptor, or the release of other neurotransmitters or modulators that can act on nearby neurons. Other mechanisms, such as changes in neurotransmitter or ion clearance rates, may also link glial/Schwann cell activation to enhanced nociceptive processing.

The release of proinflammatory cytokines by peripheral immune cells provides a critical signal for communicating with the CNS. Proinflammatory cytokines, including tumor necrosis factor (TNF), interleukin-1 (IL-1), and IL-6 are key players in the response to immune challenge, acting to recruit and activate immune cells (Watkins and Maier 2005). Indeed, proinflammatory cytokines are recognized as key mediators of communication between the immune system and the brain.

Specific trophic factors and cytokines are transported in an anterograde direction along peripheral and central axons and released to postsynaptic cells (Caleo and Cenni 2004). TNF-α is an important pro-inflammatory cytokine that may play a role in the neurodegenerative processes that accompany painful peripheral neuropathy. TNF-α elicits hyperalgesic responses in rats (Wagner and Myers 1996). It may be axonally transported and thus may contribute to the degenerative pathologies observed at both the central and peripheral nerve terminals (Schafers et al. 2002; Shubayev and Myers 2002). Immune activation may also affect neuronal function at the level of the cell bodies in the DRG and their adjoining central processes and in the spinal cord, suggesting potential sites of intervention for the treatment of painful peripheral neuropathies.

BARRIERS TO TARGET ACCESS

Treatment for neuropathic pain may require therapeutic interventions at multiple sites throughout the neuraxis. Compounds such as opioids that act both centrally and in the periphery may ultimately be the most efficacious interventions. However, it is also clear that the use of drugs restricted to the PNS may enable significant pain relief while avoiding CNS side effects (Butleman et al. 2004; Valenzano et al. 2004; Whiteside et al. 2004). Promising therapeutic targets include cannabinoid receptors, opioid receptors, metabotropic glutamate receptors, and a variety of voltage-gated channels for sodium, potassium, and calcium ions (see the chapter by Schmidt and Moreadith).

Several barriers between the blood and various tissues are critical in the regulation of homeostasis. In addition to the blood-brain barrier, these include the blood-nerve barrier, the blood–cerebrospinal fluid barrier, and the blood-retinal barrier. The tissue-nerve barrier is also important. These various blood-tissue and tissue-nerve barriers are mediated by tight junctions that seal the interface between endothelial and epithelial cells (Omura et al. 2004). The presence of these barriers presents a special challenge for treatments because it is often more difficult to develop a compound with reasonable access to a target than to develop one with exquisite specificity and affinity.

While the blood-brain barrier prevents access of hydrophilic agents to the CNS, the blood-nerve barrier serves an analogous function in the periphery, limiting access to peripheral axons. However, the blood-nerve barrier enables access to primary afferent neurons at two key sites: peripheral terminals and the sensory neuron somata (Devor 1999). Thus, agents that have no effect when applied mid-nerve can have profound effects when applied directly to the ganglia or to nerve terminals in the end organs such as the skin, or even more importantly, when applied systemically (Rechthand and Rapoport 1987; Allen and Kiernan 1994; Wadhwani and Rapoport 1994).

This potential barrier to peripherally restricted drugs is removed in the context of nerve injury. Indeed, the blood-nerve barrier breaks down at the site of traumatic injury and even along the nerve during Wallerian degeneration (Olsson 1966; Mellick and Cavanagh 1968; Poduslo and Curran 1992; Omura et al. 2004). This breakdown should allow for more efficient delivery of peripherally acting analgesics all along the injured and uninjured axons, in addition to the somata and peripheral termini, thus increasing the likelihood of efficacy of these drugs. A similar disruption occurs in the blood-nerve barrier in cases of diabetic neuropathy (Poduslo and Curran 1992).

It is important to note that the central terminals of primary afferents, while technically part of the PNS, are behind the blood-brain barrier. Therefore, although a target may be expressed in primary afferents, the precise location of this target is also of critical importance for any peripherally restricted drug strategy. On the other hand, approaches involving siRNA or antisense technology should consider that targets expressed in the peripheral primary afferent, but behind the blood-brain barrier, can still be accessed by peripherally restricted means of delivery.

CONSENSUS

1) Ectopic activity (ongoing and/or evoked) is one of the mechanisms that can contribute to neuropathic pain.

2) Central sensitization is also one of the mechanisms that can contribute to neuropathic pain.

3) Central sensitization can be induced by C-fiber input.

4) In addition to the activity in injured afferents, aberrant activity in adjacent uninjured fibers may contribute to the mechanisms of neuropathic pain.

5) Changes in neurotrophic factors and cytokines may contribute to neuropathic pain.

6) Dynamic mechanical allodynia is signaled by Aβ-fiber low-threshold mechanoreceptors.

7) The blood-nerve barrier is compromised at strategic locations including the nerve injury site and sensory ganglia.

RESEARCH QUESTIONS

1) Can injured Aβ-fiber low-threshold mechanoreceptors induce central sensitization? If so, how and under what conditions?

2) What is the role of mechanoinsensitive afferents in neuropathic pain?

3) Can depolarization of an axon in mid-nerve by itself lead to repetitive

action potential firing, or is a local change in membrane excitability required?

4) What mechanisms contribute to depolarization at ectopic sites (aberrant expression of transduction channels, transmitter actions, increased leakage current)?

TIME-DEPENDENT CHANGES: INITIATION VERSUS MAINTENANCE

Several lines of evidence indicate that there are time-dependent changes in the underlying mechanisms of neuropathic pain. For example, in mice lacking the prodynorphin gene, SNL injury results in pain behavior that develops normally over the first several days, yet it is not maintained as it is in wild-type mice (Wang et al. 2001). These observations indicate that dynorphin is necessary for the maintenance, but not for the initiation, of neuropathic pain behavior. There are dramatic differences in the efficacy of systemic infusions of lidocaine relative to the timing of a traumatic nerve injury (Araujo et al. 2003). Time-dependent changes in the activation of spinal glial cells have also been described following traumatic nerve injury (Zhuang et al. 2005). In addition, traumatic injury of human nerves initiates time-dependent changes in the relative contribution of the voltage-gated Na^+ channel $Na_V1.8$ to neuropathic pain (Coward et al. 2000).

Understanding the issue of timing is of further importance because it will reveal to what extent pain can be abrogated by the abolition (or normalization) of peripheral activity and to what degree and for how long abnormal peripheral activity must continue before the clinical features of neuropathic pain are established.

In the context of maintenance of nerve injury pain, clinical data suggest that local block of the affected nerve often quickly abolishes the sensation of pain. Because these nerve blocks may provide temporary relief, continued peripheral input seems to be a requirement for perception of pain (Gracely et al. 1992; Treede et al. 1992; Abram 2000). However, local nerve block may not abolish excessive nerve firing originating from sites other than the area of primary injury (e.g., the DRG). Thus, failure to abolish pain with a local nerve block cannot be unequivocally interpreted as a sign of pain centralization. The implication of the nerve block data is that in at least some forms of neuropathic pain, the process of central sensitization is self-limiting. However, the cessation of the excessive peripheral input may be required to allow normalization of CNS circuitry in a time frame of hours to days. Consistent with this suggestion, preclinical studies have demonstrated that central sensitization is dependent on afferent input for its maintenance because it disappears in the isolated spinal cord (Hedo et al. 1999). The extent to which "normalization" of peripheral input will serve to eliminate pain remains to be determined.

It is also unclear to what extent aberrant activity is sufficient to produce pain. Many neuropathies are painless. Nerve damage from *Varicella zoster* infection rarely yields persistent neuropathic pain. Pain in diabetic neuropathy is relatively infrequent. Painless large-fiber neuropathies have been described, and nerve fiber pathology fails to differentiate between patients with or without pain (Serra 1999; Malik et al. 2001). Thus, the extent to which anatomical changes (i.e., loss of fibers, terminal sprouting, and reorganization of Remak bundles) reflect altered electrical excitability remains largely unknown. Systematic study of abnormal peripheral firing patterns in these neuropathies needs to be performed, although preclinical studies suggest that development of neuropathic pain (and central sensitization) after injury is dependent on the specific fibers that become active (as well as those that become inactive) and on the intensity and duration of peripheral afferent barrage (Hedo et al. 1999).

CONSENSUS

1) The physiological process of central sensitization usually does not outlast peripheral provoking stimuli by more than one day.

RESEARCH QUESTIONS

1) Under what circumstances might peripheral neuropathic pain become independent of peripheral maintaining input?

2) How quickly does neuropathic pain develop after a peripheral nerve lesion?

3) Is C-fiber activity essential for the induction and/or maintenance of neuropathic pain?

CELLULAR AND MOLECULAR MECHANISMS

The majority of data concerning mechanisms have been derived from studies of animal models, most commonly of traumatic nerve injury. While some of the mechanisms described below have also been demonstrated in humans, further clinical work is still required.

SODIUM CHANNELS

Data from animal models. The fact that local anesthetics could block neuropathic pain has focused further research on voltage-gated Na^+ channels, whose net activity may be increased following nerve injury (see the chapter by Devor). These channels accumulate at the ends of injured axons (Devor et al. 1989). Nerve injury is associated with an increase in the expression of the tetrodotoxin (TTX)-sensitive voltage-gated Na^+ channel, $Na_V1.3$ (Waxman et al. 1994). Heterologous expression of this channel suggests that it has biophysical properties that support an underlying mechanism of repetitive spiking; the channel recovers from inactivation relatively rapidly and therefore may sustain higher levels of activity for longer periods of time (Cummins et al. 2001). Nerve injury also decreases the TTX-resistant Na^+ channel $Na_V1.8$ mRNA and protein (Dib-Hajj et al. 1996, 1999a; Cummins and Waxman 1997; Okuse et al. 1997; Novakovic et al. 1998; Black et al. 1999; Boucher et al. 2000; Decosterd et al. 2002; Leffler et al. 2002; Xiao et al. 2002; Eriksson and Fried 2003; Gold et al. 2003). This decrease in mRNA and protein has generally been associated with a decrease in the slowly inactivating TTX-resistant Na^+ current observed in isolated sensory neurons (Rizzo et al. 1995; Dib-Hajj et al. 1996, 1998, 1999a; Cummins and Waxman 1997; Everill et al. 2001; Lancaster and Weinreich 2001; Gold et al. 2003). However, it should be noted that a nerve injury-induced increase in the slowly inactivating TTX-resistant Na^+ current has been observed in DRG neurons (Abdulla and Smith 2002)

Several other Na^+ channels whose expression may also be decreased following nerve injury include $Na_V1.9$ (Gold 2000), $Na_V1.6$, and $Na_V1.7$ (Kim et al. 2001). Findings relevant to nerve-injury-induced changes in Na^+ currents in sensory neurons have been mixed, with investigators reporting increases (Rizzo et al. 1995; Abdulla and Smith 2002; Flake et al. 2004), slight decreases (Everill et al. 2001), or no change (Cummins and Waxman 1997) in the magnitude of TTX-sensitive Na^+ currents, as well as increases (Cummins and Waxman 1997; Everill et al. 2001) or no change (Flake et al. 2004) in the repriming of TTX-sensitive Na^+ currents. Importantly, since $Na_V1.8$ has a high threshold for activation, an increase in the proportion of a low-threshold TTX-sensitive channel relative to that of a high-threshold channel should be associated with a dramatic increase in neuronal excitability. Recent data call this assumption into question, however, as no change in excitability was observed in the cell bodies of injured afferents in vitro, at a time when TTX-resistant currents were suppressed and TTX-sensitive currents were augmented (Flake et al. 2004).

Human data. Almost all the nerve injury-induced changes in Na^+ channels observed in animal models of peripheral nerve injury have been demonstrated in human peripheral nerves following nerve injury. In patients with peripheral (but not central) axotomy, $Na_V1.3$ is upregulated in the peripheral axons (Coward et al. 2001), while $Na_V1.7$ (Coward et al. 2001) as well as $Na_V1.8$ and $Na_V1.9$ (Coward et al. 2000) are downregulated in the cell bodies of primary afferents. An increase in $Na_V1.8$ was also observed in afferents innervating hypersensitive skin in patients with distal nerve injury (Coward et al. 2000; Shembalkar et al. 2001), suggesting that the channel is upregulated in uninjured neighbors of injured afferents and that it may contribute to the hyperexcitability of intact nerve fibers. While evidence from animal models indicates that $Na_V1.8$ is not present in the cut end of axons following traumatic nerve injury (Gold et al. 2003), this channel appears to accumulate in painful peripheral neuromas months after nerve injury (Coward et al. 2000). This finding indicates that the contribution of this channel to neuropathic pain may be important and that it changes with time following nerve injury. Although increased or reduced channel expression may underlie changes in excitability following nerve injury, heritable channel mutations, such as that of $Na_V1.7$, have been shown to underlie the peripheral nerve hyperexcitability associated with painful erythromelalgia (Cummins et al. 2004).

POTASSIUM CHANNELS

Nerve injury also results in a decrease in voltage-gated K^+ channels, as assessed with immunohistochemistry (Rasband et al. 1998) and functional protein measures (Everill and Kocsis 1999). At least one of these K^+ currents has a low threshold for activation and therefore may contribute to resting membrane potential. A decrease in this current may result in membrane depolarization (Flake et al. 2004), which may inactivate TTX-sensitive Na^+ channels. Thus, it is possible that despite an increase in Na^+ channel expression, channel availability may decrease as a result of changes in other ion channels. Thus, the impact of changes in ion channels on neuronal excitability will depend on a number of factors, including relative channel density, spatial distribution of channels, and resting membrane potential.

NEUROTROPHIC FACTORS

The nerve-injury-induced changes in ion channel expression appear to reflect either decreased or increased access to various neurotrophic factors. For example, decreased access to target sources of glial-cell-line-derived neurotrophic factor (GDNF) is believed to be responsible for the increased expression of $Na_V1.3$ in fibers injured by SNL, resulting in spontaneous firing of the primary sensory neuron (Boucher et al. 2000; Cummins et al. 2000). Intrathecal administration of GDNF (Boucher et al. 2000) or systemic administration of artemin (Gardell et al. 2003) normalizes the level of $Na_V1.3$ and reverses behavioral hyperalgesia.

Injury-induced increases in NGF secretion from Schwann cells, keratinocytes, macrophages, or mast cells may lead to spontaneous activity in uninjured C-fiber nociceptors (Ali et al. 1999). These changes may also mediate the redistribution of $Na_V1.8$ channels along the axonal terminals (Gold et al. 2003). Administration of an anti-NGF antibody (Woolf et al. 1994) or of a molecule that blocks NGF signaling through TrkA (McMahon et al. 1995) attenuated behavioral hyperalgesia in several models of inflammation-induced pain, and administration of neutralizing anti-NGF antibodies reversed allodynia in models of neuropathic pain (Ro et al. 1999; Li et al. 2003). In addition, anti-NGF therapy also reduces bone cancer pain and decreases the markers of peripheral and central sensitization (Sevcik et al. 2005).

These studies emphasize that changes in the availability of trophic factors following nerve injury are associated with increase neuronal excitability and pain. Pain therapy can correct the trophic milieu by either administration or neutralization of the appropriate trophic factor.

MOLECULAR CHANGES IN "UNINJURED" AFFERENTS

While changes in injured axons have been well documented, neighboring uninjured afferents also undergo a number of marked changes, suggesting that they also contribute to neuropathic pain. These changes include increases in the expression and density of "pronociceptive" receptors, such as $P2X_3$ (Tsuzuki et al. 2001) and TRPV1 (Fukuoka et al. 2002), and a redistribution of the sodium channel $Na_V1.8$ (Gold et al. 2003). These changes are also driven by target-derived neurotrophic factors. For example, high levels of NGF cause increased expression of TRPV1 (Ji et al. 2002; Amaya et al. 2004), acid-sensing ion channel-3 (Mamet et al. 2002, 2003), the bradykinin B_2 receptor (Kasai et al. 1998), and the neuropeptides calcitonin gene-related peptide and substance P (Zhang et al. 1995; Shadiack et al. 2001), which may contribute to the increased excitability of the axonal terminals. These observations are also consistent with literature demonstrating that NGF can play a key role in driving inflammatory pain (Woolf et al. 1994; McMahon 1996; Bennett 2001) and neuropathic pain (Ramer et al. 1998; Ro et al. 1999).

PROTEIN TRAFFICKING

A growing body of evidence indicates that a diverse array of proteins are involved in the regulation of receptor trafficking and anchoring receptors to specific sites in neuronal membranes, particularly at synapses in the CNS. Such mechanisms also exist in the periphery, although they have been less well characterized. For example, $Na_V1.8$ is normally only functional in the afferent cell body (Ritter and Mendell 1992) and in the peripheral and central terminals (Jeftinija 1994; Brock et al. 1998; Khasar et al. 1998), while the distribution of $Na_V1.6$ is primarily restricted to axons and to the nodes of Ranvier in myelinated axons (Wittmack et al. 2004). This unique distribution pattern may be disrupted by interventions designed to target the trafficking of specific proteins to neuronal membranes. For example, $Na_V1.8$ channel trafficking can be blocked by disruption of the p11 annexin-anchoring protein (Okuse et al. 2002).

POINTS OF CONVERGENCE

This brief description of peripheral mechanisms in neuropathic pain illustrates the variety of potential drug targets. Research can be prioritized by focusing on targets that may serve as points of convergence for several abnormal cellular processes. For example, the mechanisms of ectopic spike initiation form a critical point of convergence (see the chapter by Devor). In primary afferents, this mechanism may involve voltage-gated Na^+ channels and resting or constitutively active K^+ channels that together establish points of membrane instability described as oscillatory behavior (Amir et al. 2002). The Na^+ channels provide the depolarizing drive of the oscillation, and the K^+ channels provide the hyperpolarizing drive. Attenuating this oscillatory behavior should prevent repetitive spiking in these neurons and block ongoing or paroxysmal pain. Another way to address repetitive firing comes from a convergence of inflammatory mechanisms that decrease an inactivating or A-type K^+ current. Under normal conditions, an A-type K^+ current appears to be critical for mediating spike adaptation in response to depolarizing stimuli (Yoshimura and de Groat 1999). Nerve injury results in a decrease in a similar A-type current (Everill and Kocsis 1999).

CONSENSUS

1) A multitude of cellular and molecular mechanisms are involved in each of the processes relevant to neuropathic pain. Therefore, "nodes" where several processes converge might be favorable targets for treatment interventions.

2) Action potential signaling (initiation and conduction), axonal transport (e.g., of neurotrophins or cytokines), and central release mechanisms (transmitters and modulators) are possible candidates.

RESEARCH QUESTION

1) Can the nodes of convergence really be addressed by a single molecular mechanism (e.g., a specific sodium channel) or will it require polypharmacy?

REQUIREMENTS OF MODELS IN NEUROPATHIC PAIN

ANIMAL MODELS

The focus of animal model development has been the generation of robust signs of clinical disease states associated with peripheral nerve injury. The ideal animal model would thus manifest ongoing pain, dynamic mechanical allodynia, and cold allodynia. As indicated above, many models have been developed, but most involve traumatic nerve injury (spinal nerve ligation, chronic constriction injury, partial nerve injury, and spared nerve injury), with fewer reflecting other clinical pathologies such as diabetic neuropathy (the streptozotocin or genetic diabetic model), postherpetic neuropathy (the *V. zoster* model), or injury models caused by cytotoxins such as vincristine or antiretroviral therapies (Joseph et al. 2004). It should also be noted that while systemic streptozotocin (resulting in the loss of pancreatic β-cells) has been used to generate a model of diabetic neuropathy and *V. zoster* administration has been used as a model of postherpetic neuropathy, it is unclear whether either model comes close to the clinical reality. Morphological changes characteristic of diabetic neuropathy have yet to be demonstrated following streptozotocin administration, and changes in nociceptive behavior observed following infection with the *V. zoster* virus are much more akin to changes observed following acute infection than to those observed in humans following resolution of the inflammatory response associated with reactivation of the latent virus. Models of central neuropathic pain are few and are not considered here.

Animal models have increased the understanding of neuropathic pain processes and hence have permitted the identification of critical cellular and molecular mechanisms (Walker et al. 1999; Le Bars et al. 2001; Malmberg and Chaplan 2002). However, it is also clear that many important limitations are associated with the animal models currently in use (see Mogil and Crager 2004). First, none are clearly associated with the most common symptom of clinical neuropathic pain, namely ongoing pain, and few are associated with a robust manifestation of dynamic mechanical allodynia. Rather, the most robust symptom observed in animal models of nerve injury is punctate mechanical hypersensitivity (assessed with von Frey hairs). While there is evidence to suggest that autotomy (self-mutilation) may be an expression of ongoing pain (Devor and Raber 1983), this view remains highly controversial. Second, most preclinical data on neuropathic pain are derived from models of traumatic nerve injuries, but mechanisms underlying pain may differ from model to model. Third, animal models using behavioral endpoints may be problematic for several reasons. Endpoints are often subjective and therefore must be recorded by blinded observers; the resulting data, though robust, may not be valid or appropriate. For example, thermal hyperalgesia is a common endpoint that appears to be less predictive of clinical translation, and it resolves with time in many animals following traumatic nerve injury. Endpoints involving reflexive withdrawal also require extensive controls for altered motor excitability.

A variety of alternative behavioral endpoints, such as ultrasound vocalization, have been used to assess nociceptive and stress responses (Calvino et al. 1996; Sanchez 2003). Furthermore, complex operant models have been developed to evaluate pain behaviors, and these may have significant utility in the identification of novel therapeutic interventions (see the chapter by Vierck). Operant models may be more appropriate for late-stage drug evaluations as they may be too labor intensive for more routine studies. Thus, an immediate challenge for model development is characterization of alternative and complex behavioral endpoints. Operant behavioral paradigms involving assessment of the presence of dynamic mechanical allodynia have yet to be developed, and there are no data on the most appropriate paradigms with which to assess ongoing pain. An alternative solution to modeling ongoing pain would be the assessment of action potential discharge from injured (or uninjured) afferents. This methodology would provide a sensitive and objective endpoint with which to evaluate new drugs. Behavioral measures, coupled with quantitative pharmacokinetic data on drug exposure, would be needed to support a mechanistic translation that would affect pain behavior.

Use of genetic models, particularly those involving constitutive manipulations (gene overexpression or gene knockout), as a means of validating potential therapeutic targets requires cautious interpretation for a number of reasons. Use of appropriate controls is critical because there is tremendous variability between mouse strains. It is also necessary to monitor the occurrence of compensatory changes that occur as a result of genetic manipulations. It is becoming clear that phenotypic characteristics due to gene alterations are not always reconstituted with selective pharmacological tools. For example, TRPV1 and P2X$_3$ knockouts have a nociceptive rather than neuro-pathic pain phenotype, while both TRPV1 and P2X$_3$ antagonists are effective against nociceptive as well as neuropathic pain behaviors. There is therefore a strong rationale for the use of mice with genetic alterations that can be controlled both spatially and temporally by the investigator (i.e., conditional knockout animals) to increase confidence in target validation.

HUMAN SURROGATE MODELS

A variety of human experimental pain models have been developed. Most clinicians agree that these models should be used to build confidence for further clinical translation in a defined disease cohort. The real utility of such models is that they provide potential mechanistic linkages (Klein et al. 2005). They also enable the generation of dosing data and could highlight potential adverse drug responses. For example, cutaneous application of capsaicin is widely used as a human surrogate model of neuropathic pain, as it is characterized by both ongoing burning pain and dynamic mechanical allodynia (Liu et al. 1998). Use of this model has provided evidence that dynamic mechanical allodynia is mediated by LTMs (Torebjork et al. 1992). Another surrogate model that may provide insight into neuropathic pain involves repetitive electrical stimulation of peripheral fibers to create central hypersensitivity (Koppert et al. 2001; Klein et al. 2004). This model may enable determination of the types of fibers and the frequency and duration of activity necessary to induce central sensitization. However, given the evidence of phenotypic switching and other time-dependent changes in the underlying mechanisms of neuropathic pain, extrapolation from these acute models to the neuropathic pain state should be made with caution.

As with animal models, human surrogate models also largely fail to model variability in the expression of neuropathic pain. An extensive body of clinical literature indicates that not all traumatic injury to the peripheral nerve and not all peripheral neuropathies are associated with pain. For example, a human surgical equivalent of the SNL model (C7 spinal root section performed following brachial plexus injuries) is rarely associated with pain (Ali et al. 2002). Since chronic experimental injuries in volunteers are undesirable for obvious reasons, drug target validation for neuropathic pain should only be conducted in well-characterized clinical populations.

MODELING IN DISEASES

In order to facilitate both forward and reverse translation of pain mechanisms and targets from animal and human data, clinical evaluations should include measures of evoked pain and ongoing pain. Evoked pain measures provide the clinical opportunity to translate animal findings using similar experimental protocols. Given that punctuate mechanical hypersensitivity is a robust paradigm in animal models, such testing in the clinic would provide invaluable data with which to validate this endpoint. The fact that dynamic mechanical allodynia is the most prominent positive sign in the clinic underscores the need to develop complementary animal endpoints.

Development and validation of methodologies for measuring human peripheral nerve excitability (microneurography) and for localized peripheral drug administration will facilitate mechanistic studies. Biomarkers for neuropathic pain have not yet been adopted (see the chapter by Urban et al.), and further work in this area is desirable. A variety of methods to collect peripheral biomarkers, including skin microdialysis, skin blisters, and skin punch biopsy, will facilitate neuropathic pain diagnosis and treatment (Cruccu et al. 2004; Leis et al. 2004).

Translation of preclinical findings with promising new mechanism-based drug targets should be hastened by the use of investigational drugs, evaluated in small but well-defined cohorts of patients. Patients with diabetic neuropathy are relatively easy to recruit due to the prevalence of this condition, but the generalization of the results from these patients may be limited. Several other easily accessible neuropathic patient populations are available, such as patients suffering from ulnar entrapment. In addition, it may be more practical to perform a proof-of-principle drug study in a single characterized patient cohort. A positive outcome would invite further evaluation in a broader range of neuropathic pain conditions. Benchmarking with reference drugs should be done where possible to characterize the sensitivity of the experimental cohorts and to identify "responders" and "nonresponders" for future follow-up studies. Importantly, more careful patient selection will be required to optimize clinical trials with small numbers of patients. Patients should be selected on the basis of evidence for the presence of the drug target and for interaction with a key cellular mechanism. For example, careful selection of capsaicin-sensitive patients will allow segregation of an appropriate clinical population (with intact C fibers) who may respond to new TRPV1 antagonists currently in preclinical development.

CONSENSUS

1) Behavioral animal and surrogate human models are only approximations of the clinical situation. Findings from these models should be interpreted with caution when predicting clinical efficacy.

2) Animal experiments should be performed in a blinded manner.

3) Clinical trials should include a reference compound.

4) Tests of evoked pain should be included in clinical trials.

5) Findings in one neuropathic pain condition cannot necessarily be extrapolated to another condition.

RESEARCH QUESTIONS

1) Why can findings in one neuropathic pain condition not necessarily extrapolated to another condition?

2) How well does efficacy of one drug predict efficacy of another drug of the same class of agents?

3) How can we improve the predictive value of human experimental models?

4) How can we improve the predictive value of animal experimental models?

5) How does one measure ongoing pain in animals?

6) How does one measure the equivalent of dynamic mechanical allodynia in animals?

7) Do non-reflex measures (e.g., operant behavior) have better construct and predictive validity for neuropathic pain?

CONCLUSIONS

Neuropathic pain in humans may arise from a variety of causes, including direct nerve trauma, infectious diseases (e.g., herpes zoster, human immunodeficiency virus), metabolic diseases (e.g., diabetes), and drug-induced neuropathies (e.g., chemotherapy, antiretroviral therapy). Nontraumatic painful neuropathies outnumber painful neuropathies caused by nerve injuries. Consequently, sympathetically maintained pain and complex regional pain syndrome, which develop in a subgroup of patients with traumatic nerve injury, are receiving less emphasis in the current clinical literature than they did 10 years ago.

While the process has been slow, data from models of neuropathic pain and evidence-based medicine are starting to change long-held beliefs about neuropathic pain. Recent experimental evidence from human and animal studies demonstrates that neuropathic pain is responsive to treatment with high doses of opioids. Furthermore, neuropathic pain appears to reflect changes in both injured afferents and their "uninjured" neighbors. Unfortunately, available data do not enable us to dispel the notion that neuropathic pain is difficult to treat.

Translational research on neuropathic pain has been hindered by the fact that basic and clinical investigators have been studying different endpoints: stimulus-evoked responses are commonly used in animal studies, whereas spontaneous pain is measured in clinical studies. While these endpoints may involve similar underlying mechanisms, clinical evidence clearly indicates that this is often not the case and that ongoing and evoked pain reflect different underlying processes. Thus, it is critical that both clinical and preclinical groups begin to study common endpoints in order to identify critical underlying mechanisms and select appropriate therapeutic targets. We must also seek an explanation for why it is often a small minority of patients who develop chronic neuropathic pain, while more than 80% of animals subjected to a traumatic nerve injury will develop neuropathic pain behavior. The genetic background emerges as an important factor in neuropathic pain susceptibility. Genetic background has been shown to affect responses to pain and analgesics in both laboratory and clinical settings, as indicated by studies examining the melanocortin-1 receptor (Mogil et al. 2003) and the catechol-*O*-methyl transferase gene (Zubieta et al. 2003). Recent prospective data also suggest that genetic background influences the likelihood of developing a chronic pain condition (Diatchenko et al. 2005).

It is generally accepted that an increase in neuronal excitability and the resulting enhanced activity in peripheral neurons play a major role in neuropathic pain. For the full expression of the most problematic neuropathic pain phenotypes (dynamic mechanical allodynia), sensitization of central neurons is also likely to be necessary. Because adequate control of these processes is likely to hold the key to adequate therapeutic interventions, the challenge of the coming decade is to elucidate the mechanisms underlying these processes, as well as the relationship between the two.

A multitude of potential peripheral mechanisms have been identified, particularly at the molecular level, that may contribute to neuropathic pain. The mechanisms most likely to yield viable therapeutic interventions are at points of convergence. The PNS has three critical nodes of convergence: neuronal electrical activity (i.e., initiation and conduction of action potentials), neuronal trafficking systems (e.g., for ion channels and neurotrophic factors), and the release of chemical mediators (neurotransmitters, neuropeptides, and axonally transported neurotrophic factors). What will be critical is the identification of underlying cellular/molecular processes that are unique to the afferents responsible for the initiation and maintenance of neuropathic pain. As noted above, reducing side effects will be at least as important as finding drugs with better primary efficacy.

REFERENCES

Abdulla FA, Smith PA. Changes in Na+ channel currents of rat dorsal root ganglion neurons following axotomy and axotomy-induced autotomy. *J Neurophysiol* 2002; 88:2518–2529.

Abram SE. Neural blockade for neuropathic pain. *Clin J Pain* 2000; 16(2 Suppl):S56–S61.

Ali Z, Ringkamp M, Hartke TV, et al. Uninjured C-fiber nociceptors develop spontaneous activity and alpha-adrenergic sensitivity following L6 spinal nerve ligation in monkey. *J Neurophysiol* 1999; 81:455–466.

Ali Z, Meyer RA, Belzberg AJ. Neuropathic pain after C7 spinal nerve transection in man. *Pain* 2002; 96:41–47.

Allen DT, Kiernan JA. Permeation of proteins from the blood into peripheral nerves and ganglia. *Neuroscience* 1994; 59:755–764.

Amaya F, Shimosato G, Nagano M, et al. NGF and GDNF differentially regulate TRPV1 expression that contributes to development of inflammatory thermal hyperalgesia. *Eur J Neurosci* 2004; 20:2303–2310.

Amir R, Liu CN, Kocsis JD, Devor M. Oscillatory mechanism in primary sensory neurones. *Brain* 2002; 125:421–435.

Araujo MC, Sinnott CJ, Strichartz GR. Multiple phases of relief from experimental mechanical allodynia by systemic lidocaine: responses to early and late infusions. *Pain* 2003; 103:21–29.

Bennett DL. Neurotrophic factors: important regulators of nociceptive function. *Neuroscientist* 2001; 7:13–17.

Black JA, Fjell J, Dib-Hajj S, et al. Abnormal expression of SNS/PN3 sodium channel in cerebellar Purkinje cells following loss of myelin in the rat. *Neuroreport* 1999; 10:913–918.

Boucher TJ, Okuse K, Bennett DL, et al. Potent analgesic effects of GDNF in neuropathic pain states. *Science* 2000; 290:124–127.

Bouhassira D, Attal N, Fermanian J, et al. Development and validation of the Neuropathic Pain Symptom Inventory. *Pain* 2004; 108:248–257.

Boureau F, Doubrere JF, Luu M. Study of verbal description in neuropathic pain. *Pain* 1990; 42:145–152.

Brock JA, McLachlan EM, Belmonte C. Tetrodotoxin-resistant impulses in single nociceptor nerve terminals in guinea-pig cornea. *J Physiol* 1998; 512:211–217.

Caleo M, Cenni MC. Anterograde transport of neurotrophic factors: possible therapeutic implications. *Mol Neurobiol* 2004; 29:179–196.

Calvino B, Besson JM, Boehrer A, Depaulis A. Ultrasonic vocalization (22–28 kHz) in a model of chronic pain, the arthritic rat: effects of analgesic drugs. *Neuroreport* 1996; 7:581–584.

Campbell JN, Raja SN, Meyer RA, Mackinnon SE. Myelinated afferents signal the hyperalgesia associated with nerve injury. *Pain* 1988; 32:89–94.

Cervero F, Laird JM. Mechanisms of touch-evoked pain (allodynia): a new model. *Pain* 1996; 68:13–23.

Cherkas PS, Huang TY, Pannicke T, et al. The effects of axotomy on neurons and satellite glial cells in mouse trigeminal ganglion. *Pain* 2004; 110:290–298.

Coward K, Plumpton C, Facer P, et al. Immunolocalization of SNS/PN3 and NaN/SNS2 sodium channels in human pain states. *Pain* 2000; 85:41–50.

Coward K, Aitken A, Powell A, et al. Plasticity of TTX-sensitive sodium channels PN1 and brain III in injured human nerves. *Neuroreport* 2001; 12:495–500.

Cruccu G, Anand P, Attal N, et al. EFNS guidelines on neuropathic pain assessment. *Eur J Neurol* 2004; 11:153–162.

Cummins TR, Waxman SG. Downregulation of tetrodotoxin-resistant sodium currents and upregulation of a rapidly repriming tetrodotoxin-sensitive sodium current in small spinal sensory neurons after nerve injury. *J Neurosci* 1997; 17:3503–3514.

Cummins TR, Black JA, Dib-Hajj SD, Waxman SG. Glial-derived neurotrophic factor upregulates expression of functional SNS and NaN sodium channels and their currents in axotomized dorsal root ganglion neurons. *J Neurosci* 2000; 20:8754–8761.

Cummins TR, Aglieco F, Renganathan M, et al. $Na_v1.3$ sodium channels: rapid repriming and slow closed-state inactivation display quantitative differences after expression in a mammalian cell line and in spinal sensory neurons. *J Neurosci* 2001; 21:5952–5961.

Cummins TR, Dib-Hajj SD, Waxman SG. Electrophysiological properties of mutant $Na_v1.7$ sodium channels in a painful inherited neuropathy. *J Neurosci* 2004; 24:8232–8236.

Daousi C, MacFarlane IA, Woodward A, et al. Chronic painful peripheral neuropathy in an urban community: a controlled comparison of people with and without diabetes. *Diabet Med* 2004; 21:976–982.

Decosterd I, Ji RR, Abdi S, Tate S, Woolf CJ. The pattern of expression of the voltage-gated sodium channels $Na_v1.8$ and $Na_v1.9$ does not change in uninjured primary sensory neurons in experimental neuropathic pain models. *Pain* 2002; 96:269–277.

Devor M. Unexplained peculiarities of the dorsal root ganglion. *Pain* 1999; Suppl 6:S27–S35.

Devor M, Raber P. Autotomy after nerve injury and its relation to spontaneous discharge originating in nerve-end neuromas. *Behav Neural Bio* 1983; 37:276–283.

Devor M, Keller CH, Deerinck TJ, Levinson SR, Ellisman MH. Na^+ channel accumulation on axolemma of afferent endings in nerve end neuromas in *Apteronotus*. *Neurosci Lett* 1989; 102:149–154.

Diatchenko L, Slade GD, Nackley AG, et al. Genetic basis for individual variations in pain perception and the development of a chronic pain condition. *Hum Mol Genet* 2005; 14:135–143.

Dib-Hajj S, Black JA, Felts P, Waxman SG. Down-regulation of transcripts for Na channel alpha-SNS in spinal sensory neurons following axotomy. *Proc Natl Acad Sci USA* 1996; 93:14950–14954.

Dib-Hajj SD, Black JA, Cummins TR, et al. Rescue of alpha-SNS sodium channel expression in small dorsal root ganglion neurons after axotomy by nerve growth factor in vivo. *J Neurophysiol* 1998; 79:2668–2676.

Dib-Hajj SD, Fjell J, Cummins TR, et al. Plasticity of sodium channel expression in DRG neurons in the chronic constriction injury model of neuropathic pain. *Pain* 1999a; 83:591–600.

Dib-Hajj SD, Tyrrell L, Cummins TR, et al. Two tetrodotoxin-resistant sodium channels in human dorsal root ganglion neurons. *FEBS Lett* 1999b; 462:117–120.

Dworkin RH, Backonja M, Rowbotham MC, et al. Advances in neuropathic pain: diagnosis, mechanisms, and treatment recommendations. *Arch Neurol* 2003; 60:1524–1534.

Eriksson J, Fried K. Expression of the sodium channel transcripts $Na_v1.8$ and $Na_v1.9$ in injured dorsal root ganglion neurons of interferon-gamma or interferon-gamma receptor deficient mice. *Neurosci Lett* 2003; 338:242–246.

Everill B, Kocsis JD. Reduction in potassium currents in identified cutaneous afferent dorsal root ganglion neurons after axotomy. *J Neurophysiol* 1999; 82:700–708.

Everill B, Cummins TR, Waxman SG, Kocsis JD. Sodium currents of large (A-beta-type) adult cutaneous afferent dorsal root ganglion neurons display rapid recovery from inactivation before and after axotomy. *Neuroscience* 2001; 106:161–169.

Flake NM, Lancaster E, Weinreich D, Gold MS. Absence of an association between axotomy-induced changes in sodium currents and excitability in DRG neurons from the adult rat. *Pain* 2004; 109:471–480.

Fukuoka T, Tokunaga A, Tachibana T, et al. VR1, but not P2X₃, increases in the spared L4 DRG in rats with L5 spinal nerve ligation. *Pain* 2002; 99:111–120.

Gardell LR, Wang R, Ehrenfels C, et al. Multiple actions of systemic artemin in experimental neuropathy. *Nat Med* 2003; 9:1383–1389.

Gold MS. Sodium channels and pain therapy. *Curr Opin Anaesthesiol* 2000; 13:565–572.

Gold MS, Weinreich D, Kim CS, et al. Redistribution of $Na_V1.8$ in uninjured axons enables neuropathic pain. *J Neurosci* 2003; 23:158–166.

Gracely RH, Lynch SA, Bennett GJ. Painful neuropathy: altered central processing maintained dynamically by peripheral input. *Pain* 1992; 51:175–194.

Hedo G, Laird JM, Lopez-Garcia JA. Time-course of spinal sensitization following carrag-eenan-induced inflammation in the young rat: a comparative electrophysiological and behavioural study in vitro and in vivo. *Neuroscience* 1999; 92:309–318.

Jeftinija S. The role of tetrodotoxin-resistant sodium channels of small primary afferent fibers. *Brain Res* 1994; 639:125–134.

Ji RR, Samad TA, Jin SX, Schmoll R, Woolf CJ. p38 MAPK activation by NGF in primary sensory neurons after inflammation increases TRPV1 levels and maintains heat hyperalge-sia. *Neuron* 2002; 36:57–68.

Joseph EK, Chen X, Khasar SG, Levine JD. Novel mechanism of enhanced nociception in a model of AIDS therapy-induced painful peripheral neuropathy in the rat. *Pain* 2004 107:147–158.

Kajander KC, Bennett GJ. Onset of a painful peripheral neuropathy in rat: a partial and differential deafferentation and spontaneous discharge in A beta and A delta primary afferent neurons. *J Neurophysiol* 1992; 68:734–744.

Kasai M, Kumazawa T, Mizumura K. Nerve growth factor increases sensitivity to bradykinin, mediated through B2 receptors, in capsaicin-sensitive small neurons cultured from rat dorsal root ganglia. *Neurosci Res* 1998; 32:231–239.

Khasar SG, Gold MS, Levine JD. A tetrodotoxin-resistant sodium current mediates inflamma-tory pain in the rat. *Neurosci Lett* 1998; 256:17–20.

Kim CH, Oh Y, Chung JM, Chung K. The changes in expression of three subtypes of TTX sensitive sodium channels in sensory neurons after spinal nerve ligation. *Brain Res Mol Brain Res* 2001; 95:153–161.

Klein T, Magerl W, Hopf HC, Sandkuhler J, Treede RD. Perceptual correlates of nociceptive long-term potentiation and long-term depression in humans. *J Neurosci* 2004; 24:964–971.

Klein T, Magerl W, Rolke R, Treede RD. Human surrogate models of neuropathic pain. *Pain* 2005; 115:227–233.

Koltzenburg M, Lundberg LE, Torebjork HE. Dynamic and static components of mechanical hyperalgesia in human hairy skin. *Pain* 1992; 51:207–219.

Koppert W, Dern SK, Sittl R, et al. A new model of electrically evoked pain and hyperalgesia in human skin: the effects of intravenous alfentanil, S+-ketamine, and lidocaine. *Anesthesi-ology* 2001; 95:395–402.

Lancaster E, Weinreich D. Sodium currents in vagotomized primary afferent neurones of the rat. *J Physiol* 2001; 536:445–458.

Le Bars D, Gozariu M, Cadden SW. Animal models of nociception. *Pharmacol Rev* 2001; 53:597–652.

Leffler A, Cummins TR, Dib-Hajj SD, et al. GDNF and NGF reverse changes in repriming of TTX-sensitive Na+ currents following axotomy of dorsal root ganglion neurons. *J Neurophysiol* 2002; 88:650–658.

Leis S, Drenkhahn S, Schick C, et al. Catecholamine release in human skin—a microdialysis study. *Exp Neurol* 2004; 188:86–93.

Li L, Xian CJ, Zhong JH, Zhou XF. Lumbar 5 ventral root transection-induced upregulation of nerve growth factor in sensory neurons and their target tissues: a mechanism in neuropathic pain. *Mol Cell Neurosci* 2003; 23:232–250.

Li Y, Dorsi MJ, Meyer RA, Belzberg AJ. Mechanical hyperalgesia after an L5 spinal nerve lesion in the rat is not dependent on input from injured nerve fibers. *Pain* 2000; 85:493–502.

Liu CN, Wall PD, Ben-Dor E, et al. Tactile allodynia in the absence of C-fiber activation: altered firing properties of DRG neurons following spinal nerve injury. *Pain* 2000; 85:503–521.

Liu M, Max MB, Robinovitz E, Gracely RH, Bennett GJ. The human capsaicin model of allodynia and hyperalgesia: sources of variability and methods for reduction. *J Pain Symptom Manage* 1998; 16:10–20.

Liu X, Chung K, Chung JM. Ectopic discharges and adrenergic sensitivity of sensory neurons after spinal nerve injury. *Brain Res* 1999; 849:244–247.

Liu X, Eschenfelder S, Blenk KH, Janig W, Habler H. Spontaneous activity of axotomized afferent neurons after L5 spinal nerve injury in rats. *Pain* 2000; 84:309–318.

Magerl W, Fuchs PN, Meyer RA, Treede RD. Roles of capsaicin-insensitive nociceptors in cutaneous pain and secondary hyperalgesia. *Brain* 2001; 124:1754–1764.

Malik RA, Veves A, Walker D, et al. Sural nerve fibre pathology in diabetic patients with mild neuropathy: relationship to pain, quantitative sensory testing and peripheral nerve electrophysiology. *Acta Neuropathol (Berl)* 2001; 101:367–374.

Malmberg AB, Chaplan SR (Eds). *Mechanisms and Mediators of Neuropathic Pain.* Basel: Birkhauser, 2002.

Mamet J, Baron A, Lazdunski M, Voilley N. Proinflammatory mediators, stimulators of sensory neuron excitability via the expression of acid-sensing ion channels. *J Neurosci* 2002; 22:10662–10670.

Mamet J, Lazdunski M, Voilley N. How nerve growth factor drives physiological and inflammatory expressions of acid-sensing ion channel 3 in sensory neurons. *J Biol Chem* 2003; 278:48907–48913.

McMahon SB. NGF as a mediator of inflammatory pain. *Philos Trans R Soc Lond B Biol Sci* 1996; 351:431–440.

McMahon SB, Bennett DL, Priestley JV, Shelton DL. The biological effects of endogenous nerve growth factor on adult sensory neurons revealed by a trkA-IgG fusion molecule. *Nat Med* 1995; 1:774–780.

Mellick RS, Cavanagh JB. Changes in blood vessel permeability during degeneration and regeneration in peripheral nerves. *Brain* 1968; 91:141–160.

Merskey H, Bogduk N. *Classification of Chronic Pain: Descriptions of Chronic Pain Syndromes and Definitions of Pain Terms,* 2nd ed. Seattle: IASP Press, 1994.

Merskey H, Albe-Fessard D, Bonica JJ, et al. Pain terms: a list with definitions and notes on usage. Recommended by the IASP subcommittee on taxonomy. *Pain* 1979; 6:249–252.

Michaelis M, Liu X, Janig W. Axotomized and intact muscle afferents but no skin afferents develop ongoing discharges of dorsal root ganglion origin after peripheral nerve lesion. *J Neurosci* 2000; 20:2742–2748.

Mogil JS, Wilson SG, Chesler EJ, et al. The melanocortin-1 receptor gene mediates female-specific mechanisms of analgesia in mice and humans. *Proc Natl Acad Sci USA* 2003; 100:4867–4872.

Mogil JS, Crager SE. What should we be measuring in behavioral studies of chronic pain in animals? *Pain* 2004; 112:12–15.

Murinson BB, Archer DR, Li Y, Griffin JW. Degeneration of myelinated efferent fibers prompts mitosis in Remak Schwann cells of uninjured C-fiber afferents. *J Neurosci* 2005; 25:1179–1187.

Nikolajsen L, Jensen TS. Phantom limb pain. *Br J Anaesth* 2001; 87:107–116.

Noguchi K, Kawai Y, Fukuoka T, et al. Substance P induced by peripheral nerve injury in primary afferent sensory neurons and its effect on dorsal column nucleus neurons. *J Neurosci* 1995; 15:7633–7643.

Novakovic SD, Tzoumaka E, McGivern JG, et al. Distribution of the tetrodotoxin-resistant sodium channel PN3 in rat sensory neurons in normal and neuropathic conditions. *J Neurosci* 1998; 18:2174–2187.

Okuse K, Chaplan SR, McMahon SB, et al. Regulation of expression of the sensory neuron-specific sodium channel SNS in inflammatory and neuropathic pain. *Mol Cell Neurosci* 1997; 10:196–207.

Okuse K, Malik-Hall M, Baker MD, et al. Annexin II light chain regulates sensory neurone-specific sodium channel expression. *Nature* 2002; 417:653–656.

Olsson Y. Studies on vascular permeability in peripheral nerves. I. Distribution of circulating fluorescent serum albumin in normal, crushed and sectioned rat sciatic nerve. *Acta Neuropathol (Berl)* 1966; 7:1–15.

Omura K, Ohbayashi M, Sano M, et al. The recovery of blood-nerve barrier in crush nerve injury—a quantitative analysis utilizing immunohistochemistry. *Brain Res* 2004; 1001:13–21.

Ørstavik K, Weidner C, Schmidt R, et al. Pathological C-fibres in patients with a chronic painful condition. *Brain* 2003; 126:567–578.

Ossipov MH, Bian D, Malan TP Jr, Lai J, Porreca F. Lack of involvement of capsaicin-sensitive primary afferents in nerve- ligation injury induced tactile allodynia in rats. *Pain* 1999; 79:127–133.

Poduslo JF, Curran GL. Increased permeability across the blood-nerve barrier of albumin glycated in vitro and in vivo from patients with diabetic polyneuropathy. *Proc Natl Acad Sci USA* 1992; 89:2218–2222.

Popovic M, Sketelj J, Bresjanac M. Changes of Schwann cell antigenic profile after peripheral nerve injury. *Pflugers Arch* 1996; 431:R287–R288.

Ramer MS, Kawaja MD, Henderson JT, Roder JC, Bisby MA. Glial overexpression of NGF enhances neuropathic pain and adrenergic sprouting into DRG following chronic sciatic constriction in mice. *Neurosci Lett* 1998; 251:53–56.

Rasband MN, Trimmer JS, Schwarz TL, et al. Potassium channel distribution, clustering, and function in remyelinating rat axons. *J Neurosci* 1998; 18:36–47.

Rasmussen PV, Sindrup SH, Jensen TS, Bach FW. Symptoms and signs in patients with suspected neuropathic pain. *Pain* 2004; 110:461–469.

Rechthand E, Rapoport SI. Regulation of the microenvironment of peripheral nerve: role of the blood-nerve barrier. *Prog Neurobiol* 1987; 28:303–343.

Ritter AM, Mendell LM. Somal membrane properties of physiologically identified sensory neurons in the rat: effects of nerve growth factor. *J Neurophysiol* 1992; 68:2033–2041.

Rizzo MA, Kocsis JD, Waxman SG. Selective loss of slow and enhancement of fast Na^+ currents in cutaneous afferent dorsal root ganglion neurones following axotomy. *Neurobiol Dis* 1995; 2:87–96.

Ro LS, Chen ST, Tang LM, Jacobs JM. Effect of NGF and anti-NGF on neuropathic pain in rats following chronic constriction injury of the sciatic nerve. *Pain* 1999; 79(2–3):265–274.

Rush RA. Immunohistochemical localization of endogenous nerve growth factor. *Nature* 1984; 312:364–367.

Sanchez C. Stress induced vocalization in adult animals. A valid model of anxiety? *Eur J Pharmacol* 2003; 463:133–143.Scadding JW, Koltzenburg M. Painful peripheral neuropathies. In: McMahon SB, Koltzenburg M (Eds). *Wall and Melzack's Textbook of Pain,* 5th ed. Philadelphia: Elsevier, 2005, pp 973–999.

Schafers M, Geis C, Brors D, Yaksh TL, Sommer C. Anterograde transport of tumor necrosis factor-alpha in the intact and injured rat sciatic nerve. *J Neurosci* 2002; 22:536–545.

Schmelz M, Schmid R, Handwerker HO, Torebjork HE. Encoding of burning pain from capsaicin-treated human skin in two categories of unmyelinated nerve fibres. *Brain* 2000; 123:560–571.

Serra J. Overview of neuropathic pain syndromes. *Acta Neurol Scand* (Suppl) 1999; 173:7–11.

Sevcik MA, Ghilardi JR, Peters CM, et al. Anti-NGF therapy profoundly reduces bone cancer pain and the accompanying increase in markers of peripheral and central sensitization. *Pain* 2005; 115:128–141.

Shadiack AM, Sun Y, Zigmond RE. Nerve growth factor antiserum induces axotomy-like changes in neuropeptide expression in intact sympathetic and sensory neurons. *J Neurosci* 2001; 21:363–371.

Shembalkar PK, Till S, Boettger MK, et al. Increased sodium channel SNS/PN3 immunoreactivity in a causalgic finger. *Eur J Pain* 2001; 5:319–323.

Sheth RN, Dorsi MJ, Li Y, et al. Mechanical hyperalgesia after an L5 ventral rhizotomy or an L5 ganglionectomy in the rat. *Pain* 2002; 96:63–72.

Shim B, Kim DW, Kim BH, et al. Mechanical and heat sensitization of cutaneous nociceptors in rats with experimental peripheral neuropathy. *Neuroscience* 2005; 132:193–201.

Shubayev VI, Myers RR. Anterograde TNF alpha transport from rat dorsal root ganglion to spinal cord and injured sciatic nerve. *Neurosci Lett* 2002; 320:99–101.

Sukhotinsky I, Ben-Dor E, Raber P, Devor M. Key role of the dorsal root ganglion in neuropathic tactile hypersensitivity. *Eur J Pain* 2004; 8:135–143.

Sun H, Ren K, Zhong CM, et al. Nerve injury-induced tactile allodynia is mediated via ascending spinal dorsal column projections. *Pain* 2001; 90:105–111.

Szallasi A, Blumberg PM. Vanilloid receptor loss in rat sensory ganglia associated with long term desensitization to resiniferatoxin. *Neurosci Lett* 1992; 140:51–54.

Taniuchi M, Clark HB, Schweitzer JB, Johnson EM Jr. Expression of nerve growth factor receptors by Schwann cells of axotomized peripheral nerves: ultrastructural location, suppression by axonal contact, and binding properties. *J Neurosci* 1988; 8:664–681.

Torebjork HE, Lundberg LE, LaMotte RH. Central changes in processing of mechanoreceptive input in capsaicin- induced secondary hyperalgesia in humans. *J Physiol (Lond)* 1992; 448:765–780.

Treede RD, Davis KD, Campbell JN, Raja SN. The plasticity of cutaneous hyperalgesia during sympathetic ganglion blockade in patients with neuropathic pain. *Brain* 1992; 115:607–621.

Treede RD, Handwerker HO, Baumgärtner U, Meyer RA, Magerl W. Hyperalgesia and allodynia: taxonomy, assessment, and mechanisms. In: Brune K, Handwerker HO (Eds). *Hyperalgesia: Molecular Mechanisms and Clinical Implications,* Progress in Pain Research and Management, Vol. 30. Seattle: IASP Press, 2004; pp 3–15.

Tsuboi Y, Takeda M, Tanimoto T, et al. Alteration of the second branch of the trigeminal nerve activity following inferior alveolar nerve transection in rats. *Pain* 2004; 111:323–334.

Tsuzuki K, Kondo E, Fukuoka T, et al. Differential regulation of $P2X_3$ mRNA expression by peripheral nerve injury in intact and injured neurons in the rat sensory ganglia. *Pain* 2001; 91:351–360.

Valder CR, Liu JJ, Song YH, Luo ZD. Coupling gene chip analyses and rat genetic variances in identifying potential target genes that may contribute to neuropathic allodynia development. *J Neurochem* 2003; 87:560–573.

Valenzano KJ, Miller W, Chen Z, et al. DiPOA ([8-(3,3-diphenyl-propyl)-4-oxo-1-phenyl-1,3,8-triazaspiro[4.5]dec-3-yl]-acetic acid), a novel, systemically available, and peripherally restricted mu opioid agonist with antihyperalgesic activity: I. In vitro pharmacological characterization and pharmacokinetic properties. *J Pharmacol Exp Ther* 2004; 310:783–792.

Wadhwani KC, Rapoport SI. Transport properties of vertebrate blood-nerve barrier: comparison with blood-brain barrier. *Prog Neurobiol* 1994; 43:235–279.

Wagner R, Myers RR. Endoneurial injection of TNF-alpha produces neuropathic pain behaviors. *Neuroreport* 1996; 7:2897–2901.

Walker K, Fox AJ, Urban LA. Animal models for pain research. *Mol Med Today* 1999; 5:319–321.

Wang Z, Gardell LR, Ossipov MH, et al. Pronociceptive actions of dynorphin maintain chronic neuropathic pain. *J Neurosci* 2001; 21:1779–1786.

Watkins LR, Maier SF. Glia: a novel drug discovery target for clinical pain. *Nat Rev Drug Discov* 2003; 2:973–985.

Watkins LR, Maier SF. Immune regulation of central nervous system functions: from sickness responses to pathological pain. *J Intern Med* 2005; 257:139–155.

Waxman SG, Kocsis JD, Black JA. Type III sodium channel mRNA is expressed in embryonic but not adult spinal sensory neurons, and is re-expressed following axotomy. *J Neurophysiol* 1994; 72:466–470.

Whiteside GT, Harrison JE, Pearson MS, et al. DiPOA ([8-(3,3-diphenyl-propyl)-4-oxo-1-phenyl-1,3,8-triazaspiro[4.5]dec-3-yl]-acetic acid), a novel, systemically available, and peripherally restricted mu opioid agonist with antihyperalgesic activity: II. In vivo pharmacological characterization in the rat. *J Pharmacol Exp Ther* 2004; 310:793–799.

Wittmack EK, Rush AM, Craner MJ, et al. Fibroblast growth factor homologous factor 2B: association with Na$_v$1.6 and selective colocalization at nodes of Ranvier of dorsal root axons. *J Neurosci* 2004; 24:6765–6775.

Woolf CJ, Safieh-Garabedian B, Ma QP, Crilly P, Winter J. Nerve growth factor contributes to the generation of inflammatory sensory hypersensitivity. *Neuroscience* 1994; 62:327–331.

Wu G, Ringkamp M, Hartke TV, et al. Early onset of spontaneous activity in uninjured C-fiber nociceptors after injury to neighboring nerve fibers. *J Neurosci* 2001; 21:RC140.

Xiao HS, Huang QH, Zhang FX, et al. Identification of gene expression profile of dorsal root ganglion in the rat peripheral axotomy model of neuropathic pain. *Proc Natl Acad Sci USA* 2002; 99:8360–8365.

Yoshimura N, de Groat WC. Increased excitability of afferent neurons innervating rat urinary bladder after chronic bladder inflammation. *J Neurosci* 1999; 19:4644–4653.

Zhang Q, Ji RR, Lindsay R, Hokfelt T. Effect of growth factors on substance P mRNA expression in axotomized dorsal root ganglia. *Neuroreport* 1995; 6:1309–1312.

Zhuang ZY, Gerner P, Woolf CJ, Ji RR. ERK is sequentially activated in neurons, microglia, and astrocytes by spinal nerve ligation and contributes to mechanical allodynia in this neuropathic pain model. *Pain* 2005; 114:149–159.

Zubieta JK, Heitzeg MM, Smith YR, et al. COMT *val158met* genotype affects mu-opioid neurotransmitter responses to a pain stressor. *Science* 2003; 299:1240–1243.

Correspondence to: Michael S. Gold, PhD, Department of Biomedical Sciences, UMB Dental School, Room 5-A-12, 666 W. Baltimore Street, Baltimore, MD 21201, USA. Tel: 410-706-0909; Fax: 410-706-0865; email: mgold@umaryland.edu.

Emerging Strategies for the Treatment of Neuropathic Pain, edited by James N. Campbell, Allan I. Basbaum, André Dray, Ronald Dubner, Robert H. Dworkin, and Christine N. Sang, IASP Press, Seattle, © 2006.

2

Peripheral Nerve Generators of Neuropathic Pain

Marshall Devor

Department of Cell and Animal Biology, Institute of Life Sciences and Center for Research on Pain, Hebrew University of Jerusalem, Jerusalem, Israel

This chapter will consider the variety of pathophysiological processes in the peripheral nervous system (PNS) that contribute to neuropathic pain, as well as mechanisms whereby PNS changes trigger and maintain relevant changes in the central nervous system (CNS). Hundreds, perhaps thousands, of distinct neural changes are triggered by nerve injury. A priori, each is a potential therapeutic target. Given the substantial resources required to test even a single target, strategies are needed to prioritize research efforts. The present analysis is guided by a single underlying principle for prioritizing—the notion that pain sensation is a function of impulse traffic reaching a conscious brain. To choose targets wisely, we need to focus on how neuropathy alters the generation and amplification of sensory signals that eventually reach the brain. The discussion in this chapter is limited to pain due to peripheral neuropathy; central pain will not be considered here.

Despite efforts by the IASP Committee on Taxonomy (Merskey and Bogduk 1994), we still lack a universally accepted definition of "neuropathic pain." For present purposes, neuropathic pain is distinguished from normal (nociceptive) pain and from pain due to inflammation as follows: In nociceptive and inflammatory pain, the neural impulses responsible for the pain experience arise from sensory endings (intact or sensitized) as part of the normal functioning of the pain detection system. Neuropathic pain results from abnormal neural discharge arising in parts of the pain system other than sensory endings (i.e., at "ectopic" locations), due to nerve injury or disease. This includes the situation where abnormal discharge due to neuropathy causes excess central amplification of signals arising in otherwise intact sensory endings. The root cause of the pain remains the neuropathy. A potential overlap with inflammatory pain is when sensory endings of intact uninjured fibers become sensitized due to damage to their neighbors (Wu et al. 2001a; Shim et al. 2005). Consistent with the current IASP definition, the bottom line is neural injury or disease (Merskey and Bogduk 1994). Think of a home alarm system: is the alarm sounding in response to an intruder or inappropriately because the circuitry has been damaged? Although a useful guide, the distinction between "intact" and "damaged" and between "sensory endings" and "ectopic locations" sometimes breaks down. For example, on a micro-level, sensory endings in burned skin, or in skin soaked in inflammatory mediators, might well be considered "damaged." Some level of ambiguity will inevitably remain in any definition as mechanisms of inflammatory and neuropathic pain partly overlap.

PRECIPITATING EVENTS

Essentially any type of neural damage or disease, whether physical, chemical, or metabolic, can induce pain-provoking pathology in a peripheral nerve (neuropathy), in a sensory or autonomic ganglion (ganglionopathy), or in a dorsal root (radiculopathy). Common precipitating events are trauma (frequently iatrogenic), viral or bacterial infection, sterile inflammation, metabolic abnormalities, malnutrition, vascular abnormalities, neurotoxins, radiation, inherited mutations, and autoimmune attack. The question of how injury causes nerve pathology is of some interest, but the key question is how pathology causes chronic pain (Fig. 1).

There are two main types of pathological change and they often occur in combination: (1) dysmyelination and demyelination, and most likely also functional disruption of the Schwann cells that embrace Remak bundles, and (2) axonal injury, from minor axonopathy to frank axotomy. There may also be other, more subtle forms of damage, such as disruption of the blood-nerve and tissue-nerve barriers or changes in endoneurial matrix molecules (Kazarinova-Noyes et al. 2001). However, to the extent that such changes cause pain, they probably do so by affecting nerve fibers and their glial

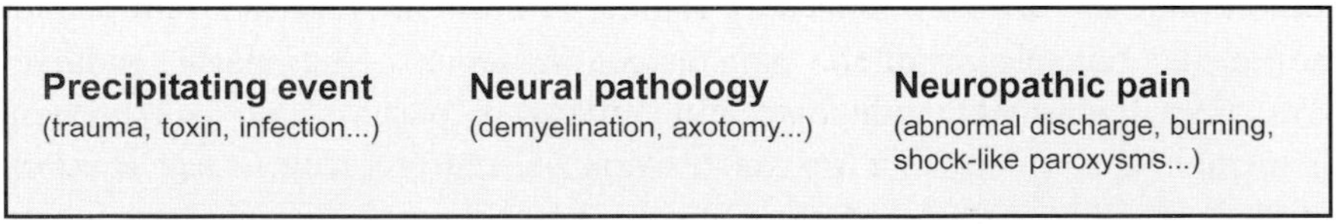

Precipitating event	Neural pathology	Neuropathic pain
(trauma, toxin, infection...)	(demyelination, axotomy...)	(abnormal discharge, burning, shock-like paroxysms...)

Fig. 1. Nerve injury and disease cause neuropathic pain due to pathological changes induced in the nerve and CNS. The relation between nerve injury and nerve pathology needs to be considered separately from the relation between nerve pathology and pain.

sheath. It is fairly obvious how disruption of the ability of axons to conduct nerve impulses causes "negative" sensory symptoms such as hypoesthesia and numbness. What needs explaining is "positive" sensory symptoms: paresthesias, dysesthesias, and pain. Sudden damage may evoke pain due to "injury discharge," but chronic neuropathic pain almost certainly results from secondary pathophysiological changes that develop over time (Devor 2005).

INDIVIDUAL VARIABILITY

Pain in neuropathy is notoriously variable from patient to patient, even when the precipitating injury or disease is essentially identical. It must be presumed that such variability is due to a combination of environmental (including psychosocial) factors and genetic predisposition (Mogil 2004). Little is currently known about genes that affect pain given a fixed neural pathology ("pain susceptibility genes"). In contrast, considerable progress has been made on the very different effort of defining mutations and polymorphisms that predispose one to acquire particular types of painful nerve pathology ("disease susceptibility genes"). Despite the clinical importance of the latter, it is the former that have the greatest potential for advancing understanding of mechanisms of pain. Disease susceptibility genes, and environmental factors that precipitate disease, primarily affect the creation of neural pathology. Pain susceptibility genes, in contrast, most likely affect the relation of pathology to pain (Fig. 1).

Quantification of relevant changes in damaged nerves in the clinical setting is unsatisfactory. A severed nerve will reliably produce functional loss, but it may or may not become an abnormal impulse generator, depending on factors discussed below. Not only is the relation of pathology to altered electrogenesis complex and variable, but we also lack good methods to detect pathology. Routine clinical nerve conduction studies and electromyography are insensitive to minor damage, especially when it affects small-diameter, slowly conducting axons. Nerve or skin-punch biopsies partly overcome this problem, but they sample only a tiny fraction of the sensory neuron, and as currently used they are unlikely to show the key molecular changes responsible for altered neural excitability and pain. We lack objective, clinically tractable indicators of abnormal electrogenesis, and are forced to rely instead on indirect measures. One should therefore keep an open mind about the possibility of chronic pains of uncertain origin perhaps being neuropathic; pains felt in deep somatic tissues or viscera, for example (Freeman 2005), or even common entities such as low back pain, fibromyalgia, and even migraine.

WHAT NEEDS EXPLAINING?

SENSORY DYSFUNCTION DUE TO NEUROPATHY

Nerve injury and disease may precipitate abnormalities of sensation including pain, motor disturbances, autonomic signs and symptoms, and trophic tissue changes. The focus here, naturally, is on sensory changes. Three categories of pain need to be distinguished. (1) *Spontaneous pain* (ongoing pain) is present at rest when no (intentional) stimulus is applied. Whether the pain is truly independent of any stimulus, or whether it is associated with internal physiological factors such as blood chemistry, autonomic nervous system activity, or hormones, is often unknown. It is a bad habit to refer to ongoing pain simply as "pain." (2) *Evoked pain* is pain on stimulation of the skin or other accessible tissues such as the oral or nasal mucosa. According to current IASP usage, pain evoked by stimuli that are normally painless (touch, warm or cool stimuli, or dilute chemicals) is called "allodynia" (tactile allodynia, heat allodynia, etc.). When a normally painful stimulus evokes more intense pain than expected, this pain is termed "hyperalgesia." (3) *Pain evoked by movement and weight bearing,* or by focal pressure to deep tissues (muscle, tendon, or visceral "tender points" or "trigger points"), might simply be mechanical allodynia due to deep tissue inflammation. Alternatively, it may reflect neuropathology, perhaps at sites where small nerve branches are pinched as they cross fascial planes (microneuroma). When the source of pain is not at the surface, it is inherently difficult to analyze.

THE SENSORY QUALITY OF NEUROPATHIC PAIN

The words that people with neural damage or disease use to describe their sensory experience can be informative. Some of these terms are generic, but some are characteristic of neuropathy in general, or even of particular neuropathic pain diagnoses (Bouhassira et al. 2004). For example, spontaneous burning pain occurs in postherpetic neuralgia (PHN) as well as after acute burns, but shooting pain and electric shock-like paroxysms are uncommon except in neuropathy. "Hyperpathia" is a constellation of pain descriptors essentially exclusive to neuropathy. In hyperpathia, sensation shows odd temporal and spatial characteristics. A gentle tap on the back of the hand may feel dull (hypoesthetic), as if felt through a boxing glove. However, with repeated tapping (say, once or twice a second for 10–20 seconds) the sensation "winds up," becoming stronger and stronger until it reaches a painful crescendo. Hyperpathic sensations also spread in space; localized touch may trigger a stinging sensation that spreads up the arm.

Even though distinctive sensory peculiarities like electric shock-like paroxysms and hyperpathia are rare compared to ongoing burning pain, they are important objects for theoretical analysis because they get to the heart of what makes a pain neuropathic.

PHANTOM LIMB PAIN AND ANESTHESIA DOLOROSA

Special mention needs to be made of neuropathic sensory experience felt in parts of the body that no longer exist or that are completely numb due to major nerve injury or traumatic avulsion of sensory roots from the spinal cord (Wynn-Parry 1980; Nikolajsen and Jensen 2001). The limb continues to be felt as a "phantom" and is painful some of the time in most patients, and most of the time in some patients. Many amputees report factors that exacerbate phantom pain (e.g., urination, emotional upset, or cold weather), or that provide temporary relief (e.g., massage or warming). What is the source of the impulses that are interpreted by the conscious brain of the amputee as phantom limb sensation and phantom limb pain? In principle, they could arise in the peripheral nerve and ganglion, in the cerebral cortex, or anywhere in between.

Beyond the sensory quality of phantom limb sensation (tingling, burning pain, etc.), amputees also report changes in the spatial aspects of phantom limb representations. There may be willed or unwilled movement of the phantom, for example, and its size and location are subject to distortion. Most amputees, for example, describe "telescoping," where over a period of months or years a full-length phantom arm draws in toward the body until only a hand is felt protruding from the stump. Sensation may also be referred to (i.e., felt in) the phantom arm upon stroking the cheek or the chest wall. As in phantom limb pain itself, there is uncertainty as to what extent these body schema distortions are due to PNS activity as opposed to plastic changes that originate in spinal and supraspinal body surface representations.

DIVERSITY OF DIAGNOSES

Neuropathic pain is fundamentally a paradox. Like cutting a telephone cable, injuring a nerve ought to make the line go dead (negative symptoms). Why, then, does neuropathy trigger paresthesias, dysesthesias, and pain (positive symptoms)? A related question concerns diversity. Many authors presume that, since different diagnoses are triggered by different precipitating events and present with different clinical pictures and natural histories, each has its own pain mechanism. Does "peripheral neuropathic pain" represent a

zoo of unrelated conditions, or a single disease with a variety of manifestations? The orthodox view is that clinical diversity reflects diversity of mechanisms. I lean toward the heresy that entities as seemingly different as amputation pain, trigeminal neuralgia, PHN, and Fabry's disease share fundamental
unifying neural mechanisms. Stated briefly, my thesis is that *chronic pain is
a disease of altered excitability in the pain system.* If it is due to tissue
inflammation, the pain is inflammatory; if due to neural damage or dysfunction, it is neuropathic. Neural inflammation is a hybrid. The term "excitability" is explained below.

The paradox of neuropathic pain is rooted in the misconception that
nerves are basically like copper telephone cables. True, primary afferents
convey electrical signals from the periphery to the CNS, but the analogy
does not go much beyond that. Axons are not wires but live, protoplasmic
extensions of specialized cells. We need to take seriously the biology of
these cells. How do they response to demyelination and axonopathy, and
how do they interact with their PNS and CNS neighbors?

NEUROPATHIC PAIN MECHANISMS

SPONTANEOUS ECTOPIC DISCHARGE

The cascade of events that lead to pain after nerve lesions, including
changes in "uninjured" neighbors and in the CNS, begins with the damaged
primary sensory neuron itself. The most striking, and on the face of it,
salient, change in neuronal phenotype is that a considerable fraction of
injured afferents (demyelinated and axotomized) are rendered prone to excess generation of electrical impulses, either spontaneously or in response to
depolarizing physical, thermal, or chemical stimuli (Devor 2005). Neurons
that previously generated impulses only at their peripheral sensory ending in
response to an adequate stimulus (such as touch or pinch) now begin to
generate impulses spontaneously at ectopic locations, primarily at the nerve
injury site and within the sensory ganglion. Ectopically generated impulses
are conveyed along the dorsal roots into the CNS, where they activate central neurons, increasing the ongoing activity of these neurons and their response to other inputs. Any discussion of elevated CNS activity (and response) must consider whether the excess activity is actually generated in
the CNS or simply reflects excessive PNS drive (Sotgiu et al. 1994).

Neurons in the PNS share a common microenvironment, and to a certain
extent they interact with one another. After nerve injury, neighboring neurons that have not been directly injured may also show phenotypic changes.
A classic example is collateral sprouting of residual afferents into the

terminal zone vacated by injured ones. Neighboring neurons may also show changes in electrogenesis. For example, Wu et al. (2001a) reported the appearance of spontaneous ectopic discharge, albeit at extremely low firing rates, in afferent C fibers that shared a nerve trunk with degenerating axons but had not been cut themselves. Shim et al. (2005), using a similar experimental design, found even more robust activity. It is not yet clear whether the electrogenic mechanism in injured and uninjured neurons is the same.

Simple logic, and a great deal of specific evidence from animal models and patients (especially that based on diagnostic nerve blocks), leads inevitably to the conclusion that spontaneous ectopic discharge arising in the periphery in large part gives rise to spontaneous paresthesias, dysesthesias, and pain in neuropathy. This includes anesthesia dolorosa and phantom limb pain (Nordin et al. 1984; Kuslich et al. 1991; Tessler and Kleiman 1994; Devor 2005). The simplest model is that the quality of sensory experience caused by spontaneous ectopic discharge is dictated by the type of afferent involved and the firing intensity (and pattern?) and kinetics. For example, thermal sensibility to heat and cold stimuli is normally due to the activation of thermosensitive C and Aδ afferents. Spontaneous burning pain in neuropathy would thus be due to ectopic activity in peripheral thermal nociceptors. Unfortunately, since it is difficult to assess sensory quality in animals, this inference will have to await better neurographic evidence from patients. It could be wrong. Given the major changes in CNS signal processing in neuropathy, sensory quality could be determined or distorted centrally. For example, a CNS pathway that signals heat and normally responds to thermal afferents might come to be driven by ectopic activity in low-threshold mechanoreceptive afferents at normal body temperature. In principle this mechanism could apply to all natural sensory qualities (qualia) including cold, pinch, flutter, etc. The simplistic and almost certainly erroneous idea that spontaneous pain in neuropathy must be driven by ectopic activity in C- and Aδ-fiber nociceptors is discussed below.

Beyond constituting a primary source of impulses underlying spontaneous neuropathic sensory experience, spontaneous ectopia probably also contributes importantly to the initiation and maintenance of central sensitization. Here too, the idea that only C- and Aδ-fiber nociceptive afferents play a role is likely to be erroneous, as discussed below.

SPONTANEOUS ECTOPIC DISCHARGE: THREE CELLULAR MECHANISMS

Axonal transection blocks the normal flow of neurotrophic signaling molecules between innervated peripheral tissues and the sensory cell body.

This event triggers a change in the quantity and disposition of proteins expressed by the cell body and exported to both peripheral and central axon endings (Boucher and McMahon 2001). Some molecules are upregulated, and others are downregulated. Data derived from oligonucleotide array analysis indicate that overall, some 5–10% of all genes expressed in axotomized dorsal root ganglion (DRG) neurons are significantly regulated, i.e., their expression is increased or decreased by 50% or more. And among genes coding for molecules of excitability (e.g., ion channels) the fraction is much higher, perhaps 100% (Costigan et al. 2002; Xiao et al. 2002). Overall, the number of regulated genes probably reaches into the thousands. Gene expression may also be affected in "uninjured" neighboring neurons (Obata et al. 2004). The potential effects on DRG cell phenotype (i.e., functional characteristics) are wide-ranging, essentially impossible to predict, and not necessarily related to pain. Fortunately, there are efficient strategies for selecting which changes affect pain response versus, say, regeneration. For example, one might compare gene regulation in pain-sensitive versus pain-resistant rodent strains, or closely examine the timing of altered pain phenotype against the timing of altered gene expression. Candidates may be verified using transgenic and pharmacological tools. A unique advantage of such array-based approaches is that they do not depend on a priori beliefs and biases about pain physiology. Therefore, in addition to confirming already suspected targets, analysis of gene regulation might reveal previously unimagined players in pain biology. Remarkably, demyelination might also affect gene expression in associated neurons (Craner et al. 2003).

The second mechanism is that neuropathy also alters neuronal trafficking and protein disposition. The most important change of this sort is the accumulation (or depletion) of molecules of excitability at sites of axonal injury, including zones of demyelination, swollen terminal endbulbs at the cut axon end, and outgrowing sprouts. The best documented example is the accumulation of Na^+ channels at injured axon ends, a process known to contribute to neuronal hyperexcitability (Fig. 2; Devor et al. 1989; England et al. 1996; Waxman 2002; Devor 2005). This factor probably does not depend on a change in gene expression. Even an unaltered flow of transported molecules, when directed to a much reduced membrane target area (e.g., neuroma endbulbs and sprouts rather than centimeters of downstream axon), can result in accumulation.

Another reason for altered trafficking is the removal of normal regulatory processes. In intact axons Na^+ channels are largely excluded from the axonal membrane underlying the myelin. When myelin is stripped off the axon, Na^+ channels begin to accumulate in the exposed axolemma (England et al. 1990). The strategies noted above regarding altered gene expression can

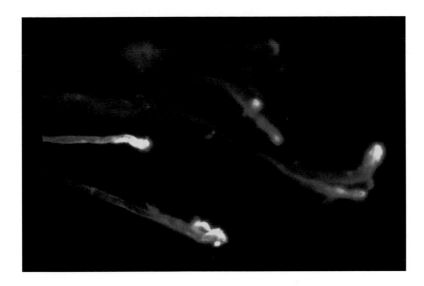

Fig. 2. Immunolabeling shows the accumulation of Na⁺ channels at the chronic cut end of injured axons in *Apteronotus* (see Devor et al. 1989).

also be used to establish *which* changes in trafficking are most important. There are many potential therapeutic targets in the axoplasmic transport process, in the trophic pathways that regulate it, in protein insertion into membranes, and in the machinery of trafficking including protein target-specific signal sequences.

The third mechanism is that, in addition to its effects on gene expression and protein trafficking, neuropathy may change the biophysical phenotype of DRG neurons by affecting the current-carrying ability of existing populations of ion channels. It is not ion channel proteins themselves that determine cell excitability, but the ionic currents they carry. Increasing mean channel open time or unitary channel conductance can have much the same effect on excitability as increasing the number of channels present. Inflammatory and other mediators associated with neuropathy can affect channel kinetics in this way. For example, cAMP-dependent phosphorylation of Na⁺ channel molecules reduces Na⁺ current, while dephosphorylation returns it to normal (e.g., Li et al. 1992; Gold et al. 1996). Because certain hormones, trophic factors, prostanoids, cytokines and other inflammatory mediators can activate protein kinases (PKA, PKC), they are positioned to affect afferent *excitability,* and not just to depolarize and excite afferents as is normally presumed. Kinase isoenzymes have tremendous diversity ($n > 500$) and considerable substrate specificity (Chen et al. 2005). They themselves could be drug targets for pain control.

PROCESSES THAT BRING ABOUT HYPEREXCITABILITY

The phenotype of a sensory neuron reflects the entire ensemble of molecules that it expresses (in partnership with glia and the extracellular matrix). It is difficult to intuit, or even to simulate, how the electrical behavior of a neuron will respond to a change in the density, disposition, and kinetics of a single such molecule. Yet the hyperexcitability observed in real-life biological systems reflects the simultaneous remodeling of many. Which are key? An inductive, genomics approach to answering this question was noted above. There are also deductive approaches. For example, when considering electrogenesis it is reasonable to focus on changes in ion channels (Waxman 2002; Chung et al. 2003). Even if the primary effect of axotomy is on a regulatory molecule, changes in electrical properties of neurons must ultimately be mediated by ion channels.

The appearance of nerve injury-evoked ectopic hyperexcitability is not simply a matter of lowered spike threshold. Pain persists over time, so relevant changes in neuronal properties must include persistent firing. Most intact DRG neurons are intrinsically *incapable* of generating sustained impulse discharge in the mid-nerve axon or in the cell soma, even in the presence of strong sustained depolarizing stimuli (e.g., by intracellular current injection or elevated extracellular K^+). Sustained discharge depends on "pacemaker capability," normally a specialized feature of sensory endings (Devor 2005). The phenotypic change resulting from neuropathic alteration of gene expression, trafficking, and kinetics is the actual creation of repetitive firing capability de novo at ectopic locations. Given the central role of repetitive firing capability in pain sensation, the cellular processes underlying it ought to deeply engage pain investigators.

Pacemaking includes two related process (Amir et al. 2002b). One is the iterative mechanism that sustains brief or prolonged spike trains (bursts). Each spike in a train *except for the first* is triggered by a rebound depolarizing afterpotential (DAP) generated by the previous spike. DAP-maintained bursts are usually brief, as they are self-limited by burst-induced hyperpolarization. Few sensory cells generate unending spike trains. The key to repetitive firing is therefore the process that generates the first spike in each train. The sudden depolarization of an electric shock can do this. However, slow ramp depolarizations characteristic of natural stimuli are generally unable to induce spikes in DRG neurons because of membrane accommodation. In order to generate sustained repetitive firing, the sine qua non of chronic pain, something must overcome accommodation.

At ectopic pacemaker sites this "something" appears to be the depolarizing phase of sinusoidal subthreshold oscillations that occur in the membrane potential of cells with pacemaker capability, or less regular fast-rising membrane potential fluctuations (Fig. 3; Amir et al. 1999). In cells that have subthreshold oscillations, slow-onset and sustained depolarizing stimuli bring the peaks of oscillation sinusoids to threshold; this is what triggers repetitive firing. Repetitive firing takes the form of sequences of single spikes in cells that do not generate DAPs, and unending trains of spike bursts in cells that do (Amir et al. 2002b). Axonopathy and demyelination cause ectopic firing and neuropathic pain because they dramatically increase the fraction of afferents that generate subthreshold oscillations in the DRG and at mid-axon sites (Kapoor et al. 1997; Amir et al. 1999).

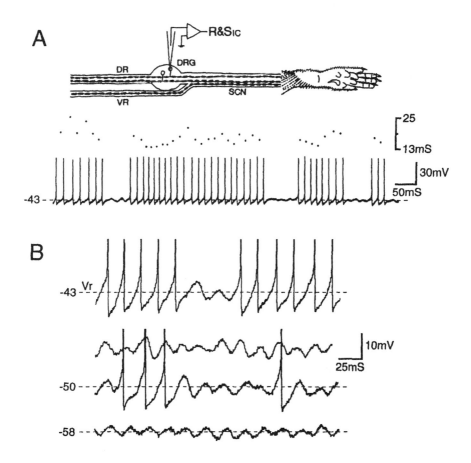

Fig. 3. Ectopic burst discharge in neuropathy is driven by subthreshold membrane potential oscillations. (A) The experimental setup for intracellular recording from the rat dorsal root ganglion (DRG), and an example of burst discharge with the associated distribution of interspike intervals. (B) A DRG neuron in which subthreshold oscillations were present at resting membrane potential (−58 mV), but with no spiking. When the cell was gradually depolarized, peaks of oscillatory sinusoids began to trigger ectopic burst discharge. (From Amir et al. 2002b.)

Resonance, reflected in the ability to generate subthreshold oscillations, is an essential requirement of pacemaker capability. The biophysical process responsible for resonance, and the reasons for its enhancement in neuropathy, are therefore of central importance to an understanding of neuropathic pain. The first steps have been taken in understanding this process (Puil et al. 1988; Wu et al. 2001b; Amir et al. 2002a; Waxman 2002). Briefly, resonance appears to reflect reciprocation between inward Na^+ current carried by fast-activating, inactivating, and repriming TTX-sensitive Na^+ channels (probably largely $Na_V1.3$ in neuropathy) and K^+ current passing through one or more voltage-insensitive K^+ leak channels (perhaps of the KCNK K2p family). These ion channels, and the processes which regulate their expression, trafficking, and kinetics, are hence prime therapeutic targets. Voltage-sensitive K^+ channels tend to hold resonance in check, and their downregulation after axotomy may be an important contributor to ectopia (Kocsis and Devor 2000). K^+ channel openers may therefore be of interest. Other channel types and conductances that might contribute to resonance characteristics of primary sensory neurons include certain Ca^{2+} channels, the hyperpolarization-activated Ih "pacemaker" channel (CNH), KCNQ potassium channels, the β_4 Na^+ channel subunit-associated resurgent current, and persistent Na^+ conductances, but their role, at this stage, is speculative.

EXCITATION VERSUS EXCITABILITY

These terms are frequently used interchangeably, but the distinction is critical to an informed choice of optimal therapeutic targets in the PNS. "Excitation" refers to transduction, the ability of a stimulus to depolarize a sensory neuron and create a *generator* current. "Excitability," in contrast, refers to the *encoding* of the generator potential into an impulse train (pacemaker capability; Fig. 4). Without careful thought, we tend to combine "excitation" and "excitability" into one, imagining that a stimulus directly evokes an impulse train. However, these processes operate using different molecules, accessible by different therapeutic agents. Excitation (transduction) depends on the stimulus itself, its physical transmission to sensory endings, and the transducer and ligand-gated receptor molecules present. Excitability (pacemaker capability), in contrast, depends primarily on certain voltage-gated ion channels.

The transduction and the pacemaker processes offer very different opportunities for therapeutic intervention. A large number of physical and chemical stimuli are able to depolarize and excite excitable neurons. The elimination of any one of them, using specific pharmacological agents for example, leaves all of the rest still in play. In contrast, if the excitability of a

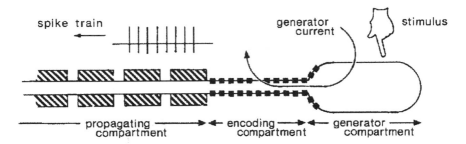

Fig. 4. Stimuli applied to sensory endings or ectopic pacemaker sites create a generator current due to transducer and receptor molecules. The generator potential is translated into a spike train in the nearby encoding compartment due to voltage-sensitive ion channels. The spike train is then propagated centrally.

cell is suppressed it loses its ability to respond to *all* depolarizing stimuli and to convey corresponding messages centrally. The encoding (pacemaker) process can be thought of as the outlet of a funnel. It is a uniquely powerful functional node, a point of access and control for pain signals (Fig. 5).

ECTOPIC SENSITIVITY TO APPLIED STIMULI

Percussion over sites of nerve injury, areas of entrapment (e.g., of the ulnar nerve) or neuromas for example, typically evokes an intense stabbing or electric shock-like sensation, the Tinel sign. Similar sensations can be evoked by other maneuvers that apply mechanical force to hyperexcitable DRG cells and spinal roots, such as straight leg lifting in sciatica (Lasègue's sign), and the signs of Spurling and L'Hermitte. When equivalent stimuli are applied to ectopic pacemaker sites in animal preparations, and in humans, they evoke corresponding discharge bursts or augment spontaneous firing (Nordin et al. 1984; Devor 2005). This is the mechanism underlying ectopic mechanosensitivity. In some conditions, diabetic neuropathy for example, paresthesias and pain may be evoked by percussion anywhere along the course of a nerve, marking out its trajectory. This situation occurs when scattered outgrowing sprouts become trapped during the course of regeneration, or when mechanosensitive ectopic generator sites become scattered along the nerve during the process of axonal dying back or disseminated dysmyelination. Pain evoked by deep palpation at tender spots, such as in the piriformis syndrome or fibromyalgia, may reflect the same sort of ectopic mechanosensitivity at locations where nerve branches cross through fascial planes, under tendons, or are otherwise at risk of local damage. These are all reflections of pathophysiological change. Tapping on normal nerves does not evoke spike discharge or sensation. Interestingly, momentary

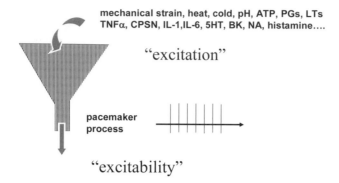

Fig. 5. The "electrogenic funnel." Many factors and molecules are able to create a generator potential in sensory endings and at ectopic pacemaker sites (excitation). A single process encodes the generator potential into a propagated spike train (excitability). Abbreviations: ATP = adenosine triphosphate; BK = bradykinin; CPSN = capsaicin; IL-1 = interleukin-1; 5HT = 5-hydroxytryptamine; LTs = leukotrienes; NA = norepinephrine; PGs = prostaglandins; TNFα = tumor necrosis factor alpha.

mechanical probing frequently evokes discharge that long outlasts the stimulus itself (Fig. 6). Such "afterdischarge" is the likely explanation of aftersensations, trigger points, and triggered pain paroxysms.

Injured neurons also develop abnormal sensitivity to other depolarizing stimuli. Notable among these are circulating epinephrine and norepinephrine released from nearby (injured) postganglionic sympathetic axons. The resulting sympathetic-sensory coupling is thought to be an important substrate of sympathetically maintained pain (SMP) states (Ali et al. 2000; Harden et al. 2001). Afferent response to local and circulating inflammatory mediators is a second example of ectopic chemosensitivity. It has been proposed, for example, that pain in sciatica is due to proinflammatory cytokines released from the nucleus pulposus of herniated intervertebral disks (Olmarker and Rydevik 2001). Abnormal discharge may also arise from other stimuli: temperature changes, ischemia, hypoxia, hypoglycemia, and indeed almost any imaginable condition that is capable of causing local membrane depolarization (Nordin et al. 1984; Devor 2005). But it needs to be stressed once again that stimulus-induced depolarization does not, in itself, provide for painful mechanosensitivity, chemosensitivity, and thermosensitivity. Ectopic spike discharge can only occur if ectopic pacemaker capability—membrane resonance—is present locally.

Ectopic mechanosensitivity, chemosensitivity, and thermosensitivity indicate that corresponding transducer and receptor proteins (such as stretch-activated mechano-channels, adrenoreceptors, receptors for prostaglandins, or transient receptor potential channels TRPV1 or TRPM8) are present near the ectopic pacemaker site. Such sensitivity does not, however, prove that expression of these transducer or receptor molecules has been upregulated, that they have accumulated locally, or that their kinetics has been altered. For example, normal DRG neurons express a variety of adrenoreceptors, and yet DRG neurons in intact animals rarely fire in response to adrenergic agonists or sympathetic stimulation (Chen et al. 1996). Firing requires membrane resonance. True, adrenoreceptor upregulation has been documented in axotomized DRG neurons (Birder and Perl 1999), but the baseline level present in these cells before upregulation might well be enough to support robust adrenosensitivity once ectopic pacemaker capability has emerged.

TACTILE ALLODYNIA

The simplest a priori explanation of pain in response to light touch is reduced response threshold in nociceptive afferents, the classical "excitable nociceptor hypothesis." For heat allodynia the data are consistent with this hypothesis. However, despite numerous studies, there is precious little evidence that mechanonociceptors ever come to respond in significant numbers to the very weak tactile stimuli that typically evoke allodynia in neuropathy, or even in inflamed tissues (Koltzenburg et al. 1994a; Banik and Brennan 2004; Tsuboi et al. 2004; Shim et al. 2005). Previously "silent" (i.e., nonresponsive) nociceptors might also be recruited, but these also rarely respond

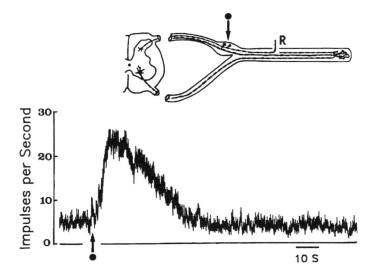

Fig. 6. Mechanical afterdischarge. A weak, momentary stimulus to the surface of the DRG (arrow) triggered a prolonged, self-sustained ectopic discharge burst.

to light brushing of the skin (Schmidt et al. 1995). Rather, tactile allodynia appears to be a sensory response to impulse activity in low-threshold mechanosensitive Aβ afferents abnormally "amplified" by central sensitization. Aβ afferents normally signal touch and vibration, but in neuropathy (and inflammation) they evoke pain, "Aβ pain" (Campbell et al. 1988; Torebjork et al. 1992; Koltzenburg et al. 1994b). Aβ pain constitutes a revolution in our understanding of the pain system, displacing Aδ and C fibers as the exclusive, and perhaps even the most important, primary afferent signaling channel for (pathophysiological) pain. Although most investigators accept the fundamental concept of Aβ pain, and the underlying data, some exhibit an odd denial of its logical consequences.

HYPERPATHIA

Causes of hyperpathic sensory peculiarities have attracted relatively little research attention, perhaps because they are relatively uncommon in patients and difficult to document in animals. They are of interest, however, as they are essentially unique to neuropathy. Hyperpathia does not necessarily reflect altered CNS processing. Pathophysiological behavior of injured peripheral sensory neurons in experimental preparations, coupled with central sensitization, echoes hyperpathic symptoms in humans (Devor 2005). For example, repeated stimulation may result in an incremental buildup of ectopic discharge in DRG cells following partial nerve injury, recalling sensory "wind-up," and excitation may spread from neuron to neuron, a likely mechanism of hyperpathic spread of sensation from the site of stimulation. Both phenomena may be due to nonsynaptic chemical communication among injured sensory neurons. Two such processes are known: ephaptic (electrical) coupling and "crossed-afterdischarge," a novel mode of neurotransmitter-mediated paracrine cross-excitation (Utzschneider et al. 1992; Fried et al. 1993; Amir and Devor 1996).

LANCINATING PAIN AND ELECTRIC SHOCK-LIKE PAROXYSMS

Crossed-afterdischarge provides a potential explanation for one of the most distinctive, peculiar, and devastating of the chronic neuropathic pain states, trigeminal neuralgia (TN, also known as tic douloureux), as well as for pain paroxysms in a wide variety of other neuropathies. Patients with TN suffer from brief, dramatic, stabbing or electric shock-like "lightning" pains felt in one or more divisions of the trigeminal distribution, either spontaneously or upon gentle tactile stimulation of a trigger point on the face or in the oral cavity (Kugelberg and Lindblom 1959). The discovery 60 years ago that TN responds to certain anticonvulsant drugs, notably carbamazepine, gave rise to the hypothesis that pain paroxysms in TN reflect seizure-like activity in the trigeminal brainstem.

More recently, however, Rappaport and Devor (1994) proposed an alternative mechanism, the "ignition hypothesis," more consistent with the known PNS pathology of TN. According to the ignition hypothesis, pain paroxysms begin with discharge in a small cluster of trigeminal nerve afferents upon cutaneous trigger-point stimulation, or spontaneously. Crossed-afterdischarge coupling in the injured trigeminal root or ganglion then "ignites" activity in passive neighboring neurons, the augmented activity ignites additional passive neighbors, and these ignite still more. The resulting positive-feedback chain reaction builds up rapidly to an intense, explosive peak. Since neurons of all types become active simultaneously, an event that otherwise occurs only with electrical stimulation, the felt sensation is electric shock-like. After a few seconds of massive firing, activity-evoked after-suppression develops (Amir and Devor 1997), damping the paroxysm and establishing a period of refractoriness. Like CNS seizure activity, the ignition mechanism is expected to be sensitive to anticonvulsant drugs that reduce membrane excitability, such as carbamazepine. Drug action, however, is supposed to be in the PNS rather than in the CNS.

HOW DOES NERVE INJURY INDUCE CENTRAL SENSITIZATION?

Central sensitization is a CNS phenomenon, but it is induced by nerve injury, and therefore cellular triggering events fall within the purview of PNS pathophysiology. The term itself deserves scrutiny. Some investigators limit "central sensitization" to functional CNS changes that are dependent on ongoing nociceptive afferent activity and reverse rapidly when the maintaining impulse activity stops (Gracely et al. 1992; Torebjork et al. 1992; Koltzenburg et al. 1994b; Ji et al. 2003). The best known mechanism of this sort is enhanced response of spinal nociceptive and wide-dynamic-range neurons to glutamate released from Aβ touch afferents as a result of enablement of N-methyl D-aspartate (NMDA)-type glutamate receptors (Willis 1992). For other investigators "central sensitization" encompasses all CNS changes that increase spinal gain and support Aβ pain, whether or not they are labile or linked to ongoing impulse traffic. Many CNS changes have been reported in addition to NMDA-receptor engagement. These include altered expression and release of neuromodulatory peptides from primary afferent terminals; enhanced non-NMDA glutamate receptor response; selective loss of inhibition by GABA, glycine, taurine, and/or endogenous opioids; altered gene expression in intrinsic spinal neurons; denervation supersensitivity; afferent terminal sprouting; release by "activated" microglia and astrocytes of proinflammatory cytokines; upregulation of postsynaptic transcription factors and transmembrane signaling molecules such as phosphorylated extracellular signal-regulated kinase (pERK), cyclic AMP-responsive element-binding protein (CREB), and mitogen-activated protein kinase (MAPK); suppression of brainstem descending inhibition; and augmentation of brainstem descending facilitation.

PNS-TO-CNS SIGNALING

Neural signaling along afferent axons takes two forms: rapid electrical impulse traffic (measured in meters/second) and relatively slow axoplasmic transport of molecules (measured in centimeters/day). These can act independently, but they also interact. Electrical impulses convey moment-to-moment sensory messages to central synaptic contacts in the dorsal horn and trigeminal nucleus. The most important change for the initiation of central sensitization is the emergence of electrical hyperexcitability and consequent abnormal impulse discharge. This mechanism both generates spurious sensory messages and triggers and maintains central sensitization. The outcome is amplification of the spurious sensory messages (augmented ongoing pain) and the emergence of stimulus-evoked pain (allodynia and hyperalgesia).

Abnormal impulse traffic probably does not affect the axoplasmic transport machinery per se, but it may well affect the induction of central sensitization by transported molecules. Specifically, impulse traffic drives the fusion and exocytosis of transported vesicles, and hence initiates both the release of transported diffusible signaling molecules (e.g., neurotrophins, cytokines) and the insertion into the presynaptic terminal of membrane proteins (Fig. 7). The latter affect terminal excitability (e.g., ion channels and presynaptic receptors) and may also directly signal to postsynaptic cells, e.g., neural cell adhesion molecules (NCAMs). Impulse traffic may also affect PNS-to-CNS signaling by altering the synthesis and processing of transported molecules in DRG neurons (Fields 1996; Devor 1999; Klein et al. 2003).

Just as impulse traffic affects the disposition of transported molecules, axoplasmic transport affects impulse traffic. Effects of neurotrophins on the regulation of primary afferent excitability in the DRG were noted above. There are also effects at the PNS-CNS interface. An example is the delivery by axoplasmic transport of neurotransmitter and ion channel-loaded vesicles to the presynaptic terminal. Transported molecules also fill structural roles (e.g., in the cytoskeleton and in membranes), control synaptic transmission

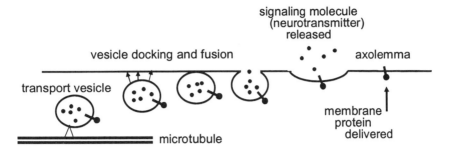

Fig. 7. Cellular trafficking. The delivery of released neurotransmitter, neuromodulator, and diffusible signaling molecules, as well as membrane-bound proteins that determine electrical excitability and cell surface recognition-signaling, depends on axoplasmic transport and exocytosis. Vesicle docking and fusion in neurons, and hence cargo delivery, are largely controlled by impulse discharge, although some occurs constitutively.

(e.g., presynaptic receptors, the exocytotic SNARE [soluble *N*-ethyl-maleimide-sensitive factor attachment protein receptor] complex, and neurotransmitter processing enzymes), and regulate postsynaptic cells (e.g., neurotrophins, cytokines, and NCAMs). Nerve injury drastically affects both spiking and axoplasmic transport, and such injury can therefore affect PNS-to-CNS signaling in many ways.

It is crucial to know which of the CNS changes that contribute to central sensitization are a direct consequence of altered impulse traffic *per se* and which (if any) are due to (non-transmitter) signaling molecules released by impulses or constitutively, independent of impulses. This information is important because different therapeutic agents are required to address impulse traffic, axoplasmic transport, and constitutive release. Surprisingly, authors who champion particular CNS changes as the key to neuropathic pain almost uniformly point to CNS targets when discussing therapeutic implications, without considering that the pain-provoking central change might be stopped before it has begun, by using a peripherally acting drug. Few, for example, have bothered to check whether their favorite change might be prevented or reversed by nerve block (Puehler et al. 2004). Still worse, few have checked whether the antiallodynic effect obtained by injecting their drug of choice intrathecally was really due to the spinal action envisioned, or alternatively to suppression of ectopic firing originating in the DRG. Dorsal root ganglia lie within the intrathecal space and are subject to the same drugs as the spinal cord on intrathecal administration. Electrogenesis in primary sensory neurons is subtle and not fully understood. Pharmacological agents, and even transgenic manipulations, can have unanticipated effects on pacemaking in the DRG.

Nerve injury does not cause one CNS change but all of them, in a funnel-like pattern like Fig. 5, but in reverse. For this reason a therapeutic attack on PNS-to-CNS signaling might be much more effective than an attack on any one of the numerous known CNS changes (Fig. 8). It is therefore of considerable importance to know the mechanism through which peripheral nerve injury brings about central change. There are three fundamental possibilities:

1) *Depolarization due to impulse traffic per se.* The resting potential of postsynaptic neurons is determined, in part, by the constant barrage of excitatory and inhibitory postsynaptic potentials impinging on their dendritic arbor (spatial and temporal summation). Ongoing ectopic afferent activity in neuropathy enhances the barrage, depolarizes the postsynaptic neuron, and brings its resting potential closer to firing threshold. This increases both spontaneous firing in the CNS and the response of CNS neurons to evoked and ectopic afferent input.

2) *Other actions of transmitters released by afferent impulse traffic.* Neurotransmitter and neuromodulator molecules released from afferent terminals during spike activity may have postsynaptic effects beyond the moment to moment modulation of the membrane potential. For example, released mediators such as substance P, brain-derived neurotrophic factor (BDNF), neuropeptide Y, and tumor necrosis factor alpha (TNF-α) might trigger relatively long-term changes in the responsiveness of postsynaptic neurons (Obata et al. 2004). Coupling may be via ligand-gated ion channels (and consequent membrane depolarization), or via transmembrane signaling pathways that are independent of membrane potential.

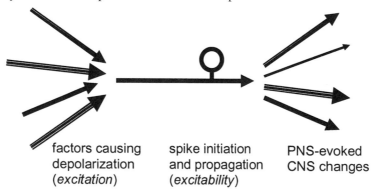

factors causing   spike initiation   PNS-evoked
depolarization   and propagation   CNS changes
(*excitation*)   (*excitability*)

Fig. 8. Nodal points in PNS-to-CNS signaling. Many independent factors can depolarize and excite sensory endings (and ectopic pacemaker sites). All of these factors converge on the process that encodes membrane potential into trains of propagated spikes (excitability). Likewise, once spike traffic reaches the CNS, it activates numerous signaling pathways with multiple divergent effects on postsynaptic neurons and glia.

In intact animals, induction of central sensitization by acute noxious events surely depends on neuro-active substances released from nociceptive C-fiber terminals (and perhaps from Aδ fibers). Even intense and prolonged activation of low-threshold mechanoreceptive Aβ afferents does not normally induce central sensitization. However, in the presence of neuropathy (and chronic inflammation), Aβ afferents begin to synthesize and release some of the very molecules suspected of being responsible for nociceptor-induced central sensitization, including substance P, CGRP, BDNF, and neuropeptide Y. Due to the release or these molecules, Aβ touch afferents may acquire the ability to directly drive spinal pain-signaling neurons, and perhaps to trigger and maintain central sensitization. Indeed, artificial activation of injured (but not of intact) Aβ afferents has been shown to trigger central changes that might be indicative of central sensitization, such as *c-fos* expression (Molander et al. 1994; Noguchi et al. 1995; Neumann et al. 1996; Allen et al. 1999; Michael et al. 1999; Malcangio et al. 2000). At least in the early stages after axotomy, the bulk of ectopic firing occurs in Aβ afferents, although the studies involved did not rule out the very low-frequency C-fiber activity later reported in uninjured neighboring C fibers (Liu et al. 2000a,b; Wu et al. 2001a). Thus, central sensitization in neuropathy might be induced by ectopic activity in injured Aβ fibers rather than, or in addition to, ectopic activity in injured or uninjured C fibers.

3) *Trophic interactions.* More speculatively, nerve injury might bring about central changes independent of impulse traffic and synaptic release. During embryonic development, the very survival of primary afferent and second-order CNS neurons is dependent on neurotrophins. Beyond a critical period these neurons lose their acute dependence on neurotrophic support, but even in adulthood neuronal phenotype is altered by changes in the provision of developmental neurotrophins (Boucher and McMahon 2001). Molecules that mediate such trophic interactions (neurotrophins, NCAMs, and perhaps ephrin) most likely are transported from the DRG and either released from the presynaptic terminal or incorporated into its membrane during spike-evoked exocytosis, or constitutively (Fields 1996; Fields et al. 2001; Battaglia et al. 2003). These molecules, and the processes that bring them to the scene, are potential therapeutic targets.

DEAFFERENTATION PAIN

In the context of PNS-triggered CNS changes, it is important to compare the frequently confused terms "neurectomy" and "deafferentation." Nerve injury denervates peripheral tissue, but in adults not only do most DRG cell somata survive (Tandrup et al. 2000), but impulses generated in them continue to be able to activate the CNS (Wall and Devor 1981) and evoke sensory experience (the Tinel sign). Deafferentation (by dorsal rhizotomy or ganglionectomy), in contrast, disconnects the PNS from the CNS and causes the rapid degeneration of central sensory terminals, with the result that electrical stimulation of corresponding nerves no longer activates dorsal horn neurons. A distinctive darkening visible in electron micrographs of central terminals in nerve-injured animals, inappropriately termed "degeneration atrophy" (Knyihar-Csillik et al. 1989), has led some observers to presume that peripheral axotomy is equivalent to deafferentation by rhizotomy. This notion is clearly incorrect.

Both neurectomy and deafferentation can trigger neuropathic pain. But while minor nerve injury sometimes produces devastating pain, modest or diffuse deafferentation does not. C2 dorsal root ganglionectomy, for example, is frequently performed for the relief of severe headache without provoking deafferentation pain, and multisegmental partial dorsal rhizotomy is routinely performed for relief of painful spasticity in children with cerebral palsy (White and Sweet 1969; Sindou et al. 1986; Gybels and Sweet 1990). On the other hand, when there is preexisting pain due to peripheral nerve or tissue pathology, pain relief following dorsal rhizotomy is transient. Pain frequently recurs after a few weeks or months (Gybels and Sweet 1990). Moreover, pain comes on rapidly when dorsal roots are avulsed from the spinal cord with consequent spinal hemorrhaging and cavitation (Wynn-Parry 1980). The mechanisms of deafferentation pain, its relation to preexisting pain of peripheral origin, and its relation to frank CNS damage (central pain) is almost entirely unknown. This subject merits more research.

STRATEGY: FROM NEURAL PROCESS
TO THERAPEUTIC TARGET

Progress in understanding peripheral neuropathic pain mechanisms has not yet been translated into improved drugs. The problem is not a dearth of targets but the massive investment required to properly test each one. Better strategic thinking may facilitate better practical choices.

FAMILIES OF TARGETS, SYSTEMS HIERARCHY,
AND NODAL POINTS

We sometimes jump too quickly from pain phenotype to specific molecules to which we have an intellectual, or perhaps financial, commitment. It is essential to consider the systems within which molecules operate. For example, efforts to find specific blockers for each Greek alphabet type and subtype of inflammatory mediator may well lead to marvelous reagents. But given the diversity of mediators, will they have practical clinical applications? Our grandchildren, of course, after coughing into a genomic scanner, may be prescribed the perfect cocktail of these highly specific agents. As for the agents designed today, patent protection will be long expired. Perhaps it is better for now to spread a wider net. The same consideration holds for CNS processes triggered by PNS injury.

Pursuing the ultimate in specificity makes more sense if the process in question is at a "node" in the pain-processing network. For example, inflammatory mediators in the skin and joints cause pain only to the extent that they enhance the generation of propagated impulses. Most evidence points to a plethora of inflammatory pathways and mediators. There are good evolutionary reasons for this. But there appears to be only one process of spike electrogenesis. Control spike electrogenesis, and will you have eliminated the pain-provoking effect of all inflammatory mediators (Fig. 5).

Some processes occur in serial order rather than as branched converging or diverging cascades. The relation of the PNS to the CNS in inflammatory and neuropathic pain is probably a case in point. All factors that cause afferent excitation must funnel through the peripheral nerve encoding and propagation pathway, and it is likely that all (or nearly all) of the CNS processes of central sensitization are activated by afferent spike activity (Fig. 8). The PNS-to-CNS link, impulse and mediator traffic along primary sensory axons, is a unique functional node. It may be possible to block this link at a variety of locations, affording the luxury of picking an optimal target. For example, peripheral pain-provoking signals and central sensitization can presumably be arrested by preventing adequate stimulation, suppressing pacemaker capability, preventing spike propagation, preventing presynaptic release of the molecules that trigger central sensitization, or preventing these molecules from accessing their postsynaptic target. As a general rule it makes sense to block the cascade as far upstream as is practical.

"DRUGABILITY": LIGANDS, ACCESS, SPECIFICITY, AND SIDE EFFECTS

The identification of a key biological processes in the pain system, ideally one at a convergent node such as spike electrogenesis, is only a first step on the path of drug development. This is so even if the molecular players can be identified with some confidence. In prioritizing targets it is logical to recognize issues of "drugability" early. Drugability includes the difficulty of generating small target-directed ligands (unique or general-purpose ones such as antibodies, siRNA, and antisense polynucleotides), pharmacody-namics (gut absorption, bioavailability, stability in the circulation, and tissue barriers), targeting (by molecular strategies or needles), selectivity, specific-ity, and predicted side-effect profile. Some of these factors play off one against the other. If the target is in the PNS, preventing CNS access may avoid a tsunami of knowable and unknowable central side effects.

CURRENTLY USED SYSTEMIC DRUGS IN THE LIGHT OF NERVE PATHOPHYSIOLOGY

The first-line analgesics recommended for the relief of neuropathic pain are "adjuvants" including (certain) anticonvulsants, antidepressants, anti-arrhythmics, and local anesthetics (McQuay and Moore 1998). As the names imply, these drugs were not developed as pain relievers. Their efficacy was discovered empirically, by chance. This is true even of gabapentin. On the face of it these agents appear to fit into highly diverse drug families. On closer consideration, however, they have a common denominator that is probably the reason for their efficacy in neuropathic pain. They are all "membrane stabilizers"; they reduce membrane excitability, and hence di-minish neuronal pacemaker capability (Catterall 1987; Deffois et al. 1996). Not *all* anticonvulsants, for example, are effective. The ones that are, such as carbamazepine, lamotrigine and gabapentin, act on ion channels and sup-press ectopia. In contrast, anticonvulsants that act by synaptic modulation (e.g., barbiturates and benzodiazepines) are ineffective against neuropathic pain. The same is true for antidepressants. Tricyclics, which are powerful Na^+ channel blockers in addition to affecting catecholamine reuptake (Wang et al. 2004), are effective against neuropathic pain, whereas serotonin-selective reuptake inhibitors (SSRIs) are largely ineffective. At clinically effective plasma concentrations, all of these adjuvant agents suppress ecto-pia selectively, without blocking axonal conduction (Fig. 9). The fact that the membrane-stabilizing adjuvant drugs are effective analgesics for essen-tially all neuropathic pain diagnoses, despite the diversity of clinical mani-festations, is a strong argument for a common neural mechanism.

Unfortunately, the effectiveness of the adjuvant drugs is usually limited by the occurrence of central side effects—sedation, vertigo, and nausea. Just as they suppress the discharge of afferent neurons, they also alter firing patterns of neurons in the brain. Indeed, their suppression of discharge in the CNS might well contribute to their efficacy as analgesics (Woolf and Wiesenfeld-Hallin 1985). But if the desired analgesic action is indeed in the PNS and the unwanted side effects are due to CNS actions, this situation might be exploited to improve clinical usefulness. For example, one might

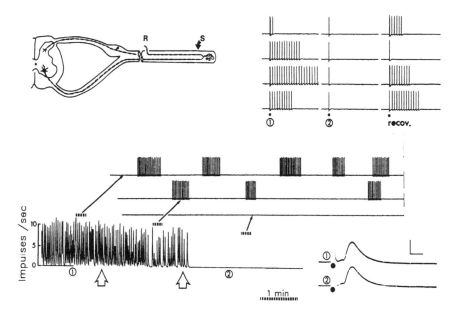

Fig. 9. Systemic administration of membrane-stabilizing drugs suppresses ectopic impulse discharge without blocking the ability of the nerve to convey impulses from the periphery into the CNS. In this experiment, ectopic burst discharge generated in a sciatic nerve end neuroma was recorded (R) from a myelinated sensory axon. Systemic infusion of a small dose of lidocaine (open arrow on left) slowed the firing, and a second bolus (open arrow on right) stopped it entirely. Nonetheless, electrical nerve stimulation (S) continued to evoke an action potential in the recorded axon just as it had prior to lidocaine injection (circled 1 and 2). Systemic concentrations of lidocaine high enough to block spike propagation are lethal (modified from Devor et al. 1992).

direct drug delivery via indwelling catheters, by molecular targeting to PNS-specific receptor types, or by reducing permeation through the blood-brain barrier (but with preservation of PNS activity).

NMDA-type glutamate receptor antagonists, in particular ketamine, have shown some promise. But it is unclear how side effects might be avoided, given the ubiquitous distribution of the targeted NMDA receptor in the CNS. Note, however, that ketamine is also a membrane-stabilizing drug, a Na^+ channel blocker, at clinically used concentrations (Brau et al. 1997; Zhou and Zhao 2000; Wagner et al. 2001). Its antinociceptive efficacy, in contrast to its side-effect profile, might actually be due to suppression of PNS ectopia rather than to CNS NMDA-receptor blockade. If so, a peripherally restricted ketamine-like compound might be of interest. Corticosteroids, including depot form agents, are also membrane stabilizers. It is not clear how much of their analgesic effect in neuropathy is due to anti-inflammation and how much to direct suppression of abnormal neural discharge. Opioid

Table I

Key neuropathic pain processes and some potential therapeutic targets

Pain Process	Potential Target Process	Potential Target Receptor or Ligand	Example of Target Molecule or Lead Compound
Inflammation (generator potential)	Substrate(s) of mediators	Membrane lipids , kininogens	Arachidonic acid, PLA_2
	Synthetic enzymes	COX, lipoxygenase, tryptase	COX-2 inhibitors, PAR_2
	Degrading enzymes	Proteases, tPA, uPA	Neutral endopeptidase
	Mediator receptors	Prostaglandin receptors, bradykinin receptors	PGE_2, diHETEs, PARs
	Mechanoreceptors	Stretch-activated channels	RR, gadolinium, amiloride
	Thermoreceptors	TRP channels	TRPV1, TRPM8
	Phenotype regulation	Neurotrophins	NGF, NT3, GDNF
Inflammation (spike encoding)	Electrogenesis	Na^+, K^+, Ca^{2+} ion channels	Channel blockers, openers
	Channel phosphorylation	Protein kinases	Specific kinase isoenzymes
	Phenotype regulation	Neurotrophins, constitutive regulators	NGF, GDNF
Ectopia: neuroma (generator potential)	Mechanoreceptors	Like sensory endings	Stretch-activated channels
	Thermoreceptors	Like sensory endings	TRPV1, TRPM8
	Chemoreceptors	Adrenoreceptors, cytokine receptors	α_{2B}, interleukin receptors
	Phenotype regulation	Neurotrophins, constitutive regulators	NGF, GDNF
Ectopia: neuroma (spike encoding)	Like DRG, sensory endings?	Ion channels	$Na_V1.3$, K2p openers, persistent Na^+ ch.
	Phenotype regulation	Ion channel disposition/density	Constitutive regulators?
		Ion channel kinetics	Hormones, protein kinases
		Channel membrane anchoring	Ankyrin, contactin
		Axoplasmic transport	Tubulin, MAPs
		Vesicle trafficking	Protein signal sequences
		Exocytosis	Synaptophysin, SNAREs,
Ectopia: demyelination	Causes of demyelination	Mutations, macrophages	MBP, P0, PMP22
	Myelin-axon signaling	Cell surface recognition	Proteoglycans, neuregulin
	Ion channel trafficking	Like neuroma?	
	Electrogenesis	Like DRG?	
	Ephaptic cross-talk	Gap junctions?	Connexins

Ectopia: DRG (generator potential)	Mechanoreceptors Thermoreceptors Chemoreceptors Phenotype regulation Paracrine cross-talk	Like sensory endings Like sensory endings Like sensory endings Like sensory endings ATP, peptides?	
Cross-talk	Ephaptic (in neuroma) Chemical (in neuroma) Chemical/paracrine in DRG	Gap junctions? Neurotransmitters, peptides, glutamate K^+, neurotransmitters and their receptors?	Connexins ATP, glutamate, α_2 receptors ATP, glutamate, SP
Ectopia: DRG (spike encoding)	Subthreshold oscillations DAPs Action potentials	Ion channels Ion channel density Ion channel kinetics Channel membrane anchoring Axoplasmic transport Vesicle trafficking Exocytosis	$Na_v1.3$, K2p openers, persistent gNa^+ Constitutive regulators? Hormones, PKAs, PKCs Ankyrin, contactin Tubulin, MAPs Signal sequences Synaptophysin, SNAREs
Ectopia: neighboring "uninjured" afferents	Like injured afferents? (not known where impulses originate)	Mechanoreceptors Thermoreceptors Chemoreceptors Ion channels	Like neuroma?
Triggers of central sensitization	Exocytosis (vesicle fusion) Postsynaptic depolarization Cell surface proteins Postsynaptic effects of released molecules on neurons or glia	Presynaptic terminal Neurotransmitter receptors Membrane signal molecules Transmitter receptors, neurotrophin receptors, transmembrane signaling cascades	N-type gCa^{2+}, SNAREs, receptors glu-R, MK-801, CNQX Ephrin, EphB, NCAM Receptors for SP, NKA, BDNF, CCK, VIP, p38MAPK, CREB, pERK, tissue plasminogen activator

Abbreviations: ATP = adenosine triphosphate; BDNF = brain-derived neurotrophic factor; CCK = cholecystokinin; COX = cyclooxygenase; CREB = cyclic AMP-responsive element-binding protein; DAPs = depolarizing afterpotentials; diHETE = dihydroxyeicosatetraenoic acid; DRG = dorsal root ganglia; GDNF = glial-derived neurotrophic factor; MAPK = mitogen-activated protein kinase; MAPs = microtubule-associated proteins; MBP = myelin basic protein; NCAM = neural cell adhesion molecule; NGF = nerve growth factor; NKA = neurokinin A; NT3 = neurotrophin 3; P0 = protein zero; pERK = phosphorylated extracellular signal-regulated kinase; PAR_2 = protease-activated receptor 2; PARs = protease-activated receptors; PGE_2 = prostaglandin E_2; PKA = protein kinase A; PKC = protein kinase C; PLA_2 = phospholipase A_2; PMP22 = peripheral myelin protein 22; RR = ruthenium red; SNARE = soluble *N*-ethyl-maleimide-sensitive factor attachment protein receptor; SP = substance P; tPA = tissue-type plasminogen activator; TRPV1 = transient receptor potential vanilloid 1; TRPM8 = transient receptor potential melastatin 8; uPA = urokinase-type plasminogen activator; VIP = vasoactive intestinal polypeptide.

analgesics are no longer viewed as ineffective in neuropathy (Rowbotham et al. 2003). They are thought to act primarily on μ-opioid receptors within the CNS by suppressing already amplified pain signals, but a significant PNS contribution is also possible, especially in the event of neuropathy.

TOPICAL AGENTS

Cutaneous allodynia requires mechanoresponsive afferents. Blocking these afferents with topical local anesthetics can therefore be effective (Davies and Galer 2004). Likewise, in patients in whom ongoing discharge of cutaneous nociceptive C-fiber endings provides painful afferent input and maintains central sensitization, agents that desensitize or silence these afferents (e.g., capsaicin, lidocaine) may provide relief.

THE FUTURE

The foregoing review of PNS pathophysiological mechanisms provides a framework for considering therapeutic targets for potential drugs of the future. For convenience I have collected the key processes from the text above and listed them in Table I, together with some underlying mechanisms and some associated molecules. In statecraft we mostly prefer democracy, equal opportunity for all. Biology does not necessarily work that way. Issues of drugability aside, some processes, mechanisms, and molecules have clear advantages over the rest, particularly the ones associated with excitability versus excitation, and the ones that act at nodal points in the pain network.

ACKNOWLEDGMENT

The author's research on neuropathic pain mechanisms has been supported by the United States–Israel Binational Science Foundation (BSF), the Israel Science Foundation, the German-Israel Foundation for Research and Development (GIF), and the Hebrew University Center for Research on Pain. I wish to acknowledge the contributions of Wm. Calvin to many of the concepts elaborated in this chapter.

REFERENCES

Ali Z, Raja SN, Wesselmann U, et al. Intradermal injection of norepinephrine evokes pain in patients with sympathetically maintained pain. *Pain* 2000; 88:161–168.

Allen BJ, Li J, Menning PM, et al. Primary afferent fibers that contribute to increased substance P receptor internalization in the spinal cord after injury. *J Neurophysiol* 1999; 81:1379–1390.

Amir R, Devor M. Chemically-mediated cross-excitation in rat dorsal root ganglia. *J Neurosci* 1996; 16:4733–4741.

Amir R, Devor M. Spike-evoked suppression and burst patterning in dorsal root ganglion neurons. *J Physiol (Lond)* 1997; 501:183–196.

Amir R, Michaelis M, Devor M. Membrane potential oscillations in dorsal root ganglion neurons: role in normal electrogenesis and in neuropathic pain. *J Neurosci* 1999; 19:8589–8596.

Amir R, Liu CN, Kocsis JD, Devor M. Oscillatory mechanism in primary sensory neurones. *Brain* 2002a; 125:421–435.

Amir R, Michaelis M, Devor M. Burst discharge in primary sensory neurons: triggered by subthreshold oscillations, maintained by depolarizing afterpotentials. *J Neurosci* 2002b; 22:1187–1198.

Banik RK, Brennan TJ. Spontaneous discharge and increased heat sensitivity of rat C-fiber nociceptors are present in vitro after plantar incision. *Pain* 2004; 112:204–213.

Battaglia AA, Sehayek K, Grist J, McMahon SB, Gavazzi I. EphB receptors and ephrin-B ligands regulate spinal sensory connectivity and modulate pain processing. *Nat Neurosci* 2003; 6:339–340.

Birder LA, Perl ER. Expression of alpha-2-adrenergic receptors in rat primary afferent neurons after peripheral nerve injury or inflammation. *J Physiol* 1999; 515.2:533–542.

Boucher TJ, McMahon SB. Neurotrophic factors and neuropathic pain. *Curr Opin Pharmacol* 2001; 1:66–72.

Bouhassira D, Attal N, Fermanian J, et al. Development and validation of the Neuropathic Pain Symptom Inventory. *Pain* 2004; 108:248–257.

Brau ME, Sander F, Vogel W, Hempelmann G. Blocking mechanisms of ketamine and its enantiomers in enzymatically demyelinated peripheral nerve as revealed by single-channel experiments. *Anesthesiology* 1997; 86:394–404.

Campbell JN, Raja SN, Meyer RA, MacKinnon SE. Myelinated afferents signal the hyperalgesia associated with nerve injury. *Pain* 1988; 32:89–94.

Catterall WA. Common modes of drug action on Na^+ channels: local anaesthetics, antiarrhythmics and anticonvulsants. *Trends Pharmacol Sci* 1987; 8:57–65.

Chen Y, Michaelis M, Jänig W, Devor M. Adrenoceptor sub-type mediating sympathetic-sensory coupling in injured sensory neurons. *J Neurophysiol* 1996; 76:3721–3730.

Chen Y, Cantrell AR, Messing RO, Scheuer T, Catterall WA. Specific modulation of Na^+ channels in hippocampal neurons by protein kinase C-epsilon. *J Neurosci* 2005; 25:507–513.

Chung JM, Dib-Hajj SD, Lawson SN. Sodium channel subtypes and neuropathic pain. In: Dostrovsky JO, Carr DB, Koltzenburg M (Eds). *Proceedings of the 10th World Congress on Pain,* Progress in Pain Research and Management, Vol. 24. Seattle: IASP Press, 2003, pp 99–114.

Costigan M, Befort K, Karchewski L, et al. Replicate high-density rat genome oligonucleotide microarrays reveal hundreds of regulated genes in the dorsal root ganglion after peripheral nerve injury. *BMC Neurosci* 2002; 3:16–28.

Craner MJ, Lo AC, Black JA, Waxman SG. Abnormal sodium channel distribution in optic nerve axons in a model of inflammatory demyelination. *Brain* 2003; 126:1552–1561.

Davies PS, Galer BS. Review of lidocaine patch 5% studies in the treatment of postherpetic neuralgia. *Drugs* 2004; 64:937–947.

Deffois A, Fage D, Carter C. Inhibition of synaptosomal veratridine-induced sodium influx by antidepressants and neuroleptics used in chronic pain. *Neurosci Lett* 1996; 220:117–120.

Devor M. Unexplained peculiarities of the dorsal root ganglion. *Pain* 1999; (Suppl)6: S27–S35.

Devor M. Response of nerves to injury in relation to neuropathic pain. In: Koltzenburg M, McMahon SB (Eds). *Wall and Melzack's Textbook of Pain.* Edinburgh: Churchill Livingstone, 2005, pp 905–927.

Devor M, Keller CH, Deerinck T, Levinson SR, Ellisman MH. Na⁺ channel accumulation on axolemma of afferents in nerve end neuromas in *Apteronotus. Neurosci Lett* 1989; 102:149–154.

Devor M, Wall PD, Catalan N. Systemic lidocaine silences ectopic neuroma and DRG discharge without blocking nerve conduction. *Pain* 1992; 48:261–268.

England JD, Gamboni F, Levinson SR, Finger TF. Changed distribution of sodium channels along demyelinated axons. *Proc Natl Acad Sci USA* 1990; 87:6777–6780.

England JD, Happel LT, Kline DG, et al. Sodium channel accumulation in humans with painful neuromas. *Neurology* 1996; 47:272–276.

Fields RD. Signaling from neural impulses to genes. *Neuroscientist* 1996; 2:315–325.

Fields RD, Eshete F, Dudek S, Ozsarac N, Stevens B. Regulation of gene expression by action potentials: dependence on complexity in cellular information processing. *Novartis Found Symp* 2001; 239:160–172.

Freeman R. Autonomic peripheral neuropathy. *Lancet* 2005; 365:1259–1270.

Fried K, Govrin-Lippmann R, Devor M. Close apposition among neighbouring axonal endings in a neuroma. *J Neurocytol* 1993; 226:663–681.

Gold MS, Reichling DB, Shuster MJ, Levine JD. Hyperalgesic agents increase a tetrodotoxin-resistant Na⁺ current in nociceptors. *Proc Natl Acad Sci USA* 1996; 93:1108–1112.

Gracely R, Lynch S, Bennett G. Painful neuropathy: altered central processing, maintained dynamically by peripheral input. *Pain* 1992; 51:175–194.

Gybels JM, Sweet WH. *Neurosurgical Treatment of Persistent Pain.* Karger: Basel, 1990.

Harden RN, Baron R, Jänig WE. *Complex Regional Pain Syndrome,* Progress in Pain research and Management, Vol. 22. Seattle: IASP Press, 2001.

Ji RR, Kohno T, Moore KA, Woolf CJ. Central sensitization and LTP: do pain and memory share similar mechanisms? *Trends Neurosci* 2003; 26:696–705.

Kapoor R, Li Y-G, Smith K. Slow sodium-dependent potential oscillations contribute to ectopic firing in mammalian demyelinated axons. *Brain* 1997; 120:647–652.

Kazarinova-Noyes K, Malhotra JD, McEwen DP, et al. Contactin associates with Na⁺ channels and increases their functional expression. *J Neurosci* 2001; 21:7517–7525.

Klein JP, Tendi EA, Dib-Hajj SD, Fields RD, Waxman SG. Patterned electrical activity modulates sodium channel expression in sensory neurons. *J Neurosci Res* 2003; 74:192–198.

Knyihar-Csillik E, Rakic P, Csillik B. Transneuronal degeneration atrophy in the Rolando substance of the primate spinal cord evoked by axotomy-induced transganglionic degenerative atrophy of central primary sensory terminals. *Cell Tissue Res* 1989; 258:515–525.

Kocsis JD, Devor M. Altered excitability of large diameter cutaneous afferents following nerve injury: consequences for chronic pain. In: Devor M, Rowbotham MC, Wiesenfeld-Hallin Z (Eds). *Proceedings of the 9th World Congress on Pain,* Progress in Pain Research and Management, Vol. 16. Seattle: IASP Press, 2000, pp 119–135.

Koltzenburg M, Kees S, Budweiser S, Ochs G, Toyka KV. The properties of unmyelinated nociceptive afferents change in a painful chronic constriction neuropathy. In: Gebhart G, Hammond D, Jensen T (Eds). *Proceedings of the 7th World Congress on Pain,* Progress in Pain Research and Management, Vol. 2. Seattle: IASP Press, 1994a, pp 511–521.

Koltzenburg M, Torebjork H, Wahren L. Nociceptor modulated central sensitization causes mechanical hyperalgesia in acute chemogenic and chronic neuropathic pain. *Brain* 1994b; 117:579–591.

Kugelberg E, Lindblom U. The mechanism of the pain in trigeminal neuralgia. *J Neurol Neurosurg Psychiatry* 1959; 22:36–43.

Kuslich S, Ulstro C, Michael C. The tissue origin of low back pain and sciatica. *Orthop Clin North Am* 1991; 22:181–187.

Li M, West JW, Lai Y, Scheuer Y, Catterall WA. Functional modulation of brain sodium channels by cAMP-dependent phosphorylation. *Neuron* 1992; 81:1151–1159.

Liu C-N, Wall PD, Ben-Dor E, et al. Tactile allodynia in the absence of C-fiber activation: altered firing properties of DRG neurons following spinal nerve injury. *Pain* 2000a; 85:503–521.

Liu X, Eschenfelder S, Blenk K-H, Jänig W, Habler H-J. Spontaneous activity of axotomized afferent neurons after L5 spinal nerve injury in rats. *Pain* 2000b; 84:309–318.

Malcangio M, Ramer MS, Jones MG, McMahon SB. Abnormal substance P release from the spinal cord following injury to primary sensory neurons. *Eur J Neurosci* 2000; 12:397–399.

McQuay M, Moore A. *An Evidence-based Resource for Pain Relief.* Oxford: Oxford University Press, 1998.

Merskey H, Bogduk N. *Classification of Chronic Pain: Descriptions of Chronic Pain Syndromes and Definitions of Pain Terms.* Seattle: IASP Press, 1994, pp 40–43.

Michael GJ, Averill S, Shortland PJ, Yan Q, Priestley JV. Axotomy results in major changes in BDNF expression by dorsal root ganglion cells: BDNF expression in large trkB and trkC cells, in pericellular baskets, and in projections to deep dorsal horn and dorsal column nuclei. *Eur J Neurosci* 1999; 11:3539–3551.

Mogil JS (Ed). *The Genetics of Pain,* Progress in Pain Research and Management, Vol. 28. Seattle: IASP Press, 2004.

Molander C, Hongpaisan J, Persson JK. Distribution of c-fos expressing dorsal horn neurons after electrical stimulation of low threshold sensory fibers in the chronically injured sciatic nerve. *Brain Res* 1994; 644:74–82.

Neumann S, Doubell TP, Leslie TA, Woolf CJ. Inflammatory pain hypersensitivity mediated by phenotypic switch in myelinated primary sensory neurons. *Nature* 1996; 384:360–364.

Nikolajsen L, Jensen TS. Phantom limb pain. *Br J Anaesth* 2001; 87:107–116.

Noguchi K, Kawai Y, Fukuoka T, Senba E, Miki K. Substance P induced by peripheral nerve injury in primary afferent sensory neurons and its effect on dorsal column nucleus neurons. *J Neurosci* 1995; 15:7633–7643.

Nordin M, Nystrom B, Wallin U, Hagbarth K-E. Ectopic sensory discharges and paresthesiae in patients with disorders of peripheral nerves, dorsal roots and dorsal columns. *Pain* 1984; 20:231–245.

Obata K, Yamanaka H, Dai Y, et al. Differential activation of MAPK in injured and uninjured DRG neurons following chronic constriction injury of the sciatic nerve in rats. *Eur J Neurosci* 2004; 20:2881–2895.

Olmarker K, Rydevik B. Selective inhibition of tumor necrosis factor-alpha prevents nucleus pulposus-induced thrombus formation, intraneural edema, and reduction of nerve conduction velocity: possible implications for future pharmacologic treatment strategies of sciatica. *Spine* 2001; 26:863–869.

Puehler W, Zollner C, Brack A, et al. Rapid upregulation of mu opioid receptor mRNA in dorsal root ganglia in response to peripheral inflammation depends on neuronal conduction. *Neuroscience* 2004; 129:473–479.

Puil E, Gimbarzevsky B, Spigelman I. Primary involvement of K^+ conductance in membrane resonance of trigeminal root ganglion neurons. *J Neurophysiol* 1988; 59:77–89.

Rappaport ZH, Devor M. Trigeminal neuralgia: the role of self sustaining discharge in the trigeminal ganglion. *Pain* 1994; 56:127–138.

Rowbotham MC, Twilling L, Davies PS, et al. Oral opioid therapy for chronic peripheral and central neuropathic pain. *N Engl J Med* 2003; 348:1223–1232.

Schmidt R, Schmelz M, Forster C, et al. Novel classes of responsive and unresponsive C nociceptors in human skin. *J Neurosci* 1995; 15:333–341.

Shim B, Kim DW, Kim BH, et al. Mechanical and heat sensitization of cutaneous nociceptors in rats with experimental peripheral neuropathy. *Neuroscience* 2005; 132:193–201.

Sindou M, Mifsud JJ, Boisson D, Goutelle A. Selective posterior rhizotomy in the dorsal root entry zone for treatment of hyperspasticity and pain in the hemiplegic upper limb. *Neurosurgery* 1986; 18:587–595.

Sotgiu M, Biella G, Castagna A, Lacerenza M, Marchettini P. Differential time-course of i.v. lidocaine effects on ganglionic and spinal units in neuropathic rats. *Neuroreport* 1994; 5:873–876.

Tandrup T, Woolf CJ, Coggeshall RE. Delayed loss of small dorsal root ganglion cells after transection of the rat sciatic nerve. *J Comp Neurol* 2000; 422:172–180.

Tessler MJ, Kleiman SJ. Spinal anaesthesia for patients with previous lower limb amputations. *Anaesthesia* 1994; 49:439–441.

Torebjork H, Lundberg L, LaMotte R. Central changes in processing of mechanoreceptive input in capsaicin-induced secondary hyperalgesia in humans. *J Physiol (Lond)* 1992; 448:765–780.

Tsuboi Y, Takeda M, Tanimoto T, et al. Alteration of the second branch of the trigeminal nerve activity following inferior alveolar nerve transection in rats. *Pain* 2004; 111:323–334.

Utzschneider D, Kocsis J, Devor M. Mutual excitation among dorsal root ganglion neurons in the rat. *Neurosci Lett* 1992; 146:53–56.

Wagner LE II, Gingrich KJ, Kulli JC, Yang J. Ketamine blockade of voltage-gated sodium channels: evidence for a shared receptor site with local anesthetics. *Anesthesiology* 2001; 95:1406–1413.

Wall P, Devor M. The effect of peripheral nerve injury on dorsal root potentials and on the transmission of afferent signals into the spinal cord. *Brain Res* 1981; 209:95–111.

Wang GK, Russell C, Wang SY. State-dependent block of voltage-gated Na$^+$ channels by amitriptyline via the local anesthetic receptor and its implication for neuropathic pain. *Pain* 2004; 110:166–174.

Waxman SG (Ed). *Sodium Channels and Neuronal Hyperexcitability,* Novartis Foundation Symposia. Chichester: Wiley, 2002.

White J, Sweet W. *Pain and the Neurosurgeon.* Springfield: Thomas, 1969, pp 123–256.

Willis W. *Hyperalgesia and Allodynia.* New York: Raven Press, 1992.

Woolf CJ, Wiesenfeld-Hallin Z. The systemic administration of local anaesthetics produces a selective depression of C-afferent fibre evoked activity in the spinal cord. *Pain* 1985; 23:361–374.

Wu G, Ringkamp M, Hartke TV, et al. Early onset of spontaneous activity in uninjured C-fiber nociceptors after injury to neighboring nerve fibers. *J Neurosci* 2001a; RC140.

Wu N, Hsiao C-F, Chandler S. Membrane resonance and subthreshold membrane oscillations in mesencephalic V neurons: participants in burst generation. *J Neurosci* 2001b; 21:3729–3739.

Wynn-Parry CB. Pain in avulsion lesions of the brachial plexus. *Pain* 1980; 9:41–53.

Xiao HS, Huang QH, Zhang FX, et al. Identification of gene expression profile of dorsal root ganglion in the rat peripheral axotomy model of neuropathic pain. *Proc Natl Acad Sci USA* 2002; 99:8360–8365.

Zhou ZS, Zhao ZQ. Ketamine blockage of both tetrodotoxin (TTX)-sensitive and TTX-resistant sodium channels of rat dorsal root ganglion neurons. *Brain Res Bull* 2000; 52:427–433.

Correspondence to: Marshall Devor, PhD, Department of Cell and Animal Biology, Institute of Life Sciences, Hebrew University of Jerusalem, Jerusalem 91904, Israel. Email: marshlu@vms.huji.ac.il.

Emerging Strategies for the Treatment of Neuropathic Pain, edited by James N. Campbell, Allan I. Basbaum, André Dray, Ronald Dubner, Robert H. Dworkin, and Christine N. Sang, IASP Press, Seattle, © 2006.

3

Peripheral Receptors in Neuropathic Pain

Robert W. Gereau IV

Washington University Pain Center, Departments of Anesthesiology and Anatomy and Neurobiology, Washington University School of Medicine, St. Louis, Missouri, USA

Neuropathic pain, defined as pain arising from disease in or damage to the peripheral or central nervous system, is an extremely complex problem. Neuropathy results in some of the most severe and disturbing pain conditions, which can be very difficult to treat (Zimmermann 2001). While some patients experience significant pain relief with a given treatment, others will not respond to the same therapy. The reasons for this lack of consistency in clinical response are not entirely clear, but they are certain to involve the diversity of insults that lead to the generation of neuropathic pain and the resulting wide variety of cellular and molecular mechanisms by which the pain is induced and maintained. In addition, individual genetic variability in pain responsiveness and drug sensitivity can account for additional variation in clinical responses.

The generation and maintenance of neuropathic pain involve both peripheral and central mechanisms. Many changes in the functioning of peripheral primary afferent fibers in response to injury are known to mediate the peripheral component of neuropathic pain (Sawynok 2003). These include, but are not limited to, the regulation of ion channel expression and distribution, resulting in increased excitability and ectopic activity of primary afferents; the engagement of the sympathetic nervous system; and the enhanced expression or activation of receptor molecules on primary afferent neurons (Devor and Seltzer 1999).

This chapter reviews the roles played by plasma membrane receptors expressed on primary afferent neurons in the generation and maintenance of neuropathic pain conditions. Some thoughts on how these receptors might be selectively targeted for the treatment of neuropathic pain are also presented.

PERIPHERAL OPIOID RECEPTORS

Morphine and other opioids are among the most effective medications for the majority of pain conditions. Despite some disagreement in the literature regarding the efficacy of opioids in animal models and in humans, the prevailing current view is that in many instances, opioids can be beneficial in the treatment of neuropathic pain conditions (Przewlocki and Przewlocka 2001; Gordon and Love 2004; Mansikka et al. 2004; Zhao et al. 2004). Opioid analgesia in neuropathic pain involves peripheral, spinal, and supraspinal sites of action. The potential for avoiding central nervous system -(CNS) side effects associated with opioids makes the selective targeting of peripheral opioid receptors an attractive option.

Neurons in the dorsal root ganglion (DRG) express μ-, δ-, and κ-opioid receptors, all of which are transported to both the central and peripheral terminals. At the central terminals, opioids can act to reduce transmitter release from primary afferent nociceptors, whereas in the periphery, opioid receptor activation can reverse peripheral sensitization induced by pronociceptive compounds and can directly hyperpolarize the DRG neuron, thereby inhibiting its firing. Opioid receptors are also present on other peripheral targets, including sympathetic postganglionic neurons and immune cells. However, analgesic actions of opioids appear to be primarily mediated by direct actions on sensory neurons (Sawynok 2003).

Of particular interest to the possible use of peripherally acting opioids in the management of neuropathic pain is the finding that peripherally mediated morphine analgesia may be enhanced following nerve injury. Thus, Pertovaara and Wei (2001) showed that morphine analgesia in neuropathic rats was achieved at a lower dose when an intraplantar injection was given in the injured limb than in the contralateral limb. Moreover, the analgesic effect of morphine injected in the injured limb was blocked by a peripherally restricted opioid receptor antagonist, whereas the analgesia in the contralateral limb was not. These results suggest that opioid receptor upregulation or hypersensitivity in peripheral targets occurs in the context of some neuropathies. Consistent with this possibility, a recent study demonstrated an increased expression of μ-opioid receptors in injured DRG in the chronic constriction injury model, and the investigators observed μ-opioid receptors in the neuroma and in sprouting axons of the injured nerve (Truong et al. 2003). These studies suggest that peripherally applied opioids might provide effective analgesia in the area of neuropathic pain while keeping systemic levels of the drugs low enough to prevent CNS side effects. Indeed, a number of clinical studies have shown efficacy of peripherally applied opioids, although not in the context of neuropathic pain (for review, see Sawynok

2003). A recent report has demonstrated a novel compound, DiPOA, which is an effective μ-opioid agonist that is systemically available but is restricted to the periphery, with CNS concentrations reaching less than 4% of plasma levels (Valenzano et al. 2004). Although DiPOA was effective in the complete Freund's adjuvant model and in a model of postsurgical incision pain, it was not effective in the partial sciatic nerve ligation (SNL) model (Whiteside et al. 2004). By contrast, another systemically active but peripherally restricted opioid agonist, loperamide, reduced signs of allodynia in the SNL model (Johanek et al. 2005). The reasons for the differences in the efficacy of these two peripherally restricted opioid agonists in these models of neuropathic pain are not clear. Nonetheless, these compounds should be interesting leads for clinical development.

A major difficulty in the long-term use of opioid medications is the development of tolerance (a decrease in the efficacy of the drug with repeated dosing). Unfortunately, tolerance appears to also be a problem with peripherally applied opioids. Repeated systemic administration of the μ-opioid agonist DAMGO leads to the development of analgesic tolerance. Topical administration of morphine induces analgesia, and tolerance develops with repeated dosing. This tolerance is blocked by topical application of ketamine, an *N*-methyl-D-aspartate (NMDA) antagonist (Kolesnikov and Pasternak 1999b). Similar to the tolerance seen with systemically or topically administered morphine, tolerance to peripherally administered DAMGO was be blocked by the NMDA-receptor antagonist MK801 when administered either systemically or topically, but not intrathecally (Kolesnikov and Pasternak 1999a). Nerve injury seems to engage the endogenous opioid system, leading to an inhibition of mechanical allodynia (Mansikka et al. 2004). Some data suggest that this endogenous activation of the opioid system can promote tolerance to peripherally applied μ-opioid agonists, decreasing the efficacy of systemically applied morphine (Rashid et al. 2004). This latter finding does not agree with the studies discussed above that showed enhanced sensitivity and upregulation of peripheral μ-opioid receptors in the context of nerve injury. Whether due to endogenous or exogenously applied opioids, the development of tolerance is a critical hurdle that needs to be overcome if we are to improve the utility of peripherally applied opioids for the management of neuropathic pain.

TRP CHANNELS/VANILLOID RECEPTORS

Primary afferent neurons express a mosaic of ion channels involved in various components of thermal sensation. These channels belong to the superfamily of transient receptor potential (TRP) channels (Patapoutian et al. 2003). In the pain system, the prototypical member of this family is TRPV1. TRPV1, cloned as the capsaicin receptor and originally named VR1, is gated by heat in the noxious range (Caterina et al. 1997). TRPV1 is expressed in a subpopulation of small-diameter nociceptive C fibers, as well as in some Aδ fibers. In addition, TRPV1 function is enhanced by a variety of inflammatory mediators, and knockout mouse studies demonstrate that TRPV1 is required for inflammation-induced thermal hyperalgesia (Davis et al. 2000; Caterina et al. 2000; Bhave and Gereau 2004). A complete discussion of the expression pattern and functional aspects of TRP channels in DRG neurons is beyond the scope of this chapter. However, at least six of the TRP channels are involved in sensation of noxious cold (TRPA1), cooling (TRPM8), warming (TRPV3, TRPV4) and noxious heat (TRPV1, TRPV2) stimuli (Patapoutian et al. 2003; Story et al. 2003). These receptor channels are found in overlapping but distinct populations of DRG neurons, as well as in other neuronal populations in the CNS and in peripheral tissues, such as skin (TRPV3, TRPV4) (Patapoutian et al. 2003).

The importance of TRPV1 as a thermal transducer that is sensitized by a variety of proalgesic compounds suggests that blocking this channel may alleviate heat hyperalgesia associated with neuropathic pain syndromes. Pharmacological studies of the role of TRPV1 in neuropathic pain have been hampered by the lack of selective ligands. However, local administration of capsazepine, a TRPV1 antagonist, blocked thermal hyperalgesia in rodent models of inflammatory and neuropathic pain. Surprisingly, peripherally applied capsazepine also blocked mechanical allodynia in the partial SNL model (Walker et al. 2003). Others have reported that a novel, orally effective TRPV1 antagonist, BCTC, was also effective in reducing thermal hyperalgesia and mechanical allodynia in rat models of neuropathic pain (Pomonis et al. 2003; Valenzano et al. 2003). These and other studies outline the importance of TRPV1 in a variety of neuropathic pain conditions.

It is interesting to note that TRPV1 knockout mice did not demonstrate any change in thermal or mechanical hypersensitivity after sciatic nerve ligation (Caterina et al. 2000). The differences between the knockout data and pharmacological manipulations regarding the role of TRPV1 in neuropathic pain warrant further investigation. For example, do the TRPV1 antagonists reverse pain behavior in the TRPV1 knockout mice?

Capsaicin activation of TRPV1 results in activation followed by desensitization at low doses, and at higher doses it can be neurotoxic. In neonates, this neurotoxicity can be permanent, while in adult animals it tends to be temporary, only pruning back the peripheral terminals. It is tempting to speculate that application of high doses of capsaicin directly to affected ganglia in neuropathic conditions could be used to provide a permanent ablation of a population of nociceptive neurons, potentially providing long-term or permanent pain relief. Indeed, a recent report shows long-term efficacy of the TRPV1 agonist resiniferatoxin in rodent and canine pain syndromes (Karai et al. 2004). In mice, an upregulation of TRPV1, including novel expression in DRG neurons that normally do not express this channel, has been proposed as a mechanism for the analgesic efficacy of topical capsaicin creams in the partial SNL model and in a model of diabetic neuropathy (Rashid et al. 2003a,b). Whether topical or intraganglionic capsaicin treatment is effective in human neuropathic pain syndromes is certainly worthy of serious consideration.

In addition to TRPV1, there may be an important role for many other TRP channels in neuropathic pain syndromes. For example, antisense knockdown of TRPV4 in DRG completely blocked mechanical hypersensitivity in a model of chemotherapy-induced neuropathic pain (Alessandri-Haber et al. 2004). The expression of TRPV4 in DRG is somewhat controversial (Alessandri-Haber et al. 2003; Patapoutian et al. 2003). Analysis of the role of the many TRP channels in pain awaits the development of specific pharmacological agents or knockout animals.

The expression patters of individual TRP channels, in overlapping but distinct subpopulations of nociceptors, provides an intriguing possibility for individualized therapies using drugs that target specific TRP channels. An additional possibility lies in the potential for the delivery of targeted cytotoxic complexes, such as had been performed to specifically ablate neurokinin-1-expressing neurons in the spinal cord using substance P-saporin (Mantyh et al. 1997) or mu-opioid receptors in the rostroventromedial medulla using dermorphin-saporin (Porreca et al. 2001). Natural or synthetic ligands that act on specific TRP channels might be useful as saporin conjugates for the targeted destruction of specific subpopulations of primary afferent neurons. A better understanding of the specific physiological role of different populations of primary afferent neurons that express specific subsets of TRP channels is needed to move this idea forward.

PERIPHERAL ADRENERGIC RECEPTORS AND SYMPATHETIC MAINTENANCE OF NEUROPATHIC PAIN

Following nerve injury, a variety of changes occur in the periphery that lead to novel engagement of the sympathetic nervous system in activation or sensitization of nociceptive pathways. These changes include sprouting of sympathetic nerve endings and sympathetic/sensory coupling at the level of the DRG, at the site of injury (neuroma), and in the periphery (Shinder et al. 1999). The involvement of the sympathetic nervous system in pain etiology is referred to as "sympathetically maintained pain." Some, but not all, neuropathic pain syndromes can be ameliorated or reversed by interventions such as sympathetic blocks or surgical sympathectomy. Furthermore, the intradermal injection of norepinephrine induces pain in patients with sympathetically maintained pain, but not in patients with sympathetically independent pain, suggesting that this technique can be used as a diagnostic tool (Ali et al. 2000). Sympathetically maintained pain syndromes do not generally result from increased sympathetic efferent activity, but rather from novel sympathetic innervation due to sprouting and from peripheral sensitization to adrenergic agonists (Devor and Seltzer 1999).

Circulating epinephrine or norepinephrine released from sympathetic varicosities activates α-adrenergic receptors, leading to increased ectopic firing of primary afferent neurons. Much of the evidence suggests that peripheral α_2 receptors are primarily involved, although a role for peripheral α_1 receptors has also been suggested (Lee et al. 1999). Although α_1 and α_2 receptors are expressed in sensory neurons, it is not clear whether the sympathetic hypersensitivity lies within the primary afferent neurons themselves, since there is some evidence that α_2 receptors expressed on postganglionic sympathetic terminals are responsible for sympathetic/sensory coupling (Tracey et al. 1995). Many studies have failed to show dramatic adrenergic hypersensitivity of isolated DRG neurons from neuropathic animals, but there is evidence that injured DRG neurons are selectively sensitized to α_2 agonists in vivo (Sato and Perl 1991). Furthermore, adrenergic sensitivity is apparent in DRG neurons recorded in neuropathic rats (Zhang et al. 1997). This hypersensitivity is more easily seen in the intact ganglion preparation and in vivo than in isolated DRG neurons in culture, perhaps due to actions on α_2 receptors expressed on the termini of sympathetic efferents, which form basket-like structures around the somata of injured DRG neurons (Zhang et al. 2004).

In the clinical setting, clonidine applied locally via transdermal patches or creams has proven efficacious in a variety of neuropathic pain conditions (Davis et al. 1991; Byas-Smith et al. 1995). Given the presence of sympathetic/sensory coupling and hypersensitivity, the analgesic efficacy of peripherally applied clonidine seems paradoxical. Eisenach and colleagues recently demonstrated that clonidine decreased the excitation of a subset of cultured DRG neurons from normal or nerve-injured rats (Ma et al. 2005). However, these authors demonstrated that in nerve-injured rats, a much larger proportion of these "clonidine-inhibited" neurons expressed functional TRPV1, suggesting a change in the population of neurons coexpressing nociceptive markers (TRPV1) and α_2-adrenergic receptors (Ma et al. 2005). These results show the great complexity of the regulation of neuropathic pain by the sympathetic nervous system. There are certainly cases in which agents acting at peripheral adrenergic receptors are effective in the treatment of sympathetically maintained pain. A better understanding of the mechanisms underlying adrenergic modulation of nociception is needed to help guide rational pharmacotherapy of complex neuropathic pain conditions using adrenergic receptor ligands.

PERIPHERAL CANNABINOID RECEPTORS

The well-known analgesic properties of Δ9-tetrahydrocannabinol (THC), the active constituent in marijuana, spawned studies that have revealed the presence of a cannabinoid system that regulates the mammalian nociceptive system (Jarbe et al. 1986; Pertwee 2001; Cravatt and Lichtman 2004). The discovery of cannabinoid receptors and the identification of anandamide as an endogenous ligand demonstrated the presence of an endogenous cannabinoid transmitter system. Cannabinoid compounds exert their biological effects mainly via activation of G-protein-coupled CB1 and CB2 receptors. While CB1 receptors are widely expressed in the CNS, CB2 expression appears to be restricted to peripheral tissues. Expression of CB1, but not CB2, receptors is observed in neurons of the DRG. CB2 receptors are abundantly expressed in cells of the immune system, including mast cells (Hohmann 2002). Indeed, it is likely that some of the analgesic efficacy of CB2 activation can be attributed to inhibition of mast cells and to the resulting decrease in the generation of inflammatory mediators that sensitize nociceptors (Mazzari et al. 1996; Bhave and Gereau 2004). In animal models of neuropathic pain, cannabinoids are antihyperalgesic and antiallodynic. Importantly, the analgesic actions of cannabinoids do not diminish with repeated administration, suggesting that the development of tolerance, such as occurs with repeated opioid treatment, may not be an issue for the clinical application of cannabinoids. In human studies, agents acting at cannabinoid receptors have shown efficacy in neuropathic pain conditions, mostly for multiple sclerosis (Karst et al. 2003).

Studies of the specific roles of CB1 and CB2 receptors have been aided by the recent development of receptor subtype-selective ligands, such as the selective CB2 agonists AM1241 and HU-308, and the selective CB2 antagonist SR144528. Many studies have examined the analgesic efficacy of cannabinoids, revealing both central and peripheral mechanisms of cannabinoid analgesia (Hohmann 2002). The main difficulty associated with the clinical use of cannabinoids as analgesics is the strong adverse side effects due to activation of cannabinoid receptors in the CNS (Malan et al. 2003; Attal et al. 2004). The restricted peripheral expression of CB2 receptors gives hope for the development of CB2-selective agonists as analgesics with limited side effects. Studies utilizing systemic application of WIN55,212-2, a mixed CB1/CB2 receptor agonist, showed clear reversal of hyperalgesia and allodynia following L5 nerve ligation. However, the authors of this study found that these effects were reversed by a CB1 antagonist, but not by a CB2 antagonist, suggesting that the analgesic efficacy of cannabinoids in neuropathic pain may be mediated by CB1, rather than CB2, receptors (Bridges et al. 2001). On the other hand, systemic or local peripheral treatment with the CB2-selective agonist, AM1241, was able to reverse neuropathic pain induced by L5/L6 nerve ligation in mice (Scott et al. 2004), including mice with genetic deletion of the CB1 receptor (Ibrahim et al. 2003). Taken together, these data support a promising future for the development of cannabinoid agonists for the treatment of neuropathic pain. While there is a robust analgesic effect of CB1 agonists, the strong side effects associated with activation of CB1 receptors in the CNS limits their utility. On the other hand, the exclusion of CB2 receptors from the CNS, taken together with the promising results showing analgesic efficacy in models of neuropathic pain, point toward the clinical development of specific CB2 agonists as an exciting possibility for the development of novel analgesics with limited CNS side effects. The functional expression of CB2 receptors in mast cells and other components of the immune system may limit the utility of these agents in the long term, as is the case for anti-TNF agents, as discussed below. One possibility that could be considered is an attempt to develop novel CB1 agonists with limited blood-brain barrier penetrance. CB1 receptors are also expressed in DRG neurons, and peripherally restricted CB1 ligands might have strong analgesic efficacy with limited CNS side effects. Given that CB1 receptors may play a more limited role than CB2 receptors in the immune system (Samson et al. 2003), there may be fewer limitations to their use from an immunological standpoint.

PERIPHERAL GLUTAMATE RECEPTORS

Glutamate is the predominant excitatory neurotransmitter in the mammalian CNS. It acts through ligand-gated ion channels known as ionotropic glutamate receptors (iGluRs) and G-protein-coupled metabotropic glutamate receptors (mGluRs). Several glutamate receptors of both the ionotropic and metabotropic varieties are expressed in thin, unmyelinated nociceptive fibers in the skin (Carlton et al. 1995; Bhave et al. 2001). Subcutaneous injection of glutamate into the rodent hindpaw results in a reduction of thermal and mechanical thresholds, and localized peripheral application of iGluR and mGluR antagonists attenuate nociceptive scores during the formalin test, a model used to study inflammatory pain in rodents (Karim et al. 2001).

The mGluRs are widely expressed in the central and peripheral nervous system, where they modulate neuronal excitability and synaptic transmission (Pin and Acher 2002). Systemic application of mGlu5 antagonists reduces neuropathic pain in rats, an effect that is mimicked by local injection in the paw, suggesting that peripheral mGlu5 receptors may be targeted for the treatment of neuropathic pain (Dogrul et al. 2000; Jang et al. 2004; Zhu et al. 2004), although some data suggest that peripheral mGlu5 antagonists are effective at reversing thermal hyperalgesia, but not cold or mechanical allodynia, after nerve injury (Walker et al. 2001; Urban et al. 2003). The utility of peripherally acting mGlu5 antagonists may therefore be limited to neuropathic conditions in which thermal hyperalgesia is the prominent symptom.

Another exciting finding related to peripheral mGluRs in the treatment of neuropathic pain comes from the studies examining the effect of mGlu2/3 receptors in peripheral sensory neurons. First, Chiechio et al. (2002) demonstrated in a rat model of neuropathic pain that the slow-onset analgesic effects of L-acetyl-carnitine (LAC) are blocked by mGlu2/3 antagonists. These authors demonstrated that LAC treatment induces an upregulation of mGlu2 in the brain, in the spinal cord dorsal horn, and in DRG neurons. Further studies suggest that it is the upregulation of mGlu2 in the peripheral sensory neurons that is important for the analgesic efficacy of LAC (Chiechio et al. 2004). The exact site of mGlu2 activation that is important for the analgesic efficacy of LAC in neuropathic pain is not known. However, in inflammatory pain models, mGlu2 on peripheral nerve terminals has been shown to be a critical mediator of endogenous anti-allodynia (Yang and Gereau 2003). Accordingly, studies have demonstrated that mGlu2 activation reduces protein kinase A-mediated enhancement of tetrodotoxin-sensitive sodium channels (Yang and Gereau 2004) and of the noxious heat transduction channel TRPV1 (Yang and Gereau 2002). Because mGlu2 regulates peripheral nociceptive transduction, it is possible that peripherally expressed mGlu2 receptors could be effectively targeted for the treatment of neuropathic pain. The finding that mGlu2 is endogenously utilized to mediate analgesia (Chiechio et al. 2002; Yang and Gereau 2003) suggests that these receptors might be targeted not by direct agonists, but by agents that increase their expression (as is the case with LAC) or by novel agents that act allosterically to enhance activation of mGlu2 by endogenously released glutamate (Pinkerton et al. 2004). In the case of glutamate receptors, it is again important to stress the necessity to restrict drug action to the periphery. Because mGluRs are so widely distributed in the brain and subserve many important physiological functions, it would be advantageous to develop ligands that are highly potent and efficacious at mGluRs, but do not cross the blood-brain barrier. Such peripherally restricted ligands would certainly reduce side effects associated with their use, allowing higher dosing to more effectively block these important receptors expressed on peripheral terminals of primary afferents.

In addition to metabotropic glutamate receptors, peripheral ionotropic glutamate receptors may also be interesting targets for analgesic development. For example, peripheral administration of the iGluR agonists NMDA, AMPA, and kainate all produce thermal and mechanical hypersensitivity in naive animals (Zhou et al. 1996). Notably, a GluR5 kainate receptor antagonist was shown to have efficacy in the chronic constriction injury model of neuropathic pain (Blackburn-Munro et al. 2004).

MAS-RELATED GENES/SENSORY-NEURON-SPECIFIC RECEPTORS

Recently, a novel family of G-protein coupled receptors that are expressed only in nociceptive primary afferent neurons has been identified in mice, rats, and humans (Dong et al. 2001; Lembo et al. 2002). These receptors are known as mas-related genes (Mrgs) in mice (Dong et al. 2001) and as sensory-neuron-specific receptors (SNSRs) in rats and humans (Lembo et al. 2002). In mice, there is remarkable diversity in this gene family, with more than 50 Mrg receptor genes known. By contrast, in humans there are six SNSR genes (*SNSR1–SNSR6*) (Lembo et al. 2002). The Mrgs/SNSRs are orphan receptors, but it is likely that they function as receptors for a variety of peptide transmitters. Screening approaches led to the discovery that some of the Mrgs (*MrgA1* and *MrgC11*) are activated by RF-amide-related peptides (Han et al. 2002). Among the known ligands for the human SNSRs is bovine adrenal medulla 22 (BAM22), a cleavage product of the proenkephalin gene with known opioid- and non-opioid mechanisms of action, the latter of which may involve activation of SNSRs. Indeed, a recent study showed that BAM22 and γ_2-melanocyte-stimulating hormone (MSH), which was identified in this study as a potent agonist of rat SNSR1, induced spontaneous pain behaviors and thermal and mechanical hypersensitivity when injected intradermally (Grazzini et al. 2004).

The demonstration that SNSR activation modulates nociception opens the door to exciting new drug development possibilities that may provide a novel mechanism for antihyperalgesia/antiallodynia in neuropathic pain. The various expression patterns of individual SNSRs in subpopulations of nociceptors provides an intriguing possibility for individualized therapies using drugs that target specific SNSRs. They also show promise for the potential delivery of targeted cytotoxin complexes for the ablation of subpopulations of primary afferent neurons, as described above for the TRP channels. Although to date there have been no reported studies of the utility of targeting SNSRs for the treatment of neuropathic pain, the restricted expression of these receptors in various subpopulations of nociceptors makes them an attractive target for the development of novel analgesics.

The substantial differences in SNSR diversity observed between humans, rats, and mice will provide some serious challenges to the already difficult preclinical validation process. Ultimately, whether effects of SNSR ligands targeted for use in humans can be developed in rodent models at all is called into question by the large differences in receptor subtypes between species.

TUMOR NECROSIS FACTOR RECEPTORS

Tumor necrosis factor-alpha (TNF-α) is a proinflammatory cytokine and an important mediator of inflammatory pain (Suryaprasad and Prindiville 2003). TNF-α not only acts as an inflammatory mediator, but can also have direct effects on sensory neurons. TNF-α exerts its actions via two main receptors: TNFR1 and TNFR2, both of which are expressed in DRG neurons (Pollock et al. 2002; Ohtori et al. 2004). These effects seem to be direct, rather than through activation of other cells, and most likely involve the generation of sphingomyelin metabolites and/or activation of p38 mitogen-activated protein kinase (MAPK) (Pollock et al. 2002; Schafers et al. 2003d; Jin and Gereau 2006).

In animal models of neuropathic pain, levels of TNF-α and expression of TNF receptors TNFR1 and TNFR2 increase in both the injured and adjacent axons (Shubayev and Myers 2001; Schafers et al. 2003a,c). Accordingly, the response of injured primary afferents or adjacent uninjured neurons to application of TNF-α is enhanced following spinal nerve ligation (Schafers et al. 2003b). Furthermore, agents that decrease TNF-α activity are reported to diminish allodynia in rat models of neuropathic pain (Sommer et al. 2001a,b; Schafers et al. 2003d). In humans, a correlation was observed between elevated levels of TNF-α in sural nerve biopsies and the degree of neuropathic pain in patients with both inflammatory- and non-inflammatory neuropathies, suggesting a potential role for TNF-α in human neuropathic pain (Lindenlaub and Sommer 2003). Anti-TNF-α therapy reportedly has efficacy in treating sciatica pain, which is believed to involve both inflammatory and neuropathic mechanisms (Karppinen et al. 2003; Baron and Binder 2004; Korhonen et al. 2004). Several anti-TNF-α agents are currently used in clinical practice, primarily for the treatment of rheumatoid arthritis and Crohn's disease (Suryaprasad and Prindiville 2003). Etanercept is a fusion protein of soluble human TNF-α receptors linked to the Fc fragment of human immunoglobulin G1, whereas adalimumab is a humanized monoclonal antibody against TNF-α and infliximab is a chimeric monoclonal antibody against TNF-α. All of these agents must be delivered via intravenous injection, and all have potential adverse effects. The development of novel orally available anti-TNF-α agents may improve some aspects of their use. In the inflammatory conditions of Crohn's disease or rheumatoid arthritis, efficacy of anti-TNF-α therapy can be temporary (Suryaprasad and Prindiville 2003). Whether anti-TNF-α agents are effective in human neuropathic pain conditions, with perhaps more permanent results than for the inflammatory disease states, is worthy of consideration.

The discussion above has been limited to only a few examples of peripheral receptor systems that might be targeted for the development of novel analgesics for the treatment of neuropathic pain syndromes. Space limitations prevent a full discussion of all receptor systems that should be considered in this context. Among many others, the role of receptor systems for adenosine triphosphate, γ-aminobutyric acid, neurokinins, galanin, neuropeptide Y, orphanin FQ/nociception, and a variety of cytokines and chemokines are worthy of further consideration. In any case, a great deal of evidence suggests that peripherally administered or orally applied but peripherally restricted compounds could prove efficacious for the management of neuropathic pain syndromes. Of course, peripheral restriction of such compounds is a secondary concern when they target receptors that are expressed only in the periphery, but off-target actions of drugs are also a potential issue. While peripheral side effects are a possibility, limiting distribution of these drugs to the periphery would prevent many potential side affects associated with CNS distribution of the drugs.

Finally, these peripheral receptors, as well as a variety of other peripheral targets, might be targeted via nontraditional means. For example, I discussed above the prospect of utilizing targeted neurotoxins to selectively ablate subpopulations of DRG neurons involved in various types of neuropathic pain syndromes. In addition, one could use viral transfection of the nerve endings, nerve trunks, or ganglia as a way to introduce genetic modifying agents such as small interfering RNA molecules, dominant negative constructs, or blocking peptides to provide long-term relief, if a good target is identified. The selective expression of a variety of TRP channels and Mrgs/SNSRs in specific subpopulations of DRG neurons would allow for the targeted introduction of genes driven specifically by promoters for individual TRP channels or SNSRs. For example, inhibitory ion channels expressed on certain populations of primary afferent neurons could silence ectopically active neurons and inhibit certain populations of nociceptors. An animal model utilizing this approach to increase μ-opioid receptor expression in DRG neurons has recently been reported (Xu et al. 2003). The ability to selectively infect neurons with certain types of viruses makes this gene therapy approach an intriguing possibility.

ACKNOWLEDGMENTS

Work in the author's laboratory is funded by the National Institutes of Health (NINDS) and the McDonnell Center for Cellular and Molecular Neurobiology.

REFERENCES

Alessandri-Haber N, Yeh JJ, Boyd AE, et al. Hypotonicity induces TRPV4-mediated nociception in rat. *Neuron* 2003; 39:497–511.

Alessandri-Haber N, Dina OA, Yeh JJ, et al. Transient receptor potential vanilloid 4 is essential in chemotherapy-induced neuropathic pain in the rat. *J Neurosci* 2004; 24:4444–4452.

Ali Z, Raja SN, Wesselmann U, et al. Intradermal injection of norepinephrine evokes pain in patients with sympathetically maintained pain. *Pain* 2000; 88:161–168.

Attal N, Brasseur L, Guirimand D, et al. Are oral cannabinoids safe and effective in refractory neuropathic pain? *Eur J Pain* 2004; 8:173–177.

Baron R, Binder A. How neuropathic is sciatica? The mixed pain concept. *Orthopade* 2004; 33:568–575.

Bhave G, Gereau RW. Posttranslational mechanisms of peripheral sensitization. *J Neurobiol* 2004; 61:88–106.

Bhave G, Karim F, Carlton SM, Gereau RW. Peripheral group I metabotropic glutamate receptors modulate nociception in mice. *Nat Neurosci* 2001; 4:417–423.

Blackburn-Munro G, Bomholt SF, Erichsen HK. Behavioural effects of the novel AMPA/GluR5 selective receptor antagonist NS1209 after systemic administration in animal models of experimental pain. *Neuropharmacology* 2004; 47:351–362.

Bridges D, Ahmad K, Rice AS. The synthetic cannabinoid WIN55,212-2 attenuates hyperalgesia and allodynia in a rat model of neuropathic pain. *Br J Pharmacol* 2001; 133:586–594.

Byas-Smith MG, Max MB, Muir J, Kingman A. Transdermal clonidine compared to placebo in painful diabetic neuropathy using a two stage 'enriched enrollment' design. *Pain* 1995; 60:267–274.

Carlton SM, Hargett GL, Coggeshall RE. Localization and activation of glutamate receptors in unmyelinated axons of rat glabrous skin. *Neurosci Lett* 1995; 197:25–28.

Caterina MJ, Schumacher MA, Tominaga M, et al. The capsaicin receptor: a heat-activated ion channel in the pain pathway. *Nature* 1997; 389:816–824.

Caterina MJ, Leffler A, Malmberg AB, et al. Impaired nociception and pain sensation in mice lacking the capsaicin receptor. *Science* 2000; 288:306–313.

Chiechio S, Caricasole A, Barletta E, et al. L-Acetylcarnitine induces analgesia by selectively upregulating mGlu2 metabotropic glutamate receptors. *Mol Pharmacol* 2002; 61989–61996.

Chiechio S, Copani A, Melchiorri D, et al. Metabotropic receptors as targets for drugs of potential use in the treatment of neuropathic pain. *J Endocrinol Invest* 2004; 27:171–176.

Cravatt BF, Lichtman AH. The endogenous cannabinoid system and its role in nociceptive behavior. *J Neurobiol* 2004; 61:149–160.

Davis KD, Treede RD, Raja SN, et al. Topical application of clonidine relieves hyperalgesia in patients with sympathetically maintained pain. *Pain* 1991; 47:309–317.

Davis JB, Gray J, Gunthorpe MJ, et al. Vanilloid receptor-1 is essential for inflammatory thermal hyperalgesia. *Nature* 2000; 405:183–187.

Devor M, Seltzer Z. Pathophysiology of damaged nerves in relation to chronic pain. In: Wall PD, Melzack R (Eds). *Textbook of Pain*. London: Churchill Livingstone, 1999, pp 129–164.

Dogrul A, Ossipov MH, Lai J, Malan TP, Porreca F. Peripheral and spinal antihyperalgesic activity of SIB-1757, a metabotropic glutamate receptor (mGluR(5)) antagonist, in experimental neuropathic pain in rats. *Neurosci Lett* 2000; 292:115–118.

Dong X, Han S, Zylka MJ, Simon MI, Anderson DJ. A diverse family of GPCRs expressed in specific subsets of nociceptive sensory neurons. *Cell* 2001; 106:619–632.

Gordon DB, Love G. Pharmacologic management of neuropathic pain. *Pain Manag Nurs* 2004; 5:19–33.

Grazzini E, Puma C, Roy MO, et al. Sensory neuron-specific receptor activation elicits central and peripheral nociceptive effects in rats. *Proc Natl Acad Sci USA* 2004; 101:7175–7180.

Han SK, Dong X, Hwang JI, et al. Orphan G protein-coupled receptors MrgA1 and MrgC11 are distinctively activated by RF-amide-related peptides through the G-alpha q/11 pathway. *Proc Natl Acad Sci USA* 2002; 99:14740–14745.

Hohmann AG. Spinal and peripheral mechanisms of cannabinoid antinociception: behavioral, neurophysiological and neuroanatomical perspectives. *Chem Phys Lipids* 2002; 121:173–190.

Ibrahim MM, Deng H, Zvonok A, et al. Activation of CB2 cannabinoid receptors by AM1241 inhibits experimental neuropathic pain: pain inhibition by receptors not present in the CNS. *Proc Natl Acad Sci USA* 2003; 100:10529–10533.

Jang JH, Kim DW, Sang Nam T, et al. Peripheral glutamate receptors contribute to mechanical hyperalgesia in a neuropathic pain model of the rat. *Neuroscience* 2004; 128:169–176.

Jarbe TU, Hiltunen AJ, Lander N, Mechoulam R. Cannabimimetic activity (delta 1-THC cue) of cannabidiol monomethyl ether and two stereoisomeric hexahydrocannabinols in rats and pigeons. *Pharmacol Biochem Behav* 1986; 25:393–399.

Jin X, Gereau RW. Acute p38-mediated modulation of TTX-resistant sodium channels in mouse sensory neurons by tumor necrosis factor-α. *J Neurosci* 2006; in press.

Johanek LM, Shim B, Horasek SJ, et al. Loperamide, a peripherally acting opioid agonist, reverses hyperalgesia induced by spinal nerve ligation in rat. *Abstracts: 11th World Congress on Pain*. Seattle: IASP Press, 2005.

Karai L, Brown DC, Mannes AJ, et al. Deletion of vanilloid receptor 1-expressing primary afferent neurons for pain control. *J Clin Invest* 2004; 113:1344–1352.

Karim F, Bhave G, Gereau RW. Metabotropic glutamate receptors on peripheral sensory neuron terminals as targets for the development of novel analgesics. *Mol Psychiatry* 2001; 6:615–617.

Karppinen J, Korhonen T, Malmivaara A, et al. Tumor necrosis factor-alpha monoclonal antibody, infliximab, used to manage severe sciatica. *Spine* 2003; 28:750–753; discussion 753–754.

Karst M, Salim K, Burstein S, et al. Analgesic effect of the synthetic cannabinoid CT-3 on chronic neuropathic pain: a randomized controlled trial. *JAMA* 2003; 290:1757–1762.

Kolesnikov Y, Pasternak GW. Topical opioids in mice: analgesia and reversal of tolerance by a topical N-methyl-D-aspartate antagonist. *J Pharmacol Exp Ther* 1999a; 290:247–252.

Kolesnikov YA, Pasternak GW. Peripheral blockade of topical morphine tolerance by ketamine. *Eur J Pharmacol* 1999b; 374:R1–2.

Korhonen T, Karppinen J, Malmivaara A, et al. Efficacy of infliximab for disc herniation-induced sciatica: one-year follow-up. *Spine* 2004; 29:2115–2119.

Lee DH, Liu X, Kim HT, Chung K, Chung JM. Receptor subtype mediating the adrenergic sensitivity of pain behavior and ectopic discharges in neuropathic Lewis rats. *J Neurophysiol* 1999; 81:2226–2233.

Lembo PM, Grazzini E, Groblewski T, et al. Proenkephalin A gene products activate a new family of sensory neuron-specific GPCRs. *Nat Neurosci* 2002; 5:201–209.

Lindenlaub T, Sommer C. Cytokines in sural nerve biopsies from inflammatory and non-inflammatory neuropathies. *Acta Neuropathol (Berl)* 2003; 105:593–602.

Ma W, Zhang Y, Bantel C, Eisenach JC. Medium and large injured dorsal root ganglion cells increase TRPV-1, accompanied by increased alpha-2C-adrenoceptor co-expression and functional inhibition by clonidine. *Pain* 2005; 113:386–394.

Malan TP Jr, Ibrahim MM, Lai J, et al. CB2 cannabinoid receptor agonists: pain relief without psychoactive effects? *Curr Opin Pharmacol* 2003; 3:62–67.

Mansikka H, Zhao C, Sheth RN, et al. Nerve injury induces a tonic bilateral mu-opioid receptor-mediated inhibitory effect on mechanical allodynia in mice. *Anesthesiology* 2004; 100:912–921.

Mantyh PW, Rogers SD, Honore P, et al. Inhibition of hyperalgesia by ablation of lamina I spinal neurons expressing the substance P receptor. *Science* 1997; 278:275–279.

Mazzari S, Canella R, Petrelli L, Marcolongo G, Leon A. N-(2-hydroxyethyl)hexadecanamide is orally active in reducing edema formation and inflammatory hyperalgesia by down-modulating mast cell activation. *Eur J Pharmacol* 1996; 300:227–236.

Ohtori S, Takahashi K, Moriya H, Myers RR. TNF-alpha and TNF-alpha receptor type 1 upregulation in glia and neurons after peripheral nerve injury: studies in murine DRG and spinal cord. *Spine* 2004; 29:1082–1088.

Patapoutian A, Peier AM, Story GM, Viswanath V. Thermo-TRP channels and beyond: mechanisms of temperature sensation. *Nat Rev Neurosci* 2003; 4:529–539.

Pertovaara A, Wei H. Peripheral effects of morphine in neuropathic rats: role of sympathetic postganglionic nerve fibers. *Eur J Pharmacol* 2001; 429:139–145.

Pertwee RG. Cannabinoid receptors and pain. *Prog Neurobiol* 2001; 63:569–611.

Pin JP, Acher F. The metabotropic glutamate receptors: structure. activation mechanism and pharmacology. *Curr Drug Targets CNS Neurol Disord* 2002; 1:297–317.

Pinkerton AB, Vernier JM, Schaffhauser H, et al. Phenyl-tetrazolyl acetophenones: discovery of positive allosteric potentiators for the metabotropic glutamate 2 receptor. *J Med Chem* 2004; 47:4595–4599.

Pollock J, McFarlane SM, Connell MC, et al. TNF-alpha receptors simultaneously activate Ca2+ mobilisation and stress kinases in cultured sensory neurones. *Neuropharmacology* 2002; 42:93–106.

Pomonis JD, Harrison JE, Mark L, et al. N-(4-Tertiarybutylphenyl)-4-(3-cholorphyridin-2-yl)tetrahydropyrazine-1(2H)-carbox-amide (BCTC), a novel, orally effective vanilloid receptor 1 antagonist with analgesic properties: II. in vivo characterization in rat models of inflammatory and neuropathic pain. *J Pharmacol Exp Ther* 2003; 306:387–393.

Porreca F, Burgess SE, Gardell LR, et al. Inhibition of neuropathic pain by selective ablation of brainstem medullary cells expressing the mu-opioid receptor. *J Neurosci* 2001; 21:5281–5288.

Przewlocki R, Przewlocka B. Opioids in chronic pain. *Eur J Pharmacol* 2001; 429:79–91.

Rashid MH, Inoue M, Bakoshi S, Ueda H. Increased expression of vanilloid receptor 1 on myelinated primary afferent neurons contributes to the antihyperalgesic effect of capsaicin cream in diabetic neuropathic pain in mice. *J Pharmacol Exp Ther* 2003a; 306:709–717.

Rashid MH, Inoue M, Kondo S, et al. Novel expression of vanilloid receptor 1 on capsaicin-insensitive fibers accounts for the analgesic effect of capsaicin cream in neuropathic pain. *J Pharmacol Exp Ther* 2003b; 304:940–948.

Rashid MH, Inoue M, Toda K, Ueda H. Loss of peripheral morphine analgesia contributes to the reduced effectiveness of systemic morphine in neuropathic pain. *J Pharmacol Exp Ther* 2004; 309:380–387.

Samson MT, Small-Howard A, Shimoda LM, et al. Differential roles of CB1 and CB2 cannabinoid receptors in mast cells. *J Immunol* 2003; 170:4953–4962.

Sato J, Perl ER. Adrenergic excitation of cutaneous pain receptors induced by peripheral nerve injury. *Science* 1991; 251:1608–1610.

Sawynok J. Topical and peripherally acting analgesics. *Pharmacol Rev* 2003; 55:1–20.

Schafers M, Geis C, Svensson CI, Luo ZD, Sommer C. Selective increase of tumour necrosis factor-alpha in injured and spared myelinated primary afferents after chronic constrictive injury of rat sciatic nerve. *Eur J Neurosci* 2003a; 17:791–804.

Schafers M, Lee DH, Brors D, et al. Increased sensitivity of injured and adjacent uninjured rat primary sensory neurons to exogenous tumor necrosis factor-alpha after spinal nerve ligation. *J Neurosci* 2003b; 23:3028–3038.

Schafers M, Sorkin LS, Geis C, Shubayev VI. Spinal nerve ligation induces transient upregulation of tumor necrosis factor receptors 1 and 2 in injured and adjacent uninjured dorsal root ganglia in the rat. *Neurosci Lett* 2003c; 347:179–182.

Schafers M, Svensson CI, Sommer C, Sorkin LS. Tumor necrosis factor-alpha induces mechanical allodynia after spinal nerve ligation by activation of p38 MAPK in primary sensory neurons. *J Neurosci* 2003d; 23:2517–2521.

Scott DA, Wright CE, Angus JA. Evidence that CB-1 and CB-2 cannabinoid receptors mediate antinociception in neuropathic pain in the rat. *Pain* 2004; 109:124–131.

Shinder V, Govrin-Lippmann R, Cohen S, et al. Structural basis of sympathetic-sensory coupling in rat and human dorsal root ganglia following peripheral nerve injury. *J Neurocytol* 1999; 28:743–761.

Shubayev VI, Myers RR. Axonal transport of TNF-alpha in painful neuropathy: distribution of ligand tracer and TNF receptors. *J Neuroimmunol* 2001; 114:48–56.

Sommer C, Lindenlaub T, Teuteberg P, et al. Anti-TNF-neutralizing antibodies reduce pain-related behavior in two different mouse models of painful mononeuropathy. *Brain Res* 2001a; 913:86–89.

Sommer C, Schafers M, Marziniak M, Toyka KV. Etanercept reduces hyperalgesia in experimental painful neuropathy. *J Peripher Nerv Syst* 2001b; 6:67–72.

Story GM, Peier AM, Reeve AJ, et al. ANKTM1, a TRP-like channel expressed in nociceptive neurons, is activated by cold temperatures. *Cell* 2003; 112:819–829.

Suryaprasad AG, Prindiville T. The biology of TNF blockade. *Autoimmun Rev* 2003; 2:346–357.

Tracey DJ, Cunningham JE, Romm MA. Peripheral hyperalgesia in experimental neuropathy: mediation by alpha 2-adrenoreceptors on post-ganglionic sympathetic terminals. *Pain* 1995; 60:317–327.

Truong W, Cheng C, Xu QG, et al. Mu opioid receptors and analgesia at the site of a peripheral nerve injury. *Ann Neurol* 2003; 53:366–375.

Urban MO, Hama AT, Bradbury M, et al. Role of metabotropic glutamate receptor subtype 5 (mGluR5) in the maintenance of cold hypersensitivity following a peripheral mononeuropathy in the rat. *Neuropharmacology* 2003; 44:983–993.

Valenzano KJ, Grant ER, Wu G, et al. N-(4-tertiarybutylphenyl)-4-(3-chloropyridin-2-yl)tetrahydropyrazine-1(2H)-carbox-amide (BCTC), a novel, orally effective vanilloid receptor 1 antagonist with analgesic properties: I. in vitro characterization and pharmacokinetic properties. *J Pharmacol Exp Ther* 2003; 306:377–386.

Valenzano KJ, Miller W, Chen Z, et al. DiPOA ([8–(3,3-diphenyl-propyl)-4-oxo-1-phenyl-1,3,8-triazaspiro[4.5]dec-3-yl]-acetic acid), a novel, systemically available, and peripherally restricted mu opioid agonist with antihyperalgesic activity: I. In vitro pharmacological characterization and pharmacokinetic properties. *J Pharmacol Exp Ther* 2004; 310:783–792.

Walker K, Bowes M, Panesar M, et al. Metabotropic glutamate receptor subtype 5 (mGlu5) and nociceptive function. I. Selective blockade of mGlu5 receptors in models of acute, persistent and chronic pain. *Neuropharmacology* 2001; 40:1–9.

Walker KM, Urban L, Medhurst SJ, et al. The VR1 antagonist capsazepine reverses mechanical hyperalgesia in models of inflammatory and neuropathic pain. *J Pharmacol Exp Ther* 2003; 304:56–62.

Whiteside GT, Harrison JE, Pearson MS, et al. DiPOA ([8-(3,3-diphenyl-propyl)-4-oxo-1-phenyl-1,3,8-triazaspiro[4.5]dec-3-yl]-acetic acid), a novel, systemically available, and peripherally restricted mu opioid agonist with antihyperalgesic activity: II. In vivo pharmacological characterization in the rat. *J Pharmacol Exp Ther* 2004; 310:793–799.

Xu Y, Gu Y, Xu G-Y, et al. Adeno-associated viral transfer of opioid receptor gene to primary sensory neurons: a strategy to increase opioid antinociception. *Proc Natl Acad Sci USA* 2003; 100:6204–6209.

Yang D, Gereau RW. Peripheral group II metabotropic glutamate receptors (mGluR2/3; regulate prostaglandin E2-mediated sensitization of capsaicin responses and thermal nociception. *J Neurosci* 2002; 22:6388–6393.

Yang D, Gereau RW. Peripheral group II metabotropic glutamate receptors mediate endogenous anti-allodynia in inflammation. *Pain* 2003; 106:411–417.

Yang D, Gereau RW. Group II metabotropic glutamate receptors inhibit cAMP-dependent protein kinase-mediated enhancement of tetrodotoxin-resistant sodium currents in mouse dorsal root ganglion neurons. *Neurosci Lett* 2004; 357:159–162.

Zhang JM, Song XJ, LaMotte RH. An in vitro study of ectopic discharge generation and adrenergic sensitivity in the intact. nerve-injured rat dorsal root ganglion. *Pain* 1997; 72:51–57.

Zhang JM, Li H, Munir MA. Decreasing sympathetic sprouting in pathologic sensory ganglia: a new mechanism for treating neuropathic pain using lidocaine. *Pain* 2004; 109:143–149.

Zhao C, Tall JM, Meyer RA, Raja SN. Antiallodynic effects of systemic and intrathecal morphine in the spared nerve injury model of neuropathic pain in rats. *Anesthesiology* 2004; 100:905–911.

Zhou S, Bonasera L, Carlton SM. Peripheral administration of NMDA, AMPA or KA results in pain behaviors in rats. *Neuroreport* 1996; 7:895–900.

Zhu CZ, Wilson SG, Mikusa JP, et al. Assessing the role of metabotropic glutamate receptor 5 in multiple nociceptive modalities. *Eur J Pharmacol* 2004; 506:107–118.

Zimmermann M. Pathobiology of neuropathic pain. *Eur J Pharmacol* 2001; 42923–42937.

Correspondence to: Robert W. Gereau IV, PhD, Washington University Pain Center, Department of Anesthesiology, 660 S. Euclid Ave, Campus Box 8054, St Louis, MO 63110, USA. Tel: 314-362-8312; Fax: 314-362-8334; email: gereaur@wustl.edu.

Emerging Strategies for the Treatment of Neuropathic Pain, edited by James N. Campbell, Allan I. Basbaum, André Dray, Ronald Dubner, Robert H. Dworkin, and Christine N. Sang, IASP Press, Seattle, © 2006.

4

Does Peripheral Sensitization of Primary Afferents Play a Role in Neuropathic Pain?

Matthias Ringkamp[a] and Richard A. Meyer[a,b,c]

Departments of *[a]Neurosurgery* and *[b]Biomedical Engineering* and *[c]Applied Physics Laboratory, Johns Hopkins University, Baltimore, Maryland, USA*

Many diseases of the peripheral nervous system lead to the development of pain and hyperalgesia. For example, painful neuropathies result from nerve trauma, nerve entrapment, infections such as shingles, neurotoxic drugs, and autoimmune or metabolic diseases. The most common animal models of neuropathic pain involve a traumatic nerve injury. In patients, traumatic injuries to nerves often lead to neuromas that can be painful upon palpation. Indeed, many investigators have found that peripheral nerve fibers ending in a neuroma develop spontaneous activity as well as ectopic mechanical, thermal, and chemical sensitivity (Devor and Seltzer 1999). Ectopic spontaneous activity also develops in the dorsal root ganglion (DRG) of the injured nerve. This chapter considers another site of abnormal activity in the peripheral nervous system following nerve injury, namely the intact, uninjured fibers that commingle with the degenerating fibers. These intact fibers are exposed to an altered milieu that contains inflammatory mediators and trophic factors that could lead to sensitization of primary afferents.

Tissue inflammation is known to cause sensitization of nociceptive afferents. The responses of nociceptors to heat and mechanical stimuli are enhanced, and spontaneous activity develops. The spontaneous activity in C fibers can provide the peripheral drive for central sensitization (Cook et al. 1987). Thus, peripheral sensitization can lead to enhanced sensitivity in the peripheral and central nervous systems.

This chapter reviews the evidence from both human and animal experiments showing that peripheral sensitization is a potentially important mechanism in neuropathic pain. This evidence suggests that the peripheral nervous system is an important therapeutic target in neuropathic pain.

EVIDENCE FROM CLINICAL STUDIES

ADRENERGIC SENSITIVITY IN PATIENTS WITH SYMPATHETICALLY MAINTAINED PAIN

For certain patients with neuropathic pain, the pain depends on activity in the sympathetic nervous system. For these patients with sympathetically maintained pain (SMP), an anesthetic block of the sympathetic nervous system or an intravenous administration of phentolamine (an α-adrenergic antagonist) will provide pain relief (Raja et al. 1991). Other patients may have sympathetically independent pain, while some may have a combination of both types of pain.

Several lines of evidence point to the conclusion that SMP results from enhanced adrenergic sensitivity of primary afferent nociceptors. First, regional infusion of guanethidine by means of a Bier's block leads to prolonged pain relief in patients with SMP (Hannington-Kiff 1974). Since guanethidine is thought to deplete norepinephrine from the sympathetic terminals, this result demonstrates that the coupling between the sympathetic nervous system and the pain system occurs in the periphery. Second, in some patients with SMP, intradermal injection of norepinephrine produces pain (Torebjörk et al. 1995). The injection causes dose-dependent pain in the affected limb but not in the unaffected limb or in normal subjects (Ali et al. 2000). An increase in adrenergic sensitivity in peripheral tissues would explain the development of pain from exogenous norepinephrine. Third, topical application of clonidine leads to localized relief of hyperalgesia (Davis et al. 1991). Clonidine is an α_2-adrenergic agonist and presumably inhibits norepinephrine release from cutaneous sympathetic terminals. As we will describe later, these phenomena in patients are mirrored in animal models of neuropathic pain in which nociceptors develop sensitivity to adrenergic agents.

"IRRITABLE NOCICEPTORS" IN POSTHERPETIC NEURALGIA

Postherpetic neuralgia (PHN) is a common type of neuropathic pain that occurs following the re-emergence of the varicella zoster virus (shingles). The pain of PHN persists after the acute viral outbreak subsides. Although some patients with PHN have pronounced sensory loss, many patients with severe hyperalgesia have lowered thermal sensory thresholds in their region of greatest pain (Rowbotham and Fields 1989). This observation has led to the hypothesis that "irritable nociceptors" account for the pain in some patients with PHN (Fields et al. 1998).

PATHOLOGICAL CHANGES IN C-FIBER AFFERENTS IN ERYTHROMELALGIA

Erythromelalgia is a chronic pain condition characterized by attacks of hot, red, painful extremities. Although vascular pathology has been thought to be responsible, recent evidence indicates that erythromelalgia may have a neuropathic component (Ørstavik et al. 2004). Microneurographic recordings in patients with erythromelalgia revealed pathological changes in C-fiber afferents, including a decrease in conduction velocity and an increase in activity-dependent slowing of conduction (Ørstavik et al. 2003). In addition, C fibers that normally would be classified as mechanically insensitive afferents based on their conduction properties displayed mechanosensitivity, suggesting that sensitization of nociceptors may play a role in this disease. Similar changes have been reported for patients with diabetic neuropathy (M. Schmelz, personal communication). Activity-dependent slowing of conduction is a normal reaction to repeated electrical stimulation of C fibers. The increased activity-dependent slowing seen in patients with erythromelalgia, similar to that observed in uninjured C fibers in rats after spinal nerve injury (Shim et al. 2003), could be a sign of peripheral neuropathy.

TOPICAL THERAPIES PROVIDE LOCAL RELIEF

Topical capsaicin treatment has been reported to produce beneficial effects in a number of neuropathic conditions including PHN, complex regional pain syndrome, and traumatic nerve injury (Watson 1994; Ellison et al. 1997; Robbins et al. 1998). Since topical application of capsaicin leads to a selective desensitization of nociceptive terminals (Nolano et al. 1999), its therapeutic benefit suggests that peripheral terminals of nociceptive fibers are involved in neuropathic pain.

Topical application of lidocaine is also beneficial, particularly in PHN (Rowbotham et al. 1996). Since lidocaine does not act selectively on nociceptors, its effect could be due to anesthesia of mechanoreceptors.

EVIDENCE FROM STUDIES IN ANIMALS

A variety of different animal models are available to study the neuronal mechanisms of neuropathic pain. Many of these models use a traumatic injury along the peripheral neuraxis to produce behavioral signs of neuropathic pain. The most commonly used models include a neuroma of the sciatic nerve (Wall and Gutnick 1974), a chronic constriction injury (CCI) of the sciatic nerve (Bennett and Xie 1988), a partial ligation of the sciatic nerve (Seltzer et al. 1990), a spinal nerve ligation (SNL) (Kim and Chung 1992), and a spared nerve injury (Decosterd and Woolf 2000). Because of the localized injury, these models do not necessarily mimic clinically relevant dying-back neuropathies in humans, such as diabetic or neurotoxic neuropathies. However, these models allow investigation of some of the different mechanisms that may play a role in clinically relevant neuropathies. For example, the relative role of injured and uninjured afferents in neuropathic pain states can be studied.

BEHAVIORAL STUDIES IN ANIMAL MODELS OF NEUROPATHIC PAIN

Accumulating evidence from different behavioral studies in animals suggests a role for uninjured nerve fibers in neuropathic pain. Using the SNL model, several groups have investigated the role of injured and uninjured afferents, either by applying local anesthetics to the different dorsal roots or by performing dorsal rhizotomies at various levels. Unfortunately, the results from these studies are contradictory. On the one hand, L5/L6 dorsal rhizotomy prevented or reversed mechanical hyperalgesia following L5/L6 spinal nerve injury (Sheen and Chung 1993). Furthermore, transection of the L5 dorsal root reversed spontaneous as well as stimulus-evoked pain, whereas single L4 dorsal rhizotomy reversed stimulus-evoked, but not spontaneous, pain (Yoon et al. 1996). On the other hand, some studies failed to demonstrate an effect of dorsal rhizotomy on neuropathic pain behavior following SNL. For example, an L5 dorsal rhizotomy after an L5 SNL did not reverse neuropathic pain behavior (Eschenfelder et al. 2000; Sheth et al. 2002), and an L5 dorsal rhizotomy prior to nerve lesion failed to prevent the development of mechanical hyperalgesia (Li et al. 2000). However, a lasting mechanical hyperalgesia following L5 dorsal rhizotomy has been reported in some studies (Eschenfelder et al. 2000); this hyperalgesia may be due to the close proximity of the surgical intervention to the L5 DRG, since hyperalgesia was not observed when the laminectomy and L5 rhizotomy were performed at a more rostral level (Sheth et al. 2002).

Two other lines of behavioral evidence strongly suggest a role of uninjured afferents in neuropathic pain. First, an L5 ventral rhizotomy results in behavioral signs of mechanical and thermal hyperalgesia (Li et al. 2002; Sheth et al. 2002; Wu et al. 2002; Obata et al. 2004; but see Colburn et al. 1999). A ventral rhizotomy does not injure the afferent pathway, but does induce spontaneous neural activity in uninjured afferents (Wu et al. 2001), as well as remodeling of Schwann cells (Murinson et al. 2005). Thus, an injury to afferent nerve fibers is not a necessary condition for the development of neuropathic pain. Second, mechanical and thermal hyperalgesia are observed following ganglionectomy of the L5 DRG (Sheth et al. 2002; Obata et al. 2004). Since a ganglionectomy removes the somata of the injured neurons, neural activity from injured afferents is not required for neuropathic pain. Both studies show that neuronal activity from uninjured afferents is sufficient to produce behavioral signs of neuropathic pain.

ELECTROPHYSIOLOGICAL FINDINGS IN MODELS OF TRAUMATIC NEUROPATHIES

Many electrophysiological studies have been performed in animal models that involve ligating and/or cutting a nerve. After these traumatic nerve injuries, uninjured C fibers developed spontaneous activity, enhanced sensitivity to chemicals, increased responsiveness to mechanical and thermal stimuli, and alterations in their conductive properties.

Spontaneous activity in uninjured C fibers. Following CCI of the saphenous nerve, an increased number of unmyelinated nociceptive afferents innervating the dorsum of the hindpaw exhibited spontaneous activity (Koltzenburg et al. 1994). In some of the fibers, spontaneous activity was abolished by lidocaine applied to the cutaneous receptive field, while in others only a partial effect or no effect on spontaneous activity was observed, suggesting that such activity may originate from multiple generator sites (Koltzenburg et al. 1994).

An increased incidence of C-fiber afferents with spontaneous activity was also seen in the superficial peroneal nerve 2–3 weeks following an L6 SNL in primates (Ali et al. 1999). In rats, low-level spontaneous activity was present in about 50% of the uninjured C fibers is the L4 spinal nerve within 1 day after an L5 SNL, and the incidence of spontaneously active fibers did not significantly change during the first week after injury (Wu et al. 2001). Spontaneous activity must have been generated in the peripheral receptive field, since it could be abolished by lidocaine injection into the skin. Following L5 SNL, spontaneous activity also increased in the DRG cells of uninjured myelinated nerve fibers (Boucher et al. 2000).

The incidence of spontaneously active C fibers in the L4 spinal nerve also increased following an L5 ventral rhizotomy (Wu et al. 2002). In the same study, paw-withdrawal thresholds to mechanical stimuli were significantly correlated with the incidence of spontaneously active, high-threshold C-fiber afferents. Similar to the finding in the SNL model, spontaneous activity was abolished by lidocaine injection into the peripheral receptive field, suggesting that it was generated in peripheral cutaneous terminals (Wu et al. 2002). An increased incidence of spontaneous activity also occurs in uninjured Aδ and C fibers of the infraorbital nerve following transection of the inferior alveolar nerve (Tsuboi et al. 2004).

Enhanced chemosensitivity in nociceptors. Adrenergic sensitivity develops in uninjured nociceptive afferents after partial peripheral nerve injury or surgical sympathectomy (Sato and Perl 1991; Bossut et al. 1996) and following SNL (Ali et al. 1999; Nam et al. 2000). The development of adrenergic sensitivity by nociceptors may explain the pain evoked by norepinephrine that develops in patients with SMP, as discussed above. After an L5 SNL, L4 nociceptive afferents also show an increased sensitivity to tumor necrosis factor-alpha (TNF-α) (Schäfers et al. 2003).

Sensitization of nociceptors to natural stimuli. Whether nerve lesions result in sensitization of uninjured nociceptive afferents to mechanical and thermal stimuli is not clear. Following CCI of the saphenous nerve in rat, cutaneous unmyelinated afferents showed a nonsignificant increase in response to heat (Koltzenburg et al. 1994). In primates, unmyelinated nociceptive afferents did not exhibit a lower mechanical threshold following spinal nerve injury (Ali et al. 1999). In contrast, a recent study in rats with SNL found sensitization of uninjured nociceptive C fibers to both heat and mechanical stimuli (Shim et al. 2005). In addition, an increased percentage of uninjured L4 DRG neurons were cold-responsive; this increase could account for the cold allodynia observed in the SNL model (Djouhri et al. 2004).

Nerve injury also induces changes in receptive properties of uninjured myelinated mechanoreceptive afferents. Following lumbar SNL, "modified rapidly adapting" mechanoreceptors have been described that are characterized by an onset and offset response typical for rapidly adapting mechanoreceptors but with neuronal activity during sustained mechanical stimulation (Na et al. 1993). In an inferior alveolar nerve transection model in the rat, uninjured myelinated afferents in the infraorbital nerve showed an increased response to mechanical stimuli (Tsuboi et al. 2004). In contrast, mechanical responses in unmyelinated afferents were not affected.

Altered conductive properties of uninjured C fibers. Partial nerve injury changes the conductive properties of adjacent, uninjured afferents. As mentioned above, under normal conditions, repeated electrical stimulation of C fibers leads to a slowing of conduction. Following SNL, this activity-dependent slowing of conduction is enhanced in uninjured fibers, both myelinated (Shin et al. 1997) and unmyelinated (Shim et al. 2003), similar to the findings reported in patients with erythromelalgia, as described above.

The sensitivity of uninjured C fibers to tetrodotoxin (TTX) also changes after nerve injury (Gold et al. 2003). After an L5 SNL, about 40% of the C-fiber component of the compound action potential of the sciatic nerve (normally blocked by TTX) becomes resistant to TTX, apparently because of increased expression of the sodium channel isoform $Na_V1.8$ in the sciatic nerve (Gold et al. 2003). Treatment with antisense oligonucleotides against $Na_V1.8$ prevented the redistribution of this channel and reversed neuropathic pain behavior. While several studies found no increase in $Na_V1.8$ mRNA or in the density of TTX-resistant currents in uninjured L4 DRG neurons (Decosterd et al. 2002; Gold et al. 2003), Zhang and colleagues (2004) did report such an increase. The discrepancy may be due to different experimental conditions, such as the varying length of time for which neurons were cultured before being studied.

ELECTROPHYSIOLOGICAL FINDINGS IN MODELS OF DIABETIC AND NEUROTOXIC NEUROPATHIES

Diabetic or neurotoxic neuropathies are systemic neuropathies, and therefore a distinction between injured and uninjured afferents is difficult. However, it cannot be excluded a priori that some of the reported changes in peripheral nerve fibers are due to secondary events related to the degeneration of neighboring nerve fibers affected by the primary insult. Regardless, primary afferent nociceptors appear to become sensitized following peripheral nerve damage.

Within a few days of receiving intraperitoneal injection of streptozotocin (STZ), which kills pancreatic beta cells, animals develop diabetes as well as signs of neuropathic pain such as mechanical hyperalgesia (Ahlgren and Levine 1993). In STZ-treated animals, unmyelinated C-fiber afferents become spontaneously active (Chen and Levine 2001, 2003; Khan et al. 2002; Suzuki et al. 2002), but the reported incidences range widely (15–70%). C fibers from diabetic animals did not exhibit lowered mechanical thresholds when tested with von Frey hairs (Chen and Levine 2001, 2003), but they did show a decreased threshold in response to a step stimulus applied with an automated mechanical stimulator (Suzuki et al. 2002). However, responses to suprathreshold mechanical stimuli were enhanced in each of these studies, demonstrating that C-fiber afferents in diabetic animals are sensitized to mechanical stimuli.

In vincristine-induced peripheral neuropathy, the incidence of unmyelinated nociceptive afferents with spontaneous activity did not increase, and mechanical thresholds did not decrease, but the response to suprathreshold mechanical stimuli was again increased (Tanner et al. 1998, 2003).

CHANGES IN PROTEIN EXPRESSION IN UNINJURED NEURONS

Uninjured neurons show multiple changes in their protein expression following injury to neighboring nerve fibers. Changes in expression have been found for proteins involved in axonal conduction as well as proteins released during synaptic transmission from the central terminal and proteins involved in signal transduction at the peripheral terminal.

Following CCI or a partial transection of the sciatic nerve, spared neurons in the L4 and L5 DRG showed an increase in preprotachykinin mRNA and substance P immunoreactivity (Ma and Bisby 1998). After L5 SNL, L4 neurons exhibited an increased immunoreactivity for calcitonin gene-related peptide (CGRP) mRNA, and their content of neurotrophic growth factor (NGF) and brain-derived neurotrophic factor (BDNF) increased (Fukuoka et al. 1998, 2000, 2001). Both growth factors are also upregulated in L5 DRG neurons following L5 ventral rhizotomy and in L4 DRG neurons following L5 ganglionectomy (Obata et al. 2004). Spinal nerve injury also results in upregulation of mRNA and protein for TRPV1 (Fukuoka et al. 2000; Hudson et al. 2001); this upregulation may underlie the observed heat hyperalgesia in this model. In the spared nerve injury model, uninjured neurons show an upregulation of purinergic $P2X_3$ mRNA (Tsuzuki et al. 2001).

PERIPHERALLY ACTING DRUGS REVERSE NEUROPATHIC PAIN BEHAVIOR

Additional evidence for a role of primary afferent nociceptors in neuropathic pain comes from animal studies in which peripherally acting drugs attenuate the neuropathic behavior. Studies that demonstrate attenuation of neuropathic behavior following local drug application into the hypersensitive area provide another line of evidence for a role of primary afferents in neuropathic pain. For example, local application of a T-type calcium channel blocker or a glutamate receptor antagonist reversed mechanical and thermal hypersensitivity after SNL (Dogrul et al. 2000, 2003). In these studies, injections of the drugs in the contralateral hindpaw were without effect. Reversal of neuropathic pain behavior following application of a drug whose target receptor is only expressed in the periphery further suggests involvement of primary afferents. For example, the cannabinoid receptor 2 (CB2) is not expressed in the central nervous system (CNS), and systemic administration of AM1241, a selective CB2 agonist, reversed signs of mechanical and thermal hyperalgesia (Ibrahim et al. 2003). AM1241 releases endogenous beta-endorphins from keratinocytes, which then act on μ-opioid receptors expressed on terminals of primary afferent nociceptors (Ibrahim et al. 2005).

Peripherally acting opioids reverse neuropathic pain symptoms. Opioid receptors are expressed in the peripheral terminals of unmyelinated primary afferent fibers. Inflammation increases the number of peripheral opioid receptors and disrupts the perineural barrier that facilitates the access of opioid agonists. A number of studies suggest that peripherally acting opioids provide pain relief in inflamed tissue (Stein et al. 2003). Recent studies suggest that peripherally acting opioids attenuate neuropathic pain. For example, systemic administration of the peripherally acting opioid agonist loperamide reversed neuropathic behavior following an SNL lesion (Johanek et al. 2005). In addition, the analgesia produced by systemic administration of morphine following an SNL or CCI lesion was significantly attenuated by intraplantar injection of a peripherally acting opioid receptor antagonist (Kayser et al. 1995; Pertovaara et al. 2001). These studies point to a role of the peripheral nociceptor terminal in neuropathic pain.

Artemin reverses neuropathic pain symptoms. The members of the glial-derived neurotrophic factor (GDNF) family signal through a common tyrosine kinase receptor known as Ret and through a GDNF-family receptor (GFR)-α accessory protein. One of these accessory proteins, GFR-α3, which is predominantly expressed in nociceptive primary afferent neurons (Orozco et al. 2001), preferentially binds a member of the GDNF family called artemin (also known as neublastin). Systemic administration of artemin dose-dependently reversed the behavioral signs of neuropathic pain in rats with an SNL injury (Gardell et al. 2003). In addition, artemin normalized many of the morphological and neurochemical features of small neurons in the L5 DRG that have been observed following SNL. For example, the SNL-induced decrease in isolectin IB4 binding, the decreased expression of P2X3 and CGRP, and the increased expression of galanin and neuropeptide Y in the L5 DRG neurons was normalized following artemin treatment. Whether the observed reversal of neuropathic behavior is due to effects on the injured L5 DRG or on uninjured neurons from the L4 DRG is not known. Regardless, these results point to a role for unmyelinated fibers in neuropathic pain.

POTENTIAL MECHANISMS TO EXPLAIN THE ALTERATIONS IN UNINJURED AFFERENTS

In injured neurons, the accumulation of proteins involved in signal transduction and action potential propagation at the site of injury can account for the manifestation of spontaneous activity and ectopic mechanical, thermal, and chemical sensitivity. Obviously, such a mechanism cannot account for the sensitization seen in uninjured nerve fibers. Development of spontaneous activity and sensitization to natural stimuli in uninjured nerve fibers may, however, be due to the inflammatory mediators generated during Wallerian degeneration. Indeed, signs of neuropathic pain are reduced in animals in which Wallerian degeneration is delayed or diminished (Myers et al. 1996; Ramer et al. 1997; Wagner et al. 1998; Liu et al. 2000). Processes related to Wallerian degeneration are likely to be involved in neuropathic pain after partial peripheral nerve injuries that result in an anatomical arrangement in which injured and uninjured afferents commingle in peripheral nerves. Most animal nerve injury models including CCI, SNL, partial sciatic nerve liga-tion, and ventral and dorsal rhizotomy result in such an arrangement. A multitude of different mediators are generated during Wallerian degenera-tion, including an array of different cytokines and growth factors (for re-view, see Stoll and Muller 1999; Shamash et al. 2002; Stoll et al. 2002). Studies have shown that some of these agents, including TNF-α and NGF, have an excitatory or sensitizing effect on nociceptive afferents (Andreev et al. 1995; Rueff and Mendell 1996; Sorkin et al. 1997; Junger and Sorkin 2000; Zhang et al. 2002), and local injection of these agents causes signs of hyperalgesia in normal animals (Cunha et al. 1992; Andreev et al. 1995).

In partial nerve injury models, commingling of injured and uninjured fibers occurs not only along the course of the peripheral nerve but also in the peripheral target tissue. For example, the peripheral innervation territo-ries of spinal nerves L4 and L5 are partially overlapping (Takahashi et al. 1996), and therefore L5 SNL will lead to a zone of partially denervated skin. In response to denervation, mRNA levels for NGF were upregulated in the skin (Mearow et al. 1993). Moreover, anti-NGF treatment prevented collateral sprouting of uninjured nerve fibers into the denervated skin (Diamond et al. 1992). NGF sensitizes nociceptive afferents (Koltzenburg et al. 1999; Stucky et al. 1999), and an upregulation or excess of NGF in the remaining nerve fibers in partially denervated skin may lead to sensitization of uninjured nociceptors. In addition to NGF, other trophic factors in the skin may be in-volved in sensitization of uninjured afferents. These mechanisms could play a role in the spared nerve injury model (Decosterd and Woolf 2000), where no commingling of injured and uninjured fibers occurs in the peripheral nerve.

With the exception of the SNL model, peripheral nerve injuries may lead to an interaction between injured and uninjured afferent neurons in the DRG. Evidence for this type of paracrine interaction came from a study that demonstrated the development of spontaneous activity in DRG neurons of uninjured, myelinated muscle afferents after complete transection of several peripheral nerves (Michaelis et al. 2000). The factors involved in this inter-action are currently unknown. A chemical interaction between DRG neurons has been suggested by authors who observed cross-depolarization and cross-excitation between neurons residing in the same DRG in normal and nerve-injured animals (Devor and Wall 1990; Amir and Devor 1996). This cross-excitation occurred between A-fiber neurons as well as between A- and C-fiber neurons (Amir and Devor 2000).

NEUROPATHIC THERAPIES TARGETING THE PERIPHERAL NERVOUS SYSTEM

Many therapies available for treatment of neuropathic pain target the CNS. However, side effects associated with these drugs often limit their usefulness. For example, a primary limiting factor in the use of systemic opioids, especially in the elderly, are their CNS side effects, including sedation and cognitive dysfunction. The evidence reviewed in this chapter makes it clear that peripheral sensitization is a factor in neuropathic pain and suggests that the peripheral nervous system is an appropriate target for therapeutic drug development. Drugs developed to target this peripheral site could minimize central side effects.

One way to target peripheral receptors is to use topical drugs. The lidocaine patch is an example (Galer et al. 2002). Topical capsaicin is another example, but the pain associated with its use makes patient compliance an issue. However, co-administration of a local anesthetic may circumvent this problem (Robbins et al. 1998).

Another way to target peripheral receptors is to develop agents that do not cross the blood-brain barrier. Loperamide is a peripherally acting opioid-receptor agonist that appears to be effective in animal models of neuropathic pain. Although it lacks the CNS effects of opioids, loperamide could still cause constipation. Asimadoline is a peripherally acting κ-opioid agonist that reduces pain in patients with irritable bowel syndrome without effecting gut motility (Delvaux et al. 2004). There is some evidence that asimadoline is effective in the CCI model of neuropathic pain (Walker et al. 1999).

In summary, peripheral sensitization of primary afferents appears to be an important mechanism in neuropathic pain. This understanding could have important implications in the development of improved management strategies for clinical neuropathic pain.

ACKNOWLEDGMENTS

We thank Drs. James N. Campbell, John W. Griffin, and Beth B. Murinson for helpful discussions. This research was supported by the National Institutes of Health (NS-14447, NS-41269).

REFERENCES

Ahlgren SC, Levine JD. Mechanical hyperalgesia in streptozotocin-diabetic rats. *Neuroscience* 1993; 52:1049–1055.

Ali Z, Ringkamp M, Hartke TV, et al. Uninjured C-fiber nociceptors develop spontaneous activity and alpha-adrenergic sensitivity following L6 spinal nerve ligation in the monkey. *J Neurophysiol* 1999; 81:455–466.

Ali Z, Raja SN, Wesselmann U, et al. Intradermal injection of norepinephrine evokes pain in patients with sympathetically maintained pain. *Pain* 2000; 88:161–168.

Amir R, Devor M. Chemically mediated cross-excitation in rat dorsal root ganglia. *J Neurosci* 1996; 16:4733–4741.

Amir R, Devor M. Functional cross-excitation between afferent A- and C-neurons in dorsal root ganglia. *Neuroscience* 2000; 95:189–195.

Andreev NY, Dimitrieva N, Koltzenburg M, McMahon SB. Peripheral administration of nerve growth factor in the adult rat produces a thermal hyperalgesia that requires the presence of sympathetic post-ganglionic neurones. *Pain* 1995; 63:109–115.

Bennett GJ, Xie Y-K. A peripheral mononeuropathy in rat that produces disorders of pain sensation like those seen in man. *Pain* 1988; 33:87–107.

Bossut DF, Shea VK, Perl ER. Sympathectomy induces adrenergic excitability of cutaneous C-fiber nociceptors. *J Neurophysiol* 1996; 75:514–517.

Boucher TJ, Okuse K, Bennett DL, et al. Potent analgesic effects of GDNF in neuropathic pain states. *Science* 2000; 290:124–127.

Chen X, Levine JD. Hyper-responsivity in a subset of C-fiber nociceptors in a model of painful diabetic neuropathy in the rat. *Neuroscience* 2001; 102:185–192.

Chen X, Levine JD. Altered temporal pattern of mechanically evoked C-fiber activity in a model of diabetic neuropathy in the rat. *Neuroscience* 2003; 121:1007–1015.

Colburn RW, Rickman AJ, DeLeo JA. The effect of site and type of nerve injury on spinal glial activation and neuropathic pain behavior. *Exp Neurol* 1999; 157:289–304.

Cook AJ, Woolf CJ, Wall PD, McMahon SB. Dynamic receptive field plasticity in rat spinal cord dorsal horn following C-primary afferent input. *Nature* 1987; 325:151–153.

Cunha FQ, Poole S, Lorenzetti BB, Ferreira SH. The pivotal role of tumour necrosis factor a in the development of inflammatory hyperalgesia. *Br J Pharmacol* 1992; 107:660–664.

Davis KD, Treede R-D, Raja SN, Meyer RA, Campbell JN. Topical application of clonidine relieves hyperalgesia in patients with sympathetically maintained pain. *Pain* 1991; 47:309–317.

Decosterd I, Woolf CJ. Spared nerve injury: an animal model of persistent peripheral neuropathic pain. *Pain* 2000; 87:149–158.

Decosterd I, Ji RR, Abdi S, Tate S, Woolf CJ. The pattern of expression of the voltage-gated sodium channels Na(v)1.8 and Na(v)1.9 does not change in uninjured primary sensory neurons in experimental neuropathic pain models. *Pain* 2002; 96:269–277.

Delvaux M, Beck A, Jacob J, et al. Effect of asimadoline, a kappa opioid agonist, on pain induced by colonic distension in patients with irritable bowel syndrome. *Aliment Pharmacol Ther* 2004; 20:237–246.

Devor M, Seltzer Z. Pathophysiology of damaged nerves in relation to chronic pain. In: Wall PD, Melzack R (Eds). *Textbook of Pain*. London: Churchill Livingstone, 1999, pp 129–164.

Devor M, Wall PD. Cross-excitation in dorsal root ganglia of nerve-injured and intact rats. *J Neurophysiol* 1990; 64:1733–1746.

Diamond J, Holmes M, Coughlin M. Endogenous NGF and nerve impulses regulate the collateral sprouting of sensory axons in the skin of the adult rat. *J Neurosci* 1992; 12:1454–1466.

Djouhri L, Wrigley D, Thut PD, Gold MS. Spinal nerve injury increases the percentage of cold-responsive DRG neurons. *Neuroreport* 2004; 15:457–460.

Dogrul A, Ossipov MH, Lai J, Malan TP Jr, Porreca F. Peripheral and spinal antihyperalgesic activity of SIB-1757, a metabotropic glutamate receptor (mGLUR$_5$) antagonist, in experimental neuropathic pain in rats. *Neurosci Lett* 2000; 292:115–118.

Dogrul A, Gardell LR, Ossipov MH, et al. Reversal of experimental neuropathic pain by T-type calcium channel blockers. *Pain* 2003; 105:159–168.

Ellison N, Loprinzi CL, Kugler J, et al. Phase III placebo-controlled trial of capsaicin cream in the management of surgical neuropathic pain in cancer patients. *J Clin Oncol* 1997; 15:2974–2980.

Eschenfelder S, Häbler H-J, Jänig W. Dorsal root section elicits signs of neuropathic pain rather than reversing them in rats with L5 spinal nerve injury. *Pain* 2000; 87:213–219.

Fields HL, Rowbotham M, Baron R. Postherpetic neuralgia: irritable nociceptors and deafferentation. *Neurobiol Dis* 1998; 5:209–227.

Fukuoka T, Tokunaga A, Kondo E, et al. Change in mRNAs for neuropeptides and the $GABA_A$ receptor in dorsal root ganglion neurons in a rat experimental neuropathic pain model. *Pain* 1998; 78:13–26.

Fukuoka T, Tokunaga A, Kondo E, Noguchi K. The role of neighboring intact dorsal root ganglion neurons in a rat neuropathic pain model. In: Devor M, Rowbotham R, Wiesenfeld-Hallin Z (Eds). *Proceedings of the 9th World Congress on Pain, Progress in Pain Research and Management*, Vol. 16. Seattle: IASP Press, 2000, pp 137–146.

Fukuoka T, Kondo E, Dai Y, Hashimoto N, Noguchi K. Brain-derived neurotrophic factor increases in the uninjured dorsal root ganglion neurons in selective spinal nerve ligation model. *J Neurosci* 2001; 21:4891–4900.

Galer BS, Jensen MP, Ma T, Davies PS, Rowbotham MC. The lidocaine patch 5% effectively treats all neuropathic pain qualities: results of a randomized, double-blind, vehicle-controlled, 3-week efficacy study with use of the neuropathic pain scale. *Clin J Pain* 2002; 18:297–301.

Gardell LR, Wang R, Ehrenfels C, et al. Multiple actions of systemic artemin in experimental neuropathy. *Nat Med* 2003; 9:1383–1389.

Gold MS, Weinreich D, Kim CS, et al. Redistribution of $Na_V1.8$ in uninjured axons enables neuropathic pain. *J Neurosci* 2003; 23:158–166.

Hannington-Kiff JG. Intravenous regional sympathetic block with guanethidine. *Lancet* 1974; i:1019–1020.

Hudson LJ, Bevan S, Wotherspoon G, et al. VR1 protein expression increases in undamaged DRG neurons after partial nerve injury. *Eur J Neurosci* 2001; 13:2105–2114.

Ibrahim MM, Deng H, Zvonok A, et al. Activation of CB2 cannabinoid receptors by AM1241 inhibits experimental neuropathic pain: pain inhibition by receptors not present in the CNS. *Proc Natl Acad Sci USA* 2003; 100:10529–10533.

Ibrahim MM, Porreca F, Lai J, et al. CB2 cannabinoid receptor activation produces antinociception by stimulating peripheral release of endogenous opioids. *Proc Natl Acad Sci USA* 2005; 102:3093–3098.

Johanek LM, Shim B, Horasek SJ, et al. Loperamide, a peripherally acting opioid agonist, reverses hyperalgesia induced by spinal nerve ligation in rat. *Abstracts: 11th World Congress on Pain*. Seattle: IASP Press, 2005, p 40.

Junger H, Sorkin LS. Nociceptive and inflammatory effects of subcutaneous TNF-alpha. *Pain* 2000; 85:145–151.

Kayser V, Lee SH, Guilbaud G. Evidence for a peripheral component in the enhanced antinociceptive effect of a low dose of systemic morphine in rats with peripheral mononeuropathy. *Neuroscience* 1995; 64:537–545.

Khan GM, Chen SR, Pan H-L. Role of primary afferent nerves in allodynia caused by diabetic neuropathy in rats. *Neuroscience* 2002; 114:291–299.

Kim SH, Chung JM. An experimental model for peripheral neuropathy produced by segmental spinal nerve ligation in the rat. *Pain* 1992; 50:355–363.

Koltzenburg M, Kees S, Budweiser S, Ochs G, Toyka KV. The properties of unmyelinated nociceptive afferents change in a painful chronic constriction neuropathy. In: Gebhart GF, Hammond DL, Jensen TS (Eds). *Proceedings of the 7th World Congress on Pain, Progress in Pain Research and Management*, Vol. 2. Seattle: IASP Press, 1994, pp 511–522.

Koltzenburg M, Bennett DL, Shelton DL, McMahon SB. Neutralization of endogenous NGF prevents the sensitization of nociceptors supplying inflamed skin. *Eur J Neurosci* 1999; 11:1698–1704.

Li Y, Dorsi MJ, Meyer RA, Belzberg AJ. Mechanical hyperalgesia after an L5 spinal nerve lesion in the rat is not dependent on input from injured nerve fibers. *Pain* 2000; 85:493–502.

Li L, Xian CJ, Zhong JH, Zhou XF. Effect of lumbar 5 ventral root transection on pain behaviors: a novel rat model for neuropathic pain without axotomy of primary sensory neurons. *Exp Neurol* 2002; 175:23–34.

Liu T, van Rooijen N, Tracey DJ. Depletion of macrophages reduces axonal degeneration and hyperalgesia following nerve injury. *Pain* 2000; 86:25–32.

Ma W, Bisby MA. Increase of preprotachykinin mRNA and substance P immunoreactivity in spared dorsal root ganglion neurons following partial sciatic nerve injury. *Eur J Neurosci* 1998; 10:2388–2399.

Mearow KM, Kril Y, Diamond J. Increased NGF mRNA expression in denervated rat skin. *Neuroreport* 1993; 4:351–354.

Michaelis M, Liu X, Jänig W. Axotomized and intact muscle afferents but not skin afferents develop ongoing discharges of dorsal root ganglion origin after peripheral nerve lesion. *J Neurosci* 2000; 20:2742–2748.

Murinson BB, Archer DR, Li Y, Griffin JW. Degeneration of myelinated efferent fibers prompts mitosis in Remak Schwann cells of uninjured C-fiber afferents. *J Neurosci* 2005; 25:1179–1187.

Myers RR, Heckman HM, Rodriguez M. Reduced hyperalgesia in nerve-injured WLD mice: relationship to nerve fiber phagocytosis, axonal degeneration, and regeneration in normal mice. *Exp Neurol* 1996; 141:94–101.

Na HS, Leem JW, Chung JM. Abnormalities of mechanoreceptors in a rat model of neuropathic pain: possible involvement in mediating mechanical allodynia. *J Neurophysiol* 1993; 70:522–528.

Nam TS, Yeon DS, Leem JW, Paik KS. Adrenergic sensitivity of uninjured C-fiber nociceptors in neuropathic rats. *Yonsei Med J* 2000; 41:252–257.

Nolano M, Simone DA, Wendelschafer-Crabb G, et al. Topical capsaicin in humans: parallel loss of epidermal nerve fibers and pain sensation. *Pain* 1999; 81:135–145.

Obata K, Yamanaka H, Dai Y, et al. Contribution of degeneration of motor and sensory fibers to pain behavior and the changes in neurotrophic factors in rat dorsal root ganglion. *Exp Neurol* 2004; 188:149–160.

Orozco OE, Walus L, Sah DW, Pepinsky RB, Sanicola M. GFR-alpha-3 is expressed predominantly in nociceptive sensory neurons. *Eur J Neurosci* 2001; 13:2177–2182.

Ørstavik K, Weidner C, Schmidt R, et al. Pathological C-fibres in patients with a chronic painful condition. *Brain* 2003; 126:567–578.

Ørstavik K, Mork C, Kvernebo K, Jorum E. Pain in primary erythromelalgia—a neuropathic component? *Pain* 2004; 110:531–538.

Pertovaara A, Wei H. Peripheral effects of morphine in neuropathic rats: role of sympathetic postganglionic nerve fibers. *Eur J Pharmacol* 2001; 429:139–145.

Raja SN, Treede R-D, Davis KD, Campbell JN. Systemic alpha-adrenergic blockade with phentolamine: a diagnostic test for sympathetically maintained pain. *Anesthesiology* 1991; 74:691–698.

Ramer MS, French GD, Bisby MA. Wallerian degeneration is required for both neuropathic pain and sympathetic sprouting into the DRG. *Pain* 1997; 72:71–78.

Robbins WR, Staats PS, Levine J, et al. Treatment of intractable pain with topical large-dose capsaicin: preliminary report. *Anesth Analg* 1998; 86:579–583.

Rowbotham MC, Fields HL. Post-herpetic neuralgia: the relation of pain complaint, sensory disturbance, and skin temperature. *Pain* 1989; 39:129–144.

Rowbotham MC, Davies PS, Verkempinck C, Galer BS. Lidocaine patch: double-blind controlled study of a new treatment method for post-herpetic neuralgia. *Pain* 1996; 65:39–44.

Rueff A, Mendell LM. Nerve growth factor and NT-5 induce increased thermal sensitivity of cutaneous nociceptors in vitro. *J Neurophysiol* 1996; 76:3593–3596.

Sato J, Perl ER. Adrenergic excitation of cutaneous pain receptors induced by peripheral nerve injury. *Science* 1991; 251:1608–1610.

Schäfers M, Lee DH, Brors D, Yaksh TL, Sorkin LS. Increased sensitivity of injured and adjacent uninjured rat primary sensory neurons to exogenous tumor necrosis factor-alpha after spinal nerve ligation. *J Neurosci* 2003; 23:3028–3038.

Seltzer Z, Dubner R, Shir Y. A novel behavioral model of neuropathic pain disorders produced in rats by partial sciatic nerve injury. *Pain* 1990; 43:205–218.

Shamash S, Reichert F, Rotshenker S. The cytokine network of Wallerian degeneration: tumor necrosis factor-alpha, interleukin-1a, and interleukin-1b. *J Neurosci* 2002; 22:3052–3060.

Sheen K, Chung JM. Signs of neuropathic pain depend on signals from injured nerve fibers in a rat model. *Brain Res* 1993; 610:62–68.

Sheth RN, Dorsi MJ, Li Y, et al. Mechanical hyperalgesia after an L5 ventral rhizotomy or an L5 ganglionectomy in the rat. *Pain* 2002; 96:63–72.

Shim B, Ringkamp M, Hartke TV, Griffin JW, Meyer RA. Enhanced activity-dependent slowing of conduction in uninjured L4 C-fibers following an L5 spinal nerve injury in rat. *Soc Neurosci Abstracts* 2003; 29:262.12.

Shim B, Kim DW, Kim BII, et al. Mechanical and heat sensitization of cutaneous nociceptors in rats with experimental peripheral neuropathy. *Neuroscience* 2005; 132:193–201.

Shin H-C, Oh S-J, Jung S-C, et al. Activity-dependent conduction latency changes in A-beta fibers of neuropathic rats. *Neuroreport* 1997; 8:2813–2816.

Sorkin LS, Xiao W-H, Wagner R, Myers RR. Tumour necrosis factor-a induces ectopic activity in nociceptive primary afferent fibres. *Neuroscience* 1997; 81:255–262.

Stein C, Schafer M, Machelska H. Attacking pain at its source: new perspectives on opioids. *Nat Med* 2003; 9:1003–1008.

Stoll G, Muller HW. Nerve injury, axonal degeneration and neural regeneration: basic insights. *Brain Pathol* 1999; 9:313–325.

Stoll G, Jander S, Myers RR. Degeneration and regeneration of the peripheral nervous system: from Augustus Waller's observations to neuroinflammation. *J Peripher Nerv Syst* 2002; 7:13–27.

Stucky CL, Koltzenburg M, Schneider M, et al. Overexpression of nerve growth factor in skin selectively affects the survival and functional properties of nociceptors. *J Neurosci* 1999; 19:8509–8516.

Suzuki Y, Sato J, Kawanishi M, Mizumura K. Lowered response threshold and increased responsiveness to mechanical stimulation of cutaneous nociceptive fibers in streptozotocin-diabetic rat skin in vitro—correlates of mechanical allodynia and hyperalgesia observed in the early stage of diabetes. *Neurosci Res* 2002; 43:171–178.

Takahashi Y, Nakajima Y. Dermatomes in the rat limbs as determined by antidromic stimulation of sensory C-fibers in spinal nerves. *Pain* 1996; 67:197–202.

Tanner KD, Reichling DB, Levine JD. Nociceptor hyper-responsiveness during vincristine-induced painful peripheral neuropathy in the rat. *J Neurosci* 1998; 18:6480–6491.

Tanner KD, Reichling DB, Gear RW, Paul SM, Levine JD. Altered temporal pattern of evoked afferent activity in a rat model of vincristine-induced painful peripheral neuropathy. *Neuroscience* 2003; 118:809–817.

Torebjörk E, Wahren LK, Wallin G, Hallin R, Koltzenburg M. Noradrenaline-evoked pain in neuralgia. *Pain* 1995; 63:11–20.

Tsuboi Y, Takeda M, Tanimoto T, et al. Alteration of the second branch of the trigeminal nerve activity following inferior alveolar nerve transection in rats. *Pain* 2004; 111:323–334.

Tsuzuki K, Kondo E, Fukuoka T, et al. Differential regulation of $P2X_3$ mRNA expression by peripheral nerve injury in intact and injured neurons in the rat sensory ganglia. *Pain* 2001; 91:351–360.

Wagner R, Heckman HM, Myers RR. Wallerian degeneration and hyperalgesia after peripheral nerve injury are glutathione-dependent. *Pain* 1998; 77:173–179.

Walker J, Catheline G, Guilbaud G, Kayser V. Lack of cross-tolerance between the antinociceptive effects of systemic morphine and asimadoline, a peripherally-selective kappa-opioid agonist, in CCI-neuropathic rats. *Pain* 1999; 83:509–516.

Wall PD, Gutnick M. Ongoing activity in peripheral nerves: the physiology and pharmacology of impulses originating from a neuroma. *Exp Neurol* 1974; 43:580–593.

Watson CP. Topical capsaicin as an adjuvant analgesic. *J Pain Symptom Manage* 1994; 9:425–433.

Wu G, Ringkamp M, Hartke TV, et al. Early onset of spontaneous activity in uninjured C-fiber nociceptors after injury to neighboring nerve fibers. *J Neurosci* 2001; 21:RC140.

Wu G, Ringkamp M, Murinson BB, et al. Degeneration of myelinated efferent fibers induces spontaneous activity in uninjured C-fiber afferents. *J Neurosci* 2002; 22:7746–7753.

Yoon YW, Na HS, Chung JM. Contributions of injured and intact afferents to neuropathic pain in an experimental rat model. *Pain* 1996; 64:27–36.

Zhang J-M, Li H, Liu B, Brull SJ. Acute topical application of tumor necrosis factor alpha evokes protein kinase A-dependent responses in rat sensory neurons. *J Neurophysiol* 2002; 88:1387–1392.

Zhang XF, Zhu CZ, Thimmapaya R, et al. Differential action potentials and firing patterns in injured and uninjured small dorsal root ganglion neurons after nerve injury. *Brain Res* 2004; 1009:147–158.

Correspondence to: Matthias Ringkamp, MD, Department of Neurosurgery, Johns Hopkins University, Meyer 5-109, 600 N. Wolfe Street, Baltimore, MD 21287, USA. Tel: 410-955-2250; Fax: 410-955-1032; email: platelet@jhmi.edu.

Part II

Central Nervous System Targets

Emerging Strategies for the Treatment of Neuropathic Pain, edited by James N. Campbell, Allan I. Basbaum, André Dray, Ronald Dubner, Robert H. Dworkin, and Christine N. Sang, IASP Press, Seattle, © 2006.

5

Central Nervous System Targets: Rapporteur Report

William D. Willis, Jr.,[a] Donna L. Hammond,[b] Ronald Dubner,[c] Michael Merzenich,[d] James C. Eisenach,[e] Michael W. Salter,[f] Smriti Iyengar,[g] and Toni Shippenberg[h]

[a]Department of Neuroscience and Cell Biology, University of Texas Medical Branch, Galveston, Texas, USA; [b]Department of Anesthesia, The University of Iowa, Iowa City, Iowa, USA; [c]Department of Biomedical Sciences, University of Maryland Dental School, Baltimore, Maryland, USA; [d]Department of Otolaryngology, University of California San Francisco, San Francisco, California, USA; [e]Department of Anesthesia, Wake Forest University School of Medicine, Winston Salem, North Carolina, USA; [f]The Hospital for Sick Children, Toronto, Ontario, Canada; [g]Neuroscience Research, Lilly Research Laboratories, Eli Lilly and Company, Indianapolis, Indiana, USA; [h]Integrative Neuroscience Section, National Institute of Drug Abuse, National Institutes of Health, Bethesda, Maryland, USA

This chapter is based on the consensus of our group colloquium regarding the role of the central nervous system (CNS) in neuropathic pain. The first step was to identify a series of relevant major topics for discussion and sets of specific questions that were suggested by these topics. The discussions that ensued were focused on CNS mechanisms that contribute to neuropathic pain and on how to develop novel pharmacological and behavioral approaches to improve therapies for neuropathic pain, based on our understanding of these mechanisms. Finally, for each topic, the group proposed research questions that should be addressed for a more complete understanding of the mechanisms of neuropathic pain.

CENTRAL SENSITIZATION

DISCUSSION QUESTIONS

1) What do we mean by "central sensitization"; how is this term used? Clinical scientists and basic scientists seem to use it differently. Are there clinical tools that help us recognize the contribution of central sensitization to human neuropathic pain?

Clinicians and many basic scientists consider central sensitization to refer to all the changes in the CNS that can contribute to the hyperexcitability that occurs after tissue or nerve injury. Such changes would include alterations in the sensitivity or synaptic strength of the N-methyl-D-aspartate (NMDA) receptor, activation of neurokinin-1 (NK1) or metabotropic glutamate receptors, reduced activation of inhibitory GABAergic receptors, effects of proinflammatory cytokines such as tumor necrosis factor (TNF) α, interleukin (IL)-1β, or IL-6, the effects of anti-inflammatory cytokines such as IL-10, the role of glial-neuronal interactions, and the activation of eicosanoids.

Some define central sensitization in a more narrow sense as a form of activity-dependent plasticity that depends in large part on activation of NMDA receptors. Activity-dependent plasticity also involves activation of protein kinases secondary to an increased intracellular calcium concentration, leading to the phosphorylation of NMDA-receptor subunits and possibly of other glutamate and nonglutamate receptors that are anchored to the postsynaptic density of synapses on central nociceptive neurons. The most important aspect of these mechanisms of hypersensitivity is that the increased sensitivity of these receptors outlasts the period of the afferent barrage, thus differentiating central sensitization from temporal summation of neuronal responses to C-fiber input, known as "wind-up." To support this narrow definition, clinical studies would need to demonstrate that central sensitization in patients outlasts the afferent barrage and ascertain whether NMDA receptors are involved. For example, as a first step, it would be useful to use NMDA-receptor antagonists such as dextromethorphan or ketamine to determine whether CNS hyper-responsiveness in patients with neuropathic pain is NMDA-dependent.

2) Does central sensitization always depend upon ongoing primary afferent input, or are there changes in the nervous system over time that lead to an absence of dependence on primary afferent barrage?

Some members of our group consider that the available data indicate that many, if not all, instances of central sensitization can be shown to be dependent upon ongoing primary afferent input. Examples include long-standing cases of arthritis in which chronically inflamed tissues were removed and replaced, following which the preexisting pain disappeared. Others argue that these are instances of an intact nociceptive system that may not be relevant to cases of peripheral neuropathies in which there is damage to the nociceptive pathway. The evidence in instances of peripheral neuropathies is not as strong, according to most of the clinical scientists in our group, who indicate that "peripheral input dependence" is based on studies with small numbers of patients. There are now examples of the generation and maintenance of central sensitization that involve activation of pro-inflammatory cytokines and eicosanoid pathways in the CNS in which central sensitization is produced by mechanisms that do not necessarily involve activation or changes in the excitability of primary afferents, and although good evidence is lacking, these examples of central sensitization are unlikely to be maintained by the peripheral neuronal barrage. Thus, additional studies are needed before it can be concluded that all peripheral neuropathic pain is dependent on continued primary afferent input.

3) Does central sensitization after nerve injury differ from central sensitization produced by tissue injury?

Although few data are available that demonstrate differences in cellular and molecular mechanisms that account for central sensitization after nerve injury as compared to tissue injury, evidence is emerging that activated microglia in the spinal dorsal horn lead to mechanisms of central sensitization that are different from those that occur after tissue injury. Additional studies are needed in this area.

4) Is there central sensitization in higher centers of the central nervous system than the spinal cord dorsal horn? Are there parallel processes for activity-dependent plasticity in the spinal cord, thalamus, cerebral cortex, hippocampus, and other parts of the CNS?

Neuronal plasticity in nociceptive pathways occurs at multiple levels of the CNS. The mechanisms of activity-dependent plasticity at these sites are similar, but not necessarily the same. For example, the initiation of NMDA-dependent central sensitization in the spinal cord involves the activation of metabotropic glutamate receptors, but these receptors do not appear to be involved in the NMDA-dependent plasticity seen at the level of the rostral ventromedial medulla. Also, changes in phosphorylation of the NR2 subunit of the NMDA receptor at the spinal level involve the NR2B subunit but not the NR2A subunit. These changes are quite similar to the cellular and molecular signal transduction mechanisms seen in the hippocampus, cerebral cortex, amygdala, and nucleus accumbens that have been reported in studies of mechanisms of learning and memory, mood, and reward. The sites of plasticity in nociceptive pathways may be nodes of convergence of relevant inputs related to the survival of the organism, and the transmitters, receptors, and second-messenger systems involved might be sites for drug discovery related to the suppression of pain. However, it is possible that the ubiquitous mechanisms working at these sites in many parts of the nervous system may preclude their selectivity and thus reduce their importance for drug discovery.

RESEARCH QUESTIONS

1) Are all peripheral neuropathies dependent on primary afferent input, and is there a temporal component to this dependence?

2) What triggers the conversion of central sensitization from a physiological process that is protective to a pathological process that outlasts the duration of the physical injury?

3) What methods can be developed to elucidate central sensitization's underlying mechanisms and to demonstrate its presence in patients?

4) How does central sensitization after nerve injury differ from that produced by other types of injury?

5) Do we accept that primary hyperalgesia and secondary hyperalgesia are mechanistically different, and do we treat these states independently in our discussions of their supraspinal mechanisms?

6) Should the treatment approach be dictated by the type of injury and the length of time after injury? For example, are CNS targets relevant in the time immediately after injury or only later on?

MECHANISMS OF PLASTICITY IN CENTRAL NEUROPATHIC PAIN

DISCUSSION QUESTION

1) How can we advance our understanding of the mechanisms that initiate and sustain neuropathic pain that is central in origin, such as post-stroke pain, syringomyelia, spinal cord injury, or multiple sclerosis?

Central pain remains largely resistant to therapeutic treatment. Particularly puzzling has been the occurrence of pain at regions below the level of spinal cord injury. Several rodent models of spinal cord injury have been developed and examined for their suitability for studies of central pain (Hao et al. 1991; Yezierski et al. 1998; Hulsebosch et al. 2000). Thus, the field is now better positioned to undertake the necessary studies. The development of below-level pain after spinal cord transaction requires damage to the dorsal horn gray matter, whereas lesions restricted to the white matter are without effect. The loss of inhibitory mechanisms and exacerbation of excitatory mechanisms in dorsal horn neurons at the level of the lesion could serve as a central generator of spontaneous or "ectopic" inputs to the thalamus. Furthermore, there is elegant work showing reorganization of both thalamic and cortical representations of the extremities after deafferentation, in which loss of the representation of the affected limb is coupled with an expansion of neighboring fields (Woods et al. 2000). Thus, central "deafferentation" may result in a similar reorganization of spinothalamic inputs at the level of the thalamus in which inputs from hyperexcitable dorsal horn neurons at the level of the lesion may expand to neighboring neurons in the thalamus and therefore give rise to pain below the lesion. However, it must be noted that this proposal is very different from the situation in which the new representation moves into a silent zone and is elaborated perceptually. The central pain example cited above is the opposite in that the old representation is enabled by the hypersensitivity of the new representation; both remain powerful.

There is a different result if the spinal nerves are ligated or cut. Jones and others studied monkeys with chronic denervation of the forelimbs for 13–21 years following cervical and upper thoracic dorsal rhizotomies. There were major changes in the organization of the somatosensory cortical map, as well as of the dorsal column and ventrobasal thalamic nuclei. The cortical representation of the face expanded into an area that would normally be occupied by the hand representation (Jones and Pons 1998). There was severe transneuronal atrophy of neurons in the cuneate, external cuneate, and ventrobasal nuclei (Woods et al. 2000). The reorganization of the dorsal column and ventrobasal nuclei might account for the change in cortical representation.

RESEARCH QUESTIONS

1) Anatomical mapping studies coupled with electrophysiological recordings are needed to demonstrate the reorganization of spinothalamic inputs to thalamic nuclei and of thalamic inputs to the cortex.

2) Does intrathecal or epidural administration of agents known to suppress dorsal horn neuron excitability, such as local anesthetics or opioid receptor agonists, reduce below-level pain? If these agents are effective, is there a temporal component to their ability to suppress below-level pain?

NEURONAL-GLIAL INTERACTIONS

DISCUSSION QUESTION

1) Is there a role for neuron-glial interactions in neuropathic pain?
For more than 25 years it has been known that injury to primary afferent

neurons causes activation of microglia in the spinal cord and fosters the recruitment of circulating monocytes (Ling 1979). Activation of microglia, and also of astrocytes, following peripheral nerve injury has been documented by numerous groups (for reviews see Watkins 2001, 2003; Tsuda et al. 2003). Acute pharmacological inhibition of purinergic P2X$_4$ receptors and of p38 mitogen-activated protein kinase, which are selectively expressed in activated microglia after nerve injury, reverses the decease in paw-withdrawal threshold after peripheral nerve injury. Moreover, intrathecal delivery of P2X$_4$-stimulated microglia to naive animals lowers the paw-withdrawal threshold to a level similar to that observed after nerve injury (Tsuda et al. 2003). Thus, these molecules, and by inference activated microglia themselves, are critical for maintaining mechanical allodynia. From these findings emerge a number of key questions, as outlined below.

RESEARCH QUESTIONS

1) What are the molecular mechanisms that lead to activation of microglia in the dorsal horn?

To a certain extent this question has been answered by recent work from DeLeo and colleagues, who have found that activation of microglia following nerve injury is markedly decreased in animals engineered to lack Toll-like receptor 4 (TLR4) or in animals in which expression of TLR4 in spinal microglia is depressed by antisense oligonucleotides against this receptor (Tanga et al. 2005). This finding then raises additional questions as to whether TLR4 is directly inline in the signaling pathway leading to microglial activation or whether TLR4 is merely permissive of this activation. If the former proposal is true, then we must determine what is activating TLR4. If the latter, then pathways gated by TLR4 need to be established.

2) Microglial activation after injury to dorsal roots by dorsal rhizotomy is markedly less than after injury to peripheral nerves. Can this differential effect be used to further elucidate the mechanism by which microglia are activated? Also, does microglial activation after peripheral nerve injury require action potential propagation in primary afferents into the spinal cord?

3) How do activated microglia signal to dorsal horn nociceptive transmission neurons? Microglial-neuronal signaling could conceivably increase excitatory synaptic transmission or suppress inhibitory transmission, either of which could occur either pre- or postsynaptically. Alternatively, or in addition, microglial-neuronal signaling could modify intrinsic membrane conductances in dorsal horn nociceptive neurons.

4) What is the role of the activation of microglia that occurs in the nucleus gracilis? Findings from Porreca and colleagues have pointed to this

nucleus as being critical for maintaining mechanical allodynia, dependent upon neuropeptide Y (see the chapter by Ossipov and Porreca in this volume). Are microglia in the nucleus gracilis involved in mediating or sustaining mechanical allodynia? Is there an interaction between activated microglia and neuropeptide Y-responsive gracile neurons?

5) What is the role, if any, of activated astrocytes in sustaining mechanical allodynia after nerve injury? This question arises from findings that activation of astrocytes in the dorsal horn, as judged by enhanced expression of the astrocyte-specific glial-fibrillary acidic protein, is increased after peripheral nerve injury. Is there signaling from astrocytes to neurons or microglia, or vice versa?

6) Do microglia change after a change in activity in the hypothalamic-pituitary axis?

7) More information is needed about the role of glia and other support cells and about their interactions with neurons at supraspinal levels. Studies are needed to investigate the role of glia in the initiation and maintenance of neuropathic pain in patients.

COMPETITION IN THE BRAIN

DISCUSSION QUESTIONS

1) Is there brain plasticity that parallels chronic pain?

The representation of chronic pain can sensitize, grow, strengthen, and elaborate over time in the brain. By "sensitize," we mean that formerly non-painful inputs can be perceived as painful. By "grow," we mean here that larger populations of neurons are engaged in parallel with ongoing pain or are activated when that pain is exacerbated by physical manipulation. As it "grows," pain can be evoked by electrical stimulation from more locations covering larger subcortical and cortical areas in the chronic pain patient. By "strengthen," we mean that the evoked responses of subcortical and cortical neuronal populations whose responses are associated with the pain or its context, as revealed in magnetic recording studies or in functional magnetic resonance imaging (fMRI) studies, progressively increase. By "elaborate," we mean that the pain can progressively change its qualities from simple to progressively more complex and longer episodic forms, and that the representations of innocuous inputs associated with and predicting pain are commonly progressively strengthened and elaborated. In its chronic phase, as in other models of learned prediction, pain is exaggerated and responses signaling pain are magnified when the individual predicts pain, even when that prediction is incorrect. In the same way, as in other models of learned prediction, the perception of pain is lessened and responses signaling pain are attenuated when the individual predicts no pain, even when that prediction is incorrect.

The sensitization, growth, strengthening, and elaboration of the distributed neurological representation of chronic pains can probably be attributed to brain plasticity processes. These dimensions of change all reflect a probable product of competitive processes in which pain-related or pain-evoked brain activities come to dominate the responses of neurons formerly dominated by nonpainful inputs. The central pain system is unique in the respect that at most levels, inputs from pain and non-pain sources are convergent. On the most basic level, we could regard pain sensation as reflecting the brain plasticity-based competition between pain-evoking and other (non-pain) inputs in a convergent brain system.

2) Is modulation of the activity-dependent plasticity that alters pain representations the same as or different from plasticity recorded in other forebrain areas?

Known neuromodulators of experience-induced plasticity evoked by painful inputs appear to differ qualitatively from those engaged in other modalities. For example, dopamine neurons, which play a prominent role in modulating cortical or hippocampal plasticity, are not as effectively excited by aversive stimuli, or by their prediction. Other neuromodulators (e.g., acetylcholine, norepinephrine, and serotonin) are released, as in other cortical sectors or in the hippocampus, with a more prominent, differential release of serotonin. Because these neuromodulators all appear to have different enabling effects for driving enduring positive and negative changes in synaptic strengths in activity-dependent plasticity, the nuances of release and presumably the shaping of experience-induced plasticity are different for pain inputs compared to those generated in other systems.

3) Can these competitive brain plasticity processes be re-engaged in ways that could weaken chronic pain?

There is some suggestion that specific forms of brain stimulation or behavioral training might lead to chronic pain suppression. The most compelling of these studies have not yet been reported in peer-reviewed papers. Other studies have defined the anatomical system by which descending inputs can facilitate or inhibit pain-evoked activity in the spinal cord, and it is plausible to believe that pain suppression might be mediated via this descending system.

In patients with chronic arm or back pain, magnetic imaging data indicate that innocuous cutaneous representations are reduced in area and degraded in topography, when compared to normal representations in pain-free subjects. In an unpublished study of possible competition-based amelioration of chronic pain, investigators asked whether the restoration of more normal representations of innocuous cutaneous inputs could affect chronic pain arising from tendonitis. To re-strengthen normal inputs and expand and renormalize their differentiated representation in the primary somatosensory cortex, subjects were intensively trained to make progressively more difficult, graded distinctions about tactile stimuli. Such stimulation in this training context led to rapid pain reduction, recorded in all patients in the first 1-hour training session. With training over 14 successive days, the chronic pain faded in all trained subjects. A confounding aspect of these studies was relatively rapid reduction of the tendonitis in the hand and arm; all signs were eliminated after a few days of daily exercise. However, the initial, nearly profound reduction of this chronic pain, which had endured in all patients over at least the preceding 3 months, is not likely to be accounted for by changes related to long-standing inflammation in the arm. Rather, it is hypothesized to be due to competitive plasticity in pain representational systems in the brain.

There is increasingly strong interest in training chronic pain patients by applying strategies in which the brain more reliably predicts non-pain, when a stimulus might evoke an otherwise painful input. The documentation of this "placebo" effect in neurological terms has been the subject of important recent brain-imaging studies (Zubieta et al. 2005). The results demonstrate that the pain that you feel is, to a great extent, the pain that you *predict* you will feel. Can intensive progressive training be used to further grow and strengthen this effect—or, in other terms, to weaken the well-learned predictions that pain is imminent?

These are two of potentially many useful nondrug strategies (magnetic or other forms of cortical stimulation are a third) that might be effectively applied to alleviate chronic pain.

RESEARCH QUESTIONS

1) Therapeutic model studies using motor cortex stimulation, intense competitive training of innocuous inputs to restore more normal tactile or proprioceptive representations, or cognitive training designed to strengthen the placebo effect or weaken the ongoing positive prediction of pain are a high priority. The former two classes of study must be conducted with controls that differentiate what is contributed by the placebo effect.

2) These competition models should be studied with a consideration of whether or not they can provide general explanations for pain origin when pain arises from different chronic causes.

3) How, more specifically, is plasticity induced by nociceptive inputs

modulated in the adult brain? Do differences in the brain's control of this system's plasticity provide any new drug targets for selectively blocking it?

4) Can specific forms of training be applied to prevent pain syndromes from evolving neurologically toward deeply embedded, chronic forms?

5) Where is the critical plasticity that can account for pain amelioration occurring?

6) Is the reduction of pain recorded after these procedures accounted for by the differential engagement of descending inhibitory (or possibly excitatory) projections to the dorsal horn? Are there other ways to evoke or pharmacologically enhance these effects?

7) What, specifically, does the competition between pain and non-pain inputs contribute to hyperalgesia, allodynia, and other clinical characteristics of neuropathic pain?

DESCENDING MODULATION

DISCUSSION QUESTIONS

1) What drives the bulbospinal pain modulatory pathways, and can we identify "nodal" points for supraspinal modulation by pharmacological, behavioral, or cognitive interventions?

Much is known about the efferent projections of brainstem neurons to the spinal cord, but less is known about the inputs that regulate the activity of these neurons. It is notable that there are 10 times as many cortical-thalamic connections as thalamocortical projections. The former projections are likely to encode pain experience in some manner. Spinobulbospinal loops probably include projections from dorsal horn neurons to parabrachial neurons, which in turn project to the amygdala and can also project to the periaqueductal gray matter. This loop may code for the unpleasantness of the pain experience. Finally, neurons in the periaqueductal gray receive projections from the preoptic hypothalamus, amygdala, and prefrontal cortex. They, in turn, via their afferent projections, are involved in integration of emotive, autonomic, cardiovascular, and stress responses to pain. Thus, it is likely that cortical control is exerted over the bulbospinal-pain modulatory pathways and that the periaqueductal gray matter may represent a "nodal point" for pharmacological, behavioral, or cognitive approaches to the treatment of neuropathic pain (see the chapter by Dubner in this volume for more details).

2) How do we improve the resolution for pathway mapping in supraspinal sites in time and place?

It is now well-recognized that bulbospinal pathways that originate in the brainstem and project to the spinal cord exert powerful control over the spinal processing of pain, and this concept has recently been extended to both inflammatory pain (see the chapter by Dubner this volume) and neuropathic pain (see the chapter by Ossipov and Porreca in this volume). Moreover, these pathways may either facilitate or inhibit nociception in a temporal manner, and they appear to arise from the same brainstem regions. It is becoming clear that further understanding of the conditions under which these pathways are activated and the determination of whether they are inhibitory or facilitatory will require the ability to identify individual neurons or classes of neurons as they are activated in a manner that affords resolution in both time and place. The past few years have witnessed new methods for mapping neurocircuitry in "real time" (see the chapter by Bushnell in this volume). Positron emission tomography (PET) and fMRI imaging techniques in the rodent, particularly of spinal cord and brainstem structures, still lack the requisite resolution. However, alternative approaches being pioneered in primary afferent nerves may be applicable. One approach that may be adapted includes the generation of transgenic mice that are engineered to express activity-dependent promoters in specific populations of neurons that, when activated, express substances that visually "label" the neuron or that may be transneuronally transported to visually identify the pathways that are activated. Application of this technique will require identification of a promoter that is specific to brainstem neurons. However, this approach holds the promise that the brainstem pathways that are activated under conditions of nerve injury can be identified in a regional and temporal manner.

RESEARCH QUESTIONS

1) How can we identify neuron-specific promoters in the brainstem and forebrain that can be used to develop a means to map neurons that are activated or inhibited?

2) How can we improve methods for PET and fMRI "real-time" imaging of ascending and descending circuitry in the rodent?

3) How best can we map the neurocircuitry of the afferent and efferent interconnections of supraspinal neurons implicated in pain transmission and modulation?

4) Bulbospinal pathways play both excitatory and inhibitory roles. How can we identify or discriminate between these neurons functionally?

5) What is the circuitry that accounts for descending facilitation with low stimulus intensities or drug dosages and modulates descending inhibition with higher dosages and stimulus intensities?

PAIN EXPERIENCE

DISCUSSION QUESTIONS

1) What is the basis for the high incidence of comorbidity that suggests a complexity of the modulation of pain? What are the multiple psychological constructs that constitute the pain experience?

Pain is often associated with sleep disorders and depression. If one expects pain, one may get pain, just as prediction of reward allows a feeling of reward before dopamine is released in the reward system. The neurochemistry of depression that is comorbid with pain may differ from depression of other kinds. There may be a special kind of stressor. Alternatively, depressed patients may be more sensitive to any kind of stress. Depression depends on monoamine systems, but there still may be a different chemistry if there is also pain. On the other hand, it may not be the pain that causes the difference, but rather processes like receptor occupancy. Depression is associated with variation in TNF-α expression. Experiments can manipulate this variation. For example, the forced swim test can be used as a model of depression. An agent affecting TNF-α can be given to produce learned helplessness.

2) What are the conditions that favor or enable chronic pain?

There may be a change in pain due to early experience. For instance, neonatal colon damage in infant rats leads to a pain state that models irritable bowel syndrome (IBS). This model was developed because of the history of such damage in neonatal humans who later developed IBS. Many people with pain have multiple problems that may result in multiple alterations in pain-modulating systems. Pain amplifications of interest in humans include conditions such as fibromyalgia and IBS. These patients have more pain than one would predict. What is the mechanism? Perhaps the answer comes back to spinobulbospinal control loops. Changes in the activity of such loops could affect wide regions of the body. It would be helpful to have a simple test of such changes in people. The idea is to look for evidence of inflammation or neuropathic pain. This kind of pain amplification can be seen in spinal cord injury. Changes in the brain enable changes in the body. Enabling is a consequence of plasticity (see the section above on "Competition in the Brain").

RESEARCH QUESTIONS

1) What are the transmitter systems that are involved in pain, depression and sleep disorders? Is there convergence among these pathways?

2) How can we develop better models of such conditions as depression and fibromyalgia?

3) How can we develop simple tests indicating the involvement of facilitatory and inhibitory spinobulbospinal loops in human pain states?

ANIMAL MODELS

DISCUSSION QUESTIONS

1) To what extent has the reliance on evoked and reflexive measures of nociceptive behaviors in animal models of nerve injury hampered or provided guidance (either appropriate or inappropriate) to investigations of supraspinal mechanisms involved in the induction or maintenance of neuropathic pain? Should additional measures be encouraged, and if so, what should they entail?

Current rodent models of neuropathic pain arising from nerve injury rely largely on dependent measures that can be considered to be reflexive or nocifensive, such as withdrawal from thermal stimuli or from stroking or punctate mechanical stimuli. The use of nocifensive behaviors as the principal dependent measure has strong proponents and opponents. Proponents argue for the ability or need to test large numbers of drugs in a relatively short period of time, to undertake complex experimental designs with matching control groups, and to obtain quantitative measures of threshold and suprathreshold responses that are amenable to the generation of drug dose-effect curves. They further note that many agents that are clinically effective alleviate thermal hyperalgesia and mechanical allodynia as measured in the nocifensive animal models, and that these models have a strong predictive value. Opponents of this approach argue that, because some of these nocifensive responses persist in the decerebrate animal, they only provide information about changes in reflex pathways and not about changes in pain. They further argue that postural asymmetries produced as a consequence of nerve injury confound these measures as currently used by others, and note that the results of operant measures frequently provide results that are diametrically opposed to those obtained using nocifensive measures. An argument for the appropriateness of operant measures is provided in the accompanying chapters by Vierck and by Price and colleagues.

We propose that the choice of dependent measure may very well be dictated by the question. Thus, nocifensive or reflexive measures may be acceptable for investigations of the role of primary afferents in the induction and maintenance of neuropathic pain. They also can be appropriate for understanding the underlying mechanisms of neuropathic pain at the spinal level. However, operant measures may be more appropriate and possibly necessary when investigating the extent to which forebrain structures or brainstem pain inhibitory and pain facilitatory pathways participate in the induction or maintenance of neuropathic pain after nerve injury, as well as its state-dependence. The latter would include the influence of attention, emotion, anxiety, and sleep disruption.

2) Can we develop animal models that will elucidate the role of psychological constructs in neuropathic pain conditions?

Let us consider the possibility of modeling some of the psychological constructs, such as the true "aversiveness" of tactile allodynia induced by nerve injury. Interestingly, this question has not been addressed in the operant models, although observations of rats indicate that they show progressively greater responses to von Frey filaments as the strength of the filaments increases. However, Fuchs and colleagues (LaGraize et al. 2004) investigated the role of the anterior cingulate cortex by subjecting rats to conditioning involving mechanical stimulation of either an allodynic or contralateral non-allodynic paw depending on which side of a chamber the animals chose to occupy. It is of note that lesions of the anterior cingulate gyrus in the rats did not ameliorate tactile allodynia induced by L5 spinal nerve ligation, yet they lessened the rats' escape/avoidance responses in this conditioned place preference paradigm.

3) Another issue concerns disparities in preclinical evaluation and clinical trials of drug effects. Preclinical studies in laboratory animal models typically focus on a single drug and generate dose-effect curves that often seek a dose that will provide complete relief of tactile allodynia, thermal hyperalgesia, or spontaneous pain behaviors. Yet, in clinical trials, a decrease of 2 on a 0–10 visual analogue scale or a 30% improvement in pain is considered biologically significant, and the efficacy of the drug is likely to be determined in patients on a background of stable medications (see the chapter by Hammond in this volume).

RESEARCH QUESTIONS

1) Can we further validate the utility of operant and classical conditioning measures of neuropathic pain by testing the effects of tricyclic antidepressants, anticonvulsants, and local anesthetics, and comparing the results to those in nocifensive or reflexive models?

2) Should we incorporate sleep disturbances into nerve-injury models?

3) How can we best study the role of specific brainstem and forebrain structures in the initiation and maintenance of neuropathic pain that utilize operant and place-conditional paradigms at various times?

4) Can we develop animal models that will elucidate the role of these psychological constructs in persistent pain conditions including neuropathic pain syndromes? Will such research necessitate a return to the use of non-human primates, or should we "just" use patients?

GENOMICS AND PROTEOMICS

DISCUSSION QUESTIONS

1) What is the basis for inter-individual differences in neuropathic pain and in response to therapy (genetic versus nongenetic, for example)? Should animal studies place greater focus on strain/stock differences in response to injury and in mapping neurocircuitry?

With regard to genomic studies in patients, we considered how useful that approach would be in identifying a therapeutic target. The identification of the *APOE4* allele as a risk factor for Alzheimer disease helps to select patients at greater risk of developing the disease for potential clinical studies or trials. Likewise, in the schizophrenia field, beginning with the twin studies, investigators have been able to extend genomic studies into single nucleotide polymorphism (SNP) studies (Chumakov et al. 2002) and combine that information with imaging and cognitive tests. While it is not yet clear that new genomic information has helped in the development of new therapeutics, it may help identify specific subgroups and diagnostics.

In the pain field we have not yet adapted this approach clinically. Theoretically, trying to identify one target molecule at a time using the SNP approach may not offer any advantage over the monoclonal antibody approach, which did not prove to be very successful. An advantage with SNPs is that this approach can be used to look at polymorphisms; once a gene has been identified, investigators could conduct animal experiments to further explore whether that target is involved with neuropathic pain. One recent example is the identification of the $Na_V1.7$ gene in erythromelalgia patients; when this was translated to the spinal nerve ligation model, it held up, giving greater confidence in that target for neuropathic pain.

Max has begun to adopt this approach in patients with lumbar root pain caused by intervertebral disk herniation (M. Max, personal communication). The advantage of this pain syndrome is a large and relatively homogeneous patient population. However, microarray and anatomical studies are difficult to pursue in these patients except for the rare cases in which the dorsal root ganglion is excised for pain control, or these relatively young patients come to autopsy. Skin biopsies for neurite counts are not very informative in nerve root injuries, unlike peripheral nerve diseases, because the dorsal root ganglion cell usually remains intact and able to nourish the peripheral nerve. A neuropathic condition that may lend itself better to such genomic studies is postherpetic neuralgia, a condition offering the advantage that investigators can follow the patients over time from the onset of the disease until autopsy.

One limitation with the current database on genomic information in pain studies is that it is not large enough to identify susceptibility genes. Using previously established in vivo and in vitro methods, investigators have identified approximately 200 targets as potential mediators of pain. Given this relatively small number, it should be possible to identify whether these targets represent biomarkers or therapeutic targets for specific neuropathic pain states.

The use of proteomics in clinical studies of supraspinal mechanisms of pain is in its infancy. Although samples of cerebrospinal fluid may provide some useful information, fundamental questions exist as to whether selective or relevant information can be obtained.

2) How can we use more genetically amenable organisms for the study of pain? The field of behavioral genetics may offer an alternative approach to identification of novel genes involved in the afferent transmission and modulation of nociception. The genomes of both *Drosophila* and *C. elegans* are now known. For *Drosophila* in particular there are libraries of thousands of flies, each with a specific mutant, for which it should be possible to identify a pain phenotype if present. A potential advantage of this approach is that one works from a known mutation to a specific phenotype. This approach contrasts with genomic or proteomic chip analyses in which a phenotype is induced (e.g., nerve injury) and then one searches for what has changed. This latter approach has identified hundreds of concomitant changes, making the choice of target gene problematic.

RESEARCH QUESTIONS

1) Genomic approaches have been used to study changes in gene expression at the level of the primary afferent. Is this approach suitable and feasible for studies of supraspinal mechanisms, making it possible to identify changes in gene expression in specific neurons in the bulbospinal pathways?

2) How can genomics and proteomics help us learn more about the mechanism of action of drugs (e.g., anticonvulsants, tricyclic antidepressants, and selective serotonin norepinephrine reuptake inhibitors) or identify the susceptibility of individual patients to drug therapy?

3) How can proteomics be incorporated into studies of supraspinal mechanisms of neuropathic pain?

4) What is the epigenetics of neuropathic pain with respect to supraspinal mechanisms that are invoked by environmental influences?

5) Longitudinal studies on the epidemiology of persistent pain are needed.

THERAPEUTICS

DISCUSSION QUESTIONS

1) Given the heterogeneity of responses in patients, can we design an intelligent algorithm for therapy based on diagnostic tools?

2) Conversely, can pharmacological agents be used to identify mechanisms?

A striking factor in neuropathic pain patients is their heterogeneity in response to analgesic therapy (Wallace et al. 2000; Raja et al. 2002). Two approaches may be considered to address this clinical problem. On the one hand, it has been suggested that psychophysical testing might distinguish subgroups with a high likelihood to respond to, or to fail, treatment with a particular class of agents. For example, it has been suggested that patients with hypoalgesia or anesthesia in the areas of postherpetic neuralgia are less likely to respond to acute opioid therapy, but more likely to respond to antidepressant treatment, than those with hypersensitivity to sensory testing in this area (Raja et al. 2002). Unfortunately from a practical standpoint, few controlled trials have used sensory testing to guide therapy, and so the acute predictive value of this approach appears low, and its value for predicting long-term analgesic treatment success is untested.

Another approach tests whether response to acute drug therapy will predict efficacy of that class of drug for individual patient treatment. For example, there is a considerable inter-individual difference in the degree to which intravenous infusion of lidocaine reduces areas of allodynia in patients with complex regional pain syndrome, suggesting that patients who respond well to acute administration of the drug might achieve better analgesia with this class of drugs than patients who experience little effect. Another example is the response to intravenous phentolamine as a diagnostic tool to predict response to sympatholytic drugs and procedures (Raja et al. 1991). Unfortunately, these studies are few and include small numbers of subjects, drugs are not available for intravenous administration in all drug classes, and failure of response to acute administration may not predict response to chronic therapy.

REFERENCES

Chumakov I, Blumenfeld M, Guerassimenko O, et al. Genetic and physiological data implicating the new human gene G72 and the gene for D-amino acid oxidase in schizophrenia. *Proc Natl Acad Sci USA* 2002; 99:13675–13680.

Hao JX, Xu XJ, Aldskogius H, Seiger A, Wiesenfeld-Hallin Z. Allodynia-like effects in rat after ischaemic spinal cord injury photochemically induced by laser irradiation. *Pain* 1991; 45:175–185.

Hulsebosch CE, Xu GY, Perez-Polo JR, et al. Rodent model of chronic central pain after spinal cord contusion injury and effects of gabapentin. *J Neurotrauma* 2000; 17:1205–1217.

Jones EG, Pons TP. Thalamic and brainstem contributions to large-scale plasticity of primate somatosensory cortex. *Science* 1998; 282:1121–1125.

LaGraize SC, Labuda CJ, Rutledge MA, Jackson RL, Fuchs PN. Differential effect of anterior cingulate cortex lesion on mechanical hypersensitivity and escape/avoidance behavior in an animal model of neuropathic pain. *Exp Neurol* 2004; 188:139–148.

Ling EA. Evidence for a haematogenous origin of the macrophages appearing in the spinal cord of the rat after dorsal rhizotomy. *J Anat* 1979; 128(Pt 1):143–154.

Michiels JJ, te Morsche RH, Jansen JB, Drenth JP. Autosomal dominant erythermalgia associated with a novel mutation in the voltage-gated sodium channel alpha subunit $Na_V1.7$. *Arch Neurol* 2005; 62:1587–1590.

Raja SN, Treede R-D, Davis KD, Campbell JN. Systemic alpha-adrenergic blockade with phentolamine: a diagnostic test for sympathetically maintained pain. *Anesthesiology* 1991; 74:691–698.

Raja SN, Haythornthwaite JA, Pappagallo M, et al. Opioids versus antidepressants in postherpetic neuralgia—a randomized, placebo-controlled trial. *Neurology* 2002; 59:1015–1021.

Tanga FY, Nutile-McMenemy N, DeLeo JA. The CNS role of Toll-like receptor 4 in innate neuroimmunity and painful neuropathy. *Proc Natl Acad Sci USA* 2005; 102:5856–5861.

Tsuda M, Shigemoto-Mogami Y, Koizumi S, et al. P2X4 receptors induced in spinal microglia gate tactile allodynia after nerve injury. *Nature* 2003; 424(6950):729–730.

Wallace MS, Ridgeway BM, Leung AY, Gerayli A, Yaksh TL. Concentration-effect relationship of intravenous lidocaine on the allodynia of complex regional pain syndrome types I and II. *Anesthesiology* 2000; 92:75–83.

Watkins LR, Milligan ED, Maier SF. Glial activation: a driving force for pathological pain. *Trends Neurosci* 2001; 24:450–455.

Watkins LR, Milligan ED, Maier SF. Glial proinflammatory cytokines mediate exaggerated pain states: implications for clinical pain. *Adv Exp Med Biol* 2003; 521:1–21.

Woods TM, Cusick CG, Pons TP, Taub E, Jones EG. Progressive transneuronal changes in the brainstem and thalamus after long-term dorsal rhizotomies in adult macaque monkeys. *J Neurosci* 2000; 20:3884–3899.

Yezierski RP, Liu S, Ruenes GL, Kajander KJ, Brewer L. Excitotoxic spinal cord injury: behavioral and morphological characteristics of a central pain model. *Pain* 1998; 75:141–155.

Zubieta JK, Bueller JA, Jackson LR, et al. Placebo effects mediated by endogenous opioid activity on mu-opioid receptors. *J Neurosci* 2005; 25:7754–7762.

Correspondence to: William D. Willis, Jr., MD, PhD, Department of Neuroscience and Cell Biology, University of Texas Medical Branch, 301 University Boulevard, Galveston, TX 77555-1069, USA. Tel: 409-772-2103; Fax: 409-772-4687; email: wdwillis@utmb.edu.

Emerging Strategies for the Treatment of Neuropathic Pain, edited by James N. Campbell, Allan I. Basbaum, André Dray, Ronald Dubner, Robert H. Dworkin, and Christine N. Sang, IASP Press, Seattle, © 2006.

6

Descending Modulatory Circuitry in the Initiation and Maintenance of Neuropathic Pain

Ronald Dubner

Department of Biomedical Sciences, University of Maryland Dental School, Baltimore, Maryland, USA

Our knowledge of the existence of endogenous descending pain-modulatory systems spans at least three decades (for comprehensive reviews, see Fields and Basbaum 1999; Millan 2002). The first line of evidence to support endogenous pain control came from the study of Reynolds (1969), who demonstrated that focal brain stimulation of the periaqueductal gray (PAG) produced sufficient analgesia to permit abdominal surgery in rats. Liebeskind and colleagues confirmed this finding and concluded that stimulation of the PAG activated a normal function of the brain: pain inhibition (Mayer et al. 1971; Mayer and Liebeskind 1974). They labeled the phenomenon "stimulation-produced analgesia" (SPA). These early studies found SPA to be specifically antinociceptive, producing no generalized sensory, attentional, emotional, or motor deficits.

An important final common descending modulatory site in the brainstem is the rostral ventromedial medulla (RVM), whose major component is the nucleus raphe magnus (NRM). The RVM receives signals directly from the PAG and indirectly from forebrain sites (Bandler and Shipley 1994). The descending PAG-RVM circuit is involved in the emotional, motivational, and cognitive factors that modulate the experience of pain.

Perhaps the most important finding concerning SPA is that analgesia induced by brain stimulation shares several characteristics with analgesia from opioid drugs. Areas of the brain from which SPA can be elicited are rich in opiate receptors, and microinjection of morphine into these brain regions produces analgesia, indicating that common brain sites support both SPA and opiate analgesia. Tsou and Jang (1964) discovered that the most sensitive sites for the analgesic action of morphine are located in the PAG and the adjacent hypothalamic periventricular area. This discovery led to the hypothesis that opioid drugs like morphine act by binding to a receptor in the brain (Pert and Snyder 1973) and that there likely are endogenous ligands or chemical mediators whose actions are mimicked by opiates. These findings led to the discovery of the endogenous opioid peptides (Hughes et al. 1975; Goldstein et al. 1979) and subsequently to the cloning of the three major subtypes of opioid receptors, mu, delta, and kappa (Evans et al. 1992; Kieffer et al. 1992; Chen et al. 1993; Thompson et al. 1993).

BIDIRECTIONAL DESCENDING CONTROL

Early studies established the presence of a descending inhibitory pain modulatory circuit linking the brainstem PAG and RVM with the spinal cord (see Basbaum and Fields 1984; Gebhart 1986; Fields and Basbaum 1999; Millan 2002, for reviews). However, we now know that there are parallel descending facilitatory mechanisms (for reviews see Porreca et al. 2002; Ren and Dubner 2002; Gebhart 2004; Vanegas and Schaible 2004). Brainstem descending pathways also facilitate nociceptive transmission at the spinal cord level. Excitation and inhibition of dorsal horn neurons can be produced by stimulation of the dorsolateral funiculus of the spinal cord (Dubuisson and Wall 1979; McMahon and Wall 1988), the NRM (Dubuisson and Wall 1980), and the nucleus reticularis gigantocellularis (NGC) (Haber et al. 1980). In the NGC, low-intensity electrical stimulation or microinjection of a low dose of glutamate or neurotensin will produce facilitation of behavioral and spinal dorsal horn neuronal responses to noxious stimulation (Zhuo and Gebhart 1992; Thomas et al. 1995; Urban and Gebhart 1999; Zhuo et al. 2002). RVM neurons may exert bidirectional control of nociception through descending serotoninergic and noradrenergic pathways (Zhuo and Gebhart 1991; Holden et al. 1999). Descending inhibitory influences from the RVM travel mainly in the dorsolateral funiculus, whereas descending facilitatory effects reach the spinal cord via the ventral and ventrolateral funiculi (Zhuo et al. 2002).

FUNCTIONAL PROPERTIES OF RVM NEURONS

In the RVM, two types of cells have been identified by Fields and colleagues (1991) as pain-modulatory neurons: on-cells are characterized by a sudden increase in activity before the initiation of a nocifensive behavior, which in their studies was a tail flick to a transient noxious heat stimulus, whereas off-cells exhibit a pause in activity just prior to the initiation of the tail flick. While off-cells are usually associated with the inhibition of nocifensive behaviors, on-cells are correlated with a facilitation of nocifensive behavior. A third type of cell, the neutral-cell, was also identified, but its activity was not correlated with nocifensive behavior in response to transient stimuli.

The RVM also contains serotoninergic cell types. These cells comprise about 15% of the cells in the RVM. Most serotoninergic RVM cells send unmyelinated axons through the dorsolateral funiculus into the spinal cord. Most serotonergic cells contain at least one and often several co-transmitters, including excitatory and inhibitory amino acids, and a plethora of neuropeptides (Bowker et al. 1982).

A second neurochemically distinct monoamine descending system in volves noradrenergic neurons whose cell bodies are in the A5, A6, and A7 cell groups in the brainstem. Several studies indicate that the descending norepinephrine system can mediate analgesia and dorsal horn inhibition and that this system is critical for opiate-induced analgesia (for reviews see Dubner and Bennett 1983; Gebhart and Proudfit 2005).

PERSISTENT PAIN AND DESCENDING MODULATION

Earlier studies of descending modulation mainly focused on responses to acute or transient stimuli. In contrast, recent studies have examined the effects of persistent pain on descending modulation following tissue damage or nerve injury. These persistent, or chronic, pain conditions are associated with prolonged functional changes in the nervous system, evidenced by the development of dorsal horn hyperexcitability and activity-dependent plasticity, also commonly referred to as spinal central sensitization (for reviews see Dubner and Ruda 1992; Woolf and Salter 2000). There is evidence of enhanced net descending inhibition after inflammation at sites of primary hyperalgesia (increased sensitivity to noxious stimuli at sites of injury). Primary hyperalgesia involves increased sensitivity of primary afferent neurons (peripheral sensitization) as well as central sensitization. Descending inhibition is greater in neurons with input from an inflamed knee as compared to a non-inflamed knee (Schaible et al. 1991). In rats with hindpaw inflammation, spinal cord lidocaine block leads to an enhancement of the activity of dorsal horn nociceptive neurons that is greater in inflamed than that in non-inflamed rats (Ren and Dubner 1996). Similar findings are found using Fos protein expression as a marker of neuronal activation. There are more inflammation-induced Fos-immunoreactive neurons in the dorsal horn in spinally transected or dorsolateral funiculus-lesioned rats, when compared to sham-operated inflamed rats (Ren and Ruda 1996; Wei et al. 1998). Kauppila et al. (1998) showed that thermal but not mechanical nociceptive responses were further enhanced in hindpaw-inflamed and spinal-nerve-ligated rats after midthoracic spinalization. Finally, hyperalgesia is intensified in rats with lesions of the dorsal lateral quadrant of the spinal cord after inflammation or formalin injection (Abbott et al. 1996; Ren and Dubner 1996). These studies reveal the *net* descending inhibitory effects of activation of multiple supraspinal sites. The findings suggest that injury-induced dorsal horn hyperexcitability and primary hyperalgesia are dampened by descending pathways, due to enhancement of descending net inhibitory effects.

The source of *enhanced net inhibition* can be found in the brainstem. Local anesthesia of the RVM results in a further increase in dorsal horn nociceptive neuronal activity in hindpaw-inflamed rats (Ren and Dubner 1996). Focal lesions of the RVM and locus coeruleus produce an increase in spinal Fos expression and hyperalgesia after inflammation (Tsuruoka and Willis 1996a,b; Wei et al. 1999b). It appears that both RVM and locus coeruleus descending pathways are major sources of enhanced net inhibition in inflamed animals.

After inflammation, descending facilitation parallels inhibition, but also can dominate it, resulting in a net enhancement of activity or hyperalgesia. The selective destruction of the NGC with a soma-selective neurotoxin, ibotenic acid, attenuates hyperalgesia and reduces inflammation-induced spinal Fos expression (Wei et al. 1999a). A descending facilitatory effect may also originate from the medullary dorsal reticular nucleus (Lima and Almeida 2002) and from other brain sites such as the anterior cingulate cortex (Calejesan et al. 2000).

A descending facilitatory drive contributes to the pathogenesis of certain types of persistent pain, particularly those associated with secondary inflammatory hyperalgesia or nerve injury (Porreca et al. 2002; Ren and Dubner 2002). Secondary hyperalgesia refers to increased sensitivity to noxious stimuli at non-injured sites outside the injured zone. Spinalization blocks mustard oil-produced secondary mechanical allodynia and mechanical hyperexcitability of spinal nociceptive neurons (Mansikka and Pertovaara 1997). Hindpaw formalin-induced hyperalgesia is prevented by RVM lesions (Wiertelak et al. 1997). RVM lesions inhibit secondary hyperalgesia produced by topical application of mustard oil (Urban and Gebhart 1999). Masseter muscle inflammation produces mechanical hyperalgesia of the overlying skin, which may involve secondary hyperalgesia of the skin and primary hyperalgesia of the muscle and is blocked by RVM lesions (Sugiyo et al.

2005). The late phase of the formalin response appears to be related at least in part to central hyperexcitability (central sensitization) and can be considered an example of primary hyperalgesia that is facilitated by descending inputs. However, it is known that descending inhibitory inputs also play a role, since elimination of the inhibition by dorsolateral funiculus lesions results in more intense responses to formalin (Abbott et al. 1996).

The same phenomenon of descending facilitation occurs in models of neuropathic hyperalgesia. The tactile allodynia after nerve injury is dependent upon a tonic activation of net descending facilitation from supraspinal sites (Kauppila et al. 1998; Ossipov et al. 2000). In nerve-injured rats, lesions of the dorsolateral funiculus, local anesthetic block of the RVM, and lesions of μ-opioid-receptor-expressing cells in the RVM do not prevent the onset, but do reverse the later maintenance, of tactile and thermal hyperalgesia (Porreca et al. 2001; Burgess et al. 2002). Whether RVM on-cells are exclusively involved in descending facilitation after nerve injury is not clear. Are only on-cells destroyed by the effect of the dermorphin-saporin conjugate on μ-opioid-receptor-expressing cells? Do μ-opioid-receptor-containing NGC cells participate in descending facilitation after nerve injury, and are they on-cells? Nevertheless, these observations point to an ascending-descending loop that is activated in response to prolonged stimulation after nerve injury, resulting in facilitation at the spinal level. Although most of the studies cited above have concluded that the hyperalgesia is completely dependent on facilitatory influences from the brainstem, it should be noted that the same effects can be produced by a reduction in descending inhibition, leading to a dominance of descending facilitation. Thus, neuropathic hyperalgesia may be dependent on a net descending facilitatory effect, wherein a simultaneous descending inhibition is dominated by the facilitation. Both facilitatory and inhibitory circuitry may be activated by ascending input after injury (Herrero and Cervero 1996; Gozariu et al. 1998; Terayama et al. 2000). What appears to be important, then, is the balance between descending synaptic excitation and inhibition. It has been shown previously that the NGC plays a role in descending facilitation of nociceptive transmission after transient noxious stimuli (Zhuo and Gebhart 1992). Lesions of the NGC produce an attenuation of hyperalgesia and spinal Fos expression after inflammation (Wei et al. 1999a). However, lesions that include the NGC and NRM abolish the opposite effects induced by separate NGC or NRM lesions (Wei et al. 1999a). It appears that severe persistent pain may be enhanced when the descending facilitatory drive originating from multiple brainstem sites overrides the descending inhibitory drive.

DYNAMIC SHIFTS IN DESCENDING
MODULATION AFTER INJURY

The enhancement of descending inhibition in response to tissue injury appears to build up gradually (Schaible et al. 1991; Ren and Dubner 1996; Ren and Ruda 1996; Danziger et al. 1999; Dubner and Ren 1999; Hurley and Hammond 2000). It appears that following inflammation, brainstem descending pathways become progressively more involved in suppressing incoming nociceptive signals in primary hyperalgesic zones. Injury-related primary afferent input is probably responsible for triggering this ascending-descending feedback circuit. This enhancement of descending inhibition appears to occur when the animal is subject to continuous, persistent noxious stimulation.

Persistent inflammation induces dramatic changes in the excitability of RVM pain-modulating circuitry, suggesting dynamic temporal changes in synaptic activation in the brainstem after inflammation (Terayama et al. 2000; Guan et al. 2002). Early in the development of inflammation—for up to 3 hours—there is an increase in descending facilitation (Urban and Gebhart 1999), which reduces the net effect of the inhibition. Over time, the level of descending inhibition increases, or descending facilitation decreases, leading to a net enhancement of antinocifensive behavior.

What are the cellular mechanisms that underlie these changes? Excitatory amino acids (EAAs) have been shown to mediate descending modulation in response to transient noxious stimulation and early inflammation (Heinricher et al. 1999; Urban and Gebhart 1999 for review), and they appear to be involved in the development of RVM excitability associated with inflammation and persistent pain (Terayama et al. 2000; Guan et al. 2002; Miki et al. 2002). At 3 hours post-inflammation, low doses of N-methyl-D-aspartate (NMDA), microinjected into the RVM, facilitate the response of the inflamed hindpaw to noxious heat (Guan et al. 2002). Higher doses of NMDA at 3 hours post-inflammation produce only inhibition, and at 24 hours post-inflammation, NMDA at all doses produces only inhibition. All of these effects are blocked by administration of NMDA-receptor antagonists. AMPA (α-amino-3-hydroxy-5-methyl-4-isoxazole propionate) produces dose- and time-dependent inhibition at 3 and 24 hours post-inflammation that are blocked by an AMPA-receptor antagonist. These findings indicate an increase in the potency of the dose-response curves of NMDA- and AMPA-produced inhibition at 24 hours post-inflammation as compared to 3 hours. The leftward shift of the dose-response curves of EAA-receptor antagonists parallels the time-dependent enhancement of net descending inhibition produced by RVM electrical stimulation. The results suggest that the time-dependent functional changes in descending modulation are mediated, in part, by enhanced EAA neurotransmission.

Rats with inflammatory hyperalgesia exhibit increased sensitivity to opioid analgesics (Neil et al. 1986; Hammond 2004). Typically, there is a leftward shift of the dose-response curve for opioids for the inflamed hyperalgesic paw when compared to the non-inflamed paw (Hylden et al. 1991). Kayser et al. (1991) suggested that this increased opioid sensitivity in inflamed animals was related to a peripheral mechanism because it is significantly attenuated after local injections of very low doses (0.5–1 µg) of naloxone. Recent observations indicate that the increased opioid sensitivity after inflammation may also reflect changes in central pain-modulating pathways. Hurley and Hammond (2000, 2001) have demonstrated enhancement and plasticity of the descending inhibitory effects of μ- and δ_2-opioid receptor agonists microinjected into the RVM during the development and maintenance of inflammatory hyperalgesia. It is likely that opioid peptide activation and γ-amino-butyric acid (GABA) disinhibition (Fields and Basbaum 1999) are also important in the initiation and maintenance of RVM plasticity.

MOLECULAR MECHANISMS OF PLASTICITY IN THE RVM

What are the molecular mechanisms of this increased potency leading to enhanced synaptic activity and increases in descending net inhibition associated with primary hyperalgesia? Recent studies have demonstrated that transcriptional, translational, and post-translational changes that occur in the RVM after inflammation may underlie the observed changes in EAA-receptor sensitivity. Examination of the mRNA expression of the NR1, NR2A, and NR2B subunits of the NMDA receptor in the RVM revealed an upregulation that parallels the time course of the changes in RVM excitability (Miki et al. 2002). This upregulation is accompanied by an increase in NMDA-receptor protein. There is also an increase in receptor phosphorylation_of the NR2A subunit of the NMDA receptor in the RVM after inflammation (Turnbach et al. 2003). Western blot analysis also revealed a time-dependent increase in the AMPA-receptor GluR1 subunit levels in the RVM at 5 and 24 hours post-inflammation as compared to naive animals (Guan et al. 2004). Western blots also demonstrated that GluR1 phosphoprotein levels were increased as early as 30 minutes post-inflammation and were time-dependent, suggesting that post-translational receptor phosphorylation may also contribute to the enhanced AMPA transmission (Guan et al. 2004). These findings support the hypothesis that activity-dependent plasticity takes place at the RVM level and involves both changes in EAA-receptor gene and protein expression and increased phosphorylation of EAA receptors.

This activity-induced plasticity in pain-modulating circuitry after inflammation complements the activity-dependent neuronal plasticity in ascending pain transmission pathways (Dubner and Ruda 1992; Ren and Dubner 2002). Inflammation leads to peripheral sensitization of nociceptors and central sensitization or activity-dependent plasticity of spinal nociceptive neurons. The increased neuronal barrage at the spinal level activates spinal projection neurons, leading to activation of glutamatergic, opioidergic, and GABAergic neurons at the brainstem level and a similar, but not identical, form of activity-dependent plasticity.

PHENOTYPIC CHANGES IN THE RVM AFTER INFLAMMATION

The time-dependent plasticity in descending pain-modulatory circuitry also involves changes in the response profiles of RVM neurons. Miki et al. (2002) used paw withdrawal as a behavioral correlate to assess the relationship between nocifensive behavior and RVM neural activity after inflammation. Similar to the findings of Fields et al. (1991), who correlated tail-flick responses with RVM neural activity after transient noxious thermal stimuli, Miki et al. (2002) observed on-like, off-like, and neutral-like cells based on the relationship of their responses to paw-withdrawal behavior during the development of inflammation. They found that some neutral-like cells changed their response profile and were reclassified as on- or off-like cells during continuous recordings of 5 hours or more. The change in the response profile of RVM neurons correlated with the temporal changes in excitability in the RVM after inflammation (Terayama et al. 2000). This phenotypic switch of RVM neurons was verified in a population study that found a significant increase in the percentage of on-like and off-like cells and a decrease in the neutral-like cell population 24 hours after inflammation. There was also a greater increase in the magnitude of the responses of on-like cells after inflammation as compared to on-like responses in naive controls, suggesting an increase in facilitatory drive in the RVM. In contrast, off-like responses were reduced after inflammation, suggesting an increase in inhibitory descending activity originating in the RVM. However, it is difficult to predict the net effect of descending facilitation and inhibition from changes in single neuronal activity without recording from very large populations of neurons.

Although the on- and off-cell classification system can explain some of the existing data, a number of unanswered questions remain. For instance, cells that are excited by noxious stimulation are not inhibited by morphine in the awake animal (Martin et al. 1992). After inflammation, some cells have different response properties depending upon the site of peripheral stimulation (K. Ren and R. Dubner, unpublished data). In awake animals, the function of these neurons may be more tightly linked to behavioral state than other aspects of the stimulus conditions (Fields 2004). RVM neurons clearly participate in a number of processes in addition to pain modulation. Determining how individual RVM neurons contribute to multiple modulatory functions is part of the future challenge in this field.

CLINICAL IMPLICATIONS

Descending modulation and activity-dependent plasticity are normal functions of the brain that presumably are activated to protect the organism from further environmental injury. Ren and Dubner (2002) proposed that after inflammatory primary hyperalgesia, the early facilitation may function to enhance nocifensive escape behavior, whereas the dominant late inhibition may provide a mechanism by which movement of the injured site is suppressed or reduced to aid in healing and recuperation. In contrast, Gebhart (2004) proposed that the need to escape from a predator requires enhanced control of pain and thus more descending inhibition (as in the football player who breaks an ankle but continues to run in order to score a touchdown). The Gebhart proposal is supported by opioid and nonopioid mechanisms of acute stress-induced analgesia seen in animals (Hayes et al. 1978), but is not consistent with the enhanced descending facilitation found at sites of secondary hyperalgesia and after nerve injury and chronic stress. Gebhart hypothesizes that descending facilitation is necessary to maintain hyperalgesia as the tissue heals and to protect the injured tissue from further insult. Support for the contrasting Dubner/Ren and Gebhart hypotheses depends upon which neural system ultimately controls the behavior—the sensory or the motor system. The Dubner/Ren hypothesis assumes that the motor output, which is directly measured in the animal experiments, will ultimately be influenced by the descending modulation. The motor output is enhanced early after injury and suppressed during recuperation (Terayama et al. 2002). The Gebhart hypothesis assumes that the sensory system will ultimately control the effect of descending modulation on the behavioral outcome. Sensory inhibition will reduce pain early after injury and enhance pain during recuperation (Gebhart 2004). More data are needed to elucidate why there is evidence in support of both contrasting hypotheses. The answer may lie in an understanding of the different mechanisms associated with acute versus chronic stress.

It is clear that enhanced modulation includes shifts in the balance between inhibitory and facilitatory components. Recuperation from an injury involves the need for this balance, which may shift according to the behavioral state of the animal, which includes other survival needs besides the control of pain. Present evidence suggests that there is a different balance in neural networks receiving input from zones of secondary hyperalgesia where there is no primary injury as well as a different balance between facilitatory and inhibitory networks in models of nerve injury. The balance toward facilitatory influences appears to be maintained for longer periods after permanent types of nerve injury. Activation of these sites would lead to an enhancement of movement behavior that could also be protective.

The imbalance between these modulatory pathways may also be one mechanism underlying variability in other persistent or chronic pain conditions, especially those involving deep tissues such as muscle and viscera. Inputs from deep tissues produce more robust dorsal horn hyperexcitability and plasticity than do inputs from cutaneous tissues. Primary afferent and spinal neurons originating from muscle and viscera are often multimodal and are responsive to innocuous as well as noxious stimuli. An imbalance of descending modulatory systems in which there is an increase in endogenous facilitation could lead to innocuous input being perceived as painful. For patients suffering from deep pains such as temporomandibular disorders, fibromyalgia, irritable bowel syndrome, and low back pain, the diffuse nature and amplification of persistent pain may, in part, be the result of a net increase in endogenous descending facilitation.

THE NEED FOR NEW KNOWLEDGE

A critical question is whether descending circuitry should be a future target for neuropathic pain therapy. Before answering that question, we need to evaluate the state of knowledge in the area, describe the gaps in our understanding, and consider whether filling these gaps will lead to a significant advance in our ability to treat neuropathic pain.

ROLE OF TRANSMITTER SYSTEMS IN DESCENDING MODULATION

Although much is known about monoaminergic, opioid, glutaminergic, and GABAergic systems in descending circuitry, many questions remain unanswered. Are serotoninergic pathways important for the elaboration of neuropathic pain? Certainly, the treatment effects of serotonin reuptake inhibitors have been less than encouraging. And do they really have their effects in descending circuitry? What is the interaction between serotoninergic and noradrenergic systems, and how do they affect the hyperalgesia found in nerve injury models that is dependent upon descending inputs? What is the circuitry that accounts for the finding of descending facilitation (and hyper-algesia) with the lowest dosages of glutamate or neurotensin, and why do higher dosages lead to descending inhibition? The prevailing hypothesis from the work of Fields and colleagues would suggest that μ-opioid recep-tors are present in on-cells, yet the destruction of cells with these receptors using saporin conjugates does not always eliminate descending facilitation. How do monoaminergic and opioid systems interact in descending circuits, and are they important for hyperalgesia produced after nerve injury in any models? Perhaps we need new approaches to the study of these interacting systems and should avoid examining the effects of individual transmitter systems. Is pharmacogenomics an answer? Can we take advantage of gene and protein microarrays in revealing changes in gene and protein expression in descending circuits after nerve injury? The effects of drugs on these changes can be correlated with changes in behavioral hyperalgesia and allodynia and may provide insights into which receptor systems and trans-mitters are critically involved in neuropathic pain.

THE DESCENDING CIRCUITRY

Most of our attention has been directed toward the role of the PAG and the RVM in descending circuitry. Are they the most critical sites of action for descending facilitation and hyperalgesia produced after nerve injury? The evidence is strong that NGC activation produces facilitatory effects and hyperalgesia associated with tissue injury, although its role after nerve in-jury has not been confirmed. There is also little information on the specific effects of various forebrain structures and their modulation of the PAG-RVM circuitry. These forebrain sites provide the neural networks by which cognitive, attentional, and motivational aspects of the pain experience modu-late nociceptive transmission at brainstem and spinal targets. Although ana-tomical connections between forebrain structures such as the prefrontal cor-tex, the amygdala, and the anterior cingulate gyrus have been established, the functional role of these connections, particularly after nerve injury, is still unknown. Research to date has largely been inadequate in determining the role of these higher centers in the modulation of pain. The use of modern imaging techniques such as positron electron tomography and functional magnetic resonance imaging has revealed distributed processing of nocicep-tive information at multiple forebrain sites. The functional relationship of these sites to descending modulation via the PAG is still unclear. Further-more, evidence suggests important *direct* descending connections between the PAG and the spinal cord that are important in pain modulation, and the relative role of these direct connections versus the PAG-RVM pathway is unknown.

MECHANISMS OF NEUROPATHIC HYPERALGESIA AS COMPARED TO INFLAMMATORY HYPERALGESIA

Evidence is growing that descending facilitation dominates in some models of tissue injury leading to inflammatory hyperalgesia, especially those associated with secondary hyperalgesia, and that it also dominates after peripheral nerve injury. These descending effects appear to be critical for the manifestation of hyperalgesia. What brainstem and descending circuits are activated by these different models of nerve and tissue injury? Are different pathways activated by nerve and tissue injury? What role does inhibition play in hyperalgesia found in nerve injury models? How can we translate this information into a better understanding of the modulatory effect of these descending systems in clinical conditions of chronic pain, particularly those associated with nerve injury?

ADEQUACY OF THE FIELDS MODEL OF DESCENDING MODULATION

Fields and colleagues made major contributions to our understanding of the bimodal nature of descending modulation and highlighted the importance of descending facilitation and inhibition. Their hypothesis of the role of on-cells in descending facilitation and off-cells in descending inhibition has been confirmed in transient pain models but has not been adequately tested in persistent pain models, particularly those models involving nerve injury. It would appear from recent studies that the activity of on- and off-cells is more tightly linked to behavioral state than to the type of stimulation and that it is clearly involved in modulation that goes beyond events related to pain. The role of neutral cells in descending modulation and in the behavioral state of the animal also needs further study. The relationship of cell phenotype in descending pathways to various transmitters and receptor subtypes is also a major future challenge.

PLASTICITY IN DESCENDING SYSTEMS

The finding that activity-dependent plasticity, or central sensitization as it is commonly termed by pain researchers, contributes to changes in descending modulation in models of chronic pain supports evidence that such plasticity is common in nociceptive pathways. The functional implications are that neural pathways critical for the survival of the organism exhibit changes in sensitivity associated with persistence of input. Such changes are found after tissue or nerve injury in the peripheral nervous system, in the spinal and medullary dorsal horns, and in descending systems, but may also be present at other sites in nociceptive pathways. I would propose that sites of such plasticity in the nervous system are critical nodal points for intervention and for development of new approaches to neuropathic pain therapy. One challenge for the future is to translate basic knowledge about neuronal plasticity in nociceptive systems gained in the laboratory into new treatment approaches for patients.

ACKNOWLEDGMENTS

This work was supported by National Institutes of Health grant DA10275.

REFERENCES

Abbott FV, Hong Y, Franklin KB. The effect of lesions of the dorsolateral funiculus on formalin pain and morphine analgesia: a dose-response analysis. *Pain* 1996; 65:17–23.

Bandler R, Shipley MT. Columnar organization in the midbrain periaqueductal gray: modules for emotional expression? *Trends Neurosci* 1994; 17:379–389.

Basbaum AI, Fields HL. Endogenous pain control systems: brainstem spinal pathways and endorphin circuitry. *Annu Rev Neurosci* 1984; 7:309–338.

Bowker RM, Westlund KN, Sullivan MC, Wilber JF, Coulter JD. Transmitters of the raphe-spinal complex: immunocytochemical studies. *Peptides* 1982; 3:291–298.

Burgess SE, Gardell LR, Ossipov MH, et al. Time-dependent descending facilitation from the rostral ventromedial medulla maintains, but does not initiate, neuropathic pain. *J Neurosci* 2002; 22:5129–5136.

Calejesan AA, Kim SJ, Zhuo M. Descending facilitatory modulation of a behavioral nociceptive response by stimulation in the adult rat anterior cingulate cortex. *Eur J Pain* 2000; 4:83–96.

Chen Y, Mestek A, Liu J, Hurley JA, Yu L. Molecular cloning and functional expression of a mu-opioid receptor from rat brain. *Mol Pharmacol* 1993; 44:8–12.

Danziger N, Weil-Fugazza J, Le Bars D, Bouhassira D. Alteration of descending modulation of nociception during the course of monoarthritis in the rat. *J Neurosci* 1999; 19:2394–2400.

Dubner R, Bennett GJ. Spinal and trigeminal mechanisms of nociception. *Ann Rev Neurosci* 1983; 6:381–418.

Dubner R, Ren K. Endogenous mechanisms of sensory modulation. *Pain* 1999; Suppl 6:S45–53.

Dubner R, Ruda MA. Activity-dependent neuronal plasticity following tissue injury and inflammation. *Trends Neurosci* 1992; 15:96–103.

Dubuisson D, Wall PD. Medullary raphe influences on units in laminae 1 and 2 of cat spinal cord. *J Physiol (Lond)* 1979; 300:33P.

Dubuisson D, Wall PD. Descending influences on receptive fields and activity of single units recorded in laminae 1, 2 and 3 of cat spinal cord. *Brain Res* 1980; 199:283–298.

Evans CJ, Keith DE Jr, Morrison H, Magendzo K, Edwards RH. Cloning of a delta opioid receptor by functional expression. *Science* 1992; 258:1952–1955.

Fields HL. State-dependent opioid control of pain. *Nat Rev Neurosci* 2004; 5:565–575.

Fields HL, Basbaum AI. Central nervous system mechanisms of pain modulation. In: Wall PD, Melzack R (Eds). *Textbook of Pain.* London: Churchill Livingstone, 1999, pp 309–329.

Fields HL, Heinricher MM, Mason P. Neurotransmitters in nociceptive modulatory circuits. *Annu Rev Neurosci* 1991; 14:219–245.

Gebhart GF. Modulatory effects of descending systems on spinal dorsal horn neurons. In: Yaksh TL (Ed). *Spinal Afferent Processing.* New York: Plenum, 1986, pp 391–416.

Gebhart GF. Descending modulation of pain. *Neurosci Bio Behav Rev* 2004; 729–737.

Gebhart GF, Proudfit HK. Descending control of pain processing. In: Hunt SP, Koltzenburg M (Eds). *The Neurobiology of Pain.* Oxford: Oxford University Press, 2005.

Goldstein A, Tachibana S, Lowney LI, Hunkapiller M, Hood L. Dynorphin-(1-13), an extraordinarily potent opioid peptide. *Proc Natl Acad Sci USA* 1979; 76:6666–6670.

Gozariu M, Bouhassira D, Willer JC, Le Bars D. The influence of temporal summation on a C-fibre reflex in the rat: effects of lesions in the rostral ventromedial medulla (RVM). *Brain Res* 1998; 792:168–172.

Guan Y, Terayama R, Dubner R, Ren K. Plasticity in excitatory amino acid receptor-mediated descending pain modulation after inflammation. *J Pharmacol Exp Ther* 2002; 300:513–520.

Guan Y, Guo W, Robbins, MT, Dubner R, Ren K. Changes in AMPA receptor phosphorylation in the rostral ventromedial medulla after inflammatory hyperalgesia in rats. *Neurosci Lett* 2004; 366:201–205.

Haber LH, Martin RF, Chung JM, Willis WD. Inhibition and excitation of primate spinothalamic tract neurons by stimulation in region of nucleus reticularis gigantocellularis. *J Neurophysiol* 1980; 43:1578–1593.

Hammond DL. Persistent inflammatory nociception and hyperalgesia: implications for opioid actions in the brainstem and spinal cord. In: Brune K, Handwerker H (Eds). *Hyperalgesia: Molecular Mechanisms and Clinical Implications,* Progress in Pain Research and Management, Vol. 30. Seattle: IASP Press, 2004.

Hayes RL, Bennett GJ, Newlon PG, Mayer DJ. Behavioral and physiological studies of non-narcotic analgesia in the rat elicited by certain environmental stimuli. *Brain Res* 1978; 155(1):69–90.

Heinricher MM, McGaraughty S, Farr DA. The role of excitatory amino acid transmission within the rostral ventromedial medulla in the antinociceptive actions of systemically administered morphine. *Pain* 1999; 81:57–65.

Herrero JF, Cervero F. Supraspinal influences on the facilitation of rat nociceptive reflexes induced by carrageenan monoarthritis. *Neurosci Lett* 1996; 209:21–24.

Holden JE, Schwartz EJ, Proudfit HK. Microinjection of morphine in the A7 catecholamine cell group produces opposing effects on nociception that are mediated by alpha-1- and alpha-2-adrenoceptors. *Neuroscience* 1999; 91:979–990.

Hughes J, Smith TW, Kosterlitz HW, et al. Identification of two related pentapeptides from the brain with potent opiate agonist activity. *Nature* 1975; 258:577–580.

Hurley RW, Hammond DL. The analgesic effects of supraspinal mu and delta opioid receptor agonists are potentiated during persistent inflammation. *J Neurosci* 2000; 20:1249–1259.

Hurley RW, Hammond DL. Contribution of endogenous enkephalins to the enhanced analgesic effects of supraspinal mu opioid receptor agonists after inflammatory injury. *J Neurosci* 2001; 21:2536–2545.

Hylden JLK, Thomas DA, Iadarola MJ, Dubner R. Spinal opioid analgesic effects are enhanced in a model of unilateral inflammation/hyperalgesia: possible involvement of noradrenergic mechanisms. *Eur J Pharmacol* 1991; 194:135–143.

Kauppila T, Kontinen VK, Pertovaara A. Influence of spinalization on spinal withdrawal reflex responses varies depending on the submodality of the test stimulus and the experimental pathophysiological condition in the rat. *Brain Res* 1998; 797:234–242.

Kayser V, Chen YL, Guilbaud G. Behavioural evidence for a peripheral component in the enhanced antinociceptive effect of a low dose of systemic morphine in carrageenin-induced hyperalgesic rats. *Brain Res* 1991; 560:237–244.

Kieffer BL, Befort K, Gaveriaux-Ruff C, Hirth CG. The delta-opioid receptor: isolation of a cDNA by expression cloning and pharmacological characterization. *Proc Natl Acad Sci USA* 1992; 89:12048–12052.

Lima D, Almeida A. The medullary dorsal reticular nucleus as a pronociceptive centre of the pain control system. *Prog Neurobiol* 2002; 66:81–108.

Mansikka H, Pertovaara A. Supraspinal influence on hindlimb withdrawal thresholds and mustard oil-induced secondary allodynia in rats. *Brain Res Bull* 1997; 42:359–365.

Martin G, Montagne CJ, Oliveras JL. Involvement of ventromedial medulla "multimodal, multireceptive" neurons in opiate spinal descending control system: a single-unit study of the effect of morphine in the awake, freely moving rat. *J Neurosci* 1992; 12:1511–1522.

Mayer DJ, Liebeskind JC. Pain reduction by focal electrical stimulation of the brain: an anatomical and behavioral analysis. *Brain Res* 1974; 68:73–93.

Mayer DJ, Wolfle TL, Akil H, Carder B, Liebeskind JC. Analgesia from electrical stimulation in the brainstem of the rat. *Science* 1971; 174:1351–1354.

McMahon SB, Wall PD. Descending excitation and inhibition of spinal cord lamina I projection neurons. *J Neurophysiol* 1988; 59:1204–1219.

Miki K, Zhou QQ, Guo W, et al. Changes in gene expression and neuronal phenotype in brain stem pain modulatory circuitry after inflammation. *J Neurophysiol* 2002; 87:750–760.

Millan MJ. Descending control of pain. *Prog Neurobiol* 2002; 66:355–474.

Neil A, Kayser V, Gacel G, Besson J-M, Guilbaud G. Opioid receptor types and antinociceptive activity in chronic inflammation: both kappa and mu opiate agonistic effects are enhanced in arthritic rats. *Eur J Pharmacol* 1986; 130:203–208.

Ossipov MH, Hong Sun T, Malan P Jr, Lai J, Porreca F. Mediation of spinal nerve injury induced tactile allodynia by descending facilitatory pathways in the dorsolateral funiculus in rats. *Neurosci Lett* 2000; 290:129–132.

Pert CB, Snyder SH. Opiate receptor: demonstration in nervous tissue. *Science* 1973; 179:1011–1014.

Porreca F, Burgess SE, Gardell LR, et al. Inhibition of neuropathic pain by selective ablation of brainstem medullary cells expressing the micro-opioid receptor. *J Neurosci* 2001; 21:5281–5288.

Porreca F, Ossipov MH, Gebhart GF. Chronic pain and medullary descending facilitation. *Trends Neurosci* 2002; 25:319–325.

Ren K, Dubner R. Enhanced descending modulation of nociception in rats with persistent hindpaw inflammation. *J Neurophysiol* 1996; 76:3025–3037.

Ren K, Dubner R. Descending modulation in persistent pain: an update. *Pain* 2002: 100:1–6.

Ren K, Ruda MA. Descending modulation of Fos expression after persistent peripheral inflammation. *Neuroreport* 1996; 7:2186–2190.

Reynolds DV. Surgery in the rat during electrical analgesia induced by focal brain stimulation. *Science* 1969; 164:444–445.

Schaible HG, Neugebauer V, Cervero F, Schmidt RF. Changes in tonic descending inhibition of spinal neurons with articular input during the development of acute arthritis in the cat. *J Neurophysiol* 1991; 66:1021–1032.

Sugiyo S, Takemura M, Dubner R, Ren K. Trigeminal transition zone-rostral ventromedial medulla connections and facilitation of orofacial hyperalgesia after masseter inflammation in rats. *J Comp Neurol* 2005; 493:510–523.

Terayama R, Guan Y, Dubner R, Ren K. Activity-induced plasticity in brain stem pain modulatory circuitry after inflammation. *Neuroreport* 2000;11:1915–1919.

Terayama R, Dubner R, Ren K. The roles of NMDA receptor activation and nucleus reticularis gigantocellularis in the time-dependent changes in descending inhibition after inflammation. *Pain* 2002; 97:171–181.

Thomas DA, McGowan MK, Hammond DL. Microinjection of baclofen in the ventromedial medulla of rats: antinociception at low does and hyperalgesia at high doses. *J Pharmacol Exp Ther* 1995: 275:274–284.

Thompson RC, Mansour A, Akil, Watson SJ. Cloning and pharmacological characterization of a rat mu opioid receptor. *Neuron* 1993; 11:903–913.

Tsou K, Jang CS. Studies on the site of analgesic action of morphine by intracerebral microinjections. *Sci Sin* 1964; 13:1099–1109.

Tsuruoka M, Willis WD. Bilateral lesions in the area of the nucleus locus coeruleus affect the development of hyperalgesia during carrageenan-induced inflammation. *Brain Res* 1996a; 726:233–236.

Tsuruoka M, Willis WD. Descending modulation from the region of the locus coeruleus or nociceptive sensitivity in a rat model of inflammatory hyperalgesia. *Brain Res* 1996b; 743:86–92.

Turnbull ME, Guo W, Dubner R, Ren K. Inflammation induces tyrosine phosphorylation of the NR2A subunit and serine phosphorylation of the NR1 subunits in the rat rostral ventromedial medulla. *Soc Neurosci Abstracts* 2003; 29.

Urban MO, Gebhart GF. Supraspinal contributions to hyperalgesia. *Proc Natl Acad Sci USA* 1999; 96:7687–7692.

Vanegas H, Schaible H-G. Descending control of persistent pain: inhibitory or facilitatory? *Brain Res Rev* 2004; 46:295–309.

Wei F, Ren K, Dubner R. Inflammation-induced Fos protein expression in the rat spinal cord is enhanced following dorsolateral or ventrolateral funiculus lesions. *Brain Res* 1998; 782:136–141.

Wei F, Dubner R, Ren K. Nucleus reticularis gigantocellularis and nucleus raphe magnus in the brain stem exert opposite effects on behavioral hyperalgesia and spinal Fos protein expression after peripheral inflammation. *Pain* 1999a; 80:127–141.

Wei F, Dubner R, Ren K. Laminar-selective noradrenergic and serotoninergic modulation includes spinoparabrachial cells after inflammation. *Neuroreport* 1999b; 10:1757–1761.

Wiertelak EP, Roemer B, Maier SF, Watkins LR. Comparison of the effects of nucleus tractus solitarius and ventral medial medulla lesions on illness-induced and subcutaneous formalin–induced hyperalgesias. *Brain Res* 1997; 748:143–150.

Woolf CJ, Salter MW. Neuronal plasticity: increasing the gain in pain. *Science* 2000; 288:1765–1768.

Zhuo M, Gebhart GF. Spinal serotonin receptors mediate descending facilitation of a nociceptive reflex from the nuclei reticularis gigantocellularis and gigantocellularis pars alpha in the rat. *Brain Res* 1991; 550:35–48.

Zhuo M, Gebhart GF. Characterization of descending facilitation and inhibition of spinal nociceptive transmission from the nuclei reticularis gigantocellularis and gigantocellularis pars alpha in the rat. *J Neurophysiol* 1992; 67:1599–1614.

Zhuo M, Sengupta JN, Gebhart GF. Biphasic modulation of spinal visceral nociceptive transmission from the rostroventral medial medulla in the rat. *J Neurophysiol* 2002; 87:2225–2236.

Correspondence to: Ronald Dubner, DDS, PhD, Department of Biomedical Sciences, University of Maryland Dental School, 666 West Baltimore Street, Room 5E-08, Baltimore, MD 21201, USA. Tel: 410-706-0860; Fax: 410-706-0865; email: rnd001@dental.umaryland.edu.

Emerging Strategies for the Treatment of Neuropathic Pain, edited by James N. Campbell, Allan I. Basbaum, André Dray, Ronald Dubner, Robert H. Dworkin, and Christine N. Sang, IASP Press, Seattle, © 2006.

7

Opioids and Neuropathic Pain

Donna L. Hammond

Departments of Anesthesia and Pharmacology, The University of Iowa, Iowa City, Iowa, USA

Few topics in pain medicine have provoked as much controversy as the use of opioid drugs for the treatment of neuropathic pain. The debate crystallized with the publication in the late 1980s of two articles that reached diametrically different conclusions. One camp endorsed the use of opioid agonists, stating that adequate pain relief could be achieved provided there was systematic titration of the drug to an effective (often high) dose coupled with close monitoring of side effects (Portenoy et al. 1990). The other camp claimed that opioids were ineffective and inappropriate for the treatment of pain states that can persist for years to a lifetime due to their attendant potential for tolerance and dependence (Arnér and Meyerson 1988). These studies sparked (occasionally intemperate) discussions and disagreements among basic and clinical scientists alike, and although the storm of controversy has since abated, the topic remains of great interest. This chapter will briefly review basic tenets of opioid pharmacology, identify key issues in the debate, and review past findings and recent advances made in clinical and basic science investigations. It will also introduce a few possibly provocative issues concerning the extent to which laboratory-based research has provided sufficient guidance to clinical treatment.

OPIOID RECEPTOR AGONISTS: MECHANISMS AND SITES OF ACTION

Opioid receptors are seven-transmembrane-domain $G_{i/o}$-protein-coupled receptors. Three different types are recognized: mu, delta, and kappa. Activation of these receptors generally decreases Ca^{2+} conductances, increases K^+ conductances, and inhibits adenylyl cyclase (Dhawan et al. 1996; Kieffer 1997). Although subtypes of each receptor type are proposed to exist, the data are principally pharmacological in nature and are not necessarily strongly supported by molecular or genetic evidence.

Mu, δ-, and κ-opioid receptors are well positioned in both the periphery and the central nervous system to produce analgesia or to alleviate allodynia and hyperalgesia. Opioid receptors are present on the cell bodies of small-diameter neurons in the dorsal root ganglia (DRG) that give rise to Aδ and C primary afferent fibers that convey nociceptive information. Few are present on large-diameter neurons that give rise to Aβ fibers that convey tactile information (Arvidsson et al. 1995a,b; Ji et al. 1995). Although opioid receptor agonists do not produce analgesia when locally injected in the periphery, their antihyperalgesic effects are readily apparent under conditions of inflammation, in which the peripheral transport and availability of opioid receptors on the peripheral nerve endings are increased (Stein 1995). In the spinal cord, opioid receptor agonists inhibit the release of glutamate, substance P, and calcitonin gene-related peptide from the central terminals of primary afferent neurons (Aimone and Yaksh 1989; Pohl et al. 1989; Kangrga and Randic 1991), presumably by inhibiting Ca^{2+} conductances.

The μ-opioid receptor is the predominant opioid receptor in the spinal cord, with δ- and κ-opioid receptors making up the remaining 25% at best (Besse et al. 1990, 1991; Stevens et al. 1991b). Both μ- and κ-opioid receptors are found on dorsal horn neurons, but there is some disagreement as to whether δ-opioid receptors exist postsynaptically on dorsal horn neurons (Arvidsson et al. 1995a,b; Mennicken et al. 2003). Unlike the μ-opioid receptor, the δ-opioid receptor is largely confined to intracellular sites such as dense core vesicles and is not inserted in the plasma membrane. However, under conditions of agonist exposure or increased neural activity, the receptor is trafficked to the plasma membrane, where it would be expected to be more available to its ligand and to couple more efficiently to intracellular effectors (Cahill et al. 2001, 2003; Bao et al. 2003). Iontophoretic application of opioid receptor agonists on dorsal horn neurons causes hyperpolarization or decreases responsiveness to noxious stimuli. This action is mediated by an increase in K^+ conductance (Light and Willcockson 1999; Eckert and Light 2002). Consistent with their ability to presynaptically inhibit transmitter release from small-diameter primary afferents and to produce postsynaptic inhibition of dorsal horn neurons, μ-, δ-, and κ-opioid receptor agonists produce analgesia and alleviate hyperalgesia and allodynia after intrathecal or epidural administration (Yaksh 1993). Interestingly, recent data indicate strong phylogenetic differences in the distribution of δ-opioid receptors in the spinal cord of humans, primates, and rodents, such that δ-opioid receptors may be better positioned to modulate nociceptive transmission in humans than in rodents (Mennicken et al. 2003).

Mu-, δ-, and κ-opioid receptors are also located supraspinally in the amygdala, locus ceruleus, hypothalamus, periaqueductal gray, and rostral ventromedial medulla (Mansour et al. 1994). These nuclei are implicated in the modulation of nociception by their direct or indirect projections to the spinal cord. Direct injection of small quantities of μ-, δ-, or κ-opioid receptor agonists in any of these regions produces analgesia, which indicates that activation of these receptors in discrete nuclei is sufficient for the production of analgesia or the relief of allodynia or hyperalgesia (Porreca and Burks 1993). Two hypotheses have been put forward concerning the mechanisms by which opioids produce analgesia when administered into the periaqueductal gray or nucleus raphe magnus, two important sites for supraspinal modulation of nociception. One hypothesis is that opioids inhibit tonically active GABAergic neurons, resulting in the disinhibition or activation of pain inhibitory pathways that are normally quiescent. Another hypothesis is that opioids directly inhibit the activity of tonically active pain facilitatory neurons (reviewed by Hammond, in press).

SYNERGISM AND THE ACTIONS OF OPIOID RECEPTOR AGONISTS

Pharmacological synergism is operationally defined as the situation in which the total dose of drug required to produce a predetermined effect when administered at two (or more) sites is significantly less than the dose that is required to produce the same effect when the drug is administered to any one site alone (Wessinger 1986; Tallarida 1992). Activation of μ-, δ-, or κ-opioid receptors at any single site, such as by intraplantar injection in the hindpaw, by intrathecal administration to the spinal cord, or by microinjection into brainstem nuclei, is sufficient to produce analgesia or to alleviate allodynia or hyperalgesia. However, coincident activation of opioid receptors results in a considerable increase in analgesic potency. For example, coincident activation of μ-opioid receptors at spinal and supraspinal sites results in synergistic analgesia (Yeung and Rudy 1980; Adams et al. 1993), as does coincident activation of supraspinal and spinal δ-opioid receptors (Hurley et al. 1999; Kovelowski et al. 1999). Coincident activation of μ- and δ-opioid receptors at a single site, such as the spinal cord, also produces synergistic analgesia (Malmberg and Yaksh 1992). The concept of synergism is relevant to discussions of opioid effects in neuropathic pain states because nerve injury can lead to a loss or downregulation of receptors in various sites, with a consequent loss of synergism and a concomitant need to escalate the dose to obtain the same effect (Bian et al. 1999).

ARCHETYPE LIGANDS FOR THE OPIOID RECEPTOR

Highly selective agonists for the μ-opioid receptor include the alkaloid morphine, the peptide [D-Ala^2,NMePhe^4,Gly-ol^5]-enkephalin (DAMGO), and the phenyl piperidine sufentanil. Archetype ligands for the δ-opioid receptor include [D-Ala^2,Glu^4]-deltorphin (DELT), [D-Pen^{2,5}]-enkephalin (DPDPE), and the systemically bioavailable SNC80. Archetype ligands for the κ-opioid receptor include U69,593 and U50,488. These agonists and their corresponding archetype antagonists CTAP, naltrindole or TIPP*psi*, and nor-binaltorphimine are extensively used to probe the sites and mechanisms by which opioid agonists modulate nociception in preclinical investigations (Corbett et al. 1993), but few lend themselves to use in clinical investigations.

OPIOID RECEPTOR AGONISTS AVAILABLE
FOR CLINICAL INVESTIGATIONS

Few of the opioid receptor agonists available for clinical use approach the experimental drugs listed above in terms of receptor selectivity. Clinical investigations are essentially limited to morphine, fentanyl, alfentanil, oxycodone, and methadone, which bind to the μ-opioid receptor with high affinity. However, when the stimulus intensity is high, morphine can appear to be a partial agonist because it must occupy a large number of receptors to produce its full effect (i.e., it has a high fractional receptor occupancy requirement). Fentanyl and alfentanil are full agonists of greater potency and small fractional receptor occupancy requirements, but they have a shorter duration of action. Oxycodone and methadone are full agonists of particularly long duration. However, methadone has additional actions, including antagonism of N-methyl-D-aspartate (NMDA) receptors and inhibition of monoamine reuptake, that confound interpretation of its effects. Nalbuphine and butorphanol are clinically available κ-opioid receptor agonists. However, they are only partial agonists at the κ receptor and have coincident activity as antagonists at the μ receptor. As of yet, no δ-receptor-selective agonists are available for clinical use. Thus, clinical investigations of the utility of opioid agonists for the relief of neuropathic pain have been confined to those with affinity for the μ-opioid receptor. In this respect, oral sustained-release formulations of morphine and oxycodone, as well as a transdermal formulation of fentanyl, are important advances because they enable greater control of steady-state pharmacokinetic parameters in clinical trials.

CLINICAL INVESTIGATIONS OF OPIOID ANALGESICS
FOR THE RELIEF OF NEUROPATHIC PAIN

The reports of Arnér and Meyerson (1988) and Portenoy and colleagues (Portenoy and Foley 1986; Portenoy et al. 1990) summarized the extensive, yet very different, experiences of these investigators in the management of patients with long-term pain of nonmalignant origin. Despite the controversy, all parties recognized that treatment must be evidence-based. The continuing interest in this question, coupled with an increased sophistication in the design of clinical trials, prompted several placebo-controlled, randomized, double-blind studies that rigorously tested the hypothesis that opioids are (or are not) efficacious for the treatment of neuropathic pain. At the same time, another intense debate centered on the definition of neuropathic pain and on whether treatment (and investigation) should be based on the etiology (e.g., postherpetic neuralgia vs. diabetic neuropathy) or on the signs and symptoms as indicative of a mechanism (e.g., dynamic, stroking allodynia vs. punctate, static allodynia, vs. spontaneous pain) (Woolf et al. 1998; Jensen and Baron 2003). This latter debate has also shaped recent clinical trials of pharmacological agents in the treatment of neuropathic pain.

Several rigorous, appropriately designed clinical trials have now established the efficacy of opioids for the treatment of neuropathic pain. One approach has emphasized the use of homogeneous patient populations and examined the ability of opioids to suppress neuropathic pain of a specific etiology. Two such randomized, double-blind, placebo-controlled trials in patients with painful diabetic neuropathy established that controlled-release oxycodone administered for periods of 4–6 weeks significantly decreased pain intensity and increased pain relief; beneficial effects were detected within the first three days (Gimbel et al. 2003; Watson et al. 2003). Three randomized, double-blind, placebo-controlled trials in patients with postherpetic neuralgia established that intravenous (i.v.) morphine, controlled-release morphine, and controlled-release oxycodone afforded significant relief (Rowbotham et al. 1991; Watson and Babul 1998; Raja et al. 2002), Although a fourth study concluded otherwise (Eide et al. 1994), the dose of morphine administered (75 µg/kg i.v.) was quite low. In general, the primary outcome measures in these studies were changes in global pain intensity and pain relief as determined by visual analogue scales (VAS) and categorical scores. Concordant with the proposal of Portenoy and colleagues (1990), many of these studies involved an initial stage during which the dose of the drug was titrated to effect or until a maximally tolerated dose was identified. Although opioid medications were discontinued prior to enrollment, in many studies patients continued their non-opioid medications such as nonsteroidal anti-inflammatory drugs, tricyclic antidepressants, or anticonvulsants.

Only one randomized, double-blind, placebo-controlled trial of central pain originating from spinal cord injury or stroke has been conducted to date (Attal et al. 2002). This careful study used quantitative sensory testing to examine the effects of i.v. morphine on the symptoms of central neuropathic pain including ongoing spontaneous pain, mechanical allodynia and hyperalgesia, and thermal allodynia and hyperalgesia. The authors concluded that i.v. morphine was largely ineffective against ongoing, spontaneous pain, but that it significantly reduced stroking allodynia. There were no effects on the detection threshold or pain threshold for mechanical or thermal stimuli, or on mechanical or thermal hyperalgesia. Because this study examined a maximally tolerated dose of morphine for each patient, it cannot be argued that the lack of efficacy is secondary to a loss of potency and that efficacy could have been revealed had a suitably high dose been tested. A subsequent study of oral levorphanol in neuropathic pain, which included a subset of patients with central pain, arrived at a similar conclusion, although that study obtained a somewhat better outcome for neuropathic pain from spinal cord injury (Rowbotham et al. 2003). The results of these two rigorous trials support anecdotal reports that neuropathic pain of central origin is less responsive to opioid therapy than that involving peripheral injury (but see Dellemijn and Vanneste 1997).

In an alternate approach, other investigators examined the ability of opioids to suppress the different signs and symptoms of neuropathic pain irrespective of etiology. These studies used quantitative sensory testing to determine thresholds for the detection of thermal and mechanical stimuli, as well as pain thresholds for mechanical and thermal stimuli, and to characterize the presence of dynamic, stroking allodynia or punctate, static allodynia. The two double-blind, placebo-controlled studies of i.v. alfentanil conducted to date were concordant in their conclusions. Each ascertained that targeted plasma concentrations were reached, and one explored the concentration-dependent nature of the effect (Leung et al. 2001; Jørum et al. 2003). Alfentanil decreased dynamic, stroking allodynia and spontaneous pain, and also increased both the detection and the pain threshold for cold in a concentration-dependent manner (Leung et al. 2001). Jørum and colleagues (2003) similarly observed that i.v. alfentanil decreased spontaneous pain and dynamic, stroking allodynia. It also increased the temperature at which heat pain was detected and decreased the temperature at which cold pain was detected, without altering the threshold for detection of heat or cold. Moreover, the intensity of cold pain at threshold was lower, as determined by VAS scores.

The studies summarized above clearly established that morphine, oxycodone, alfentanil, and fentanyl, agonists that are selective for the μ-opioid receptor, are efficacious for the treatment of neuropathic pain in subpopulations of patients, particularly those with injury to peripheral nerves. Although the utility of these drugs is now firmly established, it should not be assumed that their potency and efficacy are unchanged in neuropathic pain states. In the studies summarized above, only a subpopulation of all patients met the criterion for a meaningful reduction in pain, defined as a decrease of at least 2 on a 0–10-point VAS or a 30–50% decrease in pain report (Farrar et al. 2000, 2001; Rowbotham 2001; McQuay 2002). Complete pain relief was obtained only in the occasional patient. At face value, the inability to produce complete pain relief in a large proportion of patients would suggest that opioids have decreased efficacy and so are not able to produce a full effect. However, these observations hold true not only for the partial agonist morphine, but also for full agonists such as levorphanol or alfentanil that have very high intrinsic activity and need to occupy only a very small fraction of available receptors to produce their maximal effect. Decreases in the maximal effect of such drugs are seen only when large numbers of receptors are removed or when coupling to G proteins is vastly reduced. Thus, partial relief of neuropathic pain may be an inherent characteristic of opioids as a class. An additional observation in these studies was that the effective doses were usually quite high. A significant number of patients experienced side effects such as constipation, nausea, and somnolence that led to substantial dropout rates of about 25% in every study in which these drugs were administered for longer than 4 weeks. These data suggest that the therapeutic index (the effective dose divided by the dose at which limiting side effects occur) for opioids is greatly diminished in neuropathic pain states. This finding would be concordant with a loss of potency and a rightward shift in the dose-response relationship for the analgesic effects of opioids.

Despite the common finding that opioids are efficacious in neuropathic pain, concerns remain with respect to their suitability for long-term administration (Harden 2002). A prospective study of the cognitive effects of oral administration of a sustained-release formulation of morphine over a period of 1 year reported no impairment of neuropsychological performance in a population of chronic noncancer pain patients (Tassain et al. 2003). These authors and others noted no escalation of dosages in those patients after 12 months of treatment (Dellemijn et al. 1998). This finding supports many anecdotal reports that patients with chronic pain of nonmalignant origin do not escalate their doses of opioids (Foley 2003), although it is acknowledged that concurrent maladaptive psychosocial factors can predispose patients to escalate their doses (Dellemijn 1999; Harden 2002). Despite the fact that patients will identify the opioid as a beneficial treatment at the conclusion of a study and convert to long-term, open-label use, only 10–25% are found to continue to use the opioid 6–12 months later (Dellemijn et al. 1998; Attal et al. 2002; Tassain et al. 2003). The predominant factors for termination of this medication are insufficient relief of pain or the occurrence of side effects (Dellemijn et al. 1998; Attal et al. 2002; Tassain et al. 2003). This finding suggests that rigorous prospective studies are needed in which tolerance and dependence are the primary outcome measures (and not secondary to determinations of opioid responsiveness). Studies of tolerance in cancer pain patients on opioid therapy are frequently confounded by the increase in pain that accompanies the metastatic nature of disease. In contrast, diabetic neuropathy or postherpetic neuralgia are long-term conditions with comparatively stable and well-characterized pain. Patients with these conditions could comprise a particularly suitable population in which to conduct rigorous studies of opioid tolerance with long-term use.

INVESTIGATIONS OF OPIOID RECEPTOR AGONISTS IN RODENT MODELS OF NEUROPATHIC PAIN

Many different rodent models of neuropathic pain now exist. Some models entail constriction, ligation, transection, or immune activation of the peripheral nerve (Bennett and Xie 1988; Seltzer et al. 1990; Eliav et al. 1999; Decosterd and Woolf 2000; Shields et al. 2003; Milligan et al. 2004). Other models entail injury to the nerve root (Kim and Chung 1992; Sheth et al. 2002). Some models mimic neuropathies associated with cancer chemotherapy (Aley et al. 1996; Polomano et al. 2001) or highly active antiretroviral therapy (Joseph et al. 2004). A rodent model of diabetic neuropathy involves the administration of streptozocin, a pancreatic islet beta cell toxin (Courteix et al. 1993), although, unlike clinical diabetes, it does not entail any loss of nerve fiber (Mandelbaum et al. 1983). Finally, at least two rodent models of central pain involving intraspinal lesions have been developed (Xu et al. 1992; Yezierski et al. 1998). At face value, animals in these models exhibit (to varying degrees) many of the symptoms reported by patients with neuropathic pain, including spontaneous pain behaviors, static or dynamic tactile allodynia, and thermal allodynia or hyperalgesia. The extent to which these models truly mimic the human neuropathic pain state is the subject of some controversy. Nonetheless, their availability has stimulated investigations of the molecular, pharmacological, and physiological mechanisms that contribute to the development and maintenance of neuropathic pain. They have also provided a means to test the potency and efficacy of pharmacological agents for the relief of neuropathic pain at the preclinical stage of drug development. The following paragraphs will briefly review the results of studies of opioid receptor agonists in several different rodent models of neuropathic pain. This section is not an exhaustive review of all work that has been performed, but it illustrates some of the mechanistic insights that these results provide.

Streptozocin-induced diabetes. Numerous authors report that the effects of both systemically administered (Courteix et al. 1998; Malcangio and Tomlinson 1998; Zurek et al. 2001) and intrathecally administered (Zurek et al. 2001; Chen and Pan 2003) μ-opioid receptor agonists are decreased in rats with streptozocin-induced diabetes. While these studies collectively demonstrate that opioid receptor agonists can reverse mechanical hyperalgcsia in this rodent model of diabetic neuropathy, whether opioids are truly less potent or less efficacious in diabetic states is more difficult to establish. The majority of these studies assessed mechanical hyperalgesia, none were conducted in a blinded manner, and all feature a flawed comparison of agonist potency or efficacy to nondiabetic controls (see below). However, other findings provide mechanistic evidence that opioids may be less potent or efficacious in this model. For example, both the volume of distribution and the clearance of morphine were increased in severely diabetic rats, whereas maximal plasma concentration and half-life were unchanged. These changes could effectively reduce plasma concentrations of free drug. The affinity and the number of μ-opioid receptors were unchanged in homogenates of whole brain (Courteix et al. 1998) or in the spinal cord dorsal horn of diabetic rats (Chen and Pan 2003). However, DAMGO-stimulated GTPγS binding was decreased in the spinal cord dorsal horn with no apparent change in levels of $G_{i/o}$ protein (Chen et al. 2002). Additionally, the ability of DAMGO to inhibit Ca^{2+} currents in DRG neurons also decreased in diabetic rats, although μ-opioid receptor number and affinity as well as the expression of $G_{i/o}$ protein in the DRG were unchanged (Hall et al. 2001). Collectively, these findings suggest that the opioid receptor couples less efficiently to G proteins in the diabetic state and provide a possible basis for findings that potency or efficacy of systemically or intrathecally administered μ-opioid receptor agonists are decreased in diabetic neuropathy.

Chronic constriction injury model. Systemic or intrathecal administration of μ-opioid receptor agonists can also reverse the thermal allodynia or mechanical hyperalgesia that accompanies chronic constriction injury (CCI) to the sciatic nerve in the rat. In an early blinded study, Guilbaud and colleagues determined that systemic morphine was equally, if not more, efficacious in suppressing vocalization evoked by pressure applied to the hindpaw of nerve-injured rats as compared to uninjured rats (Attal et al. 1991). When morphine was administered intrathecally, the dose-response curve in the ipsilateral hindpaw of injured rats was shifted to the right of that of sham-operated rats, suggesting a loss of potency (Yamamoto and Yaksh 1991). In contrast, the dose-effect relationship for intrathecal morphine for the contralateral, uninjured hindpaw of ligated rats in the thermally evoked paw-flick test was shifted five-fold to the *left* of that in naive rats, showing that the drug was more potent. Although they are frequently made in the literature, comparisons of the responses of ipsilateral hindpaws in injured and sham-operated rats are confounded because the baseline withdrawal latencies of the two treatment conditions differ greatly. Yamamoto and colleagues (1994) circumvented this problem in a later study by comparing the effects of intrathecally administered morphine on the ipsilateral hindpaw 1 and 5 weeks after CCI, when baseline paw-withdrawal latencies did not differ. They determined that the ability of morphine to increase thermally evoked paw-withdrawal response latencies 5 weeks after injury was much less than that at 1 week after injury, suggesting a time-dependent decrease in agonist potency after injury. Unfortunately, measurements of the contralateral hindpaw were not reported. In another approach, Mao et al. (1995) used a single intrathecal injection of the NMDA-receptor antagonist MK801 to normalize thermally evoked paw-withdrawal latencies between sham and ligated rats. These investigators demonstrated that intrathecal morphine was less potent, but not less efficacious, in both ipsilateral and contralateral hindpaws. A recent study reported that local injection of μ-opioid receptor agonists at the site of injury reversed thermal hyperalgesia and attenuated mechanical allodynia in this model (Truong et al. 2003). However, injection of opioid receptor agonists distal to the nerve injury, i.e., in the hindpaw, were ineffective (Aley and Levine 2002).

Investigations of μ-opioid receptor binding in the spinal cord after CCI have yielded conflicting results. The changes were often marginal when one considers the fractional receptor occupancy requirements of the agonists. For example, μ-opioid receptor binding increased bilaterally in lamina V and ipsilaterally in laminae I–II shortly after injury and then decreased to control values by day 10 (Stevens et al. 1991a). In contrast, δ-opioid receptor binding decreased bilaterally by day 10, with the largest decrease occurring ipsilaterally in laminae I–II. Levels of both μ- and δ-opioid receptor binding decreased 2 weeks after CCI and then subsequently recovered to control values between 4 and 15 weeks after injury (Besse et al. 1992). Mu-opioid receptor immunoreactivity increased by 28% in the ipsilateral dorsal horn after CCI, and this increase persisted for 4 weeks (Goff et al. 1997). In the DRG, the proportion of neurons that were immunoreactive for the μ-opioid receptor increased between 2 and 14 days after injury; later times were not examined (Truong et al. 2003). Collectively, these data indicate that the receptors necessary for opioid action in the spinal cord and primary afferents are not greatly affected by CCI. However, it has yet to be determined whether these receptors remain functional or exhibit changes in their phosphorylation state that result in a decrease in agonist potency or efficacy.

Spinal nerve ligation model. Several studies have concluded that intrathecally administered morphine was ineffective or substantially less effective in suppressing tactile allodynia (Lee et al. 1995; Bian et al. 1999), whereas it retained its ability to suppress thermal hyperalgesia (Wegert et al. 1997). As noted earlier, the very different response thresholds of nerve-injured and uninjured or sham-operated rats is a significant confounding factor. To circumvent this problem, Ossipov and colleagues (1995) examined the effects of intrathecal morphine on responses latencies to noxious thermal stimulus of the tail in nerve-injured and sham-operated rats. The tail-flick reflex is mediated by sacral primary afferents, and baseline tail-flick withdrawal latencies do not differ between ligated and sham-operated rats. In this model, intrathecally administered morphine retained its ability to suppress the thermally evoked tail-flick reflex, although it was significantly less potent (Wegert et al. 1997; Pertovaara and Wei 2003) or less efficacious (Ossipov et al. 1995) when paired with an intense thermal stimulus. Interestingly, the higher-efficacy μ-opioid receptor agonist DAMGO or the δ-opioid receptor agonist DELT produced a dose-dependent reversal of tactile allodynia, suggesting that poor anti-allodynic effects of intrathecal morphine may be specific to that drug or a function of its partial agonist actions (Nichols et al. 1995). The disparate efficacy of morphine (but not DAMGO) on tactile allodynia as compared to thermal hyperalgesia or thermal antinociception is intriguing. Opioid receptor agonists would not be expected to suppress tactile allodynia that is mediated by Aβ primary afferents because these large-diameter afferents do not express opioid receptors, whereas they would be expected to suppress thermal hyperalgesia or nociception due to their expression on small-diameter nociceptive afferents. However, the anti-allodynic efficacy of DAMGO and DELT do not support this interpretation. Moreover, this explanation hinges on opioid agonists having an entirely presynaptic site of action in the spinal cord, and on an assumption that nerve injury does not alter the expression of opioid receptors on the different populations of primary afferent neurons.

Multiple mechanisms could contribute to the relative lack of efficacy of intrathecal opioids in animal models. Spinal nerve ligation (SNL) is associated with a marginal and highly restricted decrease in the number of μ-opioid receptors and no apparent loss of coupling to $G_{i/o}$ proteins in the dorsal horn

(Porreca et al. 1998). It is also associated with a modest decrease in immu-nohistochemical staining of δ-opioid receptors in the spinal cord dorsal horn (Stone et al. 2004). It is not known whether these changes occur exclusively on primary afferent neurons, or whether transsynaptic effects may occur on postsynaptic dorsal horn neurons. Partial ligation of the sciatic nerve was recently reported to increase levels of immunoreactivity for the Ser357-phosphorylated form of the μ-opioid receptor in the spinal cord (Narita et al. 2004). Phosphorylation of the receptor results in its internalization and is a mechanism for its desensitization, which could contribute to the decreased effects of intrathecal morphine. Opioid receptor internalization can occur because of an increased release of endogenous opioid peptides. Thus, this finding suggests that nerve injury results in a compensatory increase in the release of endogenous opioid peptides in the spinal cord that bind preferen-tially to μ-opioid receptors, leading to their downregulation. Indeed, SNL induces greater tactile allodynia, although not greater thermal hyperalgesia, in μ-opioid receptor knockout mice than in wild-type mice, suggesting that injury results in tonic activation of spinal μ-opioid receptors (Mansikka et al. 2004).

Spinal nerve ligation was also found to increase levels of the endog-enous opioid peptide dynorphin in the spinal cord (Bian et al. 1999; Malan et al. 2000; Gardell et al. 2004). Dynorphin's actions are complex, and it may exert both pronociceptive and antinociceptive effects in the spinal cord. Dynorphin is an endogenous agonist for the κ-opioid receptor. Recent stud-ies in mice lacking the κ-opioid receptor provide evidence that nerve injury results in a sustained release of dynorphin that leads to phosphorylation and subsequent desensitization of κ-opioid receptors in the spinal cord (Xu et al. 2004). Mice lacking the κ-opioid receptor exhibited greater tactile allodynia and thermal hyperalgesia than wild-type mice (Xu et al. 2004). As a κ-opioid receptor agonist, dynorphin can also exert μ-receptor antagonist ef-fects (Pan 1998) that could contribute to the reduced effects of intrathecally administered μ-receptor agonists. In fact, intrathecal administration of anti-bodies to dynorphin restored the efficacy of intrathecally administered mor-phine in ligated rats (Nichols et al. 1997; Bian et al. 1999). Finally, dynorphin is rapidly metabolized, and its des-Tyr peptide functions as an agonist of the NMDA receptor (Lai et al. 2001), which has a well-documented pronoci-ceptive role in neuropathic and inflammatory pain. Tactile allodynia and thermal hyperalgesia are not sustained after SNL in mice that lack the gene for prodynorphin (Wang et al. 2001).

When administered systemically, morphine suppressed tactile allodynia after SNL, albeit often at doses that produce catalepsy (Lee et al. 1995; Bian et al. 1999; Pertovaara and Wei 2003). It also alleviated mechanical hyperalgesia and produced thermal antinociception (Pertovaara and Wei 2003). Given that morphine was largely ineffective by the intrathecal route, these reports suggest that a supraspinal site of action may confer the efficacy of systemically administered opioids. Consistent with this proposal, intracerebroventricular injection (Lee et al. 1995) or direct injection of morphine into the periaqueductal gray (Wei et al. 1998; Pertovaara and Wei 2003; but see Kovelowski et al. 2000) suppressed tactile allodynia or produced thermal antinociception with a potency and efficacy similar to that observed in sham-operated rats. The antiallodynic effects of morphine do not appear to involve activation or disinhibition of the conventional monoaminergic bulbospinal pathways because the effects were not reversed by intrathecal administration of monoaminergic antagonists, unlike the antinociceptive effects of supraspinally administered opioid agonists in naive rats (Lee et al. 1995).

Finally, it was recently advanced that activation of bulbospinal pain facilitatory pathways that arise in the rostral ventromedial medulla contributes to the maintenance of tactile allodynia and thermal hyperalgesia after SNL (Pertovaara 2000; Porreca et al. 2002). At least a portion of these neurons must express μ-opioid receptors, given that their destruction by microinjection of dermorphin-saporin in the rostral ventromedial medulla reversed established tactile allodynia and thermal hyperalgesia after SNL. It is interesting to note that an enhanced responsiveness to tactile and thermal stimuli, which could originate from bulbospinal influences, is observed bilaterally in both μ- and κ-opioid receptor knockout mice.

There are few studies of opioid action beyond those using behavioral measures. One study to do so used expression of the protein product of the early immediate gene *c-fos* as a marker of neuronal activation in the dorsal horn following nerve injury (Catheline et al. 2001). Although systemic morphine did not suppress the expression of Fos by dorsal horn neurons in nerve-injured rats in response to repetitive light touch, it did decrease the number of dorsal horn neurons in which Fos-like immunoreactivity was evoked by noxious thermal stimulation. Studies of the effects of intrathecally or systemically administered morphine on the responses of dorsal horn neurons in rats with SNL indicate that the effects were dependent on the stimulus modality and were time-dependent. Both an increase (Suzuki et al. 1999) and a decrease (Pertovaara and Wei 2003) in the effects of morphine have been reported.

THREE TOPICS FOR FURTHER CONSIDERATION

The development of animal models of neuropathic pain occurred in the very late 1980s, coincident with the debate on whether neuropathic pain was responsive to opioids. It is interesting to note how the idea that neuropathic pain is "opioid resistant" permeated the literature. Indeed, "insensitivity" to opioids was frequently invoked by many different investigators as evidence supporting the validity of a particular animal model of neuropathic pain. It now appears that too few basic scientists have closely followed the clinical literature or are cognizant of the findings that neuropathic pain can be effectively treated with systemic opioids. This discordance between findings made in many different basic science laboratories and reports from the clinic serves to highlight several issues that are rarely discussed. The first issue concerns the uncomfortable topic of "fulfilled expectations" in the performance of animal studies. The second issue concerns the very different criteria used to demonstrate efficacy in human and rodent studies. The third issue is a methodological confound encountered when one attempts to determine whether a drug is more or less potent or efficacious in the injured animal.

Comparatively few animal studies are conducted in a blinded manner due to the limitations of time and effort and the requirements of an often complex experimental design. If the results of unblinded or open-label clinical studies are viewed with some skepticism, should this not also be the case for unblinded preclinical studies? Indeed, many studies from my own laboratory are subject to this criticism. Whether they admit it or not, knowledgeable individuals will start a study with some form of latent expectation. Most studies are, after all, hypothesis driven. Also, most animal models of neuropathic pain involve an evoked response, the measurement of which is highly subjective. Nerve-injured rats frequently have a different posture than sham-operated rats, which will "unblind" the tester to the surgical condition of the animal. However, blinding to drug treatment within a surgical treatment group should still be possible. Raja and colleagues (Zhao et al. 2004) recently reported that morphine was highly potent and efficacious in suppressing tactile allodynia in two models of nerve injury in a dose range that was well below that associated with side effects when the drug was tested by persons blind to the treatment condition. Repeating a previous study under blinded conditions, Eisenach and Lindner (2004) came to a similar conclusion. Differences among laboratories in diet and housing conditions, in methods for assessment of thermal hyperalgesia or mechanical allodynia, in the type of nerve injury, and in animal species and strain must certainly be considered as contributing factors when comparing studies that begin with similar aims and end with different outcomes. However, given the many factors that can influence experimental outcomes, investigators should routinely seek to control experimental biases wherever possible. Effective blinding of staff to remove the *potential* for investigative bias and "fulfilled expectations" is an approach that should be encouraged where ever possible.

A second issue that merits further discussion concerns outcome measures. Outcome measures in animal studies are very different from those in clinical trials. In animal models, the primary outcome measure is the effect of the drug on specific modalities (stroking allodynia, punctate allodynia, or thermal hyperalgesia). However, relatively few clinical studies assess efficacy in terms of specific modalities. Drug effects on spontaneous pain behaviors are rarely examined in the rodent models; nearly all studies involve measurement of evoked behaviors. Yet, clinical trials frequently examine drug effects on spontaneous pain or pain at rest. Finally, in human studies, a modest change of 2 points on a VAS scale or a 30–50% reduction in pain intensity is considered a biologically significant and meaningful effect. In contrast, behavioral analyses of drug effects in rodent models usually involve measures on a continuum and tend to focus on a demonstration that the drug can produce a complete reversal or exhibit full efficacy, an expectation that may be unwarranted (or unnecessary) on the basis of clinical experiences. Should we aim for better concordance in outcome measures used in clinical trials and in laboratory investigations?

A third issue that merits attention is a methodological one. Many animal studies seek to compare drug efficacy and potency in the injured state to that in the uninjured state. However, these comparisons are inappropriate. In the uninjured state, opioids act to increase the threshold for detection of a noxious thermal, mechanical, or chemical stimulus *beyond normal values*. Their effect is to produce antinociception or analgesia. In the injured state, the thresholds at which thermal, mechanical, or chemical stimuli are perceived to be noxious are substantially decreased. Animals exhibit pain-like responses to nonpainful stimuli such as brush (i.e., allodynia) and exhibit increased pain responses to noxious stimuli (i.e., hyperalgesia). In the injured state, opioids act to *restore threshold to normative values*, to produce antiallodynia or antihyperalgesia. Hence, studies that attempt to compare the potency or efficacy of opioids in the injured state to the uninjured state are, in effect, comparing "apples" to "oranges." Uninjured animals do not exhibit spontaneous pain behaviors, allodynia, or hyperalgesia. Furthermore, attempts to compare by transformation of the data to percent control or percent maximal effect do not correct the problem, as the baseline threshold values in the treatment groups are very different. Indeed, transformation of the data can mislead the uninformed reader because the implicit assumption is that the baseline values do not differ.

CONCLUSION

It is not entirely clear that preclinical investigations to date have provided clinicians with needed guidance. For example, neuropathic pain often persists for months to years in patients, yet nearly all the behavioral analyses in laboratory rodents are short-term, focusing on the period from 3 to 21 days after injury. Few studies have examined the effects of long-term administration of opioids in rodent models of neuropathic pain. Such studies could provide mechanistic insight into the basis for the high dropout rate experienced in clinical trials over time and might identify concomitant pharmacological strategies to address this problem. The next decade should reveal many new insights into the mechanisms that mediate the onset and maintenance of neuropathic pain states. Now may be an appropriate time to evaluate how well the design of preclinical investigations has provided appropriate guidance to clinical investigations, and whether the findings of clinical investigations have been appropriately incorporated into hypothesis testing in the laboratory.

ACKNOWLEDGMENTS

This work was supported by RO1DA06736.

REFERENCES

Adams JU, Tallarida RJ, Geller EB, Adler MW. Isobolographic superadditivity between *delta* and *mu* opioid agonists in the rat depends on the ratio of compounds, the *mu* agonist and the analgesic assay used. *J Pharmacol Exp Ther* 1993; 266:1261–1267.
Aimone LD, Yaksh TL. Opioid modulation of capsaicin-evoked release of substance P from rat spinal cord in vivo. *Peptides* 1989; 10:1127–1131.
Aley KO, Levine JD. Different peripheral mechanisms mediate enhanced nociception in metabolic/toxic and traumatic painful peripheral neuropathies in the rat. *Neuroscience* 2002; 111:389–397.
Aley KO, Reichling DB, Levine JD. Vincristine hyperalgesia in the rat: a model of painful vincristine neuropathy in humans. *Neuroscience* 1996; 73:259–265.
Arnér S, Meyerson BA. Lack of analgesic effect of opioids on neuropathic and idiopathic forms of pain. *Pain* 1988; 33:11–23.
Arvidsson U, Dado RJ, Riedl M, et al. δ-opioid receptor immunoreactivity: distribution in brainstem and spinal cord, and relationship to biogenic amines and enkephalin. *J Neurosci* 1995a; 15:1215–1235.
Arvidsson U, Riedl M, Chakrabarti S, et al. Distribution and targeting of a μ-opioid receptor (MOR1) in brain and spinal cord. *J Neurosci* 1995b; 15:3328–3341.
Attal N, Chen YL, Kayser V, Guilbaud G. Behavioural evidence that systemic morphine may modulate a phasic pain-related behaviour in a rat model of peripheral mononeuropathy. *Pain* 1991; 47:65–70.

Attal N, Guirimand F, Brasseur L, et al. Effects of IV morphine in central pain: a randomized placebo-controlled study. *Neurology* 2002; 58:554–563.

Bao L, Jin SX, Zhang C, et al. Activation of delta opioid receptors induces receptor insertion and neuropeptide secretion. *Neuron* 2003; 37:121–133.

Bennett GJ, Xie YK. A peripheral mononeuropathy in rat that produces disorders of pain sensation like those seen in man. *Pain* 1988; 33:87–107.

Besse D, Lombard MC, Zajac JM, Roques BP, Besson JM. Pre- and postsynaptic distribution of μ, δ and κ opioid receptors in the superficial layers of the cervical dorsal horn of the rat spinal cord. *Brain Res* 1990; 521:15–22.

Besse D, Lombard MC, Besson JM. Autoradiographic distribution of μ, δ and κ opioid binding sites in the superficial dorsal horn, over the rostrocaudal axis of the rat spinal cord. *Brain Res* 1991; 548:287–291.

Besse D, Lombard MC, Perrot S, Besson JM. Regulation of opioid binding sites in the superficial dorsal horn of the rat spinal cord following loose ligation of the sciatic nerve: comparison with sciatic nerve section and lumbar dorsal rhizotomy. *Neuroscience* 1992; 50:921–933.

Bian D, Ossipov MH, Ibrahim M et al. Loss of antiallodynic and antinociceptive spinal/suprasinal morphine synergy in nerve-injured rats: restoration by MK-801 or dynorphin antiserum. *Brain Res* 1999; 831:55–63.

Cahill CM, Morinville A, Lee MC, et al. Prolonged morphine treatment targets delta opioid receptors to neuronal plasma membranes and enhances delta-mediated antinociception. *J Neurosci* 2001; 21:7598–7607.

Cahill CM, Morinville A, Hoffert C, O'Donnell D, Beaudet A. Up-regulation and trafficking of δ opioid receptor in a model of chronic inflammation: implications for pain control. *Pain* 2003; 101:199–208.

Catheline G, Le Guen S, Besson JM. Intravenous morphine does not modify dorsal horn touch-evoked allodynia in the mononeuropathic rat: a Fos study. *Pain* 2001; 92:389–398.

Chen SR, Pan HL. Antinociceptive effect of morphine, but not mu opioid receptor number, is attenuated in the spinal cord of diabetic rats. *Anesthesiology* 2003; 99:1409–1414.

Chen SR, Sweigart KL, Lakoski JM, Pan HL. Functional mu opioid receptors are reduced in the spinal cord dorsal horn of diabetic rats. *Anesthesiology* 2002; 97:1602–1608.

Corbett AD, Paterson SJ, Kosterlitz HW. Selectivity of ligands for opioid receptors. In: Herz A (Ed). *Handbook of Experimental Pharmacology*. Berlin: Springer-Verlag, 1993, pp 645–679.

Courteix C, Eschalier A, Lavarenne J. Streptozocin-induced diabetic rats: behavioural evidence for a model of chronic pain. *Pain* 1993; 53:81–88.

Courteix C, Bourget P, Caussade F, et al. Is the reduced efficacy of morphine in diabetic rats caused by alterations of opiate receptors or of morphine pharmacokinetics? *J Pharmacol Exp Ther* 1998; 285:63–70.

Decosterd I, Woolf CJ. Spared nerve injury: an animal model of persistent peripheral neuropathic pain. *Pain* 2000; 87:149–158.

Dellemijn P. Are opioids effective in relieving neuropathic pain? *Pain* 1999; 80:453–462.

Dellemijn PL, Vanneste JA. Randomised double-blind active-placebo-controlled crossover trial of intravenous fentanyl in neuropathic pain. *Lancet* 1997; 349:753–758.

Dellemijn PL, van Duijn H, Vanneste JA. Prolonged treatment with transdermal fentanyl in neuropathic pain. *J Pain Symptom Manage* 1998; 16:220–229.

Dhawan BN, Cesselin F, Raghubir R, et al. International union of pharmacology. XII. Classification of opioid receptors. *Pharmacol Rev* 1996; 48:567–592.

Eckert WA III, Light AR. Hyperpolarization of substantia gelatinosa neurons evoked by mu-, kappa-, delta 1-, and delta 2-selective opioids. *J Pain* 2002; 3:115–125.

Eide PK, Jorum E, Stubhaug A, Bremnes J, Breivik H. Relief of post-herpetic neuralgia with the *N*-methyl-D-aspartic acid receptor antagonist ketamine: a double-blind, cross-over comparison with morphine and placebo. *Pain* 1994; 58:347–354.

Eisenach JC, Lindner MD. Did experimenter bias conceal the efficacy of spinal opioids in previous studies with the spinal nerve ligation model of neuropathic pain? *Anesthesiology* 2004; 100:765–767.

Eliav E, Herzberg U, Ruda MA, Bennett GJ. Neuropathic pain from an experimental neuritis of the rat sciatic nerve. *Pain* 1999; 83:169–182.

Farrar JT, Portenoy RK, Berlin JA, Kinman JL, Strom BL. Defining the clinically important difference in pain outcome measures. *Pain* 2000; 88:287–294.

Farrar JT, Young JP Jr, LaMoreaux L, Werth JL, Poole RM. Clinical importance of changes in chronic pain intensity measured on an 11-point numerical pain rating scale. *Pain* 2001; 94:149–158.

Foley KM. Opioids and chronic neuropathic pain. *N Engl J Med* 2003; 348:1279–1281.

Gardell LR, Ibrahim M, Wang R, et al. Mouse strains that lack spinal dynorphin upregulation after peripheral nerve injury do not develop neuropathic pain. *Neuroscience* 2004; 123:43–52.

Gimbel JS, Richards P, Portenoy RK. Controlled-release oxycodone for pain in diabetic neuropathy: a randomized controlled trial. *Neurology* 2003; 60:927–934.

Goff JR, Burkey AR, Goff DJ, Jasmin L. Reorganization of the spinal dorsal horn in models of chronic pain: correlation with behaviour. *Neuroscience* 1997; 82:559.

Hall KE, Liu J, Sima AA, Wiley JW. Impaired inhibitory G-protein function contributes to increased calcium currents in rats with diabetic neuropathy. *J Neurophysiol* 2001; 86:760–770.

Hammond DL. Descending circuitry, opioids. In: Schmidt RF, Willis WD, (Eds). *The Encyclopedic Reference of Pain*. Berlin: Springer-Verlag, in press.

Harden RN. Chronic opioid therapy: another reappraisal. *APS Bull* 2002; 12:x–x.

Hurley RW, Grabow TS, Tallarida RJ, Hammond DL. Interaction between medullary and spinal delta-1 and delta-2 opioid receptors in the production of antinociception in the rat. *J Pharmacol Exp Ther* 1999; 289:993–999.

Jensen TS, Baron R. Translation of symptoms and signs into mechanisms in neuropathic pain. *Pain* 2003; 102:1–8.

Ji R-R, Zhang Q, Law P-Y et al. Expression of μ-, δ-, and κ-opioid receptor-like immunoreactivities in rat dorsal root ganglia after carrageenan-induced inflammation. *J Neurosci* 1995; 15:8156–8166.

Jørum E, Warncke T, Stubhaug A. Cold allodynia and hyperalgesia in neuropathic pain: the effect of N-methyl-D-aspartate (NMDA) receptor antagonist ketamine—a double-blind, cross-over comparison with alfentanil and placebo. *Pain* 2003; 101:229–235.

Joseph EK, Chen X, Khasar SG, Levine JD. Novel mechanism of enhanced nociception in a model of AIDS therapy-induced painful peripheral neuropathy in the rat. *Pain* 2004; 107:147–158.

Kangrga I, Randic M. Outflow of endogenous aspartate and glutamate from the rat spinal dorsal horn in vitro by activation of low- and high-threshold primary afferent fibers. Modulation by μ-opioids. *Brain Res* 1991; 553:347–352.

Kieffer B. Molecular aspects of opioid receptors. In: Dickenson AH, Besson JM (Eds). *The Pharmacology of Pain*. Berlin: Springer, 1997, pp 281–304.

Kim SH, Chung JM. An experimental model for peripheral neuropathy produced by segmental spinal nerve ligation in the rat. *Pain* 1992; 50:355–363.

Kovelowski CJ, Bian D, Hruby VJ, et al. Selective opioid delta agonists elicit antinociceptive supraspinal/spinal synergy in the rat. *Brain Res* 1999; 843:12–17.

Kovelowski CJ, Ossipov MH, Sun H, et al. Supraspinal cholecystokinin may drive tonic descending facilitation mechanisms to maintain neuropathic pain in the rat. *Pain* 2000; 87:265–273.

Lai J, Ossipov MH, Vanderah TW, Malan TP, Porreca F. Neuropathic pain: the paradox of dynorphin. *Mol Interv* 2001; 1:160–167.

Lee YW, Chaplan SR, Yaksh TL. Systemic and supraspinal, but not spinal, opiates suppress allodynia in a rat neuropathic pain model. *Neurosci Lett* 1995; 199:111–114.

Leung A, Wallace MS, Ridgeway B, Yaksh T. Concentration-effect relationship of intravenous alfentanil and ketamine on peripheral neurosensory thresholds, allodynia and hyperalgesia of neuropathic pain. *Pain* 2001; 91:177–187.

Light AR, Willcockson HH. Spinal laminae I-II neurons in rat recorded in vivo in whole cell, tight seal configuration: properties and opioid responses. *J Neurophysiol* 1999; 82:3316–3326.

Malan TP, Ossipov MH, Gardell LR, et al. Extraterritorial neuropathic pain correlates with multisegmental elevation of spinal dynorphin in nerve-injured rats. *Pain* 2000; 86:185–194.

Malcangio M, Tomlinson DR. A pharmacologic analysis of mechanical hyperalgesia in streptozotocin/diabetic rats. *Pain* 1998; 76:151–157.

Malmberg AB, Yaksh TL. Isobolographic and dose-response analyses of the interaction between intrathecal *mu* and *delta* agonists: effects of naltrindole and its benzofuran analog (NTB). *J Pharmacol Exp Ther* 1992; 263:264–275.

Mandelbaum JA, Felten DL, Westfall SG, Newlin GE, Peterson RG. Neuropathic changes associated with insulin treatment of diabetic rats: electron microscopic and morphometric analysis. *Brain Res Bull* 1983; 10:377–384.

Mansikka H, Zhao C, Sheth RN, et al. Nerve injury induces a tonic bilateral mu-opioid receptor-mediated inhibitory effect on mechanical allodynia in mice. *Anesthesiology* 2004; 100:912–921.

Mansour A, Fox CA, Burke S, et al. Mu, delta and kappa opioid receptor mRNA expression in the rat CNS: an in situ hybridization study. *J Comp Neurol* 1994; 350:412–438.

Mao J, Price DD, Mayer DJ. Experimental mononeuropathy reduces the antinociceptive effects of morphine: implications for common intracellular mechanisms involved in morphine tolerance and neuropathic pain. *Pain* 1995; 61:353–364.

McQuay HJ. Neuropathic pain: evidence matters. *Eur J Pain* 2002; 6(Suppl A):11–18.

Mennicken F, Zhang J, Hoffert C, et al. Phylogenetic changes in the expression of delta opioid receptors in spinal cord and dorsal root ganglia. *J Comp Neurol* 2003; 465:349–360.

Milligan ED, Maier SF, Watkins LR. Sciatic inflammatory neuropathy in the rat: surgical procedures, induction of inflammation, and behavioral testing. *Methods Mol Med* 2004; 99:67–89.

Narita M, Kuzumaki N, Suzuki M, et al. Increased phosphorylated-mu-opioid receptor immunoreactivity in the mouse spinal cord following sciatic nerve ligation. *Neurosci Lett* 2004; 354:148–152.

Nichols ML, Bian D, Ossipov MH, Lai J, Porreca F. Regulation of morphine antiallodynic efficacy by cholecystokinin in a model of neuropathic pain in rats. *J Pharmacol Exp Ther* 1995; 275:1339–1345.

Nichols ML, Lopez Y, Ossipov MH, Bian D, Porreca F. Enhancement of the antiallodynic and antinociceptive efficacy of spinal morphine by antisera to dynorphin A (1-13) or MK-801 in a nerve-ligation model of peripheral neuropathy. *Pain* 1997; 69:317–322.

Ossipov MH, Lopez Y, Nichols ML, Bian D, Porreca F. Inhibition by spinal morphine of the tail-flick response is attenuated in rats with nerve ligation injury. *Neurosci Lett* 1995; 199:83–86.

Pan ZZ. μ-Opposing actions of the κ-opioid receptor. *Trends Pharmacol Sci* 1998; 19:94–98.

Pertovaara A. Plasticity in descending pain modulatory systems. *Prog Brain Res* 2000; 129:231–242.

Pertovaara A, Wei H. A dissociative change in the efficacy of supraspinal versus spinal morphine in the neuropathic rat. *Pain* 2003; 101:237–250.

Pohl M, Lombard MC, Bourgoin S, et al. Opioid control of the in vitro release of calcitonin gene-related peptide from primary afferent fibres projecting in the rat cervical cord. *Neuropeptides* 1989; 14:151–159.

Polomano RC, Mannes AJ, Clark US, Bennett GJ. A painful peripheral neuropathy in the rat produced by the chemotherapeutic drug, paclitaxel. *Pain* 2001; 94:293–304.

Porreca F, Burks T. Supraspinal opioid receptors in antinociception. In: Herz A (Ed). *Opioids II*. Berlin: Springer Verlag, 1993, pp 21–51.

Porreca F, Tang QB, Bian D, et al. Spinal opioid mu receptor expression in lumbar spinal cord of rats following nerve injury. *Brain Res* 1998; 795:197–203.

Porreca F, Ossipov MH, Gebhart GF. Chronic pain and medullary descending facilitation. *Trends Neurosci* 2002; 25:319–325.

Portenoy RK, Foley KM. Chronic use of opioid analgesics in non-malignant pain: report of 38 cases. *Pain* 1986; 25:171–186.

Portenoy RK, Foley KM, Inturrisi CE. The nature of opioid responsiveness and its implications for neuropathic pain: new hypotheses derived from studies of opioid infusions. *Pain* 1990; 43:273–286.

Raja SN, Haythornthwaite JA, Pappagallo M, et al. Opioids versus antidepressants in postherpetic neuralgia: a randomized, placebo-controlled trial. *Neurology* 2002; 59:1015–1021.

Rowbotham MC. What is a 'clinically meaningful' reduction in pain? *Pain* 2001; 94:131–132.

Rowbotham MC, Reisner-Keller LA, Fields HL. Both intravenous lidocaine and morphine reduce the pain of postherpetic neuralgia. *Neurology* 1991; 41:1024–1028.

Rowbotham MC, Twilling L, Davies PS, et al. Oral opioid therapy for chronic peripheral and central neuropathic pain. *N Engl J Med* 2003; 348:1223–1232.

Seltzer W, Dubner R, Shir Y. A novel behavioral model of neuropathic pain disorders produced in rats by partial sciatic nerve injury. *Pain* 1990; 43:205–218.

Sheth RN, Dorsi MJ, Li Y, et al. Mechanical hyperalgesia after an L5 ventral rhizotomy or an L5 ganglionectomy in the rat. *Pain* 2002; 96:63–72.

Shields SD, Eckert WA III, Basbaum AI. Spared nerve injury model of neuropathic pain in the mouse: a behavioral and anatomic analysis. *J Pain* 2003; 4:465–470.

Stein C. The control of pain in peripheral tissue by opioids. *New Engl J Med* 1995; 332:1685–1690.

Stevens CW, Kajander KC, Bennett GJ, Seybold VS. Bilateral and differential changes in spinal mu, delta and kappa opioid binding in rats with a painful, unilateral neuropathy. *Pain* 1991a; 46:315–326.

Stevens CW, Lacey CB, Miller KE, Elde RP, Seybold VS. Biochemical characterization and regional quantification of mu, delta and kappa opioid binding sites in rat spinal cord. *Brain Res* 1991b; 550:77–85.

Stone LS, Vulchanova L, Riedl MS, et al. Effects of peripheral nerve injury on delta opioid receptor (DOR) immunoreactivity in the rat spinal cord. *Neurosci Lett* 2004; 361:208–211.

Suzuki R, Chapman V, Dickenson AH. The effectiveness of spinal and systemic morphine on rat dorsal horn neuronal responses in the spinal nerve ligation model of neuropathic pain. *Pain* 1999; 80:215–228.

Tallarida RJ. Statistical analysis of drug combinations for synergism. *Pain* 1992; 49:93–97.

Tassain V, Attal N, Fletcher D, et al. Long term effects of oral sustained release morphine on neuropsychological performance in patients with chronic non-cancer pain. *Pain* 2003; 104:389–400.

Truong W, Cheng C, Xu QG, Li XQ, Zochodne DW. Mu opioid receptors and analgesia at the site of a peripheral nerve injury. *Ann Neurol* 2003; 53:366–375.

Wang Z, Gardell LR, Ossipov MH, et al. Pronociceptive actions of dynorphin maintain chronic neuropathic pain. *J Neurosci* 2001; 21:1779–1786.

Watson CP, Babul N. Efficacy of oxycodone in neuropathic pain: a randomized trial in postherpetic neuralgia. *Neurology* 1998; 50:1837–1841.

Watson CP, Moulin D, Watt-Watson J, Gordon A, Eisenhoffer J. Controlled-release oxycodone relieves neuropathic pain: a randomized controlled trial in painful diabetic neuropathy. *Pain* 2003; 105:71–78.

Wegert S, Ossipov MH, Nichols ML, et al. Differential activities of intrathecal MK-801 or morphine to alter responses to thermal and mechanical stimuli in normal or nerve-injured rats. *Pain* 1997; 71:57–64.

Wei H, Panula P, Pertovaara A. A differential modulation of allodynia, hyperalgesia and nociception by neuropeptide FF in the periaqueductal gray of neuropathic rats: interactions with morphine and naloxone. *Neuroscience* 1998; 86:311–319.

Wessinger WD. Approaches to the study of drug interactions in behavioral pharmacology. *Neurosci Biobehav Rev* 1986; 10:103–113.

Woolf CJ, Bennett GJ, Doherty M, et al. Towards a mechanism-based classification of pain? *Pain* 1998; 77:227–229.

Xu M, Petraschka M, McLaughlin JP, et al. Neuropathic pain activates the endogenous kappa opioid system in mouse spinal cord and induces opioid receptor tolerance. *J Neurosci* 2004; 24:4576–4584.

Xu XJ, Hao JX, Aldskogius H, Seiger A, Wiesenfeld-Hallin Z. Chronic pain-related syndrome in rats after ischemic spinal cord lesion: a possible animal model for pain in patients with spinal cord injury. *Pain* 1992; 48:279–290.

Yaksh TL. The spinal action of opioids. In: Herz A (Ed). *Handbook of Experimental Pharmacology.* Berlin: Springer-Verlag, 1993, pp 53–90.

Yamamoto T, Yaksh TL. Spinal pharmacology of thermal hyperesthesia induced by incomplete ligation of sciatic nerve. I. Opioid and nonopioid receptors. *Anesthesiology* 1991; 75:817–826.

Yamamoto T, Shimoyama N, Asano H, Mizuguchi T. Time-dependent effect of morphine and time-independent effect of MK-801, an NMDA antagonist, on the thermal hyperesthesia induced by unilateral constriction injury to the sciatic nerve in the rat. *Anesthesiology* 1994; 80:1311–1319.

Yeung JC, Rudy TA. Multiplicative interaction between narcotic agonisms expressed at spinal and supraspinal sites of antinociceptive action as revealed by concurrent intrathecal and intracerebroventricular injections of morphine. *J Pharmacol Exp Ther* 1980; 215.

Yezierski RP, Liu S, Ruenes GL, Kajander KJ, Brewer KL. Excitotoxic spinal cord injury: behavioral and morphological characteristics of a central pain model. *Pain* 1998; 75:141–155.

Zhao C, Tall JM, Meyer RA, Raja SN. Antiallodynic effects of systemic and intrathecal morphine in the spared nerve injury model of neuropathic pain in rats. *Anesthesiology* 2004; 100:905–911.

Zurek JR, Nadeson R, Goodchild CS. Spinal and supraspinal components of opioid antinociception in streptozotocin induced diabetic neuropathy in rats. *Pain* 2001; 90:57–63.

Correspondence to: Donna L. Hammond, PhD, Department of Anesthesia, The University of Iowa, 200 Hawkins Drive, 6 JCP, Iowa City, IA 52242, USA. Tel: 319-384-7127; Fax: 319-356-2940; email: donna-hammond@uiowa.edu.

Emerging Strategies for the Treatment of Neuropathic Pain, edited by James N. Campbell, Allan I. Basbaum, André Dray, Ronald Dubner, Robert H. Dworkin, and Christine N. Sang, IASP Press, Seattle, © 2006.

8

The Role of Neuroimmune Activation in Chronic Neuropathic Pain and New Targets for Therapeutic Intervention

Donald C. Manning

Department of Anesthesiology and Pain Management, University of Virginia Health Sciences Center, Charlottesville, Virginia; Clinical Research and Development, Celgene Corporation, Summit, New Jersey, USA

Therapies for neuropathic pain directed at receptors and channels on neurons have been disappointing, with many suffering patients achieving only partial relief. This chapter will address an alternate and complimentary approach to thinking about and treating neuropathic pain involving the immune system. It will highlight the role of cytokines and neuroimmune activation in neuropathic pain or nerve trauma and offer a list of therapeutic strategies to address these mechanisms. In keeping with the spirit of the conference that inspired this volume, some of the therapeutic avenues will be unconventional.

Neuroinflammation is defined as the infiltration of immune cells into the site of injury in response to damage of the peripheral or central nervous system. Neuroimmune activation involves endothelial cells, microglia, and astrocytes, which when activated produce cytokines and chemokines and induce the expression of surface antigens to enhance the immune cascade independently of immune cell infiltration to the site of injury (DeLeo and Yezierski 2001). Peripheral nerve stimulation alone is insufficient to induce neuroimmune activation unless the stimulation is sufficient to result in damage to the nerve (Molander et al. 1997). The involvement of cytokines as chemical messengers of tissue trauma or illness is required. Wallerian degeneration can be viewed as the inflammatory response to axonal injury and is primarily attributable to the production of cytokines and chemokines from Schwann cells (Shamash et al. 2002). These cytokines and chemokines regulate macrophage responses and may facilitate myelin breakdown and clearance

(Perrin et al. 2005). Thermal hyperalgesia in mice following a chronic constriction injury (CCI) is temporally related to the onset of Wallerian degeneration, to macrophage infiltration, and to the presence of endoneurial tumor necrosis factor (TNF)-α, whereas mechanical allodynia is temporally related to nerve fiber regeneration. This point is emphasized in a strain of mice demonstrating delayed Wallerian degeneration, which display diffuse alterations in cytokine production and an abnormal onset and duration of neuropathic pain behaviors in response to nerve injury (Sommer and Schafers 1998; Shamash et al. 2002).

Damage to a peripheral nerve can initiate the recruitment of inflammatory cells to the site of injury. Macrophages can remove debris and secrete chemokines to recruit other immune cells and stimulate tissue regeneration (Stoll and Jander 1999). The predominant subtype of T cell defines the type of immune response to injury. Upon activation, CD4[+] T cells can differentiate into T-helper (Th) cells of two types. Type 1 (Th-1) cells generally produce proinflammatory cytokines, such as interferon (IFN)-γ, interleukin (IL)-1β, and TNF-α, that can augment the cellular immune response. Type 2 (Th-2) T-helper cells produce anti-inflammatory cytokines such as IL-4 and IL-10 that mediate humoral immunity, suppress macrophage function, and inhibit the production of pro-inflammatory cytokines. Following injury, T cells can infiltrate the injured sciatic nerve and contribute to thermal hyperalgesia and mechanical allodynia. Experiments utilizing passive transfer of Th-1 cells markedly enhanced pain hypersensitivity, while passive transfer of Th-2 cells had a modest inhibitory effect on pain hypersensitivity. The long-term presence of T cells in the injured nerve has been found to coincide with neuropathic pain behavior (Moalem et al. 2004). Th-1 and Th-2 subsets differentially affect sensitivity to neuropathic pain, which suggests that manipulation of the T-cell subsets and their response to injury could be a target for pain therapy.

Cytokines are not typically stored in cells but are regulated by gene transcription following a stimulus. In addition, the messages for most cytokines are unstable, and cytokine synthesis is therefore transient. Cytokines are pleiotropic in multiple ways. One cytokine can act on different cell types, limiting the utility of therapeutic administration of cytokines due to the development of many unwanted effects. Cytokines also are redundant in that multiple cytokines can exhibit the same functional effects. Antagonists to a single cytokine or alteration of a cytokine gene may have limited effects because other cytokines may be capable of compensating for the resulting loss of function. Cytokine production can promote the synthesis of other cytokines in a cascade mechanism. This secondary cytokine production can antagonize the first cytokine or act in synergy to enhance the effect. Often the outcome will depend upon the milieu surrounding the site of injury or trauma. Cytokines can exert their actions in a local autocrine or paracrine manner or act systemically in an endocrine fashion. Cytokines typically act by binding to ultra-high-affinity receptors on the cell surface such that only a few molecules are needed to effect a response. The concentration of cytokines in a tissue or in the plasma is often low, and thus the inability to detect a particular cytokine does not mean that it is not acting in a given situation. With the exception of TNF-α and chemokines (molecules that stimulate the migration of other immune cells such as macrophages), cytokines exert their actions by causing changes in gene expression, by triggering production of new molecules, or by altering the function of the target cell (Abbas and Lichtman 2003).

INTERLEUKIN–1

IL-1β levels increase early in both inflammatory and nerve injury animal models of pain (Murphy et al. 1995; Lee et al. 2004). Injection of exogenous IL-1β can induce thermal hyperalgesia and mechanical allodynia in the rat paw (Wagner and Myers 1996a; Sorkin et al. 1997; Sachs et al. 2002). However, direct nerve injury to the spinal root induces glial activation and enhances expression of IL-1β bilaterally in the dorsal and ventral horns of the spinal cord. This finding suggests a central neuroimmune reaction (Hashizume et al. 2000a) that is not confined to the innervation pattern of the nerve root. IL-1β is found in dorsal root ganglion (DRG) neurons and in Schwann cells. Intraneural injections of IL-1β can produce thermal hyperalgesia and mechanical allodynia, exhibiting a bell-shaped curve with dose-dependent activation at physiological concentrations and reduced firing rates at higher concentrations (Zelenka et al. 2005).

The type-I IL-1β receptor is highly expressed in intrinsic neurons of the dorsal horn in superficial laminae (Samad et al. 2001). Following peripheral inflammation, central injection of the naturally occurring IL-1β-receptor antagonist (IL-1RA) or an inhibitor of the IL-1β-converting enzyme blocked the induction of cyclooxygenase (COX)-2 protein and prevented mechanical hyperalgesia. IL-1β produced in peripheral tissues can enter the central nervous system (CNS) through a specific, saturable transport system in the blood-brain barrier (Pan and Kastin 2004) and induce central COX-2 isoenzyme expression. Indirect inhibition of COX-2 expression through disruption of IL-1β production or action may lead to safer anti-inflammatory approaches to pain than those which directly target the COX-2 isoenzyme.

IL-1β can attenuate the analgesic effects of morphine and may be to morphine tolerance mechanisms. Mice rendered genetically nonresponsive to IL-1β (through overexpression of IL-1RA or loss of the IL-1β receptor) have enhanced analgesia from morphine (Shavit et al. 2005). This finding is consistent with reports of IL-1β elevation in the cerebrospinal fluid of animals following chronic morphine administration. Shavit and colleagues (2005) suggest that the analgesic effect of chronic morphine administration could be enhanced through inhibition of IL-1b function within the spinal cord. Dynorphin-induced hyperalgesia and allodynia involve the action of IL-1b and activation of nuclear factor (NF)-kB and are reversed by IL-10 and IL-1RA (Laughlin et al. 2000).

TUMOR NECROSIS FACTOR ALPHA

TNF-α activity depends on its expression levels, on its activation from an inactive precursor, and on the availability of its receptors. The zinc-dependent protease family of matrix metalloproteinases (MMPs) releases TNF-α from its precursor and facilitates TNF receptor sequestration (Shubayev and Myers 2000). Within this group of proteases are the basal lamina-degrading gelatinases that play a role in Wallerian degeneration by (1) allowing macrophage transit though the Schwann cell basal lamina, the blood vessels, and the blood-nerve barrier; (2) inducing axonal degeneration; and (3) inducing local edema. Following CCI, two peaks of TNF-α are noted corresponding to peaks in pain behavior (Shubayev and Myers 2000). The first peak is derived from Schwann cells, local resident macrophages, and mast cells and corresponds with an increase in MMP-9 activity. The second peak, appearing 5 days after injury, probably represents TNF-α release from hematogenously derived macrophages and corresponds with an increase in MMP-2 activity. Therapeutically, MMP inhibitors and TNF-α protease inhibitor show variable abilities to downregulate TNF-α and TNF-receptor protein levels (Williams et al. 1996; Chandler et al. 1997; Sommer et al. 1997; Glaser et al. 1999).

At high concentrations, TNF-α can trimerize and form a membrane-inserted channel (Baldwin et al. 1996). The importance of this process in vivo has yet to be determined. Specific antibodies to one or more of the TNF-α receptors can block many TNF-α actions, so the mass action membrane insertion appears to be of minor importance.

TNF-α acts predominantly through two main receptors. The type 1 TNF receptor (TNFR1) is constitutively expressed, while the type 2 TNF receptor (TNFR2) can be induced (Vandenabeele et al. 1995). Within a few days after a crush-type or CCI injury to the murine sciatic nerve, TNFR1 expression modestly increases transiently at the site of injury (George et al. 2005) and mediates thermal hyperalgesia (Sommer et al. 1998b). TNFR2, on the other hand, is markedly increased immediately after injury and remained elevated for at least 28 days. When TNF-α binds to TNFR1 it is preferentially internalized, while interaction with TNFR2 leads to shedding of the complex. Thermal hyperalgesia has been attributed to TNFR1 only (Sommer et al. 1998b). The large increase in TNFR2 and shedding after TNF-α binding suggests that it can act as a TNF-α antagonist because the soluble TNF-α/TNFR2 complex is inactive (George et al. 2005). Antibodies against TNFR1 (but not TNFR2) reduce thermal hyperalgesia and mechanical allodynia in mice that have undergone CCI (George et al. 1999). The predominant subtype of receptor expressed on the target cells, either constitutively or induced by other cytokines, shapes the cellular response to TNF-α (Fontaine et al. 2002; Yang et al. 2002).

The main sources of TNF-α are glial cells and resident macrophages; it is not clear to what extent it is expressed by DRG neurons. TNF-α is constitutively expressed in the sciatic nerve tissue and is induced along with IL-1β in resident macrophages after injury (Brown et al. 1991; Griffin et al. 1993; George et al. 1999). Peripheral nerve injury or endotoxin challenge induces a large increase in TNF-α in non-neuronal DRG cells (possibly including macrophages, Schwann cells, endoneurial fibroblasts, and mast cells) (Ohtori et al. 2004). TNF-α and TNFR1-expressing microglial cells or astrocytes surround TNFR1-positive neurons (Ohtori et al. 2004). TNFR1 (but not TNFR2) mRNA is constitutively expressed in DRG neurons, in the dorsal root, in afferent fibers, in the dorsal root entry zone, and in laminae I and II of the dorsal horn (Holmes et al. 2004). After endotoxin challenge, TNFR1 was upregulated in neuronal and non-neuronal cells, but TNFR2 is only induced in non-neuronal cells (Li et al. 2004). The near-ubiquitous presence of TNFR1 in sensory neurons may belie their role as immunosensors (Weihe et al. 1991). A linkage to immune-competent cells in the periphery may allow activation during inflammation and immune reactions and may drive illness behavior and fatigue syndromes (Li et al. 2004). TNF-α may act in an autocrine fashion among microglia, inducing its own production and that of microglial IL-10, potentially acting in a negative autocrine feedback loop (Kuno et al. 2005). TNF-α is anterogradely transported in sensory fibers to innervated muscle, consistent with the observation that axotomized and intact muscle afferents develop ongoing activity following a peripheral nerve lesion (Michaelis et al. 2000). While TNF-α may be present in small neurons at baseline, its increase following injury has been observed exclusively in medium to large DRG neurons (Schafers et al. 2002). In this study, DRG cells were considered the primary source of the anterogradely transported TNF-α. TNF-α may also be taken up through the participation of TNFR1 and TNFR2 receptor systems (Shubayev and Myers 2001). Conflicting data regarding retrograde transport of TNF-α (Shubayev and Myers 2001; Schafers et al. 2002) may be related to the tracer used.

TNF-α immunoreactivity is greater in Schwann cells of patients with painful neuropathy compared to those with nonpainful neuropathy (Empl et al. 2001). Soluble TNFR1 is also elevated in the serum of patients with mechanical allodynia as compared to patients without allodynia (Empl et al. 2001). TNF-α is associated with phagocytosing macrophages, most intensely in acute vasculitis (Oka et al. 1998) and chronic inflammatory demyelinating neuropathies, but not in non-inflammatory neuropathies (Lindenlaub and Sommer 2003). In animal studies, TNF-α applied to the sciatic nerve (Wagner and Myers 1996a) or the dorsal root (Sorkin et al. 1997) increases firing in both C and Aδ fibers and reduces the mechanical threshold for paw withdrawal when injected intradermally (Cunha et al. 1992). TNF-α production in Schwann cells after nerve injury (Wagner and Myers 1996b) may mediate injury-associated signals to afferent fibers and could ultimately lead to neurodegeneration. Within hours of nerve injury, resident Schwann cells, fibroblasts, and endothelial cells in the endoneurium upregulate the production of TNF-α (Wagner et al. 1998). Anti-TNF-α antibodies reduce thermal hyperalgesia in both CCI and partial nerve transection mouse models of painful neuropathy, but mechanical allodynia is only reduced by intraoperative administration (Sommer et al. 2001). The TNF-α inhibitor etanercept inhibits both allodynia and p38 phosphorylation only when given before injury and intrathecally (Svensson et al. 2005). Systemic delivery of etanercept is only 50% effective. However, mice deficient in TNFR1 develop mechanical allodynia, but not thermal hyperalgesia, after CCI (Sommer et al. 2001). Enhanced mechanical allodynia is also observed in transgenic mice (with astrocytic targeted chronic expression of TNF-α) following peripheral nerve injury (DeLeo et al. 2000), suggesting a central role of TNF-α in neuropathic pain.

Several animal studies have implicated TNF-α and other cytokines in the etiology of radiculopathic pain and herniated nucleus pulposus-induced nerve damage (Igarashi et al. 2000; Olmarker and Rydevik 2001). Direct application of nucleus pulposus cells or of TNF-α or other cytokines is associated with increased and spontaneous neural activity in spinal root afferent fibers and pain behavior in animals (Olmarker and Larsson 1998). Human herniated disk samples can produce several inflammatory mediators such as TNF-α, IL-1α, IL-1β, IL-6, and granulocyte-monocyte colony-stimulating factor (Takahashi et al. 1996). TNF-α, when applied to exposed nerve roots, has effects that are even more pronounced than those of nucleus pulposus material (Aoki et al. 2002). TNF-α will produce myelin injury (Olmarker et al. 1993, 1994; Kayama et al. 1996), axonal degeneration (Kayama et al. 1996), nerve conduction block (Olmarker and Rydevik 2001), thrombus formation (Olmarker and Rydevik 2001), increased vascular permeability (Olmarker and Rydevik 2001), thermal hyperalgesia (Olmarker et al. 1996; Sorkin et al. 1997), mechanical allodynia, and ectopic discharges when applied in low physiological concentrations to the nerve root (Onda et al. 2002). In studies of nucleus pulposus material applied to exposed nerve roots with extracellular recordings of wide-dynamic-range neurons, TNF-α antibodies markedly reduce after-responses following noxious stimulation, while evoked responses are not inhibited (Onda et al. 2003). Application of TNF-α antibodies to a rat nerve root can partially prevent the nucleus pulposus-induced abnormal nerve discharges (Onda et al. 2003) and nucleus pulposus-induced histological changes (Murata et al. 2004). Nerve roots injured by compression are sensitized to the excitatory effects of TNF-α application (Liu et al. 2002; Schafers et al. 2003).

TNF-α is localized in neurons in several norepinephrine-rich areas of the brain including the locus ceruleus and the hippocampus (Covey et al. 2002). TNF-α in these regions acts in concert with α_2-adrenergic receptors to inhibit norepinephrine release. During persistent neuropathic pain induced by CCI, TNF-α levels increase in these brain regions, and there is greater α_2-adrenergic receptor/TNF-α-induced inhibition of norepinephrine release, resulting in decreased norepinephrine function (Covey et al. 2000). Infusion of anti-TNF-α antibodies reverses the thermal hyperalgesia and hyperalgesia. In naive rats, intracerebroventricular infusion of recombinant TNF-α can induce thermal hyperalgesia and mechanical allodynia (Ignatowski et al. 1999). Activation of α_2-adrenergic receptors increases TNF-α production in primary hippocampal neurons (Renauld and Spengler 2002). Administration of a tricyclic antidepressant, either desipramine or amitriptyline, reduces neuron-localized TNF-α (Ignatowski et al. 1997). After chronic administration of desipramine, zimelidine (Nickola et al. 2000), or amitriptyline (Reynolds et al. 2004a), the TNF-α inhibition of norepinephrine release reverses to facilitation. TNF-α has also been implicated in the antidepressant activity of desipramine in the forced swim model of depression (Reynolds et al. 2004b). These findings suggest that TNF-α is involved in therapeutic actions of tricyclic antidepressants in pain and depression. In the periphery, α_2-adrenergic receptor stimulation increases the endotoxin-stimulated production and release of TNF-α in macrophages (Spengler et al. 1990), whereas β-adrenergic receptor stimulation decreases TNF-α production in macrophages and microglia (Spengler et al. 1994; Kaneko et al. 2005). Thus, the sympathetic system may influence the somatosensory system through a cytokine mechanism.

Neuronal apoptosis or cell death has been reported in the dorsal horn of rats after CCI or axotomy (Sugimoto et al. 1990; Whiteside and Munglani 2001). Such apoptosis may occur in a small subpopulation of cells because the total cell count does not significantly decrease (Polgar et al. 2004). Selective dorsal horn neuronal loss may contribute to pain hypersensitivity in these animals through a temporary loss of inhibitory neurons (Ibuki et al. 1997), although this conclusion has recently been challenged (Polgar et al. 2003). An understanding of this apoptotic response and a means to prevent it could have potential value in treating neuropathic pain and its consequences. TNF-α enhances AMPA/kainate-receptor-mediated neuronal injury and plasticity by inducing a rapid upregulation of calcium-permeable AMPA/ kainate channels (Ogoshi et al. 2005) and an increase in cell-surface AMPA receptors (Beattie et al. 2002). TNF-α may also be indirectly involved in neurodegeneration and plasticity by inducing the release (Bezzi et al. 2001) and inhibiting the uptake (Fine et al. 1996) of glutamate by astrocytes and microglia. Astrocytes normally take up glutamate to reduce neuronal exposure, but this uptake is inhibited in a dose-dependent manner by TNF-α (Hu et al. 2000; Shaked et al. 2005). Glutamate is also released by activated microglia to act via microglial NMDA receptors in an autocrine fashion to stimulate release of TNF-α (Piani et al. 1992; Bezzi and Volterra 2001). Combined deletion of the genes for TNF-α receptors 1 and 2 almost completely prevents motor neuron cell death after facial axotomy in the adult mouse. These data highlight the role of TNF-α and both subtypes of TNF receptor in the early phase of neuronal cell loss following traumatic neuronal injury (Raivich et al. 2002). The degree of neurodegeneration may be more extensive if the supply of TNF-α is sustained for longer periods.

INTERLEUKIN-6

TNF-α and IL-1β play important roles in the initiation of persistent neuropathic pain, whereas delayed IL-6 production is a factor in the maintenance of such pain. This pattern is reversed in axotomy models, with IL-1β and IL-6 peaking earlier than TNF-α (Murphy et al. 1995). Interleukin-6 is one of a family of several similar molecules that act in both paracrine and endocrine fashion. Members of the IL-6 family are grouped according to their three-dimensional shape; they can interact with unique receptors, but they all act through a common mediator, gp130 (Gadient and Otten 1997). When dimerized by an activated receptor, gp130 can activate intracellular kinases and influence gene transcription. Members of the IL-6 family include leukemia inhibitory factor, ciliary neurotrophic factor, IL-6, and IL-11 (De Jongh et al. 2003). Members of the IL-6 family, like other cytokines, are pluripotent, with broad effects on hematopoiesis, immune response, and inflammation as well as on the induction of acute-phase reactants. Acute-phase reactants are plasma proteins, primarily synthesized in the liver, whose plasma concentrations increase in response to trauma, infection, or direct action of cytokines. These proteins play a role in the innate immune response (Abbas and Lichtman 2003).

IL-6 acts through a specific receptor that is expressed on lymphocytes, macrophages, and other immune cells. Within the nervous system, mRNA for both IL-6 and its receptor are expressed in the hippocampus, neocortex, cerebellum, neurons, and astrocytes (Gadient and Otten 1997). The IL-6 receptor is easily shed by proteolysis; however, the resulting soluble receptor can still complex with many cell types. Thus, the influence of the IL-6 complex is expanded by the immune cell supply of IL-6 receptor. Most soluble receptors act as antagonists, but those for IL-6 function as agonists when coupled with IL-6, a process known as "trans-signaling" (Heinrich et al. 2003). IL-6 mRNA is expressed at low levels in spinal cord neurons in the dorsal horn and is upregulated following peripheral nerve injury, where it may play a role in nociceptive processing at the spinal level (Arruda et al. 1998). IL-6 mRNA is not detected in the normal rat sciatic nerve, but it can be induced in Schwann cells distal to a sciatic nerve crush (Bolin et al. 1995). Upregulation of the IL-6 and IL-6 receptor message is observed in medium to large sensory neurons following nerve injury or axotomy (Bolin et al. 1995; Lee et al. 2004). While gp130 is found in nearly all DRG neurons and is constitutively expressed (Obreja et al. 2002), only 33% of such neurons in one study were able to form functional receptor complexes (Segond et al. 2005). IL-6 is localized in human DRG in more than 75% of cells and co-localized with substance P and CGRP in more than 60% of cells (Nordlind et al. 2000). Membrane depolarization and neuronal activity itself can induce IL-6 in neurons (Sallmann et al. 2000). The depolarization-responsive factor appears to be the glucocorticoid response element-2, possibly accounting for the net inhibitory effect of glucocorticoids on IL-6 transcription (Ray et al. 1990).

IL-6 can exert both neuroprotective and neurodegenerative actions (Gadient and Otten 1997; Okada et al. 2004). IL-6 expression in neurons contributes to activation of glial cells (Klein et al. 1997) and supports the regeneration of peripheral nerves after injury (Zhong et al. 1999); however, chronic exposure can lead to neurodegeneration (Campbell et al. 1993; Qiu et al. 1998). Intrathecal or intraplantar administration of IL-6 in rats with a

CCI mononeuropathy increases cold allodynia (Vissers et al. 2005). Intrathecal injection of IL-6 soluble receptor or IL-6 neutralizing antibody attenuates nerve-injury-induced mechanical allodynia (DeLeo et al. 1996). In other settings, exogenously applied IL-6 reduces neural firing in a model of mechanical allodynia (Flatters et al. 2003). IL-6 does not directly stimulate neurons, but the IL-6 receptor complex can potentiate heat-activated ionic currents in nociceptors through the phosphorylation of TRPV1 molecules (Obreja et al. 2005). Some of the variability of response to IL-6 may stem from the lack of baseline IL-6 receptors in neurons and from the need to stimulate these neurons with a combination of IL-6 and its receptor. In IL-6 knockout animals, mechanical hyperalgesia is attenuated without an effect on thermal hyperalgesia (Ramer et al. 1998). The pleiotropic nature of the IL-6 family is both a challenge and an opportunity. In the same chronic pain condition, several of the family members are present but may act in opposing manners. In certain arthritis models, for example, IL-11 is anti-inflammatory and IL-6 is pro-inflammatory (Gadient and Patterson 1999). The actions of IL-6 may be state dependent and, as Flatters and colleagues (2003, 2004) have proposed, may intriguingly be both pro-inflammatory and antinociceptive under certain conditions. IL-6 (Borner et al. 2004) and other cytokines (Ruzicka et al. 1996; Kraus et al. 2001) can induce the expression of μ-opioid receptors, and morphine can increase IL-6 levels in the plasma (Houghtling et al. 2000) and spinal cord (Raghavendra et al. 2002).

IL-6, whether induced by injury or exogenously applied, forms sympathetic baskets in the DRG (Ramer et al. 1999); IL-6 knockout mice have greatly reduced sympathetic basket formation (Ramer et al. 1998). The invasion of DRG by sympathetic nerves has been linked to mechanical allodynia (Ramer et al. 1999). IL-6 may contribute to human pain states. Herniated lumbar disks produce increased amounts of IL-6 relative to nonherniated disks (Kang et al. 1996) and are associated with mechanical hyperalgesia following surgery. An IL-6 gene variation associated with increased expression and plasma levels of IL-6 has been identified in patients with herniated disks characterized by sciatica (Noponen-Hietala et al. 2005). Patients with persistent pain 8 weeks after diskectomy have a significantly elevated IL-6 level compared to pain-free volunteers (Geiss et al. 1997).

INTERLEUKIN-10

IL-10 is the prototypical anti-inflammatory cytokine. It can act in an antagonistic manner to reverse or oppose many of the actions of pro-inflammatory cytokines. IL-10 can inhibit the production, release, and activity of

TNF-α, IL-1β, and IL-6; it can inhibit p38 MAP kinase and NF-κB activation and can downregulate the receptors for pro-inflammatory cytokines (reviewed in Watkins and Maier 2003). IL-10 can be secreted from infiltrating macrophages and lymphocytes to suppress ongoing inflammation. Augmentation of IL-10 appears to be attractive for managing neuropathic pain associated with glial activation because IL-10 inhibits only the pathological functions and increased cytokine activity and does not alter basal activity. Gene therapy methods have been developed to augment IL-10 release, but the delivery system is awkward. IL-10 therapy may be complicated because this cytokine can downregulate the expression of its own receptor in an autocrine or paracrine negative feedback system (Ledeboer et al. 2002). Studies with IL-10 knockout animals or administration of anti-IL-10 antibodies have demonstrated decreased thermal hyperalgesia, suggesting that endogenous IL-10 contributes to nociception (Tu et al. 2003). Clearly, more work is needed to elucidate this area.

FRACTALKINE

Another potential signal for glial activation comes from the neuron itself. The chemokine fractalkine is exclusively expressed on neurons, particularly spinal neurons and sensory afferents, and is clipped off during high levels of neural stimulation to act on fractalkine receptors located exclusively on microglial cells (Verge et al. 2004). Thus, fractalkine represents a true neuron-to-glia messenger (Bacon and Harrison 2000; Hatori et al. 2002). Intrathecal administration of a fractalkine-neutralizing antibody prevents the onset of mechanical allodynia in sciatic inflammatory neuropathy and is even effective when administered 5–7 days after the injury. Intrathecal administration of fractalkine produces dose-dependent mechanical allodynia and thermal hyperalgesia (Milligan et al. 2004).

BEHAVIORAL ISSUES

Cytokine involvement in chronic pain derives from a much broader view of injury-related behavior termed the "sickness response." This response is composed of a wide range of changes initiated by a peripheral immune or inflammatory challenge (Maier and Watkins 1998). The sickness response includes fever, increased white blood count, activation of the hypothalamic-pituitary-adrenal axis, sympathetic nervous system arousal, decreased social interaction, decreased food and water intake, and increased sensitivity to pain (Wieseler-Frank et al. 2005). Chronic pain is often associated with behavioral and cognitive alterations. A marked dysregulation (increased levels and shifted circadian cycle) of IL-6 secretion has been reported in patients with major depressive disorder (Alesci et al. 2005). Increased levels of IL-6 following diskectomy are associated with depressed mood, increased self-reported stress, and altered morning cortisol secretion (Geiss et al. 1997). This finding is consistent with other reports of behavioral changes associated with prolonged elevated IL-6 levels (Geiss et al. 1997; Papanicolaou et al. 1998). Infusion of IL-1β or TNF-α for adjuvant cancer chemotherapy is associated with an incidence of nearly 50% of pain syndromes or complaints of pain and tenderness at the injection site (Kemeny et al. 1990; Del Mastro et al. 1995; Elkordy et al. 1997). Immune activation also is associated with a decrease in mood and cognitive function, a common adverse effect of cytokine administration for cancer (Meyers 1999). IL-6 is also associated with inhibition of certain types of learning and memory (Balschun et al. 2004). These findings suggest that some of the behavioral consequences of chronic pain may have an origin in increased IL-6 levels. Conclusions from exogenous cytokine administrations are limited due to the general illness of the patients and the large doses of cytokines that are given, which may contribute to physical illness and could account in part for the behavioral and cognitive changes observed. To address this problem, Reichenberg and colleagues (2001) administered doses of endotoxin to trigger an inflammatory response just short of physical symptoms in normal subjects. After the administration of endotoxin, the subjects reported significantly increased levels of anxiety and depressed mood and decreases in verbal and nonverbal memory. All these behavioral symptoms were significantly correlated with elevated levels of cytokines including TNF-α, IL-1RA, IL-6, and soluble TNF-α receptor (Reichenberg et al. 2001).

GLIA

Glia are recognized as essential participants in the initial and sustained response to injury and in the generation of neuropathic pain (reviewed in Covey et al. 2000; Watkins and Maier 2003; Wieseler-Frank et al. 2004). DeLeo and associates have shown over several studies that microglia are involved in the initial phase of pain hypersensitivity followed by astrocytic involvement in the maintenance phase (Raghavendra et al. 2003; Tanga et al. 2004).

Microglia are the principle sources of the pro-inflammatory cytokines IL-1β, IL-6, and TNF-α as well as the anti-inflammatory cytokines IL-10 and IL-1RA (Aloisi 2001). Microglia, part of the innate immune system, can initiate the response to injury that can be shaped and controlled by T cells, part of the adaptive immune system. The disruption of this highly controlled and balanced system of interaction between the innate and adaptive immune systems could lead to unregulated inflammation and neurodegeneration and chronic pain. The pluripotentiality of microglia allows these cells to engage in a neuroimmune dialogue (Shaked et al. 2005) that is regulated by the adaptive immune system in physiological conditions but converts to a destructive phenotype in pathological situations. Microglia can therefore be either protective or destructive, depending upon the immune and chemical microenvironment.

What is the link between nerve injury and microglial activation? Partial but significant reduction in hyperalgesia and allodynia behavior can be accomplished by interfering with the function of Toll-like receptor-4 (TLR-4) in microglia (Tanga et al. 2005). TLR-4 functions in the innate immune system as a stable pattern recognition receptor for invariant structures of pathogens. TLR-4 are transmembrane receptors with a cytoplasmic signaling domain; they are similar to the cytoplasmic portion of the IL-1 receptor and have the ability to activate the same pathways as IL-1β. Activation of TLR-4 is linked to activation of nuclear transcription factor kappa B (NF-κB) and to induction of COX-2 and other inflammatory mediators. TLR-4 occurs exclusively on microglia in the rat CNS (Lehnardt et al. 2003). TLR-4 can be activated by bacterial wall molecules such as endotoxins or lipopolysaccharide and by endogenous ligands such as heat shock proteins, proteoglycans, and saturated fatty acids released after neural injury and degeneration (Hwang 2001; Lee et al. 2001). In addition, Toll-like receptors control the activation of antigen-specific Th-1 and Th-2 immune responses. Mice lacking TLR4 function either through genetic alteration or through the use of a TLR-4 antisense oligodeoxynucleotide display significantly reduced (but not absent) pain hypersensitivity and reduced expression of mRNA for microglial markers of activation and proinflammatory cytokines (IFNγ, IL-1β, and TNF-α) following L5 nerve transection (Tanga et al. 2005).

Leukocyte trafficking into the spinal cord increases over time following nerve root injury (Rutkowski et al. 2002). Intercellular cell adhesion molecule 1 (ICAM-1) and platelet endothelial cell adhesion molecule (PECAM) can facilitate hematogenously derived leukocyte infiltration to the CNS. Peripheral inflammation mediated by proinflammatory cytokine activation of the NF-κB signaling pathway can trigger ICAM and PECAM expression, whereas nerve injury precipitates expression of ICAM and PECAM as well as major histocompatibility complex (MHC) class II, coincident with the development of bilateral mechanical hypersensitivity (Sweitzer et al. 2002). Infiltrating leukocytes can interact with microglia expressing MHC class II molecules and can act as antigen-presenting cells. Following presentation of antigen in the context of the appropriate MHC molecule, full T-cell activation depends upon the presence of a second positive stimulus or costimulatory factor. The B7 family of costimulators is upregulated in neural tissue damaged through trauma or inflammation. B7.1 and B7.2 are both single-chain glycoproteins, with two extracellular Ig-like domains, a transmembrane segment, and a cytoplasmic tail (Abbas and Lichtman 2003). The B7.2 molecule has been associated with protective immunity, whereas B7.1, another costimulatory molecule, has been associated with destructive immunity such as that observed in multiple sclerosis. Inhibition or elimination of microglial MHC class II expression can reduce pain following nerve transection (Sweitzer et al. 2002). Nociceptive transmitters, substance P, and glutamate can differentially modulate glial MHC expression in a tissue-specific manner (McCluskey and Lampson 2001). The B7.2 molecule is expressed in microglia and not in astrocytes (Menendez et al. 1997); it is strongly upregulated by painful peripheral nerve injury (Rutkowski et al. 2004), axotomy (Bohatschek et al. 2004), endotoxin, IL-1β, TNF-α, and IFNγ and is inhibited by IL-10, PGE$_2$, and cyclic AMP-elevating agents (Menendez et al. 1997). Increased B7.2 expression can be prevented by genetic deletion of receptors for IL-1β or TNF-α (R1 or R2) (Bohatschek et al. 2004). This neuroimmune activation is accompanied by microglial activation and by the release of pro-inflammatory cytokines. The challenge to pain therapeutics is to inhibit the destructive immunity and pro-inflammatory cytokines without compromising the protective immunity elicited by B7.2 and associated molecules. Glutamate can inhibit antigen presentation (Angelini et al. 2002). Consequently, reduction of environmental glutamate by microglia can lead to improved antigen presentation and subsequent activation of T cells, leading to the production of IFNγ and further glutamate uptake (Shaked et al. 2005). Microglia can increase glutamate transporter I expression after nerve axotomy (Lopez-Redondo et al. 2000) and can play an early role in reestablishing glutamate homeostasis. Metabotropic glutamate receptors, present on both microglia and T cells, can sense the environmental levels of glutamate (Heuss et al. 1999; Storto et al. 2000) and synergize with IL-1β to enhance IL-6 release (Aronica et al. 2005). This regulation occurs at the transcriptional level and provides an additional means of regulation of the inflammatory response (Aronica et al. 2005).

　　Astrocytes.　　Activated microglia release proinflammatory substances, including cytokines, and activate astrocytes. Once activated, astrocytes can maintain hyperalgesia and allodynia independent of microglia. The point of conversion to astrocyte-driven sensitization appears to occur within the first 24 hours following injury. Virtually all synapses are enclosed by an astrocyte casing and allow for a bidirectional excitatory interchange (Araque et al. 1999; Vesce et al. 1999). Astrocytes have a "cellular memory" in that intracellular calcium responses are greatly amplified when astrocytes have previously been repetitively stimulated or exposed to strong synaptic activity (Pasti et al. 1997; Carmignoto 2000). This finding could account for the reports of pain reactivation with new injury, especially in cases of complex regional pain syndrome.

Spinal cord astrocytes exhibit extensive gap junction networks that become more extensive in response to high-intensity or high-frequency neural activity, as seen in chronic pain associated with nerve injury. Microglia do not have these connections at baseline, but they can develop them under pathological conditions (Eugenin et al. 2001). A network of signaling among glia could lead to release of glial-derived substances such as cytokines, glutamate, and adenosine triphosphate at distances far removed from the initial site of excitation and in patterns not predicted by neuroanatomy. In models of inflammatory and traumatic neuropathic pain, low doses of carbenoxolone, a nonspecific, reversible uncoupler of gap junctions (Davidson et al. 1986; Davidson and Baumgarten 1988), dramatically suppresses contralateral or mirror-image allodynia and suppresses IL-1β and IL-6 production (Spataro et al. 2004). The ipsilateral pain is reduced only at higher carbenoxolone doses. The density of astrocytes and gap junction protein levels is high in the superficial dorsal horn, across the breadth of the spinal cord, and around the circumference of the spinal cord, thus providing a near-continuous signaling path for astrocyte communication and for the potential activation of distant neuronal systems. Astrocyte networks may account for the increased cytokine expression in non-operated nerves found in a transected sciatic nerve model in rats (Ruohonen et al. 2002), casting doubt on studies that have used the nonoperated nerve as an internal experimental control.

MOLECULAR MECHANISMS OF CYTOKINE FUNCTION AND GLIAL ACTIVATION

The link between cytokine binding, glial cell activation, and new cytokine production starts with activation of intracellular protein kinases, especially the mitogen-activated protein kinases (MAPKs) (Watkins and Maier 2003). The MAPK family has at least three groups: extracellular signal-related kinases (ERKs) (Grewal et al. 1999); p38 kinases (Ono and Han 2000); and c-Jun, N-terminal protein kinases (JNKs), also known as stress-activated protein kinases (Gupta et al. 1996). ERKs are primarily activated by neuronal activity, p38 kinases are mainly activated by cytokines, and JNKs are activated by cytokines and by cellular stress or injury. All may contribute to the various post-injury responses of a nerve.

Activated p38 MAPK is present in spinal microglia and in small TNF-α-positive DRG neurons (Schafers et al. 2003), but not in spinal cord neurons or astrocytes (Tsuda et al. 2004). It is elevated in DRG neurons and in dorsal horn microglia after peripheral inflammation, peripheral nerve injury, and spinal nerve injury (Watkins and Maier 2003). A specific inhibitor of p38 kinase (SB203580), given intrathecally at the time of nerve injury and for 7 to 14 days thereafter, inhibits the development of tactile allodynia (Schafers et al. 2003; Tsuda et al. 2004). CNI-1493, another p38 kinase inhibitor, can reverse established allodynia induced by inflammation of the sciatic nerve (Milligan et al. 2003).

Stimulation of microglia by TLR-4 activation or by TNF-α induces a rapid and lasting activation of the JNK2 isoform. JNK2 may also be responsible for differentiation of T cells into the Th-1 lineage (Yang et al. 1998). Direct inhibition of all JNKs by SP600125, a nonspecific JNK inhibitor, reduces endotoxin induction of activator protein (AP)-1 target genes coding for several inflammatory mediators such as COX-2, TNF-α, and IL-6 (Waetzig et al. 2005).

Transcription factors are the link between receptor-driven cytoplasmic signaling events and changes in gene expression. The transcription factors NF-κB and AP-1 are essential for the induction of genes involved in inflammation. NF-κB is an inducible transcription factor that regulates the expression of various genes involved in the inflammatory and immune responses. Many of the pro-inflammatory cytokine genes contain binding sites for NF-κB (De Bosscher et al. 2003). In the resting state, NF-κB is inactivated by the endogenous inhibitor I-κB. Upon cellular stimulation, I-κB is phosphorylated by I-κB kinase (IKK) and degrades, freeing NF-κB to enter the nucleus. Activation of NF-κB has been described in models of traumatic spinal cord injury (Bethea et al. 1998), nerve injury, and neuropathic pain (Ma and Bisby 1998). Activated NF-κB is localized to DRG neurons and Schwann cells following partial sciatic nerve injury (Ma and Bisby 1998). Employing an endoneurially applied DNA decoy strategy, Sakue et al. (2001) inhibited NF-κB activation immediately following L5 spinal nerve ligation and prevented the development of thermal hyperalgesia and the expression of cytokines TNF-α, IL-1β, IL-6, IFNγ, and of ICAM-1 mRNAs in the injured DRG for up to 2 weeks. Tegeder and colleagues (2004) used a potent inhibitor of IKK (S1627) to block the IL-1β activation of NF-κB. S1627 had no effect on baseline nociception or on acute inflammatory hyperalgesia due to formalin, but it did reverse the thermal and mechanical hyperalgesia in inflammatory pain and tactile and cold allodynia in a CCI model of neuropathic pain. Inhibition of IKK was more effective than nonsteroidal anti-inflammatory drugs and was effective in both reversing and preventing hyperalgesia and allodynia. S1627 did not fully inhibit NF-κB, which may be advantageous because complete inhibition of NF-κB might cause too high a rate of adverse effects.

THERAPEUTIC INTERVENTIONS

The systems and mechanisms above represent a departure from the traditional thinking about neuropathic pain. Targeting therapies toward cytokines, glia, or infiltrating immune cells is a new approach for pain therapy, although it has already been employed with some success in oncology and rheumatology. Many neuroimmune mediators participate in a synergy of action and production such that inhibition of one compound will influence the production and action of others. This complex spider web of interactions holds both a promise and challenge for pain therapeutics. In addition, many mediators are involved in activities well beyond pain, including nerve regeneration, control of infection, behavior, and cognitive/memory functions. Therapeutic manipulation of these complex interactions holds promise for addressing the total symptom complex associated with nerve injury and chronic pain. Many of the examples below are from drugs currently on the market but not yet applied to pain conditions. Some may have too narrow a therapeutic index to be routinely used, but in selected patients they may represent an effective strategy. If these targets prove useful, the incentive to develop safer analogues will increase.

Glucocorticoid treatment. The therapeutic value of glucocorticoids has been known for over 60 years, but their utility is tempered by the wide range of adverse events triggered by their prolonged use, including development of tachyphylaxis to steroids, diabetes, impaired wound healing, skin and muscle atrophy, susceptibility to infections, metabolic derangements, and mineral loss from bone (Schacke et al. 2002). Glucocorticoids counteract the production of pro-inflammatory mediators and stimulate the production of anti-inflammatory mediators, including cytokines, through interference in the signaling pathways employing NF-κB and AP-1. In addition to glucocorticoids, several drugs used to treat chronic inflammatory diseases such as gold salts and high-dose salicylates inhibit NF-κB activation (Auphan et al. 1995; Yin et al. 1998). When released as part of the stress system, glucocorticoids can serve a negative feedback role to keep in check the immune and inflammatory reactions to trauma.

Glial and immune response inhibitors. Propentofylline, a methylxanthine derivative, was developed to treat Alzheimer's disease but failed to gain approval in Europe. It has a complex set of effects including reduced production of IL-1β and TNF-α, increased extracellular adenosine, inhibition of glial activation, and release of TNF-α and IL-1β (Watkins and Maier 2003). When given either systemically or centrally, it both prevents and reverses the development of allodynia in a rat L5 ligation model of neuropathic pain, and it also reduces both microglial and astrocytic activation (Sweitzer et al. 2001). Central administration is more effective, consistent with an effect on spinal glial function.

Intrathecal administration of the tetracycline derivative minocycline can attenuate the induction of mechanical allodynia in the sciatic inflammation model of chronic pain, but it is ineffective if administered after the allodynia is manifest for 7 days (Ledeboer et al. 2005).

The p38 MAPK inhibitor CNI-1493 is structurally similar to an agent clinically available in Japan, gabexate mesylate, a synthetic protease inhibitor that has anticoagulant properties and is used to treat patients with disseminated intravascular coagulation associated with sepsis (Yuksel et al. 2003). Gabexate can also inhibit endotoxin-induced TNF-α production in human monocytes, an effect that is due to an inhibition of both NF-κB and AP-1 activation (Yuksel et al. 2003). Its utility in chronic pain has yet to be assessed.

In neurodegenerative conditions such as spinal cord injury, the adaptive immune system can be augmented by T-cell-based therapeutic vaccination, literally allowing the body to heal itself (Hauben and Schwartz 2003). Notably, in animal studies the regenerative action of the immune system can be augmented without triggering autoimmune disease (Hauben et al. 2001).

Immunosuppression. Immunosuppressive agents such as methotrexate (Hashizume et al. 2000b) and leflunomide (Sweitzer and DeLeo 2002) attenuate tactile hypersensitivity at doses that inhibit MHC class II expression in rodent radiculopathy and neuropathy models. Leflunomide is approved for clinical use in rheumatoid arthritis and has several anti-inflammatory actions, including inhibition of IL-1β, TNF-α, TNF-α-activated NF-κB, and the expression of nitric oxide and COX-2 genes. The drug's potent immunosuppressive effects temper its clinical utility in chronic pain. In a rat mononeuropathy model the active metabolite of leflunomide (A771726), when administered either centrally or peripherally, reduced glial activation and lowered the expression of MHC class II markers at doses that attenuated mechanical allodynia. It did not, however, affect IL-6 levels (Sweitzer and DeLeo 2002). No data were presented for leflunomide's ability to reduce established allodynia.

Methotrexate can inhibit the production of pro-inflammatory cytokines and increase the release of the anti-inflammatory cytokine IL-10. It both prevents and reverses established allodynia and reduces indices of glial activation. One problem is that methotrexate can cause direct astrocytic neurotoxicity. Cyclosporine A, the clinical immunosuppressant, administered at the time of sciatic CCI in the rat, dramatically inhibited the development of heat hyperalgesia (Bennett 2000). Cyclosporine A administration is complicated by weight loss and diarrhea.

Inhibitors of cytokine production and function. Anakinra is a recombinant human IL-1-receptor antagonist approved for use in rheumatoid arthritis (Hallegua and Weisman 2002). No studies have looked at its ability to alter the development or maintenance of other chronic pain states. Successful use of TNF-α monoclonal antibodies or TNF-α-receptor fusion protein has changed the therapy for rheumatoid arthritis and several other chronic inflammatory diseases. The TNF-α monoclonal antibody infliximab has been reported in an open-label study to improve acute sciatica after a single systemic administration, with a reported instant and dramatic reduction in leg pain (Karppinen et al. 2003). Open-label clinical reports have claimed rapid resolution of acute sciatica (involving spinal root irritation) using TNF-α antibodies. One study of 10 patients used intravenous infliximab (Karppinen et al. 2003), and another used subcutaneous etanercept administered once every three days (Genevay et al. 2004) in a different set of 10 patients. All patients had been diagnosed with herniation-induced sciatica. The successful outcomes suggest TNF-α involvement in radiculopathy. In the etanercept study, all outcome variables improved, and the outcome was better than that of a comparison group of 10 patients enrolled in an intravenous steroid treatment study (Genevay et al. 2004).

The presence of IL-6 in several inflammatory conditions has generated much interest in selective inhibition of IL-6 or its receptor. A humanized anti-IL-6 antibody has completed clinical trials in rheumatoid arthritis in Japan and Europe with demonstrated efficacy (Naka et al. 2002; Okada et al. 2004). A fusion protein of soluble IL-6 receptor and IL-6 antagonist (Sporeno et al. 1996) has been employed to bind and inactivate the gp130 molecule (Renne et al. 1998), thereby inhibiting all members of the IL-6 family that use gp130 for signaling. One of the difficulties in using exogenous antibodies or soluble receptors is the need for continuous administration, eventually causing immune-mediated resistance to the treatment. One intriguing way around this problem, at least for IL-6, is to vaccinate an animal against an engineered IL-6 antagonist to induce neutralizing autoantibodies to IL-6 (Ciapponi et al. 1997; De Benedetti et al. 2001). Recently, non-peptide and presumably less antigenic IL-6 antagonists have been reported (Hayashi et al. 2002). Development of small-molecule antagonists or cytokine mimetics for IL-6 is an ongoing and promising venture because there are few receptor recognition epitopes for the IL-6 family (Bravo and Heath 2000).

Thalidomide was developed as a sedative and antinausea drug, but its teratogenic effects and propensity to cause peripheral neuropathy with prolonged use have limited its utility. It is orally active, readily crosses the blood-brain barrier And functions as an immunomodulator by inhibiting the production of a broad range of pro-inflammatory mediators including TNF-α, IL-1β, IL-6, and IL-8 and by increasing the level of IL-10, IL-2, and IFNγ (Corral et al. 1999). It is also a potent co-stimulator of T-cell function and can mediate a shift to a Th-2 type of immune profile (Haslett et al. 1998). Thalidomide inhibits the activation of NF-κB (Lokensgard et al. 2000) through the suppression of I-κB kinase activity (Keifer et al. 2001). It also inhibits the production of TNF-α from human microglial cells (Peterson et al. 1995). Thalidomide can reduce allodynia- and hyperalgesia-related behaviors when given at the time of sciatic nerve injury, but it was found to be ineffective when administered postoperatively (Sommer et al. 1998a). It has poor bioavailability in rats, however, and the dose and duration of therapy may not have been sufficient to reverse allodynia or hyperalgesia. Thalidomide reduces endoneurial TNF-α and increases endoneurial IL-10 and dorsal horn levels of met-enkephalin, but it does not alter IL-1β or IL-6 levels (George et al. 2000). It can reduce the expression of COX-2 in endotoxin- and cytokine-stimulated peripheral blood monocytes in a partially IL-10 dependent manner (Payvandi et al. 2004). Thalidomide can attenuate the development of vincristine-induced mechanical hyperalgesia in rats (Cata et al. 2004). Clinically, thalidomide has been reported to reduce pain and hyperalgesia in complex regional pain syndrome (CRPS) type I (Schwartzman et al. 2003). More potent, presumably less toxic, analogues, might reduce pain in subjects with CRPS type I as well as other painful conditions (Schwartzman 2005; D.C. Manning, unpublished observations 2005).

Suppression of neuroinflammation has been an active strategy in multiple sclerosis for many years. Much of our knowledge about cytokine and glial therapeutics has derived from treatment of CNS inflammatory immune conditions such as multiple sclerosis. IFNβ-1b can downregulate expression of MHC class II (Ransohoff et al. 1991) and adhesion molecules and upregulate IL-10 production (Chabot and Yong 2000). The utility of this and other multiple sclerosis therapies is unexplored in neuropathic pain.

Nutrition and fatty acid therapies. A somewhat unexpected drug class for immunomodulation are the statins or 3-hydroxy-3-methylglutaryl coenzyme A (HMGCoA) reductase inhibitors. Following reports that statin treatment produces improvement in a model of multiple sclerosis (Youssef et al.

2002), great interest is now being directed toward this class of drugs (Menge et al. 2005). Treatment with atorvastatin induces the secretion of Th-2 cytokines (IL-4, IL-5, and IL-10) and inhibits the secretion of Th-1 pro-inflammatory cytokines (IL-2, IL-12, IFNγ, and TNF-α). Atorvastatin inhibits MMP-9 (Wong et al. 2001) and reduces CNS penetration of leukocytes and well as reducing the expression of MHC class II molecules (Youssef et al. 2002). This effect on MHC expression is also noted on microglia (Menge et al 2005). Atorvastatin also reduces the expression of the costimulatory molecules B7.1 and B7.2 (Youssef et al. 2002; Stuve et al. 2003), reduces pro-inflammatory cytokine production, and improves the functional outcome in a rat model of spinal cord injury (Pannu et al. 2005). Another statin, lovastatin, inhibits endotoxin activation of NF-κB and diminishes the expression of TNF-α, IL-1β, and IL-6 in rat astrocytes, microglia, and macrophages (Pahan et al. 1997). Statins decrease the migration of leukocytes in the CNS, inhibit MHC class II and costimulatory signals required for activation of pro-inflammatory T cells, induce a Th-2 phenotype in T cells, and decrease the expression of inflammatory mediators in the CNS, including nitric oxide and TNF-α (Stuve et al. 2003). The potential benefit of statins in neuropathic pain is unexplored, but these agents may be effective in preemptive use. How many postoperative or traumatic neuropathic pain states have been avoided by concomitant use of statins?

Shir and colleagues have reported that dietary fat can reduce the neuropathic pain-related behaviors resulting from partial sciatic nerve ligation (Perez et al. 2004). The consumption of unsaturated corn or soy oils suppresses tactile allodynia and heat hyperalgesia, and this effect is accentuated by dietary protein from multiple sources (Perez et al. 2004). Dietary fats can modulate both innate and adaptive immune responses through TLR-4 receptors. Saturated fatty acids activate Toll-like receptors, but omega-3 polyunsaturated fatty acids inhibit agonist-induced TLR activation (Weatherill et al. 2005). Saturated fatty acids increase, and omega-3 polyunsaturated fatty acids decrease, or inhibit endotoxin activation of, B7.1, B7.2, MHC class II, and IL-6 expression in bone-marrow-derived dendritic cells (Weatherill et al. 2005). The effects of these nutritive agents on nerve-injury-induced pain are unexplored. Using nutritional therapies to prevent and possibly treat neuropathic pain raises intriguing therapeutic possibilities.

CONCLUSION

To ease the suffering of our patients, we need to find new approaches to the treatment of chronic neuropathic pain. By changing our perspective and looking beyond traditional neuroanatomy and neurophysiology to understand the body's response to injury, we may uncover new therapeutic strategies. An appreciation of the role played by the immune system in injury-induced pain states, as summarized in this chapter, represents a new opportunity. Currently available immunomodulatory and immunosuppressive agents need to be cautiously evaluated for their pain-modulating ability. The results of these initial studies will certainly foster more extensive therapeutic development efforts.

REFERENCES

Abbas A, Lichtman A. *Cellular and Molecular Immunology*, 5th ed. Philadelphia: Saunders, 2003.

Alesci S, Martinez PE, Kelkar S, et al. Major depression is associated with significant diurnal elevations in plasma interleukin-6 levels, a shift of its circadian rhythm, and loss of physiological complexity in its secretion: clinical implications. *J Clin Endocrinol Metab* 2005; 90:2522–2530.

Aloisi F. Immune function of microglia. *Glia* 2001; 36:165–179.

Angelini G, Gardella S, Ardy M, et al. Antigen-presenting dendritic cells provide the reducing extracellular microenvironment required for T lymphocyte activation. *Proc Natl Acad Sci USA* 2002; 99:1491–1496.

Aoki Y, Rydevik B, Kikuchi S, Olmarker K. Local application of disc-related cytokines on spinal nerve roots. *Spine* 2002; 27:1614–1617.

Araque A, Parpura V, Sanzgiri RP, Haydon PG. Tripartite synapses: glia, the unacknowledged partner. *Trends Neurosci* 1999; 22:208–215.

Aronica E, Gorter JA, Rozemuller AJ, Yankaya B, Troost D. Activation of metabotropic glutamate receptor 3 enhances interleukin (IL)-1-beta-stimulated release of IL-6 in cultured human astrocytes. *Neuroscience* 2005; 130:927–933.

Arruda JL, Colburn RW, Rickman AJ, Ruthowski MD, DeLeo JA. Increase of interleukin-6 mRNA in the spinal cord following peripheral nerve injury in the rat: potential role of IL-6 in neuropathic pain. *Mol Brain Res* 1998; 62:228–235.

Auphan N, DiDonato JA, Rosette C, Helmberg A, Karin M. Immunosuppression by glucocorticoids: inhibition of NF-kappa B activity through induction of I kappa B synthesis. *Science* 1995; 270:286–290.

Bacon KB, Harrison, JK. Chemokines and their receptors in neurobiology: perspectives in physiology and homeostasis. *J Neuroimmunol* 2000; 104:92–97.

Baldwin RL, Stolowitz ML, Hood L, Wisnieski BJ. Structural changes of tumor necrosis factor alpha associated with membrane insertion and channel formation. *Proc Natl Acad Sci USA* 1996; 93:1021–1026.

Balschun D, Wetzel W, Del Rey A, et al. Interleukin-6: a cytokine to forget. *FASEB J* 2004; 18:1788–1790.

Beattie EC, Stellwagen D, Morishita W, et al. Control of synaptic strength by glial TNF-alpha. *Science* 2002; 295:2282–2285.

Bennett GJ. A neuroimmune interaction in painful peripheral neuropathy. *Clin J Pain* 2000; 16:S139–S143.

Bethea JR, Castro M, Keane RW, et al. Traumatic spinal cord injury induces nuclear factor-kappa B activation. *J Neurosci* 1998; 18:3251–3260.

Bezzi P, Volterra A. A neuron-glia signalling network in the active brain. *Curr Opin Neurobiol* 2001; 11:387–394.

Bezzi P, Domercq, M, Brambilla L, et al. CXCR4-activated astrocyte glutamate release via TNF-alpha: amplification by microglia triggers neurotoxicity. *Nat Neurosci* 2001; 4:702–710.

Bohatschek M, Kloss CU, Pfeffer K, Bluethmann H, Raivich G. B7.2 on activated and phagocytic microglia in the facial axotomy model: regulation by interleukin-1 receptor type 1, tumor necrosis factor receptors 1 and 2 and endotoxin. *J Neuroimmunol* 2004; 156:132–145.

Bolin LM, Verity AN, Silver JE, Shooter EM, Abrams JS. Interleukin-6 production by Schwann cells and induction in sciatic nerve injury. *J Neurochem* 1995; 64:850–858.

Borner C, Kraus J, Schroder H, Ammer H, Hollt V. Transcriptional regulation of the human mu-opioid receptor gene by interleukin-6. *Mol Pharmacol* 2004; 66:1719–1726.

Bravo J, Heath JK. Receptor recognition by gp130 cytokines. *EMBO J* 2000; 19:2399–2411.

Brown MC, Perry VH, Lunn ER, Gordon S, Heumann R. Macrophage dependence of peripheral sensory nerve regeneration: possible involvement of nerve growth factor. *Neuron* 1991; 6:359–370.

Campbell IL, Abraham CR, Masliah E, et al. Neurologic disease induced in transgenic mice by cerebral overexpression of interleukin 6. *Proc Natl Acad Sci USA* 1993; 90.10061–10065.

Carmignoto G. Reciprocal communication systems between astrocytes and neurones. *Prog Neurobiol* 2000; 62:561–581.

Cata JP, Weng HR, Dougherty PM. Cyclooxygenase inhibitors and thalidomide ameliorate vincristine-induced hyperalgesia in rats. *Cancer Chemother Pharmacol* 2004; 54:391–397.

Chabot S, Yong VW. Interferon beta-1b increases interleukin-10 in a model of T cell-microglia interaction: relevance to MS. *Neurology* 2000; 55:1497–1505.

Chandler S, Miller KM, Clements JM, et al. Matrix metalloproteinases, tumor necrosis factor and multiple sclerosis: an overview. *J Neuroimmunol* 1997; 72:155–161.

Ciapponi L, Maione D, Scoumanne A, et al. Induction of interleukin-6 (IL-6) autoantibodies through vaccination with an engineered IL-6 receptor antagonist. *Nat Biotechnol* 1997; 15:997–1001.

Corral LG, Haslett PAJ, Muller GW, et al. Differential cytokine modulation and T-cell activation by two distinct classes of thalidomide analogues that are potent inhibitors of TNF-alpha. *J Immunol* 1999; 163:380–386.

Covey WC, Ignatowski TA, Knight PR, Spengler RN. Brain-derived TNF-alpha: involvement in neuroplastic changes implicated in the conscious perception of persistent pain. *Brain Res* 2000; 859:113–122.

Covey WC, Ignatowski TA, Renauld AE, et al. Expression of neuron-associated tumor necrosis factor alpha in the brain is increased during persistent pain. *Reg Anesth Pain Med* 2002; 27:357–366.

Cunha FQ, Poole S, Lorenzetti BB, Ferreira SH. The pivotal role of tumour necrosis factor alpha in the development of inflammatory hyperalgesia. *Br J Pharmacol* 1992; 107:660–664.

Davidson JS, Baumgarten IM. Glycyrrhetinic acid derivatives: a novel class of inhibitors of gap-junctional intercellular communication. Structure-activity relationships. *J Pharmacol Exp Ther* 1988; 246:1104–1107.

Davidson JS, Baumgarten IM, Harley EH. Reversible inhibition of intercellular junctional communication by glycyrrhetinic acid. *Biochem Biophys Res Commun* 1986; 134:29–36.

De Benedetti F, Pignatti P, Vivarelli M, et al. In vivo neutralization of human IL-6 (hIL-6) achieved by immunization of hIL-6-transgenic mice with a hIL-6 receptor antagonist. *J Immunol* 2001; 166:4334–4340.

De Bosscher K, Vanden Berghe W, Haegeman G. The interplay between the glucocorticoid receptor and nuclear factor-kappa B or activator protein-1: molecular mechanisms for gene repression. *Endocr Rev* 2003; 24:488–522.

De Jongh RF, Vissers KC, Meert TF, et al. The role of interleukin-6 in nociception and pain. *Anesth Analg* 2003; 96:1096–1103.

Del Mastro L, Venturini M, Giannessi PG, et al. Intraperitoneal infusion of recombinant human tumor necrosis factor and mitoxantrone in neoplastic ascites: a feasibility study. *Anticancer Res* 1995; 15:2207–2212.

DeLeo JA, Yezierski RP. The role of neuroinflammation and neuroimmune activation in persistent pain. *Pain* 2001; 90:1–6.

DeLeo JA, Colburn RW, Nichols M, Malhotra A. Interleukin-6-mediated hyperalgesia/allodynia and increased spinal IL-6 expression in a rat mononeuropathy model. *J Interferon Cytokine Res* 1996; 16:695–700.

DeLeo JA, Rutkowski MD, Stalder AK, Campbell IL. Transgenic expression of TNF by astrocytes increases mechanical allodynia in a mouse neuropathy model. *Pain* 2000; 11:599–602.

Elkordy M, Crump M, Vredenburgh JJ, et al. A phase I trial of recombinant human interleukin-1 beta (OCT-43) following high-dose chemotherapy and autologous bone marrow transplantation. *Bone Marrow Transplant* 1997; 19:315–322.

Empl M, Renaud S, Erne B, et al. TNF-alpha expression in painful and nonpainful neuropathies. *Neurology* 2001; 56:1371–1377.

Eugenin EA, Eckardt D, Theis M, et al. Microglia at brain stab wounds express connexin 43 and in vitro form functional gap junctions after treatment with interferon-gamma and tumor necrosis factor-alpha. *Proc Natl Acad Sci USA* 2001; 98:4190–4195.

Fine SM, Angel RA, Perry SW, et al. Tumor necrosis factor alpha inhibits glutamate uptake by primary human astrocytes. Implications for pathogenesis of HIV-1 dementia. *J Biol Chem* 1996; 271:15303–15306.

Flatters SJ, Fox AJ, Dickenson AH. Spinal interleukin-6 (IL-6) inhibits nociceptive transmission following neuropathy. *Brain Res* 2003; 984:54–62.

Flatters SJ, Fox AJ, Dickenson AH. Nerve injury alters the effects of interleukin-6 on nociceptive transmission in peripheral afferents. *Eur J Pharmacol* 2004; 484:183–191.

Fontaine V, Mohand-Said S, Hanoteau N, et al. Neurodegenerative and neuroprotective effects of tumor necrosis factor (TNF) in retinal ischemia: opposite roles of TNF receptor 1 and TNF receptor 2. *J Neurosci* 2002; 22:RC216.

Gadient RA, Otten UH. Interleukin-6 (IL-6)—a molecule with both beneficial and destructive potentials. *Prog Neurobiol* 1997; 52:379–390.

Gadient RA, Patterson PH. Leukemia inhibitory factor, interleukin 6, and other cytokines using the GP130 transducing receptor: roles in inflammation and injury. *Stem Cells* 1999; 17:127–137.

Geiss A, Varadi E, Steinbach K, Bauer HW, Anton F. Psychoneuroimmunological correlates of persisting sciatic pain in patients who underwent discectomy. *Neurosci Lett* 1997; 237:65–68.

Genevay S, Stingelin S, Gabay C. Efficacy of etanercept in the treatment of acute, severe sciatica: a pilot study. *Ann Rheum Dis* 2004; 63:1120–1123.

George A, Schmidt C, Weishaupt A, Toyka KV, Sommer C. Serial determination of tumor necrosis factor-alpha content in rat sciatic nerve after chronic constriction injury. *Exp Neurol* 1999; 160:124–132.

George A, Marziniak M, Schafers M, Toyka KV, Sommer C. Thalidomide treatment in chronic constrictive neuropathy decreases endoneurial tumor necrosis factor-alpha, increases interleukin-10 and has long-term effects on spinal cord dorsal horn met-enkephalin. *Pain* 2000; 88:267–275.

George A, Buehl A, Sommer C. Tumor necrosis factor receptor 1 and 2 proteins are differentially regulated during Wallerian degeneration of mouse sciatic nerve. *Exp Neurol* 2005; 192:163–166.

Glaser KB, Pease L, Li J, Morgan DW. Enhancement of the surface expression of tumor necrosis factor alpha (TNF-alpha) but not the p55 TNF-alpha receptor in the THP-1 monocytic cell line by matrix metalloprotease inhibitors. *Biochem Pharmacol* 1999; 57:291–302.

Grewal SS, York RD, Stork PJ. Extracellular-signal-regulated kinase signalling in neurons. *Curr Opin Neurobiol* 1999; 9:544–553.

Griffin JW, George R, Ho T. Macrophage systems in peripheral nerves: a review. *J Neuropathol Exp Neurol* 1993; 52:553–560.

Gupta S, Barrett T, Whitmarsh AJ, et al. Selective interaction of JNK protein kinase isoforms with transcription factors. *EMBO J* 1996; 15:2760–2770.

Hallegua DS, Weisman MH. Potential therapeutic uses of interleukin 1 receptor antagonists in human diseases. *Ann Rheum Dis* 2002; 61:960–967.

Hashizume H, DeLeo JA, Colburn RW, Weinstein JN. Spinal glial activation and cytokine expression after lumbar root injury in the rat. *Spine* 2000a; 25:1206–1217.

Hashizume H, Rutkowski MD, Weinstein JN, DeLeo JA. Central administration of methotrexate reduces mechanical allodynia in an animal model of radiculopathy/sciatica. *Pain* 2000b; 87:159–169.

Haslett PAJ, Corral LG, Albert M Kaplan G. Thalidomide costimulates primary human T lymphocytes, preferentially inducing proliferation, cytokine production, and cytotoxic responses in the CD8+ subset. *J Exp Med* 1998; 187:1885–1892.

Hatori K, Nagai A, Heisel R, Ryu JK, Kim SU. Fractalkine and fractalkine receptors in human neurons and glial cells. *J Neurosci Res* 2002; 69:418–426.

Hauben E, Schwartz M. Therapeutic vaccination for spinal cord injury: helping the body to cure itself. *Trends Pharmacol Sci* 2003; 24:7–12.

Hauben E, Agranov E, Gothilf A, et al. Posttraumatic therapeutic vaccination with modified myelin self-antigen prevents complete paralysis while avoiding autoimmune disease. *J Clin Invest* 2001; 108:591–599.

Hayashi M, Rho MC, Fukami A, et al. Biological activity of a novel nonpeptide antagonist to the interleukin-6 receptor 20S, 21-epoxy-resibufogenin-3-formate. *J Pharmacol Exp Ther* 2002; 303:104–109.

Heinrich PC, Behrmann I, Haan S, et al. Principles of interleukin (IL)-6-type cytokine signalling and its regulation. *Biochem J* 2003; 374:1–20.

Heuss C, Scanziani M, Gahwiler BH, Gerber U. G-protein-independent signaling mediated by metabotropic glutamate receptors. *Nat Neurosci* 1999; 2:1070–1077.

Holmes GM, Hebert SL, Rogers RC, Hermann GE. Immunocytochemical localization of TNF type 1 and type 2 receptors in the rat spinal cord. *Brain Res* 2004; 1025:210–219.

Houghtling RA, Mellon RD, Tan RJ, Bayer BM. Acute effects of morphine on blood lymphocyte proliferation and plasma IL-6 levels. *Ann NY Acad Sci* 2000; 917:771–777.

Hu S, Sheng WS, Ehrlich LC, et al. Cytokine effects on glutamate uptake by human astrocytes. *Neuroimmunomodulation* 2000; 7:153–159.

Hwang D. Modulation of the expression of cyclooxygenase-2 by fatty acids mediated through toll-like receptor 4-derived signaling pathways. *FASEB J* 2001; 15:2556–2564.

Ibuki T, Hama AT, Wang XT, et al. Loss of GABA-immunoreactivity in the spinal dorsal horn of rats with peripheral nerve injury and promotion of recovery by adrenal medullary grafts. *Neuroscience* 1997; 76:845–858.

Igarashi T, Kikuchi S, Shubayev V, Myers RR. Exogenous tumor necrosis factor-alpha mimics nucleus pulposus-induced neuropathology. Molecular, histologic, and behavioral comparisons in rats. *Spine* 2000; 25:2975–2980.

Ignatowski TA, Noble BK, Wright JR, et al. Neuronal-associated tumor necrosis factor (TNF alpha): its role in noradrenergic functioning and modification of its expression following antidepressant drug administration. *J Neuroimmunol* 1997; 79:84–90.

Ignatowski TA, Covey WC, Knight PR, et al. Brain-derived TNF-alpha mediates neuropathic pain. *Brain Res* 1999; 841:70–77.

Kaneko YS, Mori K, Nakashima A, et al. Peripheral injection of lipopolysaccharide enhances expression of inflammatory cytokines in murine locus coeruleus: possible role of increased norepinephrine turnover. *J Neurochem* 2005; 94:393–404.

Kang JD, Georgescu HI, McIntyre-Larkin L, et al. Herniated lumbar intervertebral discs spontaneously produce matrix metalloproteinases, nitric oxide, interleukin-6, and prostaglandin E2. *Spine* 1996; 21:271–277.

Karppinen J, Korhonen T, Malmivaara A, et al. Tumor necrosis factor-alpha monoclonal antibody, infliximab, used to manage severe sciatica. *Spine* 2003; 28:750–753.

Kayama S, Konno S, Olmarker K, Yabuki S, Kikuchi S. Incision of the anulus fibrosus induces nerve root morphologic, vascular, and functional changes. An experimental study. *Spine* 1996; 21:2539–2543.

Keifer, JA, Guttridge, DC, Ashburner BP, Baldwin J. Inhibition of NF-kappa-B activity by thalidomide through suppression of I-kappa-B kinase activity. *J Biol Chem* 2001; 1–28.

Kemeny N, Childs B, Larchian W, Rosado K, Kelsen D. A phase II trial of recombinant tumor necrosis factor in patients with advanced colorectal carcinoma. *Cancer* 1990; 66:659–663.

Klein MA, Moller JC, Jones LL, et al. Impaired neuroglial activation in interleukin-6 deficient mice. *Glia* 1997; 19:227–233.

Kraus J, Borner C, Giannini E, et al. Regulation of mu-opioid receptor gene transcription by interleukin-4 and influence of an allelic variation within a STAT6 transcription factor binding site. *J Biol Chem* 2001; 276:43901–43908.

Kuno R, Wang J, Kawanokuchi J, et al. Autocrine activation of microglia by tumor necrosis factor-alpha. *J Neuroimmunol* 2005; 162:89–96.

Laughlin TM, Bethea JR, Yezierski RP, Wilcox GL. Cytokine involvement in dynorphin-induced allodynia. *Pain* 2000; 84:159–167.

Ledeboer A, Breve JJ, Wierinckx A, et al. Expression and regulation of interleukin-10 and interleukin-10 receptor in rat astroglial and microglial cells. *Eur J Neurosci* 2002; 16:1175–1185.

Ledeboer A, Sloane EM, Milligan ED, et al. Minocycline attenuates mechanical allodynia and proinflammatory cytokine expression in rat models of pain facilitation. *Pain* 2005; 115:71–83.

Lee HL, Lee KM, Son SJ, Hwang SH, Cho HJ. Temporal expression of cytokines and their receptors mRNAs in a neuropathic pain model. *Neuroreport* 2004; 15:2807–2811.

Lee JY, Sohn KH, Rhee SH, Hwang D. Saturated fatty acids, but not unsaturated fatty acids, induce the expression of cyclooxygenase-2 mediated through Toll-like receptor 4. *J Biol Chem* 2001; 276:16683–16689.

Lehnardt S, Massillon L, Follett P, et al. Activation of innate immunity in the CNS triggers neurodegeneration through a Toll-like receptor 4-dependent pathway. *Proc Natl Acad Sci USA* 2003; 100:8514–8519.

Li Y, Ji A, Weihe E, Schafer MK. Cell-specific expression and lipopolysaccharide-induced regulation of tumor necrosis factor alpha (TNF-alpha) and TNF receptors in rat dorsal root ganglion. *J Neurosci* 2004; 24:9623–9631.

Lindenlaub T, Sommer C. Cytokines in sural nerve biopsies from inflammatory and non-inflammatory neuropathies. *Acta Neuropathol (Berl)* 2003; 105:593–602.

Liu B, Li H, Brull SJ, Zhang JM. Increased sensitivity of sensory neurons to tumor necrosis factor alpha in rats with chronic compression of the lumbar ganglia. *J Neurophysiol* 2002; 88:1393–1399.

Lokensgard JR, Hu S, van Fenema EM, et al. Effect of thalidomide on chemokine production by human microglia. *J Infect Dis* 2000; 182:983–987.

Lopez-Redondo Г, Nakajima K, Honda S, Kohsaka S. Glutamate transporter GLT-1 is highly expressed in activated microglia following facial nerve axotomy. *Brain Res Mol Brain Res* 2000; 76:429–435.

Ma W, Bisby MA. Increased activation of nuclear factor kappa B in rat lumbar dorsal root ganglion neurons following partial sciatic nerve injuries. *Brain Res* 1998; 797:243–254.

Maier SF, Watkins LR. Cytokines for psychologists: implications of bidirectional immune-to-brain communication for understanding behavior, mood, and cognition. *Psychol Rev* 1998; 105:83–107.

McCluskey LP, Lampson LA. Local immune regulation in the central nervous system by substance P vs. glutamate. *J Neuroimmunol* 2001; 116:136–146.

Menendez IB, Cerase J, Ceracchini C, Levi G, Aloisi F. Analysis of B7-1 and B7-2 costimulatory ligands in cultured mouse microglia: upregulation by interferon-gamma and lipopolysaccharide and downregulation by interleukin-10, prostaglandin E2 and cyclic AMP-elevating agents. *J Neuroimmunol* 1997; 72:83–93.

Menge T, Hartung HP, Stuve O. Statins—a cure-all for the brain? *Nat Rev Neurosci* 2005; 6:325–331.

Meyers C. Mood and cognitive disorders in cancer patients receiving cytokine therapy. In: Dantzer R (Ed). *Cytokines, Stress and Depression*. New York: Plenum, 1999, pp 75–82.

Michaelis M, Liu X, Jänig W. Axotomized and intact muscle afferents but no skin afferents develop ongoing discharges of dorsal root ganglion origin after peripheral nerve lesion. *J Neurosci* 2000; 20:2742–2748.

Milligan ED, Twining C, Chacur M, et al. Spinal glia and proinflammatory cytokines mediate mirror-image neuropathic pain in rats. *J Neurosci* 2003; 23:1026–1040.

Milligan ED, Zapata V, Chacur M, et al. Evidence that exogenous and endogenous fractalkine can induce spinal nociceptive facilitation in rats. *Eur J Neurosci* 2004; 20:2294–2302.

Moalem G, Xu K, Yu L. T lymphocytes play a role in neuropathic pain following peripheral nerve injury in rats. *Neuroscience* 2004; 129:767–777.

Molander C, Hongpaisan J, Svensson M, Aldskogius H. Glial cell reactions in the spinal cord after sensory nerve stimulation are associated with axonal injury. *Brain Res* 1997; 747:122–129.

Murata Y, Onda A, Rydevik B, Takahashi K, Olmarker K. Selective inhibition of tumor necrosis factor-alpha prevents nucleus pulposus-induced histologic changes in the dorsal root ganglion. *Spine* 2004; 29:2477–2484.

Murphy PG, Grondin J, Altares M, Richardson PM. Induction of interleukin-6 in axotomized sensory neurons. *J Neurosci* 1995; 15:5130–5138.

Naka T, Nishimoto N, Kishimoto T. The paradigm of IL-6: from basic science to medicine. *Arthritis Res* 2002; 4 Suppl 3:S233–S242.

Nickola TJ, Ignatowski TA, Spengler RN. Antidepressant drug administration modifies the interactive relationship between alpha(2)-adrenergic sensitivity and levels of TNF in the rat brain. *J Neuroimmunol* 2000; 107:50–58.

Noponen-Hietala N, Virtanen I, Karttunen R, et al. Genetic variations in IL6 associate with intervertebral disc disease characterized by sciatica. *Pain* 2005; 114:186–194.

Nordlind K, Eriksson L, Seiger A, Bakhiet M. Expression of interleukin-6 in human dorsal root ganglion cells. *Neurosci Lett* 2000; 280:139–142.

Obreja O, Schmelz M, Poole S, Kress M. Interleukin-6 in combination with its soluble IL-6 receptor sensitizes rat skin nociceptors to heat, in vivo. *Pain* 2002; 96:57-62.

Obreja O, Biasio W, Andratsch M, et al. Fast modulation of heat-activated ionic current by proinflammatory interleukin 6 in rat sensory neurons. *Brain* 2005; 128:1634–1641.

Ogoshi F, Yin HZ, Kuppumbatti Y, et al. Tumor necrosis-factor-alpha (TNF-alpha) induces rapid insertion of Ca^{2+}-permeable alpha-amino-3-hydroxy-5-methyl-4-isoxazole-propionate (AMPA)/kainate (Ca-A/K) channels in a subset of hippocampal pyramidal neurons. *Exp Neurol* 2005; 193:384–393.

Ohtori S, Takahashi K, Moriya H, Myers RR. TNF-alpha and TNF-alpha receptor type 1 upregulation in glia and neurons after peripheral nerve injury: studies in murine DRG and spinal cord. *Spine* 2004; 29:1082–1088.

Oka N, Akiguchi I, Kawasaki T, et al. Tumor necrosis factor-alpha in peripheral nerve lesions. *Acta Neuropathol (Berl)* 1998; 95:57–62.

Okada S, Nakamura M, Mikami Y, et al. Blockade of interleukin-6 receptor suppresses reactive astrogliosis and ameliorates functional recovery in experimental spinal cord injury. *J Neurosci Res* 2004; 76:265–276.

Olmarker K, Larsson K. Tumor necrosis factor alpha and nucleus-pulposus-induced nerve root injury. *Spine* 1998; 23:2538–2544.

Olmarker K, Rydevik B. Selective inhibition of tumor necrosis factor-alpha prevents nucleus pulposus-induced thrombus formation, intraneural edema, and reduction of nerve conduction velocity: possible implications for future pharmacologic treatment strategies of sciatica. *Spine* 2001; 26:863–869.

Olmarker K, Rydevik B, Nordborg C. Autologous nucleus pulposus induces neurophysiologic and histologic changes in porcine cauda equina nerve roots. *Spine* 1993; 18:1425–1432.

Olmarker K, Byrod G, Cornetjord M, Nordborg C, Rydevik B. Effects of methylprednisolone on nucleus pulposus-induced nerve root injury. *Spine* 1994; 19:1803–1808.

Olmarker K, Nordborg C, Larsson K, Rydevik B. Ultrastructural changes in spinal nerve roots induced by autologous nucleus pulposus. *Spine* 1996; 21:411–414.

Onda A, Hamba M, Yabuki S, Kikuchi S. Exogenous tumor necrosis factor-alpha induces abnormal discharges in rat dorsal horn neurons. *Spine* 2002; 27:1618–1624.

Onda A, Yabuki S, Kikuchi S. Effects of neutralizing antibodies to tumor necrosis factor-alpha on nucleus pulposus-induced abnormal nociresponses in rat dorsal horn neurons. *Spine* 2003; 28:967–972.

Ono K, Han J. The p38 signal transduction pathway: activation and function. *Cell Signal* 2000; 12:1–13.

Pahan K, Sheikh FG, Namboodiri AM, Singh I. Lovastatin and phenylacetate inhibit the induction of nitric oxide synthase and cytokines in rat primary astrocytes, microglia, and macrophages. *J Clin Invest* 1997; 100:2671–2679.

Pan W, Kastin AJ. Transport of cytokines and neurotrophins across the blood-brain barrier and their regulation after spinal cord injury. In: Sharma HS, Westman J (Eds). *Blood-Spinal Cord and Brain Barriers in Health and Disease,* San Diego: Elsevier Academic Press, 2004, pp 395–407.

Pannu R, Barbosa E, Singh AK, Singh I. Attenuation of acute inflammatory response by atorvastatin after spinal cord injury in rats. *J Neurosci Res* 2005; 79:340–350.

Papanicolaou DA, Wilder RL, Manolagas SC, Chrousos GP. The pathophysiologic roles of interleukin-6 in human disease. *Ann Intern Med* 1998; 128:127–137.

Pasti L, Volterra A, Pozzan T, Carmignoto G. Intracellular calcium oscillations in astrocytes: a highly plastic, bidirectional form of communication between neurons and astrocytes in situ. *J Neurosci* 1997; 17:7817–7830.

Payvandi F, Wu L, Haley M, et al. Immunomodulatory drugs inhibit expression of cyclooxygenase-2 from TNF-alpha, IL-1-beta, and LPS-stimulated human PBMC in a partially IL-10-dependent manner. *Cell Immunol* 2004; 230:81–88.

Perez J, Ware MA, Chevalier S, et al. Dietary fat and protein interact in suppressing neuropathic pain-related disorders following a partial sciatic ligation injury in rats. *Pain* 2004; 111:297–305.

Perrin FE, Lacroix S, Aviles-Trigueros M, David S. Involvement of monocyte chemoattractant protein-1, macrophage inflammatory protein-1-alpha and interleukin-1-beta in Wallerian degeneration. *Brain* 2005; 128:854–866.

Peterson PK, Hu S, Sheng WS, et al. Thalidomide inhibits tumor necrosis factor-α production by lipopolysaccharide- and lipoarabinomannan-stimulated human microglial cells. *J Infect Dis* 1995; 172:1137–1140.

Piani D, Spranger M, Frei K, Schaffner A, Fontana A. Macrophage-induced cytotoxicity of *N*-methyl-D-aspartate receptor positive neurons involves excitatory amino acids rather than reactive oxygen intermediates and cytokines. *Eur J Immunol* 1992; 22:2429–2436.

Polgar E, Hughes DI, Riddell JS, et al. Selective loss of spinal GABAergic or glycinergic neurons is not necessary for development of thermal hyperalgesia in the chronic constriction injury model of neuropathic pain. *Pain* 2003; 104:229–239.

Polgar E, Gray S, Riddell JS, Todd AJ. Lack of evidence for significant neuronal loss in laminae I-III of the spinal dorsal horn of the rat in the chronic constriction injury model. *Pain* 2004; 111:144–150.

Qiu Z, Sweeney DD, Netzeband JG, Gruol DL. Chronic interleukin-6 alters NMDA receptor-mediated membrane responses and enhances neurotoxicity in developing CNS neurons. *J Neurosci* 1998; 18:10445–10456.

Raghavendra V, Rutkowski MD, DeLeo JA. The role of spinal neuroimmune activation in morphine tolerance/hyperalgesia in neuropathic and sham-operated rats. *J Neurosci* 2002; 22:9980–9989.

Raghavendra V, Tanga F, DeLeo JA. Inhibition of microglial activation attenuates the development but not existing hypersensitivity in a rat model of neuropathy. *J Pharmacol Exp Ther* 2003; 306:624–630.

Raivich G, Liu ZQ, Kloss CU, et al. Cytotoxic potential of proinflammatory cytokines: combined deletion of TNF receptors TNFR1 and TNFR2 prevents motoneuron cell death after facial axotomy in adult mouse. *Exp Neurol* 2002; 178:186–193.

Ramer MS, Murphy PG, Richardson PM, Bisby MA. Spinal nerve lesion-induced mechanoallodynia and adrenergic sprouting in sensory ganglia are attenuated in interleukin-6 knockout mice. *Pain* 1998; 78:115–121.

Ramer MS, Thompson SW, McMahon SB. Causes and consequences of sympathetic basket formation in dorsal root ganglia. *Pain* 1999; Suppl 6: S111–S120.

Ransohoff RM, Devajyothi C, Estes ML, et al. Interferon-beta specifically inhibits interferon-gamma-induced class II major histocompatibility complex gene transcription in a human astrocytoma cell line. *J Neuroimmunol* 1991; 33:103–112.

Ray A, LaForge KS, Sehgal PB. On the mechanism for efficient repression of the interleukin-6 promoter by glucocorticoids: enhancer, TATA box, and RNA start site (Inr motif) occlusion. *Mol Cell Biol* 1990; 10:5736–5746.

Reichenberg A, Yirmiya R, Schuld A. Cytokine-associated emotional and cognitive disturbances in humans. *Arch Gen Psychiatry* 2001; 58:445–452.

Renauld AE, Spengler RN. Tumor necrosis factor expressed by primary hippocampal neurons and SH-SY5Y cells is regulated by alpha(2)-adrenergic receptor activation. *J Neurosci Res* 2002; 67:264–274.

Renne C, Kallen KJ, Mullberg J, et al. A new type of cytokine receptor antagonist directly targeting gp130. *J Biol Chem* 1998; 273:27213–27219.

Reynolds JL, Ignatowski TA, Gallant S, Spengler RN. Amitriptyline administration transforms tumor necrosis factor-alpha regulation of norepinephrine release in the brain. *Brain Res* 2004a; 1023:112–120.

Reynolds JL, Ignatowski TA, Sud R, Spengler RN. Brain-derived tumor necrosis factor-alpha and its involvement in noradrenergic neuron functioning involved in the mechanism of action of an antidepressant. *J Pharmacol Exp Ther* 2004b; 310:1216–1225.

Ruohonen S, Jagodi M, Khademi M, et al. Contralateral non-operated nerve to transected rat sciatic nerve shows increased expression of IL-1-beta, TGF-beta-1, TNF-alpha, and IL-10. *J Neuroimmunol* 2002; 132:11–17.

Rutkowski MD, Winkelstein BA, Hickey WF, Pahl JL, DeLeo JA. Lumbar nerve root injury induces central nervous system neuroimmune activation and neuroinflammation in the rat: relationship to painful radiculopathy. *Spine* 2002; 27:1604–1613.

Rutkowski MD, Lambert F, Raghavendra V, DeLeo JA. Presence of spinal B7.2 (CD86) but not B7.1 (CD80) co-stimulatory molecules following peripheral nerve injury: role of nondestructive immunity in neuropathic pain. *J Neuroimmunol* 2004; 146:94–98.

Ruzicka BB, Thompson RC, Watson SJ, Akil H. Interleukin-1 beta-mediated regulation of mu-opioid receptor mRNA in primary astrocyte-enriched cultures. *J Neurochem* 1996; 66:425–428.

Sachs D, Cunha FQ, Poole S, Ferreira SH. Tumour necrosis factor-alpha, interleukin-1-beta and interleukin-8 induce persistent mechanical nociceptor hypersensitivity. *Pain* 2002; 96:89–97.

Sakaue G, Shimaoka M, Fukuoka T, et al. NF-kappa B decoy suppresses cytokine expression and thermal hyperalgesia in a rat neuropathic pain model. *Neuroreport* 2001; 12:2079–2084.

Sallmann S, Juttler E, Prinz S, et al. Induction of interleukin-6 by depolarization of neurons. *J Neurosci* 2000; 20:8637–8642.

Samad TA, Moore KA, Sapirstein A, et al. Interleukin-1-beta-mediated induction of Cox-2 in the CNS contributes to inflammatory pain hypersensitivity. *Nature* 2001; 410:471–475.

Schacke H, Docke WD, Asadullah K. Mechanisms involved in the side effects of glucocorticoids. *Pharmacol Ther* 2002; 96:23–43.

Schafers M, Geis C, Brors D, Yaksh TL, Sommer C. Anterograde transport of tumor necrosis factor-alpha in the intact and injured rat sciatic nerve. *J Neurosci* 2002; 22:536–545.

Schafers M, Svensson CI, Sommer C, Sorkin LS. Tumor necrosis factor-alpha induces mechanical allodynia after spinal nerve ligation by activation of p38 MAPK in primary sensory neurons. *J Neurosci* 2003; 23:2517–2521.

Schwartzman R, Chevlen E, Bengtson K. Thalidomide has activity in treating complex regional pain syndrome. *Arch Intern Med* 2003; 163:1487–1488.

Schwartzman R, Irving G, Wallace M, et al. A multicenter, open-label, 12-week study with extension to evaluate the safety and efficacy of lenalidomide (CC5013) in the treatment of complex regional pain syndrome type-I. In: *Abstracts: 11th World Congress on Pain.* Seattle: IASP Press, 2005, p 580.

Segond VB, Kiehl M, Schaible HG. Acute and long-term effects of IL-6 on cultured dorsal root ganglion neurones from adult rat. *J Neurochem* 2005; 94:238–248.

Shaked I, Tchoresh D, Gersner R, et al. Protective autoimmunity: interferon-gamma enables microglia to remove glutamate without evoking inflammatory mediators. *J Neurochem* 2005; 92:997–1009.

Shamash S, Reichert F, Rotshenker S. The cytokine network of Wallerian degeneration: tumor necrosis factor-alpha, interleukin-1-alpha, and interleukin-1-beta. *J Neurosci* 2002; 22:3052–3060.

Shavit Y, Wolf G, Goshen I, Livshits D, Yirmiya R. Interleukin-1 antagonizes morphine analgesia and underlies morphine tolerance. *Pain* 2005; 115:50–59.

Shubayev VI, Myers RR. Upregulation and interaction of TNF-alpha and gelatinases A and B in painful peripheral nerve injury. *Brain Res* 2000; 855:83–89.

Shubayev VI, Myers RR. Axonal transport of TNF-alpha in painful neuropathy: distribution of ligand tracer and TNF receptors. *J Neuroimmunol* 2001; 114:48–56.

Sommer C, Schafers M. Painful mononeuropathy in C57BL/Wld mice with delayed Wallerian degeneration: differential effects of cytokine production and nerve regeneration on thermal and mechanical hypersensitivity. *Brain Res* 1998; 784:154–162.

Sommer C, Schmidt C, George A, Toyka KV. A metalloprotease-inhibitor reduces pain associated behavior in mice with experimental neuropathy. *Neurosci Lett* 1997; 237:45–48.

Sommer C, Marziniak M, Myers RR. The effect of thalidomide treatment on vascular pathology and hyperalgesia caused by chronic constriction injury of rat nerve. *Pain* 1998a; 74:83–91.

Sommer C, Schmidt C, George A. Hyperalgesia in experimental neuropathy is dependent on the TNF receptor 1. *Exp Neurol* 1998b; 151:138–142.

Sommer C, Lindenlaub T, Teuteberg P, et al. Anti-TNF-neutralizing antibodies reduce pain-related behavior in two different mouse models of painful mononeuropathy. *Brain Res* 2001; 913:86–89.

Sorkin LS, Xiao WH, Wagner R, Myers RR. Tumour necrosis factor-alpha induces ectopic activity in nociceptive primary afferent fibres. *Neuroscience* 1997; 81:255–262.

Spataro LE, Sloane EM, Milligan ED, et al. Spinal gap junctions: potential involvement in pain facilitation. *J Pain* 2004; 5:392–405.

Spengler RN, Allen RM, Remick DG, Strieter RM, Kunkel SL. Stimulation of alpha-adrenergic receptor augments the production of macrophage-derived tumor necrosis factor. *J Immunol* 1990; 145:1430–1434.

Spengler RN, Chensue SW, Giacherio DA, Blenk N, Kunkel SL. Endogenous norepinephrine regulates tumor necrosis factor-alpha production from macrophages in vitro. *J Immunol* 1994; 152:3024–3031.

Sporeno E, Savino R, Ciapponi L, et al. Human interleukin-6 receptor super-antagonists with high potency and wide spectrum on multiple myeloma cells. *Blood* 1996; 87:4510–4519.

Stoll G, Jander S. The role of microglia and macrophages in the pathophysiology of the CNS. *Prog Neurobiol* 1999; 58:233–247.

Storto M, de Grazia U, Battaglia G, et al. Expression of metabotropic glutamate receptors in murine thymocytes and thymic stromal cells. *J Neuroimmunol* 2000; 109:112–120.

Stuve O, Youssef S, Steinman L, Zamvil SS. Statins as potential therapeutic agents in neuroinflammatory disorders. *Curr Opin Neurol* 2003; 16:393–401.

Sugimoto T, Bennett GJ, Kajander KC. Transsynaptic degeneration in the superficial dorsal horn after sciatic nerve injury: effects of a chronic constriction injury, transection, and strychnine. *Pain* 1990; 42:205–213.

Svensson CI, Schafers M, Jones TL, Powell H, Sorkin LS. Spinal blockade of TNF blocks spinal nerve ligation-induced increases in spinal P-p38. *Neurosci Lett* 2005; 379:209–213.

Sweitzer SM, DeLeo JA. The active metabolite of leflunomide, an immunosuppressive agent, reduces mechanical sensitivity in a rat mononeuropathy model. *J Pain* 2002; 3:360–368.

Sweitzer SM, Schubert P, DeLeo JA. Propentofylline, a glial modulating agent, exhibits antiallodynic properties in a rat model of neuropathic pain. *J Pharmacol Exp Ther* 2001; 297:1210–1217.

Sweitzer SM, White KA, Dutta C, DeLeo JA. The differential role of spinal MHC class II and cellular adhesion molecules in peripheral inflammatory versus neuropathic pain in rodents. *J Neuroimmunol* 2002; 125:82–93.

Takahashi H, Suguro T, Okazima Y, et al. Inflammatory cytokines in the herniated disc of the lumbar spine. *Spine* 1996; 21:218–224.

Tanga FY, Raghavendra V, DeLeo JA. Quantitative real-time RT-PCR assessment of spinal microglial and astrocytic activation markers in a rat model of neuropathic pain. *Neurochem Int* 2004; 45:397–407.

Tanga FY, Nutile-McMenemy N, DeLeo JA. The CNS role of Toll-like receptor 4 in innate neuroimmunity and painful neuropathy. *Proc Natl Acad Sci USA* 2005; 102:5856–5861.

Tegeder I, Niederberger E, Schmidt R, et al. Specific Inhibition of I kappa B kinase reduces hyperalgesia in inflammatory and neuropathic pain models in rats. *J Neurosci* 2004; 24:1637–1645.

Tsuda M, Mizokoshi A, Shigemoto-Mogami Y, Koizumi S, Inoue K. Activation of p38 mitogen-activated protein kinase in spinal hyperactive microglia contributes to pain hypersensitivity following peripheral nerve injury. *Glia* 2004; 45:89–95.

Tu H, Juelich T, Smith EM, et al. Evidence for endogenous interleukin-10 during nociception. *J Neuroimmunol* 2003; 139:145–149.

Vandenabeele P, Declercq W, Beyaert R, Fiers W. Two tumour necrosis factor receptors: structure and function. *Trends Cell Biol* 1995; 5:392–399.

Verge GM, Milligan ED, Maier SF, et al. Fractalkine (CX3CL1) and fractalkine receptor (CX3CR1) distribution in spinal cord and dorsal root ganglia under basal and neuropathic pain conditions. *Eur J Neurosci* 2004; 20:1150–1160.

Vesce S, Bezzi P, Volterra A. The active role of astrocytes in synaptic transmission. *Cell Mol Life Sci* 1999; 56:991–1000.

Vissers KC, De Jongh RF, Hoffmann VL, Meert TF. Exogenous interleukin-6 increases cold allodynia in rats with a mononeuropathy. *Cytokine* 2005; 30:154–159.

Waetzig V, Czeloth K, Hidding U, et al. c-Jun N-terminal kinases (JNKs) mediate proinflammatory actions of microglia. *Glia* 2005; 50:235–246.

Wagner R, Myers RR. Endoneurial injection of TNF-alpha produces neuropathic pain behaviors. *Neuroreport* 1996a; 7:2897–2901.

Wagner R, Myers RR. Schwann cells produce tumor necrosis factor alpha: expression in injured and non-injured nerves. *Neuroscience* 1996b; 73:625–629.

Wagner R, Janjigian M, Myers RR. Anti-inflammatory interleukin-10 therapy in CCI neuropathy decreases thermal hyperalgesia, macrophage recruitment, and endoneurial TNF-alpha expression. *Pain* 1998; 74:35–42.

Watkins LR, Maier SF. Glia: a novel drug discovery target for clinical pain. *Nat Rev Drug Discov* 2003; 2:973–985.

Weatherill AR, Lee JY, Zhao L, et al. Saturated and polyunsaturated fatty acids reciprocally modulate dendritic cell functions mediated through TLR4. *J Immunol* 2005; 174:5390–5397.

Weihe E, Nohr D, Michel S, et al. Molecular anatomy of the neuro-immune connection. *Int J Neurosci* 1991; 59:1–23.

Whiteside GT, Munglani R. Cell death in the superficial dorsal horn in a model of neuropathic pain. *J Neurosci Res* 2001; 64:168–173.

Wieseler-Frank J, Maier SF, Watkins LR. Glial activation and pathological pain. *Neurochem Int* 2004; 45:389–395.

Wieseler-Frank J, Maier SF, Watkins LR. Immune-to-brain communication dynamically modulates pain: physiological and pathological consequences. *Brain Behav Immun* 2005; 19:104–111.

Williams LM, Gibbons DL, Gearing A, et al. Paradoxical effects of a synthetic metalloproteinase inhibitor that blocks both p55 and p75 TNF receptor shedding and TNF alpha processing in RA synovial membrane cell cultures. *J Clin Invest* 1996; 97:2833–2841.

Wong B, Lumma WC, Smith AM, et al. Statins suppress THP-1 cell migration and secretion of matrix metalloproteinase 9 by inhibiting geranylgeranylation. *J Leukoc Biol* 2001; 69:959–962.

Yang DD, Conze D, Whitmarsh AJ, et al. Differentiation of CD4+ T cells to Th1 cells requires MAP kinase JNK2. *Immunity* 1998; 9:575–585.

Yang L, Lindholm K, Konishi Y, Li R, Shen Y. Target depletion of distinct tumor necrosis factor receptor subtypes reveals hippocampal neuron death and survival through different signal transduction pathways. *J Neurosci* 2002; 22:3025–3032.

Yin MJ, Yamamoto Y, Gaynor RB. The anti-inflammatory agents aspirin and salicylate inhibit the activity of I(kappa)B kinase-beta. *Nature* 1998; 396:77–80.

Youssef S, Stuve O, Patarroyo JC, et al. The HMG-CoA reductase inhibitor, atorvastatin, promotes a Th2 bias and reverses paralysis in central nervous system autoimmune disease. *Nature* 2002; 420:78–84.

Yuksel M, Okajima K, Uchiba M, Okabe H. Gabexate mesilate, a synthetic protease inhibitor, inhibits lipopolysaccharide-induced tumor necrosis factor-alpha production by inhibiting activation of both nuclear factor-kappa-B and activator protein-1 in human monocytes. *J Pharmacol Exp Ther* 2003; 305:298–305.

Zelenka M, Schafers M, Sommer C. Intraneural injection of interleukin-1-beta and tumor necrosis factor-alpha into rat sciatic nerve at physiological doses induces signs of neuropathic pain. *Pain* 2005; 116:257–263.

Zhong J, Dietzel ID, Wahle P, Kopf M, Heumann R. Sensory impairments and delayed regeneration of sensory axons in interleukin-6-deficient mice. *J Neurosci* 1999; 19:4305–4313.

Correspondence to: Donald C. Manning, MD, PhD, Clinical Research and Development, Celgene Corporation, 86 Morris Avenue, Summit, NJ 07901, USA. Tel: 908-673-9529; Fax: 908-673-2778; email: dmanning@celgene.com.

Emerging Strategies for the Treatment of Neuropathic Pain, edited by James N. Campbell, Allan I. Basbaum, André Dray, Ronald Dubner, Robert H. Dworkin, and Christine N. Sang, IASP Press, Seattle, © 2006.

9

Signaling Pathways in Pain Neuroplasticity in the Spinal Dorsal Horn

Michael W. Salter

University of Toronto Centre for the Study of Pain and The Hospital for Sick Children, Toronto, Ontario, Canada

In nociceptive pathways in the dorsal horn of the spinal cord, synaptic inputs from primary afferent nociceptors are principally mediated at fast glutamatergic synapses onto second-order neurons. This excitatory transmission occurs primarily through the AMPA/kainate and NMDA-receptor subtypes of ionotropic glutamate receptors. These glutamatergic synapses exhibit multiple forms of short-lasting and long-lasting synaptic plasticity, and within the dorsal horn they produce a form of long-lasting enhancement of nociceptive transmission known as "central sensitization." This form of persistent enhancement of synaptic transmission shares features of long-term potentiation of glutamatergic transmission in other regions of the central nervous system (CNS). Central sensitization is an expression of increased gain of glutamatergic transmission in central nociceptive transmission neurons and is dependent upon the activity of NMDA receptors. NMDA-receptor activity in dorsal horn neurons is facilitated by nociceptive peripheral inputs as a result of various convergent mechanisms that make important contributions to pain hypersensitivity. In addition to this role of neurons, a rapidly growing body of evidence indicates that following peripheral injury, glia within the spinal cord play important roles in initiating and maintaining the enhancement of nociceptive transmission. In particular, a role has emerged for microglia in pain hypersensitivity following nerve injury. Thus, a comprehensive understanding of cellular signaling mechanisms in the dorsal horn, which may be used to create new strategies for the diagnosis and management of neuropathic pain, must include both neurons and glia.

Acute nociceptive pain is an important defense mechanism that warns of recent or imminent damage to the body and is produced by the physiological functioning of normal peripheral and central nervous systems. In contrast, chronic pain is typically not directly related to tissue damage, and it may persist long after the resolution of any tissue damage that may have caused acute pain. Thus, chronic pain subserves no known defensive, or other help-ful, function. Rather, it reflects aberrant functioning of a nervous system that has been pathologically altered by one or more cellular signaling processes (Woolf and Salter 2000, 2005). The pathological changes may occur in the peripheral nervous system or in numerous sites within the CNS.

The ultimate effect of the intracellular signaling processes in the dorsal horn that is relevant to chronic pain is alteration of the activity of neurons in the nociceptive processing network in the dorsal horn such that the output of this network, for a given input, is facilitated. A prominent cellular substrate for this effect is the alteration of synaptic connectivity, either between the input primary afferent neurons and nociceptive neurons in the dorsal horn, or between dorsal horn neurons themselves. Over the past two decades it has become apparent that, throughout the nervous system, synaptic connections between neurons are subject to great modifiability, or neuroplasticity. The modifications in synaptic connectivity are highly dependent upon the imme-diate, and longer-term, history of the electrical activity and on the state of multiple intracellular biochemical signaling processes in the pre- and postsyn-aptic neurons. In the adult, the continual interplay of these intracellular signaling processes serves to produce synaptic modifications that underlie physiological processes such as learning and memory and pathological pro-cesses including epilepsy, neurodegeneration, and pain. In this chapter I will briefly review synaptic physiology within the dorsal horn, describing types of synaptic plasticity that may contribute to neuropathic pain. I will then describe recently emerging work that suggests a crucial role for glia, and by inference neuronal-glial-neuronal signaling, in nerve-injury-induced pain.

SYNAPTIC TRANSMISSION AND INTEGRATION
IN DORSAL HORN NEURONS

Synaptic input from all types of primary afferents onto second-order neurons in the dorsal horn is excitatory and, with few exceptions, is medi-ated by release of glutamate. Individual presynaptic action potentials in the presynaptic terminals cause the release of individual quanta of glutamate, which produce an excitatory postsynaptic potential (EPSP) primarily by ac-tivation of the α-amino-3-hydroxy-5-methyl-4-isoxazole propionate (AMPA) (Jessell and Jahr 1985) and kainate (Li et al. 1999) subtypes of glutamate receptor. The N-methyl-D-aspartate (NMDA) subtype of glutamate receptor, which is also localized at excitatory synapses, contributes little to the responses to single presynaptic action potentials by a combination of two factors: (1) at the resting membrane potential, current flow through NMDA receptors is tonically suppressed by extracellular Mg^{2+}, which blocks the channel pore; and (2) the activity per se of the channels is tonically downregulated by biasing of kinase/phosphatase signaling toward dephosphorylation. Fast glutamatergic transmission occurs even at synapses of primary afferents that may be typically considered slow, from the perspective of axonal conduction velocity, and which are predominantly nociceptors (Moore et al. 2000). Activation of individual nociceptors produces unitary EPSPs in dorsal horn neurons. However, because each individual primary afferent makes few synapses with a given dorsal horn neuron, EPSPs from multiple primary afferent nociceptors must normally summate temporally and spatially in order to evoke an action potential in the dorsal horn neuron. Likewise, temporal and spatial summation of EPSPs from nociceptive and non-nociceptive primary afferents is required for action potential generation in the case of dorsal horn neurons with multi-convergent inputs. With mild noxious stimuli in the periphery, low-frequency action potential activity evoked by nociceptors produces EPSPs, and action potentials, in dorsal horn neurons that may signal the onset, duration, and intensity of the stimulation.

While action potential discharge by dorsal horn neurons is driven by glutamatergic EPSPs, the discharge activity of these neurons is powerfully sculpted by inhibitory inputs (Malcangio and Bowery 1996; Dickenson et al. 1997). The dominant type of inhibition is that produced by release of γ-aminobutyric acid (GABA) and/or glycine, leading to fast inhibitory postsynaptic potentials (IPSPs) mediated by $GABA_A$ and glycine receptors, respectively, which are ligand-gated Cl^- channels. Activation of these receptors suppresses the generation of action potentials by hyperpolarizing and by "shunting" the postsynaptic cell membrane (Prescott and De Koninck 2003). Postsynaptic inhibition may also be produced by activation of metabotropic receptors, i.e., G-protein-coupled receptors, such as $GABA_B$, adenosine, and opioid receptors, which typically produce postsynaptic hyperpolarization by means of activating K^+ channels. In addition, to postsynaptic inhibition, discharge of dorsal horn neurons may be inhibited by presynaptically suppressing release of glutamate. This presynaptic inhibition involves many of the same chemical mediators that cause postsynaptic inhibition.

The efficacy of excitatory synaptic transmission and of the coupling between EPSPs and action potential generation are thus fundamentally important for the working of the nociceptive network within the dorsal horn. There are various cellular and molecular mechanisms for increasing, or decreasing, the strength of glutamatergic synapses and the efficiency by which this synaptic input produces action potentials. As described below, these mechanisms range from those that are very rapid in onset, and typically also rapidly reversible, to those that are more slowly developing and persistent. It is the integration of these various mechanisms, based on the prior short- and long-term electrical and biochemical history of the dorsal horn neurons, that controls the output of the nociceptive dorsal horn network.

"WIND-UP" VERSUS CLASSICAL "CENTRAL SENSITIZATION"

Noxious peripheral stimulation that is more intense or sustained than that mentioned above induces primary afferent nociceptors to discharge at higher frequencies, resulting in release of peptide neuromodulators such as substance P and calcitonin gene-related peptide, together with glutamate, from central nociceptor terminals (Duggan et al. 1995). The resulting slow, depolarizing synaptic potentials, lasting up to tens of seconds (De Koninck and Henry 1991), provide substantial opportunities for temporal summation of fast EPSPs (Sivilotti et al. 1993). The cumulative depolarization of the dorsal horn neurons is accentuated by feedforward recruitment of NMDA-receptor current through progressive relief of the Mg^{2+} blockade of the channels. The sustained depolarization may also recruit voltage-gated Ca^{2+} currents, causing a further boost in the level of intracellular Ca^{2+} and triggering plateau potentials mediated by calcium-activated nonselective cation channels (Morisset and Nagy 1999). The end result of these intracellular signaling cascades is "wind-up" (Mendell 1984), which is a progressive increase in the action potential discharge in second-order nociceptive transmission neurons elicited during a train of peripheral stimuli (Woolf and Salter 2000).

Nociceptive neurons in the dorsal horn exhibit a form of enhanced responsiveness to nociceptive inputs—often referred to as "central sensitization"—that is mechanistically distinct from wind-up (Woolf 1983). Although the cellular and molecular mechanisms producing central sensitization are different from those that produce wind-up, each is initiated by peripheral nociceptor input; activating low-threshold primary afferents produces neither of these phenomena. In contrast to wind-up, sensitization of central nociceptive pathway neurons outlasts, by up to many hours, the duration of the nociceptor inputs that initiates it. These inputs initiate multiple intracellular signaling cascades, leading to a concerted modification of neuronal network behavior consisting of enhancement of excitatory postsynaptic responses and depression of inhibition. The consequence of this signaling is an increase in the gain of nociceptive pathway neurons, resulting in amplified responses, not only to noxious but also to innocuous inputs. Most nociceptive transmission neurons have a large excitatory subliminal fringe, and thus the increased gain also results in unmasking of subthreshold inputs, causing the neurons to become sensitive to stimuli in surrounding regions of the periphery (Woolf and Salter 2005). Thus, responses of individual nociceptive neurons are amplified, and there is an increase in the overall number of nociceptive transmitting neurons activated by a given peripheral input.

The primary means by which central sensitization is initiated and sustained over the short term is through post-translational modification of the repertoire of gene products expressed by nociceptive transmission neurons (Woolf and Salter 2000). Importantly, these post-translational modifications are readily reversible, allowing the dorsal horn network to return to the basal state. However, gain of nociceptive pathways can increase over a much longer time course through activation of additional signaling cascades, which leads to alteration in the repertoire of genes expressed in neurons and glia in the dorsal horn. These changes in gene expression alter the functional and structural phenotype of central nociceptive transmission neurons and may lead to disruption or death of inhibitory neurons.

PERSISTENT ENHANCEMENT OF EXCITATORY SYNAPTIC TRANSMISSION

It is well known that glutamatergic synapses in many cell types in the CNS show a long-lasting increase in efficacy in response to a brief period of high-frequency presynaptic activity. This widespread phenomenon has come to be denoted "long-term potentiation" (LTP) (for reviews see Collingridge et al. 2004; Malenka and Bear 2004). Before discussing persistent enhancement of glutamatergic synaptic transmission in the dorsal horn, I will give a brief overview of some of the unifying themes about LTP that have been established through studies primarily in the brain areas, especially the hippocampus.

Mechanistically, LTP is diverse and may involve pre- and postsynaptic processes that can vary at different synapses, may differentially depend upon the pattern of presynaptic activity, and may vary over time after the brief period of high-frequency activity. Despite this great diversity, a number of simplifying principles have been discovered. First, it has been found that selective blockade of particular processes at or just after the high-frequency stimulation prevents the development of LTP. However, blockade of these same processes is unable to reverse established LTP. This finding has led to the concept that "induction" of LTP is mechanistically distinct from its "maintenance." The processes responsible for induction of LTP are rapidly engaged following the high-frequency synaptic activity and activate the processes by which LTP is ultimately expressed and maintained. Because most of the current at glutamatergic synapses is mediated via AMPA (or kainate) receptors, all of the mechanisms for expression of LTP ultimately lead to increased efficacy of synaptic transmission mediated by these receptor subtypes.

A second broad principle follows from findings that at some synapses, induction of LTP is prevented by blocking NMDA receptors, whereas at other synapses it is independent of NMDA-receptor function. Thus, LTP falls into two broad classes: NMDA-receptor-dependent and NMDA-receptor-independent (Malenka and Bear 2004). Many types of neurons in various regions of the CNS show NMDA-receptor-dependent LTP. Because the relevant NMDA receptors are located on the postsynaptic neuron, NMDA-receptor-dependent LTP is initiated postsynaptically, but the expression of NMDA-receptor-dependent LTP could conceivably be either pre- or postsynaptic. At the most intensively studied synapse in the mammalian CNS—the Schaffer synapse onto CA1 neurons in the hippocampus—the preponderance of evidence is that the potentiation is expressed postsynaptically by an increase in cell-surface expression or in the function of AMPA receptors. A key consideration about NMDA-receptor-dependent LTP relates to the tonic basal suppression of synaptic NMDA-receptor currents. In order to initiate this type of LTP, synaptic NMDA-receptor currents must be acutely increased. This acute increase is accomplished by partial relief of Mg^{2+} blockade (Malenka and Nicoll 1999; Malenka and Bear 2004), as is widely appreciated, and by Src-kinase-mediated enhancement currents (Ali and Salter 2001; Salter and Kalia 2004), which is less well known. A new wrinkle was added to this story with the recent discovery that at CA1-Schaffer collateral synapses, NMDA receptors containing the NR2A subunit must be activated for induction of LTP (Liu et al. 2004). Conversely, NMDA-receptor-dependent long-term depression (LTD), the functional opposite of LTP, depends on activation of NMDA receptors containing the NR2B subunit. Thus, not only must NMDA-receptor-mediated current be enhanced in order for LTP to occur, but NMDA receptors of the correct molecular composition need to be activated.

A third general principle is that induction of LTP requires a rise in postsynaptic Ca^{2+} concentration. The increase in Ca^{2+} may be provided by NMDA-receptor activation, but other types of Ca^{2+}-permeable channels such as voltage-gated Ca^{2+} channels or Ca^{2+}-permeable AMPA receptors may also contribute at particular synapses or under certain conditions of stimulation or activity. The rise in postsynaptic Ca^{2+} initiates signaling cascades that increase AMPA-receptor-mediated synaptic transmission and hence lead to the varied mechanisms through which LTP is expressed. It is perhaps curious that, like NMDA-receptor-dependent LTP, NMDA-receptor-dependent LTD also requires a postsynaptic rise in Ca^{2+}. Previously, it was thought differing levels of intracellular Ca^{2+} were the critical variable determining whether LTP or LTD is induced, with higher levels causing LTP and lower levels producing LTD. However, the discovery that differing NMDA-receptor subunits subserve LTP versus LTD raises a new possibility—the key difference may be that the Ca^{2+}-dependent intracellular enzymes associated with NR2A may be distinct from those associated with NR2B. Thus, Ca^{2+} may activate different intracellular signaling cascades depending upon whether this ion enters through NR2A- or NR2B-containing receptors.

In terms of lasting potentiation of synaptic responses at primary afferent nociceptor synapses, numerous studies have shown that primary afferent-evoked responses of nociceptive dorsal horn neurons are enhanced by a wide variety of conditioning stimuli. However, it is usually not possible to ascertain precisely whether the increased responses are mediated by enhanced efficacy at primary-afferent-to-second-order synapses because often the neurons studied receive long-latency monosynaptic responses that overlap temporally with polysynaptic responses, or else the responses are evoked by stimuli producing asynchronous discharge of primary afferents where the requisite timing information is lost. Nevertheless, with the most rigorous studies of monosynaptic responses, which have by necessity been done using superficial dorsal horn neurons, it is clear that brief, high-frequency primary afferent stimulation may induce potentiation of AMPA-receptor-mediated responses at synapses onto second-order neurons (Randic et al. 1993; Ikeda et al. 2003). The potentiation is prevented by blocking NMDA receptors and thus falls into the general class of NMDA-receptor-dependent LTP. As described elsewhere in detail (Woolf and Salter 2000; Ji et al. 2003), the lasting enhancement of excitatory synaptic responses at primary afferent-second order synapses in nociceptive pathways may share the common signaling cascade elucidated in most depth in the hippocampus, including dependency on activation of Src tyrosine kinases and of mitogen-activated protein (MAP) kinase.

LTP is a form of homosynaptic plasticity in that the potentiation occurs at the synapses that are activated by high-frequency stimulation. Dorsal horn nociceptive neurons also show heterosynaptic potentiation (McMahon and Wall 1983; Woolf 1983; Cook et al. 1987), in that synapses not activated by the high-frequency stimulation also become potentiated. Heterosynaptic potentiation, which is in fact more prominent than homosynaptic potentiation, may manifest as an increase in synaptic efficacy at central synapses of non-nociceptive afferents as well as at those of nociceptive afferents. This process increases the overall excitatory drive to the nociceptive dorsal horn neurons and broadens out their dynamic range. When subthreshold EPSPs from afferents in the subliminal fringe are sufficiently facilitated, heterosynaptic potentiation may also increase the size of the receptive field of the dorsal horn neurons. The intracellular biochemical cascades converge on those common mechanisms by which AMPA and/or kainate receptor-mediated transmission is enhanced, through increased number and/or activity of the receptors. Thus, heterosynaptic enhancement may use many of the same signaling cascades as those used in homosynaptic LTP, including initiation of NMDA-receptor-mediated synaptic plasticity by activation of the diacylglycerol-inositol trisphosphate pathway and release of calcium for intracellular stores (Guo et al. 2004), but these processes are not spatially restricted in the postsynaptic neuron as they are in LTP.

While AMPA receptors are generally impermeable to Ca^{2+}, by virtue of containing the edited form of the GluR2 subunit of the glutamate receptor (Seeburg et al. 1998; Dingledine et al. 1999), AMPA receptors lacking edited GluR2 do have a high permeability to Ca^{2+}, which provides a source for postsynaptic Ca^{2+} that may mediate synaptic plasticity. Neurons expressing Ca^{2+}-permeable AMPA receptors are preferentially localized in the superficial dorsal horn (Albuquerque et al. 1999). Lasting enhancement of synaptic transmission mediated by GluR2-less AMPA receptors by a postsynaptic mechanism has been demonstrated at dorsal horn synapses (Gu et al. 1996). Thus, through both NMDA-receptor-dependent and -independent mechanisms, such enhancement may contribute to the amplification of responsiveness of dorsal horn nociceptive neurons.

Sustained facilitation of release of glutamate from primary afferent nociceptors would result in sustained increase in the gain of nociceptive transmission. This facilitation could be produced by direct enhancement of transmitter release or by suppression of tonic presynaptic inhibition and provides profound control of the release of glutamate from primary afferents. Release of glutamate could be enhanced by stimulating receptors on primary afferent terminals, including purinergic $P2X_3$ receptors (Gu and MacDermott 1997) and NMDA receptors (Liu et al. 1994). However, the effects of such receptor stimulation appear to be relatively short-lived after the receptor stimulation, and do not result in LTP. Nevertheless, tonic activation of these receptors could maintain persistent facilitation, but it would be mechanistically dissimilar from the "induction" and "maintenance" paradigm of LTP.

PERSISTENT SUPPRESSION OF INHIBITION

Because of the critical importance of inhibition in controlling the output of the nociceptive network in the dorsal horn, persistent suppression of inhibitory mechanisms may be as important as facilitation of excitatory transmission. Inhibitory neurons in the dorsal receive excitatory input from primary afferents, and other sources, and thus one mechanism for reducing inhibition is to decrease the excitatory drive onto the inhibitory neurons. For example, LTD of glutamatergic transmission at primary afferent synapses onto inhibitory dorsal horn neurons is elicited by activation of Aδ-fiber primary afferents (Randic et al. 1993). The depression, which requires NMDA-receptor activation and a subsequent rise in postsynaptic Ca^{2+}, is mechanistically similar to LTD in other regions of the CNS. A prominent mechanism for LTD is clathrin-mediated endocytosis of synaptically localized AMPA receptors (for review see Collingridge et al. 2004). Thus, it is likely that LTD at primary afferent synapses onto inhibitory dorsal horn neurons is due to internalization of cell-surface AMPA receptors.

Considering the inhibitory synapses themselves, where the predominant transmitters are GABA and glycine, one general mechanism for dis-inhibition would be to suppress the sensitivity of the postsynaptic neurons. By analogy to what has been reported in the hippocampus, it is conceivable that the function of $GABA_A$ receptors could be suppressed by post-translational mechanisms initiated by Ca^{2+} rise secondary to NMDA-receptor activation (Lu et al. 2000; Wang et al. 2003). In this way, a single initiating postsynaptic event, activation of NMDA receptors, may lead in parallel to two mechanisms—facilitation of AMPA/kainate transmission and suppression of GABA transmission—both boosting net excitation. Another mechanism for suppressing glycine/GABA transmission in central nociceptive neurons is downregulation of postsynaptic glycine and GABA receptors. Evidence indicates that glycine α_3 receptors may be downregulated by PGE_2, contributing to inflammatory pain hypersensitivity (Harvey et al. 2004).

An additional mechanism by which GABA/glycine inhibition may be suppressed, or even converted to net excitation, has been recently been discovered (Coull et al. 2003). This mechanism relates to changing the equilibrium potential for Cl⁻ in lamina I neurons in the dorsal horn following peripheral nerve injury. Normally in lamina I neurons in the adult spinal cord the intracellular concentration of Cl⁻ is kept low by the action of the K^+-Cl⁻ transporter KCC2. However, after nerve injury the expression of KCC2 is dramatically decreased, leading to a rise in intracellular Cl⁻ concentration. The resultant depolarizing shift in the equilibrium potential for Cl⁻ means that chloride-mediated postsynaptic responses to GABA and glycine become much less depolarizing (causing dis-inhibition). In up to about a third of lamina I neurons, the shift in Cl⁻ equilibrium potential is sufficiently large that opening of $GABA_A$, or glycine, receptors causes depolarization, which switches the function of these receptors from inhibition to excitation.

GABA may also act presynaptically on the terminals of primary afferent nociceptors to produce primary afferent depolarization (PAD). While classically PAD was considered a mechanism for producing presynaptic inhibition (Eccles and Krnjevic 1959; Eccles et al. 1961), it has since been found that depolarization may be sufficient to cause generation of action potentials producing both orthodromic and antidromic discharges in primary afferents (for review, see Cervero et al. 2003). The orthodromic discharges can evoke the release of glutamate, thereby facilitating excitation rather than causing presynaptic inhibition. The antidromic discharges propagate out through the dorsal roots, causing the so-called "dorsal root reflex," and may cause release of chemical mediators at the peripheral terminals. Recent genetic evidence indicates that the Na^+-K^+-Cl^- cotransporter NKCC1 may be crucial for maintaining the depolarizing Cl^- equilibrium potential in the terminals of primary afferents (Laird et al. 2004).

A final mechanism for producing disinhibition is through loss of inhibitory neurons, through selective death of GABAergic inhibitory interneurons following nerve injury. Within a week after nerve injuries that produce pain hypersensitivity, inhibitory neurons begin to undergo apoptosis in the dorsal horn (Moore et al. 2002). This process may be excitotoxic, due to excessive glutamate release, a failure of glutamate uptake, or a result of cell death-inducing signals such as TNF-α. Thus, together there is a very broad range of mechanisms by which sustained loss of inhibition may contribute importantly to pain hypersensitivity.

MICROGLIA HAVE A KEY ROLE IN NERVE-INJURY PAIN PLASTICITY

In the CNS, neurons are outnumbered approximately 10:1 by glial cells. Traditionally, glia have been viewed as cells that serve primarily housekeeping roles, but this view has changed dramatically over the past decade. Glia are known to play key roles in regulating synaptic transmission and participating in synaptic plasticity (Fields and Stevens-Graham 2002; Auld and Robitaille 2003; Pascual and Haydon 2003; Zhang and Haydon 2005). For pain resulting from peripheral nerve injury, a growing body of evidence indicates that hyperalgesia, allodynia, and ongoing pain involve active participation of glia in the spinal dorsal horn. The CNS contains three types of glia—astrocytes, oligodendrocytes, and microglia—and it is the microglia that have emerged as a central character in nerve-injury pain. Microglia comprise 5–10% of the total glial population in the CNS (Kreutzberg 1996; Stoll and Jander 1999). Under basal conditions microglia are at said to be in a resting state—a surveillance mode where they act as "sensors" to various stimuli that threaten physiological homeostasis. When activated by one of more of these stimuli, microglia show a stereotypic program of changes in morphology, gene expression, function, and number (Perry 1994). Activated microglia are competent to perform phagocytosis, giving rise to the view that these cells are resident macrophages of the CNS.

Activated microglia change their morphology from a resting, ramified shape into an active, ameboid shape (Kreutzberg 1996; Stoll and Jander 1999; Streit et al. 1999; Nakajima and Kohsaka 2001). They upregulate expression of a variety of cell-surface molecules including the complement receptor 3 (CR3), which is recognized by the antibody OX-42 (Robinson et al. 1986). Activated microglia also express immune molecules such as major histocompatibility complex (MHC) class I and II (Kreutzberg 1996; Stoll and Jander 1999; Streit et al. 1999), which play a role in antigen presentation to T lymphocytes. Activated microglia produce and release various chemical mediators, including proinflammatory cytokines, that can produce immunological actions and can also act on neurons to alter their function (Stoll and Jander 1999; Nakajima and Kohsaka 2001; Hanisch 2002). Various cytokines have activating and others inhibitory effects, such that microglial activation is reversible and tightly regulated.

The activation state of spinal microglia in the spinal cord has been examined in nerve injury models involving compression, ligation, or transaction of the sciatic nerve (Bennett and Xie 1988), spinal nerves (Kim and Chung 1992), or peripheral branches of the sciatic nerve (Decosterd and Woolf 2000). A common feature of these models is that after nerve injury, nociceptive withdrawal behaviors are evoked by stimuli that are normally perceived as innocuous, such as gentle mechanical stimulation of the skin. These models thereby mirror the allodynia suffered by humans with neuropathic pain (Zimmermann 2001; Jensen and Baron 2003; Woolf 2004). Following peripheral nerve injury a series of changes take place in microglia within spinal dorsal horn (Eriksson et al. 1993; Liu et al. 1995; Coyle 1998; Tanga et al. 2004), although the extent and time course of the changes varies in these models (Colburn et al. 1997, 1999). Within the first 24 hours after peripheral nerve injury, the first signs of microglial activation can be observed: the small soma become hypertrophic, and the long and thin processes withdraw (Eriksson et al. 1993). There is then a proliferation of microglia, peaking around 3 days after nerve injury (Gehrmann and Banati 1995). The microglia show an increased level of a number of activation "marker" proteins including CR3 (Eriksson et al. 1993; Liu et al. 1995; Coyle 1998; Tsuda et al. 2003), toll-like receptor 4 (TLR4) (Tanga et al. 2004), cluster determinant 14 (CD14) (Tanga et al. 2004), CD4 (Sweitzer et al. 2002), and MHC class II protein (Sweitzer et al. 2002; Sweitzer and DeLeo 2002). Many reports have shown a correlation between activation of microglia and signs of pain hypersensitivity. But only recently was it demonstrated that microglia have a causal role in these nerve-injury-evoked pain behaviors in studies implicating p38 MAP kinase (Jin et al. 2003) and P2X$_4$ receptors (Tsuda et al. 2003).

The P2X$_4$ receptor is a subtype of the P2X family of ligand-gated ion channels activated by adenosine triphosphate (ATP) (North 2002). Mechanical allodynia following spinal nerve ligation is acutely reversed by means of intrathecally administering a P2X$_4$ antagonist. P2X$_4$ receptors are found neither in neurons nor astrocytes (Tsuda et al. 2003). Rather, expression of P2X$_4$ receptors, which is low in the naive spinal cord, progressively increases in microglia during the days following nerve injury, paralleling the development of mechanical allodynia. Inhibiting the rise in P2X$_4$ level prevents the development of allodynia. Thus, microglial P2X$_4$ receptors are necessary for mechanical allodynia after nerve injury. Moreover, in otherwise naive animals, mechanical allodynia develops following the intrathecal administration of microglia in which P2X$_4$ receptors had been stimulated in vitro. Unstimulated microglia do not cause allodynia, nor does administering vehicle or ATP-only controls (Tsuda et al. 2003). Thus, stimulating P2X$_4$ receptors in activated microglia is both necessary and sufficient for producing mechanical allodynia.

For p38 MAP kinase, it was found that inhibiting this enzyme pharmacologically reversed mechanical allodynia following spinal nerve ligation (Jin et al. 2003). Beginning intrathecal infusion of a p38 inhibitor prior to the nerve injury prevented allodynia from developing. The nerve lesion leads to persistent activation of p38 MAP kinase, as assessed by phospho-p38 MAP kinase labeling, which is entirely restricted to microglia. Together, the findings from these two studies suggest a model in which activation of microglia, P2X$_4$ receptors, and p38 MAP kinase are central to allodynia and neuropathic pain following nerve injury. Because P2X$_4$ receptors are nonspecific cation channels that are permeable to Ca^{2+}, it is possible that ATP stimulation of these receptors leads to Ca^{2+} influx that indirectly activates p38 MAP kinase, and possibly also other downstream signaling proteins, leading to release of one or more factors that enhance transmission through the spinal nociceptive network. This enhanced transmission might be due to facilitation of glutamatergic synaptic transmission (Woolf and Salter 2000) or due to reversal of GABA/glycinergic inhibition (Coull et al. 2003).

The trigger by which a peripheral nerve injury initiates activation of spinal microglia has yet to be established, although very recent evidence suggests that TLR4 expression by these microglia is critical (Tanga et al. 2005). Nevertheless, these newly activated microglia change the properties of the spinal neurons in their vicinity to bring the ongoing maintenance of nerve-injury pain behaviors. Activated microglia are known to be functionally and phenotypically heterogenous, with various microglial proteins being altered at different times and to various degrees, depending upon the stimulus that produces the activation (Streit and Graeber 1993; Kreutzberg 1996; Stoll and Jander 1999; Nakajima and Kohsaka 2001). Evidence indicates that there is heterogeneity in the responses of spinal microglia to stimulation in the periphery that may depend upon the type of nociceptive stimulus. For example, expression of CR3 is elevated in the spinal cord following various types of peripheral nerve injury (see above and Raghavendra et al. 2003; Zhang et al. 2003). Increases in CR3 levels are also observed following stimulation that produces inflammation peripherally (Sweitzer et al. 1999; Raghavendra et al. 2004), although this finding is not uniform; there are reports that peripheral inflammatory stimulation may not lead to an increase in CR3 (Honore et al. 2000; Zhang et al. 2003). TLR4 and CD14 are also increased following peripheral nerve injury (Tanga et al. 2004) or peripheral inflammation by complete Freund's adjuvant (Raghavendra et al. 2004). In contrast, expression of $P2X_4R$ (Tsuda et al. 2003), CCR2 (Abbadie et al. 2003), CB2 (Zhang et al. 2003), and MHC class II (Sweitzer et al. 2002) is increased in spinal microglia following peripheral nerve injury but not following peripheral inflammation. Thus, while there are some similarities in the spinal microglial proteins that are upregulated following peripheral nerve injury compared with peripheral inflammation, there are also differences in microglial responses that depend upon the type of stimulus in the periphery. The differential microglial activation may explain why drugs that are clinically effective as analgesics for inflammatory pain are typically ineffective for neuropathic pain. Understanding of the key role of microglia may lead to new strategies for the diagnosis and management of neuropathic pain, strategies not previously anticipated by a view of pain plasticity focused solely on neurons.

CONCLUSION

An overall picture is emerging in which peripheral nerve damage stimulates changes in the spinal cord that evoke multiple forms of neuronal plasticity and cause activation of glial cells with subsequent glial-neuronal signaling that is critical for maintaining pain behaviors. These forms of synaptic plasticity are mechanistically similar to persistent enhancement of excitatory synaptic transmission found in most regions of the CNS. Enhancement of excitatory responses, directly or through suppression of inhibition, is a key process that increases the gain of nociceptive transmission and leads to pain hypersensitivity.

ACKNOWLEDGMENTS

The author's work is supported by grants from the Canadian Institutes of Health Research and from Neuroscience Canada. Dr. Salter holds a Canada Research Chair (Tier I) in Neuroplasticity and Pain.

REFERENCES

Abbadie C, Lindia JA, Cumiskey AM, et al. Impaired neuropathic pain responses in mice lacking the chemokine receptor CCR2. *Proc Natl Acad Sci USA* 2003; 100:7947–7952.

Albuquerque C, Lee CJ, Jackson AC, MacDermott AB. Subpopulations of GABAergic and non-GABAergic rat dorsal horn neurons express Ca^{2+}-permeable AMPA receptors. *Eur J Neurosci* 1999; 11:2758–2766.

Ali DW, Salter MW. NMDA receptor regulation by Src kinase signalling in excitatory synaptic transmission and plasticity. *Curr Opin Neurobiol* 2001; 11:336–342.

Auld DS, Robitaille R. Glial cells and neurotransmission: an inclusive view of synaptic function. *Neuron* 2003; 40:389–400.

Bennett GJ, Xie YK. A peripheral mononeuropathy in rat that produces disorders of pain sensation like those seen in man. *Pain* 1988; 33:87–107.

Cervero F, Laird JM, Garcia-Nicas E. Secondary hyperalgesia and presynaptic inhibition: an update. *Eur J Pain* 2003; 7:345-351.

Colburn RW, DeLeo JA, Rickman AJ, et al. Dissociation of microglial activation and neuropathic pain behaviors following peripheral nerve injury in the rat. *J Neuroimmunol* 1997; 79:163–175.

Colburn RW, Rickman AJ, DeLeo JA. The effect of site and type of nerve injury on spinal glial activation and neuropathic pain behavior. *Exp Neurol* 1999; 157:289–304.

Collingridge GL, Isaac JT, Wang YT. Receptor trafficking and synaptic plasticity. *Nat Rev Neurosci* 2004; 5:952–962.

Cook AJ, Woolf CJ, Wall PD, McMahon SB. Dynamic receptive field plasticity in rat spinal cord dorsal horn following C-primary afferent input. *Nature* 1987; 325:151–153.

Coull JA, Boudreau D, Bachand K, et al. Trans-synaptic shift in anion gradient in spinal lamina I neurons as a mechanism of neuropathic pain. *Nature* 2003; 424:938–942.

Coyle DE. Partial peripheral nerve injury leads to activation of astroglia and microglia which parallels the development of allodynic behavior. *Glia* 1998; 23:75–83.

De Koninck Y, Henry JL. Substance P-mediated slow excitatory postsynaptic potential elicited in dorsal horn neurons in vivo by noxious stimulation. *Proc Natl Acad Sci USA* 1991; 88:11344–11348.

Decosterd I, Woolf CJ. Spared nerve injury: an animal model of persistent peripheral neuropathic pain. *Pain* 2000; 87:149–158.

Dickenson AH, Chapman V, Green GM. The pharmacology of excitatory and inhibitory amino acid-mediated events in the transmission and modulation of pain in the spinal cord. *Gen Pharmacol* 1997; 28:633–638.

Dingledine R, Borges K, Bowie D, Traynelis SF. The glutamate receptor ion channels. *Pharmacol Rev* 1999; 51:7–61.

Duggan AW, Riley RC, Mark MA, MacMillan SJ, Schaible HG. Afferent volley patterns and the spinal release of immunoreactive substance P in the dorsal horn of the anaesthetized spinal cat. *Neuroscience* 1995; 65:849–858.

Eccles JC, Eccles RM, Magni F. Central inhibitory action attributable to presynaptic depolarization produced by muscle afferent volleys. *J Physiol (Paris)* 1961; 159:147–166.

Eccles JC, Krnjevic K. Potential changes recorded inside primary afferent fibres within the spinal cord. *J Physiol* 1959; 149:250–273.

Ehlers MR. CR3: a general purpose adhesion-recognition receptor essential for innate immunity. *Microbes Infect* 2000; 2:289–294.

Eriksson NP, Persson JK, Svensson M, et al. A quantitative analysis of the microglial cell reaction in central primary sensory projection territories following peripheral nerve injury in the adult rat. *Exp Brain Res* 1993; 96:19–27.

Fields RD, Stevens-Graham B. New insights into neuron-glia communication. *Science* 2002; 298:556–562.

Gehrmann J, Banati RB. Microglial turnover in the injured CNS: activated microglia undergo delayed DNA fragmentation following peripheral nerve injury. *J Neuropathol Exp Neurol* 1995; 54:680–688.

Gu JG, MacDermott AB. Activation of ATP P2X receptors elicits glutamate release from sensory neuron synapses. *Nature* 1997; 389:749–753.

Gu JG, Albuquerque C, Lee CJ, MacDermott AB. Synaptic strengthening through activation of Ca^{2+}-permeable AMPA receptors. *Nature* 1996; 381:793–796.

Guo W, Wei F, Zou S, et al. Group I metabotropic glutamate receptor NMDA receptor coupling and signaling cascade mediate spinal dorsal horn NMDA receptor 2B tyrosine phosphorylation associated with inflammatory hyperalgesia. *J Neurosci* 2004; 24:9161–9173.

Hanisch UK. Microglia as a source and target of cytokines. *Glia* 2002; 40:140–155.

Harvey RJ, Depner UB, Wassle H, et al. GlyR alpha3: an essential target for spinal PGE$_2$-mediated inflammatory pain sensitization. *Science* 2004; 304:884–887.

Honore P, Rogers SD, Schwei MJ, et al. Murine models of inflammatory, neuropathic and cancer pain each generates a unique set of neurochemical changes in the spinal cord and sensory neurons. *Neuroscience* 2000; 98:585–598.

Ikeda H, Heinke B, Ruscheweyh R, Sandkuhler J. Synaptic plasticity in spinal lamina I projection neurons that mediate hyperalgesia. *Science* 2003; 299:1237–1240.

Jensen TS, Baron R. Translation of symptoms and signs into mechanisms in neuropathic pain. *Pain* 2003; 102:1–8.

Jessell TM, Jahr CE. Fast and slow excitatory transmitters at primary afferent synapses in the dorsal horn of the spinal-cord. In: Fields HL, Dubner R, Cervero R (Eds). *Proceedings of the Fourth World Congress on Pain,* Advances in Pain Research and Therapy, Vol. 9. New York: Raven Press, 1985, pp 31–39.

Ji RR, Kohno T, Moore KA, Woolf CJ. Central sensitization and LTP: do pain and memory share similar mechanisms? *Trends Neurosci* 2003; 26:696–705.

Jin SX, Zhuang ZY, Woolf CJ, Ji RR. p38 mitogen-activated protein kinase is activated after a spinal nerve ligation in spinal cord microglia and dorsal root ganglion neurons and contributes to the generation of neuropathic pain. *J Neurosci* 2003; 23:4017–4022.

Kim SH, Chung JM. An experimental model for peripheral neuropathy produced by segmental spinal nerve ligation in the rat. *Pain* 1992; 50:355–363.

Kreutzberg GW. Microglia: a sensor for pathological events in the CNS. *Trends Neurosci* 1996; 19:312–318.

Laird JM, Garcia-Nicas E, Delpire EJ, Cervero F. Presynaptic inhibition and spinal pain processing in mice: a possible role of the NKCC1 cation-chloride co-transporter in hyperalgesia. *Neurosci Lett* 2004; 361:200–203.

Li P, Wilding TJ, Kim SJ, et al. Kainate-receptor-mediated sensory synaptic transmission in mammalian spinal cord. *Nature* 1999; 397:161–164.

Liu H, Wang H, Sheng M, et al. Evidence for presynaptic N-methyl-D-aspartate autoreceptors in the spinal cord dorsal horn. *Proc Natl Acad Sci USA* 1994; 91:8383–8387.

Liu L, Tornqvist E, Mattsson P, et al. Complement and clusterin in the spinal cord dorsal horn and gracile nucleus following sciatic nerve injury in the adult rat. *Neuroscience* 1995; 68:167–179.

Liu L, Wong TP, Pozza MF, et al. Role of NMDA receptor subtypes in governing the direction of hippocampal synaptic plasticity. *Science* 2004; 304:1021–1024.

Lu YM, Mansuy IM, Kandel ER, Roder J. Calcineurin-mediated LTD of GABAergic inhibition underlies the increased excitability of CA1 neurons associated with LTP. *Neuron* 2000; 26:197–205.

Malcangio M, Bowery NG. GABA and its receptors in the spinal cord. *Trends Pharmacol Sci* 1996; 17:457–462.

Malenka RC, Bear MF. LTP and LTD: an embarrassment of riches. *Neuron* 2004; 44:5–21.

Malenka RC, Nicoll RA. Long-term potentiation—a decade of progress? *Science* 1999; 285:1870–1874.

McMahon SB, Wall PD. A system of rat spinal cord lamina 1 cells projecting through the contralateral dorsolateral funiculus. *J Comp Neurol* 1983; 214:217–223.

Mendell LM. Modifiability of spinal synapses. *Physiol Rev* 1984; 64:260–324.

Moore KA, Baba H, Woolf CJ. Synaptic transmission and plasticity in the superficial dorsal horn. *Prog Brain Res* 2000; 129:63–80.

Moore KA, Kohno T, Karchewski LA, et al. Partial peripheral nerve injury promotes a selective loss of GABAergic inhibition in the superficial dorsal horn of the spinal cord. *J Neurosci* 2002; 15:6724–6731.

Morisset V, Nagy F. Ionic basis for plateau potentials in deep dorsal horn neurons of the rat spinal cord. *J Neurosci* 1999; 19:7309–7316.

Nakajima K, Kohsaka S. Microglia: activation and their significance in the central nervous system. *J Biochem (Tokyo)* 2001; 130:169–175.

North RA. Molecular physiology of P2X receptors. *Physiol Rev* 2002; 82:1013–1067.

Pascual O, Haydon PG. Synaptic inhibition mediated by glia. *Neuron* 2003; 40:873–875.

Perry VH. Modulation of microglia phenotype. *Neuropathol Appl Neurobiol* 1994; 20:177–

Prescott SA, De Koninck Y. Gain control of firing rate by shunting inhibition: roles of synaptic noise and dendritic saturation. *Proc Natl Acad Sci USA* 2003; 100:2076–2081.

Raghavendra V, Tanga F, DeLeo JA. Inhibition of microglial activation attenuates the development but not existing hypersensitivity in a rat model of neuropathy. *J Pharmacol Exp Ther* 2003; 306:624–630.

Raghavendra V, Tanga FY, DeLeo JA. Complete Freund's adjuvant-induced peripheral inflammation evokes glial activation and proinflammatory cytokine expression in the CNS. *Eur J Neurosci* 2004; 20:467–473.

Randic M, Jiang MC, Cerne R. Long-term potentiation and long-term depression of primary afferent neurotransmission in the rat spinal cord. *J Neurosci* 1993; 13:5228–5241.

Robinson AP, White TM, Mason DW. Macrophage heterogeneity in the rat as delineated by two monoclonal antibodies MRC OX-41 and MRC OX-42, the latter recognizing complement receptor type 3. *Immunology* 1986; 57:239–247.

Salter MW, Kalia LV. Src kinases: a hub for NMDA receptor regulation. *Nat Rev Neurosci* 2004; 5:317–328.

Seeburg PH, Higuchi M, Sprengel R. RNA editing of brain glutamate receptor channels: mechanism and physiology. *Brain Res Brain Res Rev* 1998; 26:217–229.

Sivilotti LG, Thompson SW, Woolf CJ. Rate of rise of the cumulative depolarization evoked by repetitive stimulation of small-caliber afferents is a predictor of action potential windup in rat spinal neurons in vitro. *J Neurophysiol* 1993; 69:1621–1631.

Stoll G, Jander S. The role of microglia and macrophages in the pathophysiology of the CNS. *Prog Neurobiol* 1999; 58:233–247.

Streit WJ, Graeber MB. Heterogeneity of microglial and perivascular cell populations: insights gained from the facial nucleus paradigm. *Glia* 1993; 7:68–74.

Streit WJ, Walter SA, Pennell NA. Reactive microgliosis. *Prog Neurobiol* 1999; 57:563–581.

Sweitzer SM, DeLeo JA. The active metabolite of leflunomide, an immunosuppressive agent, reduces mechanical sensitivity in a rat mononeuropathy model. *J Pain* 2002; 3:360–368.

Sweitzer SM, Colburn RW, Rutkowski M, DeLeo JA. Acute peripheral inflammation induces moderate glial activation and spinal IL-1-beta expression that correlates with pain behavior in the rat. *Brain Res* 1999; 829:209–221.

Sweitzer SM, White KA, Dutta C, DeLeo JA. The differential role of spinal MHC class II and cellular adhesion molecules in peripheral inflammatory versus neuropathic pain in rodents. *J Neuroimmunol* 2002; 125:82–93.

Tanga FY, Nutile-McMenemy N, DeLeo JA. The CNS role of Toll-like receptor 4 in innate neuroimmunity and painful neuropathy. *Proc Natl Acad Sci USA* 2005; 102:5856–5861.

Tanga FY, Raghavendra V, DeLeo JA. Quantitative real-time RT-PCR assessment of spinal microglial and astrocytic activation markers in a rat model of neuropathic pain. *Neurochem Int* 2004; 45:397–407.

Tsuda M, Shigemoto-Mogami Y, Koizumi S, et al. P2X4 receptors induced in spinal microglia gate tactile allodynia after nerve injury. *Nature* 2003; 424:778–783.

Wang J, Liu S, Haditsch U, et al. Interaction of calcineurin and type-A GABA receptor gamma 2 subunits produces long-term depression at CA1 inhibitory synapses. *J Neurosci* 2003; 23:826–836.

Woolf CJ. Dissecting out mechanisms responsible for peripheral neuropathic pain: implications for diagnosis and therapy. *Life Sci* 2004; 74:2605–2610.

Woolf CJ. Evidence for a central component of post-injury pain hypersensitivity. *Nature* 1983; 306:686–688.

Woolf CJ, Salter MW. Neuronal plasticity: increasing the gain in pain. *Science* 2000; 288:1765–1769.

Woolf CJ, Salter MW. Plasticity and pain: role of the dorsal horn. In: McMahon, Koltzenburg M (Eds). *Textbook of Pain.* Edinburgh: Churchill Livingstone, 2005, in press.

Zhang J, Hoffert C, Vu HK, et al. Induction of CB2 receptor expression in the rat spinal cord of neuropathic but not inflammatory chronic pain models. *Eur J Neurosci* 2003; 17:2750–2754.

Zhang Q, Haydon PG. Roles for gliotransmission in the nervous system. *J Neural Transm* 2005; 112:121–125.

Zimmermann M. Pathobiology of neuropathic pain. *Eur J Pharmacol* 2001; 429:23–37.

Correspondence to: Michael W. Salter, MD, PhD, The Hospital for Sick Children, 555 University Avenue, Toronto, Ontario, Canada M5G 1X8. Tel: 416-813-6272; Fax: 416-813-7921; email: mike.salter@utoronto.ca.

Emerging Strategies for the Treatment of Neuropathic Pain, edited by James N. Campbell, Allan I. Basbaum, André Dray, Ronald Dubner, Robert H. Dworkin, and Christine N. Sang, IASP Press, Seattle, © 2006.

10

Ascending and Descending Facilitatory Circuits in Neuropathic Pain States

Michael H. Ossipov and Frank Porreca

Department of Pharmacology, College of Medicine, University of Arizona, Tucson, Arizona, USA

Chronic pain states, typically represented as inflammatory or neuropathic in origin, are characterized by enhanced perception of pain to a nociceptive stimulus (i.e., hyperalgesia) and by the novel perception of a normally innocuous stimulus as being painful (i.e., allodynia). Our knowledge of the mechanisms that drive these enhanced pain states has grown considerably over the last three decades, and we now understand that chronic pain states depend in part on sensitization of the spinal cord, on activation of nociceptive pathways projecting to medullary and midbrain sites, and on activation of descending pain-facilitatory systems. The latter appear to be essential in maintaining a sensitized state of the spinal cord.

SENSITIZATION OF THE SPINAL DORSAL HORN BY PRIMARY AFFERENT INPUTS

Injury or inflammation of peripheral nerves results, clinically, in hyperalgesia and allodynia, and is closely related to sensitization of the spinal cord. Spinal sensitization has been thought to be a direct result of increased primary afferent discharges into the spinal cord that maintain a state of excitation. Injured nerves show spontaneous, ectopic discharges from injury-induced neuromas, and mechanical stimulation of the neuromas elicit sensations ranging from minor dysesthesias to intense pain (Wall and Gutnick 1974a,b; Devor 1991). Spontaneous ectopic discharge has been shown to be generated in the dorsal root ganglion (DRG) of the injured nerves that remained after excision of the neuroma (Kirk 1974; Bennett 1993; Koltzenburg et al. 1994; Wilcox et al. 2004). Electrophysiological studies with sciatic nerve bundles or DRG neurons demonstrated that spontaneous ectopic discharges occurred not only in the injured nerves, but also in adjacent uninjured nerve bundles (Tal and Eliav 1996; Chen and Devor 1998; Michaelis et al. 2000). It was suggested that Wallerian degeneration of the injured, spontaneously active myelinated fibers may excite unmyelinated fibers through the commingling of fibers or by the release of cytokines and other excitatory factors, resulting in a sensitized peripheral nerve (Li et al. 2000; Wu et al. 2001, 2002). However, research has demonstrated little temporal correlation between injury-induced ectopic discharges and the development of behavioral signs of neuropathic pain. Ectopic action potentials and spontaneous discharges from injured peripheral nerves increased within the immediate post-injury period to maximal levels within 1 week of injury, but they declined very rapidly, diminishing by approximately one-half within 3 weeks, and were essentially lost within 10 weeks (Han et al. 2000; C.N. Liu et al. 2000; X. Liu et al. 2000). In contrast, behavioral manifestations of nerve injury endure for months after the initial injury (Chaplan et al. 1994; Malan et al. 2000; Burgess et al. 2002). Current evidence indicates that the initial discharges initiate a state of central sensitization, but neuroplastic changes within the central nervous system maintain the long-term sensitized status of the spinal dorsal horn (Burgess et al. 2002; Porreca et al. 2002; Heinricher et al. 2003). This chapter describes the neuroplastic activation of ascending and descending components of the pain-facilitatory system.

PRIMARY AFFERENT INPUTS AND SPINAL SENSITIZATION: A PRELUDE TO NEUROPATHIC PAIN STATES

The augmented primary afferent activity in the immediate aftermath of nerve injury produces a state similar to long-term potentiation, commonly referred to as spinal sensitization (Ma and Woolf 1995b; Ji et al. 2003). A specific type of sensitization may be suggested by the phenomenon of wind-up, which is observed as progressively increasing responses of spinal dorsal horn neurons following repetitive electrical stimulation of C fibers (Mendell 1966; Li et al. 1999a). This phenomenon implies that an initial stimulus produces sufficient excitation of postsynaptic cells and that these cells are not fully repolarized before the next stimulus arrives, and thus are primed to produce an enhanced response. Importantly, wind-up is not elicited by repeated stimulation of $A\beta$ fibers and is nociceptive-specific (Mendell 1966; Woolf 1996; Li et al. 1999a). A more generalized and long-lasting type of sensitization occurs when conditioning stimuli elicited as electrically evoked trains of C fibers produce a long-term responsiveness of dorsal horn units to later stimuli, ultimately resulting in a prolonged afterdischarge (Ma and Woolf 1995b; Ji et al. 2003). The slow depolarizations of these dorsal horn neurons allow the development of temporal summation to inputs from primary afferent C fibers, which may translate as increased pain (Woolf and Thompson 1991; Ren 1994).

These observations correlate well with studies performed with natural stimuli. Noxious stimuli applied to the skin enhance the excitability of dorsal horn units such that responses to subsequent stimuli are exaggerated and repetitive C-fiber conditioning stimuli cause prolonged flexion reflexes in rats (Woolf 1983; Woolf and Thompson 1991). The persistent spontaneous afferent discharges after peripheral nerve injury are also believed to produce a similar sensitized state, leading to the enhanced pain observed in the neuropathic state (Woolf and Wiesenfeld-Hallin 1985; Ma and Woolf 1995b; Ziegler et al. 1999; Zimmermann 2001). Both the spontaneous and C-fiber-evoked activities of wide-dynamic-range (WDR) neurons in the dorsal horn were enhanced in rats with nerve injury (Rygh et al. 2000). Nerve injury caused increased spontaneous activity and afterdischarges of spinothalamic tract (STT) neurons to noxious thermal or mechanical stimuli and enhanced responses to innocuous light brush (Palecek et al. 1992; Leem et al. 1995; Suzuki and Dickenson 2000). The stimulus-response function of WDR neurons in response to tactile, but not thermal, stimuli applied within their receptive field was shifted to the left in nerve-injured rats (Pertovaara et al. 1997). C-fiber-evoked sensitization renders these neurons excitable by Aβ-fiber inputs, to which they are unreactive in the resting state, and may contribute to touch-evoked allodynia in chronic pain states (Ma and Woolf 1995b; Ji et al. 2003). The latter observations also suggest that thermal and tactile dysesthesias may be mediated, at least partly, through different pathways, as discussed further below.

Evidence of spinal sensitization in the nerve-injured state also comes from the augmented evoked expression of the proto-oncogene product Fos, which is a reliable indicator for neurons that are activated by noxious stimulation (Hunt et al. 1987; Molander et al. 1992; Harris 1998; Shortland and Molander 1998). Natural noxious stimuli and electrical stimulation of C fibers provokes the expression of Fos, predominantly in laminae I, II, and V of the spinal dorsal horn, whereas stimulation at Aβ intensity does not evoke the expression of Fos (Hunt et al. 1987; Willis and Coggeshall 1991; Shortland and Molander 1998). The level of Fos expression increases with the intensity of nociceptive stimuli (Presley et al. 1990; Gogas et al. 1991). The expression of Fos in the spinal cord is enhanced in states of peripheral nerve injury and correlates with increased nociceptive responses (Hunt et al. 1987; Molander et al. 1992, 1994, 1998; Shortland and Molander 1998). The expression of Fos in response to light tactile stimulation is increased in the spinal and medullary dorsal horns after peripheral nerve injury (Molander et al. 1992, 1994; Shortland and Molander 1998; Nomura et al. 2002). Moreover, light tactile stimulation that does not evoke FOS expression in normal rats causes significant increases in Fos expression after nerve injury, which is observed throughout the spinal dorsal horn (Catheline et al. 1999, 2001). Similarly, electrical stimulation of peripheral nerves at Aβ intensity evokes novel Fos expression predominantly in laminae I and V, but also in laminae III and IV, although to a lesser extent (Molander et al. 1992, 1994; Shortland and Molander 1998; Nomura et al. 2002). Spinal sensitization may result in novel responsiveness to light tactile stimuli, which may be interpreted behaviorally as tactile hyperesthesia, in addition to the increased responsiveness of nociceptors, yielding hyperalgesia.

ENHANCED PRIMARY AFFERENT ACTIVITY PROMOTES SENSITIZATION

Evidence for increased primary afferent activity is supported by microdialysis studies showing that the release of glutamate and aspartate from primary afferents is increased in response to intradermal capsaicin or formalin or to repeated electrical stimulation of C fibers (Skilling et al. 1988; Paleckova et al. 1992; Sluka and Willis 1998). A recent study employing microdialysis found that spinal administration of N-methyl-D-aspartate (NMDA) elicited a long-lasting release of prostaglandin E_2 (PGE_2) and, subsequently, of excitatory amino acids (Koetzner et al. 2004). Spontaneous and stimulus-evoked release of substance P and calcitonin gene-related peptide (CGRP) from primary afferent terminals is increased after peripheral nerve injury (Wallin and Schott 2002; Gardell et al. 2003). The increased release of excitatory neurotransmitters from primary afferents, including glutamate, substance P, and CGRP, promotes the sensitization of target neurons and can lead to hyperalgesia by virtue of the enhanced responsiveness of the excited cells (Ma and Woolf 1995a; Sun et al. 2004). For example, the increased WDR activity in response to light brush caused by intradermal capsaicin was blocked by a CGRP-receptor antagonist, and superfusion of the spinal cord with CGRP induced hypersensitivity, leading to the conclusion that increased CGRP release from primary afferents sensitizes dorsal horn neurons (Sun et al. 2004). Moreover, the superfusion of dorsal spinal cord section with CGRP potentiated the release of substance P, and spinal injection of CGRP enhanced behavioral responses to noxious mechanical stimuli (Oku et al. 1987). Primary afferent outflow is also boosted by glutamate acting at excitatory presynaptic NMDA autoreceptors of the primary afferent terminals (Liu et al. 1994; Ohishi et al. 1995). This increase in primary afferent outflow amplifies the activity of the second-order neurons, which release nitric oxide and PGE_2, which then promote further release of glutamate and excitatory neuropeptides from primary afferent terminals (Liu et al. 1997; Kawamata and Omote 1999). The selective activation of central terminals of C-fiber nociceptors with capsaicin resulted in the release of PGE_2 from the postsynaptic cells (Malmberg and Yaksh 1994). In turn, PGE_2 enhanced capsaicin-evoked release of substance P and CGRP through presynaptic excitation (Hingtgen and Vasko 1994; Vasko 1995; Southall and Vasko 2001). Taken together, these studies indicate that repeated or persistent noxious stimuli can enhance the outflow of excitatory neurotransmitters and may potentiate their excitatory functions, setting the stage for the development of central sensitization.

POSTSYNAPTIC TARGETS OF PRIMARY AFFERENTS: SPINOTHALAMIC TRACT NEURONS OF LAMINA I THAT EXPRESS NK1 RECEPTORS

The development of behavioral hypersensitivity to sensory stimuli is partly dependent on the long-term sensitization of the projection neurons of lamina I that express neurokinin-1 (NK1) receptors (Ikeda et al. 2003). Spinal NMDA administration evoked an increase in release of substance P and caused a marked internalization of the NK1 receptor of dorsal horn neurons that was abolished by capsaicin-induced desensitization of nociceptors or by administration of CGRP antagonists (Liu et al. 1997). Peripheral nerve injury is associated with an upregulation of NK1 receptors in the spinal dorsal horn (Taylor and McCarson 2004). Normally, only noxious stimulation causes the internalization of the NK1 receptor, which occurs in lamina I (Abbadie et al. 1997). However, after nerve injury or inflammation, substantial internalization of the NK1 receptor occurs not only in the superficial dorsal horn, but also in laminae III through V, even in response to light brush, clearly indicating a sensitized state (Abbadie et al. 1997; Allen et al. 1999). Although stimulation of Aβ fibers alone was insufficient to provoke NK1 internalization even after nerve injury, the possibility of Aβ-mediated sensitization is not eliminated because a novel Aβ-induced "windup" has been observed after chronic inflammation (Allen et al. 1999; Hedo et al. 1999). Substance P is co-released with CGRP from primary afferent terminals, and the release of both neuropeptides is enhanced with nerve injury, even though the content of these transmitters decreases in the nerve-injured state (Kajander and Xu 1995; Gardell et al. 2003; Ma and Eisenach 2003). Recent evidence showed that activation of the CGRP receptor stimulates expression of the NK1 receptor, providing for augmented responsiveness of the postsynaptic neurons to substance P (Seybold et al. 2003). Activation of the NK1 receptor acts synergistically with activation of the NMDA/calcium channel complex to facilitate firing of the NK1-expressing cells of lamina I, thus promoting central sensitization (Ikeda et al. 2003). Antagonists blocking the NK1 and NMDA receptors abolished augmented release of excitatory neurotransmitters from postsynaptic neurons (Sluka and Westlund 1993). In addition, recent studies indicate that the potassium-chloride exporter KCC2 is downregulated in the chronic nerve-injured state, thus altering anionic currents such that normally inhibitory currents become excitatory, resulting in an increased excitability, or sensitization, of the lamina I neuron (Coull et al. 2003).

Although the NK1-expressing neurons constitute less than 5% of the population of dorsal horn cells, they account for more than 77% of the nociceptive-responsive cells of lamina I that project through the STT and are the principal targets of the primary afferent nociceptors that release substance P (Nichols et al. 1999; Cheunsuang and Morris 2000; Suzuki et al. 2002). Importantly, only the neurons that project supraspinally exhibit sensitization, whereas those with local terminations show no signs of sensitization (Khasabov et al. 2002; Mantyh and Hunt 2004). Morphologically distinct populations of NK1-expressing neurons of laminae I have axonal projections to the thalamus and parabrachial regions, and one group demonstrates axonal arborizations that project to deeper laminae of the spinal cord and are able to promote sensitization of the deeper WDR neurons in a chronic pain state (Cheunsuang and Morris 2000). A selective ablation of neurons that express the NK1 receptor was accomplished by the spinal administration of substance P conjugated to saporin (SP-SAP) (Nichols et al. 1999; Suzuki et al. 2002). The selective knock-down of the NK1-expressing neurons abolished behavioral signs of tactile and thermal hyperesthesias in rats with peripheral nerve injury or inflammation of the hindpaw, but did not alter responses to acute nociceptive stimuli (Nichols et al. 1999). In a more recent study, ablation of NK1-expressing neurons of laminae I with SP-SAP resulted in a loss of the augmented behavioral responses and electrophysiological responses of WDR neurons to tactile and thermal stimuli after inflammation and abolished both the tonic phase of formalin-induced flinching and C-fiber-induced wind-up (Suzuki et al. 2002). The electrophysiological responses of postsynaptic cells in the superficial and deep laminae of the spinal dorsal horns to intradermal capsaicin and the resulting hypersensitivity to mechanical and thermal stimuli were abolished by the selective destruction of NK1-expressing lamina I neurons by SP-SAP (Khasabov et al. 2002). The activation of this ascending limb relays persistent nociceptive messages to the parabrachial and thalamic regions, and appears to ultimately induce an activation of descending pain facilitatory systems from the rostroventromedial medulla (RVM) (Suzuki et al. 2002, 2004b).

AN ALTERNATE PATHWAY: PROJECTIONS TO THE DORSAL COLUMN NUCLEI

The dorsal column pathway is a major ascending pathway to the nucleus gracilis and nucleus cuneatus of the caudal medulla and transmits primarily tactile sensation. This pathway consists of direct projections from the large-diameter myelinated primary afferent $A\beta$ fibers as well as from the postsynaptic dorsal column (PSDC) neurons, which receive afferent inputs and terminate in the dorsal column nuclei (Wang et al. 1999). The PSDC neuronal cell bodies are distributed within laminae III–VI of the dorsal horn of the spinal cord, with some neurons dispersed about the central canal (Bennett et al. 1983, 1984; Giesler et al. 1984; Wang et al. 1999). This distribution coincides with the terminal arborizations of the $A\beta$, but not C, fibers (Todd 2002). Although the role of the PSDC neurons, and of the dorsal column pathway overall, in nociceptive transmission is not established, some evidence shows that a subpopulation of PSDC cells can mediate nociceptive signals from viscera and bone (Willis and Westlund 1997). Dorsal column lesions relieved intractable pelvic cancer pain (Hirshberg et al. 1996; Nauta et al. 1997). Likewise, dorsal column lesions abolished behavioral and electrophysiological nociceptive responses to experimental pancreatitis (Houghton et al. 1997, 2001). Furthermore, neuronal excitation of the n. gracilis or of the ventroposterolateral nucleus of the thalamus in response to colorectal distension were blocked by dorsal column lesions (Al-Chaer et al. 1996a,b). Noxious pinch, but not light touch, applied over 4 hours evoked Fos expression in retrogradely labeled PSDC cells within laminae III and IV of the spinal dorsal horn (Day et al. 2001b).

The dorsal column pathway may play a role with regard to neuropathic pain. The n. gracilis demonstrates significant neuroplastic changes in response to peripheral nerve injury, including de novo expression of substance P, CGRP, and neuropeptide Y (Noguchi et al. 1995; Miki et al. 1998; Li et al. 1999b). Upregulation of neuropeptide Y in the n. gracilis was abolished by dorsal rhizotomy and by ipsilateral, but not contralateral, lesions of the dorsal column, as was tactile hyperesthesia, but not thermal hyperalgesia (Sun et al. 2001; Ossipov et al. 2002). Similarly, tactile, but not thermal, behavioral signs of neuropathic pain were abolished by lidocaine or neuropeptide Y antagonists given into the ipsilateral, but not the contralateral, n. gracilis (Sun et al. 2001; Ossipov et al. 2002).

Electrical stimulation of the sciatic nerve does not evoke Fos expression in the n. gracilis in the normal state, whereas after nerve injury, stimulation at only Aβ intensities evoked substantial Fos expression in the n. gracilis (Persson et al. 1993; Molander et al. 1994; Shortland and Molander 1998). Approximately 80% of the Fos-labeled neurons projected to the thalamus (Persson et al. 1993). Similarly, Aβ stimulation of the median nerve elicited Fos expression in neurons of the n. cuneatus that project to the thalamus, but only after injury (Day et al. 2001a). Additionally, electrical stimulation of Aβ fibers evoked Fos expression in retrogradely labeled PSDC neurons, but only after sciatic nerve injury (Molander et al. 1994; Shortland and Molander 1998). Sciatic injury caused sensitization of WDR neurons of the ventroposterolateral nucleus of the thalamus that was abolished by lesions of the dorsal columns or the n. gracilis, suggesting an excitatory input through this ascending pathway (Miki et al. 2000). Evidence indicates that tactile inputs mediated through the dorsal column/medial lemniscal pathways converge with nociceptive inputs from the STT in the ventrobasal complex of the thalamus, which may serve as a site of interaction between noxious and innocuous sensory inputs (Ma et al. 1987). Moreover, sciatic nerve injury is associated with enhanced responses of low-threshold mechanoreceptive and WDR neurons of the ventroposterolateral nucleus of the thalamus and evokes FOS expression there as well (Miki et al. 2000; Narita et al. 2003). Thus, a sensitized spinothalamic system may be more receptive to tactile inputs from the dorsal column pathway and may therefore allow the interpretation of innocuous tactile sensory input as being nociceptive, or aversive. This converged information may then be processed through the descending pain-modulatory systems from the periaqueductal gray and RVM to ultimately produce a tonic descending pain-facilitatory system.

ACTIVATION OF DESCENDING PAIN FACILITATORY PATHWAYS FROM THE RVM MAINTAIN CENTRAL SENSITIZATION

The rostroventromedial medulla, considered to be the final common relay with respect to nociceptive processing and modulation, receives inputs from the spinal dorsal horn and also from rostral sites (Fields et al. 1983; Fields and Heinricher 1985; Fields and Basbaum 1999). Whereas its role in modulating a spinopetal pain inhibitory system has long been recognized, it is now realized that the RVM also acts as a source of descending facilitation of nociceptive inputs at the level of the spinal dorsal horn (Fields 1992; Zhuo and Gebhart 1997; Urban and Gebhart 1999; Calejesan et al. 2000; Porreca et al. 2002; Gebhart 2004). Early studies identified reciprocal excitatory connections between the spinal cord and the area corresponding to the RVM in cats (Cervero and Wolstencroft 1984). Electrical stimulation applied in the n. raphe magnus and surrounding tissue elicited excitatory responses in neurons of the spinal dorsal horns (Cervero and Wolstencroft 1984). Although focal electrical stimulation of the RVM at high current intensities inhibits behavioral and electrophysiological responses to nociceptive stimuli, stimulation at low intensities actually promotes nociceptive responses (Zhuo and Gebhart 1990, 1992). Similarly, microinjection of glutamate or neurotensin into the RVM also produced biphasic effects on dorsal horn unit activity in response to noxious heat and on visceromotor responses to noxious colorectal distension (Zhuo and Gebhart 1990, 1992; Urban et al. 1999). Manipulations that attenuate RVM activity have blocked enhanced nociception caused by a variety of methods. Hyperalgesia induced by naloxone-precipitated opioid withdrawal was blocked by the microinjection of lidocaine into the RVM (Kaplan and Fields 1991). Taken together, these observations indicate the existence of an endogenous pain-facilitatory system that arises from the RVM (Urban and Gebhart 1997).

DESCENDING FACILITATION FROM THE ROSTROVENTROMEDIAL MEDULLA: ON-CELLS

Electrophysiological studies of responses of RVM neurons to noxious thermal stimulation have identified the existence of "on"-cells and "off"-cells (Fields 1992; Fields and Basbaum 1999; Heinricher et al. 2003). By definition, the off-cells are tonically active and pause in firing immediately before a withdrawal response from a noxious thermal stimulus, whereas the on-cells accelerate firing immediately before the nociceptive reflex occurs (Fields 1992; Fields and Basbaum 1999; Heinricher et al. 2003). In addition, a class of "neutral" cells was initially characterized by the absence of response to noxious thermal stimulation. The activity of off-cells correlates with inhibition of nociceptive input and nocifensive responses, and these neurons are essential for the antinociceptive effect of opioids (Fields 1992; Fields and Basbaum 1999; Heinricher et al. 2003). In contrast, the response characteristics of the on-cells suggest that these neurons are the source of descending facilitation of nociception (Fields 1992; Fields and Basbaum 1999; McNally 1999; Heinricher et al. 2003). Nociceptive tail-flick latency was longer during periods of increased off-cell activity and shorter when the on-cells were active, leading to the conclusion that the off-cells inhibit and the on-cells facilitate transmission of, and responses to, spinal nociceptive input (Heinricher et al. 1989). Accordingly, manipulations that increase on-cell activity also increase nociceptive responsiveness, which is consistent with descending facilitation. The enhanced nociceptive behavior that is observed during naloxone-precipitated withdrawal from morphine has been associated with increased spontaneous activity of the RVM on-cells (Bederson et al. 1990; Kim et al. 1990). Furthermore, both naloxone-induced hyperalgesia and on-cell activity were abolished by microinjection of lidocaine into the RVM (Kaplan and Fields 1991). It has been suggested that supraspinal sites can contribute to either the development or maintenance of chronic pain states, and that the RVM is a critical component of a spino-bulbospinal loop important to the development and maintenance of exaggerated pain behaviors produced by noxious and non-noxious peripheral stimuli (Morgan and Fields 1994; Suzuki et al. 2002; see Fig. 1).

DESCENDING FACILITATION MEDIATES
THE NEUROPATHIC PAIN STATE

Converging lines of evidence suggest that the development of abnormal pain states depends on the establishment of descending facilitatory mechanisms arising from the RVM. For example, the application of a noxious thermal conditioning stimulus applied to the tail facilitated the hindpaw withdrawal reflex and increased on-cell activity (Morgan and Fields 1994). Both the enhanced on-cell activity and facilitation of nociception were abolished by lidocaine microinjected into the RVM (Morgan and Fields 1994). The heightened responses to mechanical or cold, but not noxious thermal, stimuli in rats with peripheral nerve injury were abolished by a transection or hemisection of the thoracic spinal cord (Bian et al. 1998; Kauppila et al. 1998a; Sung et al. 1998; Sun et al. 2001). The selective disruption of the dorsolateral funiculus (DLF) made ipsilateral, but not contralateral, to peripheral nerve injury abolished tactile allodynia without altering normal behaviors (Ossipov et al. 2000a). These results are consistent with the hypothesis that behavioral manifestations of chronic pain states are dependent on descending facilitation of spinal nociceptive input from the RVM, given that this region is a principal source of descending DLF projections (Fields and Basbaum 1999; Gebhart 2004). Importantly, DLF lesions in normal rats did not increase or decrease basal responses to acute noxious stimuli, indicating that the RVM does not exert a tonic modulation of nociception in normal

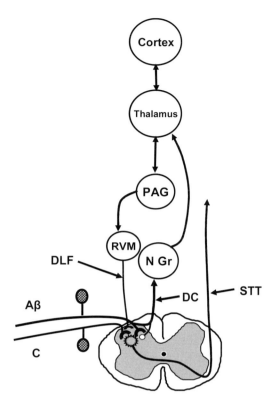

Fig. 1. Large-diameter primary afferent (Aβ) fibers project directly through the dorsal columns (DC) to the nucleus gracilis (N Gr). These primary afferents may also terminate in the intermediate laminae of the spinal dorsal horn and synapse with second-order neurons that might include postsynaptic dorsal column (PSDC) cells that project along the DC to the n. gracilis. The n. gracilis communicates with thalamic nuclei via the medial lemniscus. The unmyelinated C-fiber nociceptors transmit nociceptive inputs to the outer laminae of the spinal dorsal horn, where they may synapse with neurons of the spinotha-lamic tract (STT), which projects to supraspinal sites, including the thalamus, and to the periaqueductal gray (PAG). Descending projections from the PAG mediate nociception by activating spinopetal inhibitory projections from the rostral ventromedial medulla (RVM). These projections course along the dorsal lateral funiculus (DLF) and inhibit nociceptive inputs either by inhibiting release of excitatory transmitters from afferent terminals or by inhibiting the response of ascending second-order neurons to noxious inputs.

conditions (Ossipov et al. 2000a; Porreca et al. 2002). Early observations indicated that electrical stimulation of the DLF elicits an excitation of dorsal horn units in lamina I through activation of descending fibers, and not through antidromic activation of ascending fibers (McMahon and Wall 1983, 1988).

Considerable evidence now exists to show that the activation of de-scending facilitation from the RVM is essential to maintain the behavioral features of the neuropathic pain state (Ossipov et al. 2001; Porreca et al.

2002; Heinricher et al. 2003). Hyperesthetic responses to cold or tactile stimuli, but not to noxious heat, in animals with peripheral nerve injuries were abolished by transection or hemisection of the spinal cord (Kauppila 1997, 1998b; Bian et al. 1998; Sung et al. 1998). Behavioral signs of neuropathic pain were blocked by lidocaine microinjected into the RVM (Pertovaara et al. 1996; Mansikka and Pertovaara 1997; Calejesan et al. 2000; Kovelowski et al. 2000; Burgess et al. 2002). The selective activation of on-cells by microinjection of cholecystokinin (CCK) into the RVM caused hypersensitivity to noxious and innocuous mechanical and thermal stimuli (Kovelowski et al. 2000; Heinricher and Neubert 2004). Electrophysiological evidence strongly suggests that the population of RVM neurons that express the μ-opioid receptor are likely to drive descending facilitation (Pan et al. 1990; Heinricher et al. 1992, 1994). It was possible to selectively destroy a large part of this population of RVM neurons by using the μ-opioid receptor as a "portal of entry" into these cells for dermorphin conjugated with the cytotoxin saporin (Porreca et al. 2001; Burgess et al. 2002). The microinjection of the dermorphin-saporin conjugate into the RVM either 7 days prior to spinal nerve ligation (SNL) or once tactile and thermal hyperesthesias were well established respectively prevented and reversed the behavioral signs of neuropathic pain, demonstrating that activity of descending pain facilitation cells is a critical component of neuropathic pain (Porreca et al. 2001; Burgess et al. 2002). Both the selective ablation of descending pain facilitation cells of the RVM and disruption of descending facilitatory tracts from the RVM by lesioning the DLF abolished the behavioral signs of neuropathic pain about 1 week after the nerve injury, and not earlier (Porreca et al. 2001; Burgess et al. 2002). Moreover, the microinjection of lidocaine into the RVM within 3 days of SNL did not block either tactile or thermal hyperesthesias, whereas the same injections made 6, 9, or 12 days after SNL were fully active (Burgess et al. 2002). These observations indicate that the maintenance phase of the neuropathic pain state is dependent on certain neuroplastic changes that activate descending pain facilitation from the RVM (Porreca et al. 2001; Burgess et al. 2002; Heinricher et al. 2003). The development and maintenance of neuropathic pain states may be linked to the increased expression or availability of CCK in the RVM.

DESCENDING FACILITATION FROM THE ROSTROVENTROMEDIAL MEDULLA MAY REQUIRE CHOLECYSTOKININ

Cholecystokinin has long been recognized as an endogenous pronociceptive agent that counters the antinociceptive effect of exogenous opioids (Faris et al. 1983; Stanfa et al. 1994). It was recently shown that CCK opposes the antinociceptive activity of morphine by attenuating the morphine-induced activation of off-cells (Heinricher et al. 2001). The microinjection of CCK into the RVM has produced behavioral hypersensitivities to innocuous and noxious tactile and thermal stimuli reminiscent of nerve injury, and the CCK_2 antagonist L365,260 given into the RVM reversed these behavioral signs in rats with peripheral nerve injury (Kovelowski et al. 2000; Xie et al. 2005). The behavioral hyperesthesias and hyperalgesia elicited by CCK administered to the RVM were abolished by DLF lesions or by microinjection of L365,260 (Kovelowski et al. 2000; Xie et al. 2005). In addition to its activities in inhibiting morphine-induced activation of off-cells, CCK also provokes a direct and selective activation of on-cells of the RVM that is directly related to the production of hyperalgesia (Heinricher and Neubert 2004).

SEROTONERGIC COMPONENT OF DESCENDING FACILITATION FROM THE ROSTROVENTROMEDIAL MEDULLA

The RVM and surrounding region include the nuclei of prominent spinopetal serotonergic projections that constitute both inhibitory and facilitatory pathways (Zhuo and Gebhart 1991; Calejesan et al. 1998; Robinson et al. 2002; Suzuki et al. 2004b). Facilitation of nociceptive reflexes elicited by electrical stimulation or by glutamate applied into the RVM was abolished by spinal methysergide (Calejesan et al. 1998). Moreover, the same dose of methysergide that blocked RVM-induced facilitation also blocked enhanced nociception elicited by intradermal formalin (Calejesan et al. 1998). It has recently become evident that serotonin (5HT) receptors of the $5HT_{1A}$ subtype mediate inhibition, whereas $5HT_3$ receptors mediate facilitation (reviewed in Suzuki et al. 2004b). Noxious thermal stimulation and intradermal formalin evoked the expression of Fos, a neurochemical marker for neuronal activation, in the nucleus raphe magnus (Suzuki et al. 2002). Importantly, double-labeling studies revealed that a subpopulation of these neurons also expressed 5HT, indicating that nociceptive inputs indirectly activate descending serotonergic fibers (Suzuki et al. 2002). The spinal administration of the $5HT_3$ antagonist ondansetron mimicked the behavioral and electrophysiological consequences of spinal SP-SAP (Suzuki et al. 2002, 2004b). The responses of dorsal horn WDR neurons to thermal and mechanical stimuli were attenuated, and the behavioral responses during the first and second phases of formalin-induced nociception were diminished, by both spinal ondansetron and SP-SAP (Ali et al. 1996; Suzuki et al. 2002). Spinal ondansetron also produced a dose-dependent attenuation of neuronal responses to tactile and thermal stimuli in rats with carrageenan-induced inflammation, although there was no difference in the magnitude of the activity of ondansetron in these rats compared to naive animals (Ali et al. 1996; Rahman et al. 2004). In contrast, ondansetron produced a dose-dependent reduction in the spontaneous firing rate of spinal dorsal horn neurons during both the first and second phases after formalin injection (Ali et al. 1996; Green et al. 2000; Rahman et al. 2004). The spinal administration of a selective $5HT_3$ agonist enhanced the activity of spinal dorsal horn neurons to noxious thermal stimuli, but did not change behavioral responses (Ali et al. 1996). Genetically altered mice that do not express subunit A of the $5HT_3$ receptor have normal responses to acute nociceptive stimuli, but they demonstrate significantly reduced behavioral and electrophysiological responses to subdermal formalin injection (Zeitz et al. 2002). Recent studies demonstrated that ondansetron produced a greater attenuation of the facilitated responses of spinal dorsal horn neurons evoked by tactile stimuli compared to noxious stimuli in nerve-injured rats (Suzuki et al. 2004a). Taken together, these studies indicate that descending serotonergic facilitation of nociception mediated through the $5HT_3$ receptor becomes tonically active during conditions of chronic pain (Suzuki et al. 2004b).

The characterization of the descending serotonergic projections that may mediate antinociceptive or pronociceptive functions remains elusive. In a study employing electrophysiology and immunohistological examination of nine off-cells, eight on-cells, and eight neutral cells revealed that only one-half of the neutral cells demonstrated intracellular labeling for 5HT (Potrebic et al. 1994). It was considered unlikely that the neutral cells contribute to nociceptive processing, given that the activity of these neurons is not altered by noxious stimuli applied at several sites over the body, nor does it change in response to opioid administration (Potrebic et al. 1994). These results contrast with the observations of Pan and colleagues (1993) in a brain slice preparation indicating that although the "secondary" RVM cells do not express 5HT, nearly all of the "primary" cells examined were labeled for 5HT. More recently, it was found that serotonergic neurons in the RVM respond to noxious heat, but the responses are qualitatively different from those of the classic on-cells and off-cells and represent an alternate group, and it has been suggested that perhaps the concept of on-cells and off-cells should be reconsidered with regard to nociception (Potrebic et al. 1994; Gao and Mason 2000). For example, the response characteristics of the RVM neurons change considerably when recorded in unanesthetized animals (Oliveras et al. 1990; McGaraughty et al. 1993). Finally, it was recently established that RVM neurons that express the neurotensin-1 receptor are serotonergic and mediate descending inhibition of nociception from the RVM (Buhler et al. 2005). Activation of these neurons with a selective neurotensin-1 receptor agonist did not induce facilitation of nociception at any dose (Buhler et al. 2005). Clearly, the role of spinopetal serotonergic projections from the RVM in the modulation of nociception remains to be determined.

DESCENDING FACILITATION AND SPINOTHALAMIC TRACT PROJECTION NEURONS: CLOSING THE LOOP

The idea that peripheral inputs may activate supraspinal sites that then excite spinal neurons had been proposed in studies that showed that electrical stimulation applied in the spinal cord of decerebrate cats caused excitation of neurons in the nucleus raphe magnus and surrounding tissue (Cervero and Wolstencroft 1984). Conversely, electrical stimulation of the supraspinal sites excited spinal neurons (Cervero and Wolstencroft 1984; Cervero and Tattersall 1986). It is now suggested that a postsynaptic target of the descending serotonergic pain-facilitatory projections may be the NK1-expressing projection neurons of lamina I (Suzuki et al. 2002, 2004b). The projection neurons that express NK1 are selectively innervated by serotonergic axons from the RVM and form basket-like structures and dense synaptic contacts (Stewart and Maxwell 2000; Polgar et al. 2002). Behavioral signs of neuropathic pain were abolished by ablation of NK1 neurons, as were sensitized responses of WDR neurons and high-threshold dorsal horn neurons to touch and heat after capsaicin (Nichols et al. 1999; Khasabov et al. 2002; Mantyh and Hunt 2004). These actions are virtually identical to the effects observed with spinal ondansetron (Suzuki et al. 2002, 2004b). It is asserted that because the lamina I projection neurons have very little communication with other spinal dorsal horn neurons, then subsequent sensitization mediated by these cells must occur through a spinal-supraspinal-spinal loop in order to facilitate nociception (Cheunsuang and Morris 2000; Suzuki et al. 2002, 2004b; Mantyh and Hunt 2004). In support of this interpretation is the observation that ondansetron did not further depress the diminished second phase of formalin-induced sensitization after SP-SAP treatment (Suzuki et al. 2002, 2004b). Fos expression evoked by formalin injection was significantly reduced in the RVM, but not in lamina I, by SP-SAP treatment (Suzuki et al. 2002, 2004b). Finally, SP-SAP treatment abolished diffuse noxious inhibitory control in the spinal dorsal horn (Suzuki et al. 2002, 2004b). Taken together, these observations indicate that the neurons of lamina I that express NK1 are the targets of primary afferent nociceptors, become sensitized with persistent nociceptive inputs, and project to supraspinal structures including the parabrachial and thalamic nuclei, ultimately provoking su-praspinal neuroplasticity of the RVM and evoking descending facilitation (Mantyh and Hunt 2004).

Based on the studies presented above, we may conclude that the projection neurons of lamina I are a critical link in a spinal supraspinal loop that coordinates spinal sensitization with activation of descending facilitation of nociceptive inputs, resulting in the maintenance of a sensitized spinal cord and enhanced pain states. Nearly all the projection neurons of lamina I express NK1 receptors, and this population is sensitized with nociceptive inputs (Suzuki et al. 2002; Mantyh and Hunt 2004). These lamina I projection neurons send terminations to thalamic nuclei, thus integrating sensory inputs and serving as a relay to the somatosensory and insular cortices and the amygdala (Gauriau and Bernard 2004a,b). There is also a significant projection from lamina I to the parabrachial region, which receives sensory and nociceptive inputs from mechanical, thermal, and cold stimuli (Bester et al. 2000). It is thought that the parabrachial region is a site of integration and discrimination of noxious inputs that are then passed on to the hypothalamus and amygdala (Bester et al. 2000). The parabrachial region and STT activate descending processes from the cortical and limbic regions to stimulate the periaqueductal gray and ultimately the RVM, which is considered the final relay in the processing of descending control of nociceptive inputs (Suzuki et al. 2002; Gebhart 2004; Mantyh and Hunt 2004). Over time, persistent noxious stimuli result in neuroplastic adaptations that manifest as increased CCK release in the RVM and tonic activation of a descending pain-facilitatory system that is mediated in part through the $5HT_3$ receptors on spinal dorsal horn neurons. Descending serotonergic projections have been identified in close contact with interneurons of laminae III and IV and in close proximity to cell bodies and primary afferent terminals of lamina I (Stewart and Maxwell 2000; Miquel et al. 2002; Todd 2002; Zeitz et al. 2002). The descending projections from the RVM also include CCK-expressing neurons, which represent another excitatory system (Mantyh and Hunt 1984). These excitatory descending projections can maintain the sensitized state of dorsal horn neurons throughout the dorsal horns of the spinal cord. Conditions that alter the normal functioning of this pain-regulatory loop such that it becomes hyperactive or tonically maintained may lead to a chronic pain state. Conversely, disruption of this positive reinforcement cycle may abolish chronic pain states. It is important to emphasize that this loop describes a chronic, abnormal pain state. Abolishing the NK1 lamina I neurons, or administering spinal ondansetron, does not abolish normal nociceptive reflexes to acute noxious stimuli such as applied heat or pinch (Suzuki et al. 2002, 2004b; Mantyh and Hunt 2004). This observation indicates that there are alternate pathways, such as projections from lamina V, that mediate normal nociceptive stimuli.

ENHANCED EXCITATORY TRANSMITTER RELEASE

Peripheral nerve injury augments the release of substance P in response to electrical stimulation of peripheral nerve fibers in vitro (Malcangio et al. 2000) or in response to potassium introduced through a microdialysis probe in vivo (Wallin and Schott 2002). Similarly, peripheral nerve injury enhances the capsaicin-evoked release of CGRP from primary afferent terminals, although CGRP content itself may be decreased (Ma and Bisby 1998, 1999; Gardell et al. 2003). Importantly, enhanced evoked CGRP release was not present 2 days after the nerve injury, but occurred 10 days after injury, consistent with the development of neuroplastic changes and activation of descending facilitatory systems (Gardell et al. 2003). The disruption of descending facilitation from the RVM, either through the microinjection of dermorphin-saporin conjugate into the RVM or through ablation of the DLF in rats with SNL, also blocked capsaicin-evoked enhancement of CGRP release without blocking normal release in sham-operated animals (Gardell et al. 2003). These manipulations abolished signs of neuropathic pain without changing behavioral responses to acute nociceptive stimuli (Burgess et al. 2002; Gardell et al. 2003). These observations are consistent with the hypothesis that persistent nociceptive inputs elicit supraspinal neuroplastic changes that activate descending facilitation of nociceptive inputs, leading to increased release of excitatory transmitters. This enhanced release of transmitters mimics primary afferent drive and keeps the spinal cord in a sensitized state.

SPINAL DYNORPHIN UPREGULATION
MAINTAINS THE PAIN STATE

Spinal sensitization and enhanced Fos expression may lead to a critical post-translational event by promoting the upregulation of dynorphin, an event closely associated with central sensitization (Ji et al. 2002, 2003). The transcription of prodynorphin is regulated by Fos complexed with Jun, which binds to the AP-1 binding site of the promoter region for prodynorphin (Hunter et al. 1995). Consequently, prevention of FOS expression by antisense oligodeoxynucleotide techniques also prevented the upregulation of spinal dynorphin (Hunter et al. 1995). Dynorphin upregulation occurs in the same postsynaptic lamina I cells that also express Fos in response to nociceptive inputs (Ji et al. 2002; Kawasaki et al. 2004). Serotonin added to a culture of dorsal horn neurons produces a concentration-dependent increase in the expression of both Fos and prodynorphin (Wang et al. 2003). Increased spinal 5HT levels due to activation of tonic descending from the RVM may contribute to Fos and prodynorphin expression (Wang et al. 2003). These observations suggest a link through which the activation of descending facilitation might elicit the upregulation of spinal dynorphin, which would serve to maintain the sensitized state.

Peripheral nerve injury has been consistently associated with increased levels of immunoreactivity for dynorphin or mRNA for prodynorphin in neurons of the dorsal horn of the spinal cord or in the trigeminal nuclei (Kajander et al. 1990; Draisci et al. 1991; Malan et al. 2000). It was suggested that spinal dynorphin, along with substance P and CGRP, elicits an enhancement of neuronal excitability at NMDA-receptor sites, leading first to dorsal horn hyperexcitability and then to excessive depolarization and excitotoxicity (Ossipov et al. 2000b; Przewlocki and Przewlocka 2001). Peripheral nerve injury results in significant ipsilateral increases in immunoreactivity for dynorphin or prodynorphin in laminae I–II and V–VII of the dorsal horn within 5 days of injury, with peak elevations at day 10 (Kajander et al. 1990; Draisci et al. 1991; Malan et al. 2000). The time-course of dynorphin upregulation after nerve injury was found to be consistent with the maintenance phase of neuropathic pain. For example, tactile and thermal hypersensitivity in mice with nerve injury was blocked by spinal MK-801 but not by antiserum to dynorphin 2 days after nerve injury, whereas both MK-801 and dynorphin antiserum blocked hypersensitivity 10 days after injury (Wang et al. 2001). Genetically altered mice that do not express spinal dynorphin (prodynorphin knockout mice) develop tactile and thermal hypersensitivities immediately after nerve injury, but these signs resolve spontaneously over the following 4 to 6 days, whereas those that express dynorphin upregulation maintain behavioral signs of neuropathic pain throughout the observation sessions (Wang et al. 2001; Gardell et al. 2004).

Manipulations that disrupt descending facilitation from the RVM, including ablation of μ-opioid-expressing cells with dermorphin-saporin or by lesions of the DLF also blocked the upregulation of spinal dynorphin (Burgess et al. 2002; Gardell et al. 2003). Studies employing in vivo microdialysis of spinal cerebrospinal fluid showed that administration of NMDA, dynorphin A_{1-17}, or dynorphin A_{2-17} into the lumbar spinal cord elicited a long-lasting release of prostaglandin E_2, glutamate, and aspartate (Koetzner et al. 2004). Dynorphin may thus promote spinal sensitization by enhancing PGE_2 release, which may subsequently enhance release of excitatory transmitters from primary afferent terminals (Koetzner et al. 2004). The capsaicin-stimulated release of CGRP was potentiated by dynorphin in spinal cord slices in vitro (Gardell et al. 2003). Similarly, dynorphin facilitated capsaicin-evoked substance P release from brainstem slices (Arcaya et al. 1999). Moreover, the addition of antiserum to dynorphin in the perfusate abolished the enhanced capsaicin-evoked release of CGRP from spinal tissue obtained from rats with nerve injury (Burgess et al. 2002; Gardell et al. 2003). Enhancement of evoked CGRP release was not observed in nerve-injured rats with prior lesions of the DLF in which dynorphin upregulation did not occur (Burgess et al. 2002; Gardell et al. 2003). Taken together, these studies suggest that elevated pathophysiological levels of spinal dynorphin continue to provide nociceptive inputs and maintain an enhanced pain state.

SYNTHESIS

The processing and interpretation of pain signals is a complex process that entails excitation of peripheral nerves, local interactions within the spinal dorsal horn, the activation of ascending and descending circuits that comprise a loop from the spinal cord to supraspinal structures, and finally excitation of nociceptive inputs at the spinal level. Although the "circuits" described here appear to be part of normal pain processing, the system demonstrates a remarkable ability to undergo neuroplastic transformations when nociceptive inputs are extended over time, and such adaptations function as a pronociceptive positive feedback loop. Manipulations directed to disrupt any of the nodes of this pain-facilitatory loop may effectively disrupt the maintenance of the sensitized pain state and diminish or abolish neuropathic pain. Some of the points that may be considered for intervention include: (1) substance P, CGRP, and glutamate and/or their receptors in the spinal dorsal horn, where these transmitters act together to potentiate nociceptive inputs; (2) PGE_2 and nitric oxide in the spinal cord, which promote release of the excitatory neurotransmitters; (3) CCK in the RVM to block tonic descending facilitation at the source; and (4) the $5HT_3$ receptor in the spinal dorsal horn to block descending facilitation at its terminus. Other structures and transmitter systems participate in this reverberating loop, but the transmitters and receptors involved are less well characterized. Importantly, disruption of the circuit that maintains the chronic pain state does not alter the normal sensorium, nor does it block behavioral responses to acute nociceptive stimuli, since these responses are mediated through other pathways projecting from deeper laminae of the dorsal horn. Understanding the ascending and descending pain-facilitatory circuit may permit the design of rational therapies that do not interfere with normal sensory processing.

The fundamental processes of central sensitization may promote chronic pain states that are not of neuropathic origin. For example, inflammatory pain may also evoke enhanced afferent inputs and activation of descending facilitatory systems to maintain an enhanced pain state. However, an important consideration is that the inflammatory process, including heightened nociception, serves a protective function in that the injured region is immobilized and protected while healing takes place. Once the traumatic insult has healed, the inflammatory processes and the enhanced pain state are terminated. Neuropathic pain represents a maladaptive process. Initially it may have served a protective function, but the initiating excitatory systems activate a spinal-supraspinal loop that becomes self-sustaining and maintains the enhanced pain state, perhaps indefinitely. Moreover, it may be possible that neuropathic pain is further maintained by neuroplastic changes such as alteration in neuropeptide expression, receptor function, and distribution of ion channels related to neuronal function, and it would therefore be less amenable to spontaneous reversal.

REFERENCES

Abbadie C, Trafton J, Liu H, Mantyh PW, Basbaum AI. Inflammation increases the distribution of dorsal horn neurons that internalize the neurokinin-1 receptor in response to noxious and non-noxious stimulation. *J Neurosci* 1997; 17:8049–8060.

Al-Chaer ED, Lawand NB, Westlund KN, Willis WD. Pelvic visceral input into the nucleus gracilis is largely mediated by the postsynaptic dorsal column pathway. *J Neurophysiol* 1996a; 76:2675–2690.

Al-Chaer ED, Lawand NB, Westlund KN, Willis WD. Visceral nociceptive input into the ventral posterolateral nucleus of the thalamus: a new function for the dorsal column pathway. *J Neurophysiol* 1996b; 76:2661–2674.

Ali Z, Wu G, Kozlov A, Barasif S. The role of 5HT3 in nociceptive processing in the rat spinal cord: results from behavioural and electrophysiological studies. *Neurosci Lett* 1996; 208:203–207.

Allen BJ, Li J, Menning PM, et al. Primary afferent fibers that contribute to increased substance P receptor internalization in the spinal cord after injury. *J Neurophysiol* 1999; 81:1379–1390.

Arcaya JL, Cano G, Gomez G, Maixner W, Suarez-Roca H. Dynorphin A increases substance P release from trigeminal primary afferent C-fibers. *Eur J Pharmacol* 1999; 366:27–34.

Bederson JB, Fields HL, Barbaro NM. Hyperalgesia during naloxone-precipitated withdrawal from morphine is associated with increased on-cell activity in the rostral ventromedial medulla. *Somatosens Mot Res* 1990; 7:185–203.

Bennett GJ. An animal model of neuropathic pain: a review. *Muscle Nerve* 1993; 16:1040–1048.

Bennett GJ, Seltzer Z, Lu GW, Nishikawa N, Dubner R. The cells of origin of the dorsal column postsynaptic projection in the lumbosacral enlargements of cats and monkeys. *Somatosens Res* 1983; 1:131–149.

Bennett GJ, Nishikawa N, Lu GW, Hoffert MJ, Dubner R. The morphology of dorsal column postsynaptic spinomedullary neurons in the cat. *J Comp Neurol* 1984; 224:568–578.

Bester H, Chapman V, Besson JM, Bernard JF. Physiological properties of the lamina I spinoparabrachial neurons in the rat. *J Neurophysiol* 2000; 83:2239–2259.

Bian D, Ossipov MH, Zhong C, Malan TP Jr, Porreca F. Tactile allodynia, but not thermal hyperalgesia, of the hindlimbs is blocked by spinal transection in rats with nerve injury. *Neurosci Lett* 1998; 241:79–82.

Buhler AV, Choi J, Proudfit HK, Gebhart GF. Neurotensin activation of the NTR1 on spinally-projecting serotonergic neurons in the rostral ventromedial medulla is antinociceptive. *Pain* 2005; 114:285–294.

Burgess SE, Gardell LR, Ossipov MH, et al. Time-dependent descending facilitation from the rostral ventromedial medulla maintains, but does not initiate, neuropathic pain. *J Neurosci* 2002; 22:5129–5136.

Calejesan AA, Chang MH, Zhuo M. Spinal serotonergic receptors mediate facilitation of a nociceptive reflex by subcutaneous formalin injection into the hindpaw in rats. *Brain Res* 1998; 798:46–54.

Calejesan AA, Kim SJ, Zhuo M. Descending facilitatory modulation of a behavioral nociceptive response by stimulation in the adult rat anterior cingulate cortex. *Eur J Pain* 2000; 4:83–96.

Catheline G, Le Guen S, Honore P, Besson JM. Are there long-term changes in the basal or evoked Fos expression in the dorsal horn of the spinal cord of the mononeuropathic rat? *Pain* 1999; 80:347–357.

Catheline G, Le Guen S, Besson JM. Intravenous morphine does not modify dorsal horn touch-evoked allodynia in the mononeuropathic rat: a Fos study. *Pain* 2001; 92:389–398.

Cervero F, Tattersall JE. Somatic and visceral sensory integration in the thoracic spinal cord. *Prog Brain Res* 1986; 67:189–205.

Cervero F, Wolstencroft JH. A positive feedback loop between spinal cord nociceptive pathways and antinociceptive areas of the cat's brain stem. *Pain* 1984; 20:125–138.

Chaplan SR, Bach FW, Pogrel JW, Chung JM, Yaksh TL. Quantitative assessment of tactile allodynia in the rat paw. *J Neurosci Methods* 1994; 53:55–63.

Chen Y, Devor M. Ectopic mechanosensitivity in injured sensory axons arises from the site of spontaneous electrogenesis. *Eur J Pain* 1998; 2:165–178.

Cheunsuang O, Morris R. Spinal lamina I neurons that express neurokinin 1 receptors: morphological analysis. *Neuroscience* 2000; 97:335–345.

Coull JA, Boudreau D, Bachand K, et al. Trans-synaptic shift in anion gradient in spinal lamina I neurons as a mechanism of neuropathic pain. *Nature* 2003; 424:938–942.

Day AS, Lue JH, Sun WZ, Shieh JY, Wen CY. A-beta-fiber intensity stimulation of chronically constricted median nerve induces c-fos expression in thalamic projection neurons of the cuneate nucleus in rats with behavioral signs of neuropathic pain. *Brain Res* 2001a; 895:194–203.

Day AS, Wen CY, Shieh JY, Sun WZ, Lue JH. Somatic noxious mechanical stimulation induces Fos expression in the postsynaptic dorsal column neurons in laminae III and IV of the rat spinal dorsal horn. *Neurosci Res* 2001b; 40:343–350.

Devor M. Sensory basis of autotomy in rats. *Pain* 1991; 45:109–110.

Draisci G, Kajander KC, Dubner R, Bennett GJ, Iadarola MJ. Up-regulation of opioid gene expression in spinal cord evoked by experimental nerve injuries and inflammation. *Brain Res* 1991; 560:186–192.

Faris PL, Komisaruk BR, Watkins LR, Mayer DJ. Evidence for the neuropeptide cholecystokinin as an antagonist of opiate analgesia. *Science* 1983; 219:310–312.

Fields HL. Is there a facilitating component to central pain modulation? *APS J* 1992; 1:71–78.

Fields HL, Basbaum AI. Central nervous system mechanisms of pain modulation. In: Wall PD, Melzack R (Eds). *Textbook of Pain*. Edinburgh: Churchill Livingstone, 1999, pp 309–329.

Fields HL, Heinricher MM. Anatomy and physiology of a nociceptive modulatory system. *Philos Trans R Soc Lond B Biol Sci* 1985; 308:361–374.

Fields HL, Bry J, Hentall I, Zorman G. The activity of neurons in the rostral medulla of the rat during withdrawal from noxious heat. *J Neurosci* 1983; 3:2545–2552.

Gao K, Mason P. Serotonergic raphe magnus cells that respond to noxious tail heat are not ON or OFF cells. *J Neurophysiol* 2000; 84:1719–1725.

Gardell LR, Vanderah TW, Gardell SE, et al. Enhanced evoked excitatory transmitter release in experimental neuropathy requires descending facilitation. *J Neurosci* 2003; 23:8370–8379.

Gardell LR, Ibrahim M, Wang R, et al. Mouse strains that lack spinal dynorphin upregulation after peripheral nerve injury do not develop neuropathic pain. *Neuroscience* 2004; 123:43–52.

Gauriau C, Bernard JF. A comparative reappraisal of projections from the superficial laminae of the dorsal horn in the rat: the forebrain. *J Comp Neurol* 2004a; 468:24–56.

Gauriau C, Bernard JF. Posterior triangular thalamic neurons convey nociceptive messages to the secondary somatosensory and insular cortices in the rat. *J Neurosci* 2004b; 24:752–761.

Gebhart GF. Descending modulation of pain. *Neurosci Biobehav Rev* 2004; 27:729–737.

Giesler GJ Jr, Nahin RL, Madsen AM. Postsynaptic dorsal column pathway of the rat. I. Anatomical studies. *J Neurophysiol* 1984; 51:260–275.

Gogas KR, Presley RW, Levine JD, Basbaum AI. The antinociceptive action of supraspinal opioids results from an increase in descending inhibitory control: correlation of nociceptive behavior and c-fos expression. *Neuroscience* 1991; 42:617–628.

Green GM, Scarth J, Dickenson A. An excitatory role for 5-HT in spinal inflammatory nociceptive transmission; state-dependent actions via dorsal horn 5-HT3 receptors in the anaesthetized rat. *Pain* 2000; 89:81–88.

Han HC, Lee DH, Chung JM. Characteristics of ectopic discharges in a rat neuropathic pain model. *Pain* 2000; 84:253–261.

Harris JA. Using c-fos as a neural marker of pain. *Brain Res Bull* 1998; 45:1–8.

Hedo G, Laird JM, Lopez-Garcia JA. Time-course of spinal sensitization following carrageenan-induced inflammation in the young rat: a comparative electrophysiological and behavioural study in vitro and in vivo. *Neuroscience* 1999; 92:309–318.

Heinricher MM, Neubert MJ. Neural basis for the hyperalgesic action of cholecystokinin in the rostral ventromedial medulla. *J Neurophysiol* 2004; 92:1982–1989.

Heinricher MM, Barbaro NM, Fields HL. Putative nociceptive modulating neurons in the rostral ventromedial medulla of the rat: firing of on- and off-cells is related to nociceptive responsiveness. *Somatosens Mot Res* 1989; 6:427–439.

Heinricher MM, Morgan MM, Fields HL. Direct and indirect actions of morphine on medullary neurons that modulate nociception. *Neuroscience* 1992; 48:533–543.

Heinricher MM, Morgan MM, Tortorici V, Fields HL. Disinhibition of off-cells and antinociception produced by an opioid action within the rostral ventromedial medulla. *Neuroscience* 1994; 63:279–288.

Heinricher MM, McGaraughty S, Tortorici V. Circuitry underlying antiopioid actions of cholecystokinin within the rostral ventromedial medulla. *J Neurophysiol* 2001; 85:280–286.

Heinricher MM, Pertovaara A, Ossipov MH. Descending modulation after injury. In: Dostrovsky DO, Carr DB, Koltzenburg M (Eds). *Proceedings of the 10th World Congress on Pain*, Progress in Pain Research and Management, Vol. 24. Seattle: IASP Press, 2003, pp 251–260.

Hingtgen CM, Vasko MR. Prostacyclin enhances the evoked-release of substance P and calcitonin gene-related peptide from rat sensory neurons. *Brain Res* 1994; 655:51–60.

Hirshberg RM, Al-Chaer ED, Lawand NB, Westlund KN, Willis WD. Is there a pathway in the posterior funiculus that signals visceral pain? *Pain* 1996; 67:291–305.

Houghton AK, Kadura S, Westlund KN. Dorsal column lesions reverse the reduction of homecage activity in rats with pancreatitis. *Neuroreport* 1997; 8:3795–3800.

Houghton AK, Wang CC, Westlund KN. Do nociceptive signals from the pancreas travel in the dorsal column? *Pain* 2001; 89:207–220.

Hunt SP, Pini A, Evan G. Induction of c-fos-like protein in spinal cord neurons following sensory stimulation. *Nature* 1987; 328:632–634.

Hunter JC, Woodburn VL, Durieux C, et al. c-Fos antisense oligodeoxynucleotide increases formalin-induced nociception and regulates preprodynorphin expression. *Neuroscience* 1995; 65:485–492.

Ikeda H, Heinke B, Ruscheweyh R, Sandkuhler J. Synaptic plasticity in spinal lamina I projection neurons that mediate hyperalgesia. *Science* 2003; 299:1237–1240.

Ji R-R, Befort K, Brenner GJ, Woolf CJ. ERK MAP kinase activation in superficial spinal cord neurons induces prodynorphin and NK-1 upregulation and contributes to persistent inflammatory pain hypersensitivity. *J Neurosci* 2002; 22:478–485.

Ji RR, Kohno T, Moore KA, Woolf CJ. Central sensitization and LTP: do pain and memory share similar mechanisms? *Trends Neurosci* 2003; 26:696–705.

Kajander KC, Sahara Y, Iadarola MJ, Bennett GJ. Dynorphin increases in the dorsal spinal cord in rats with a painful peripheral neuropathy. *Peptides* 1990; 11:719–728.

Kajander KC, Xu J. Quantitative evaluation of calcitonin gene-related peptide and substance P levels in rat spinal cord following peripheral nerve injury. *Neurosci Lett* 1995; 186:184–188.

Kaplan H, Fields HL. Hyperalgesia during acute opioid abstinence: evidence for a nociceptive facilitating function of the rostral ventromedial medulla. *J Neurosci* 1991; 11:1433–1439.

Kauppila T. Spinalization increases the mechanical stimulation-induced withdrawal reflex threshold after a sciatic cut in the rat. *Brain Res* 1997; 770:310–312.

Kauppila T, Kontinen VK, Pertovaara A. Influence of spinalization on spinal withdrawal reflex responses varies depending on the submodality of the test stimulus and the experimental pathophysiological condition in the rat. *Brain Res* 1998a; 797:234–242.

Kauppila T, Kontinen VK, Pertovaara A. Influence of spinalization on spinal withdrawal reflex responses varies depending on the submodality of the test stimulus and the experimental pathophysiological condition in the rat. *Brain Res* 1998b; 797:234–242.

Kawamata T, Omote K. Activation of spinal *N*-methyl-D-aspartate receptors stimulates a nitric oxide/cyclic guanosine 3,5-monophosphate/glutamate release cascade in nociceptive signaling. *Anesthesiology* 1999; 91:1415–1424.

Kawasaki Y, Kohno T, Zhuang ZY, et al. Ionotropic and metabotropic receptors, protein kinase A, protein kinase C, and Src contribute to C-fiber-induced ERK activation and cAMP response element-binding protein phosphorylation in dorsal horn neurons, leading to central sensitization. *J Neurosci* 2004; 24:8310–8321.

Khasabov SG, Rogers SD, Ghilardi JR, et al. Spinal neurons that possess the substance P receptor are required for the development of central sensitization. *J Neurosci* 2002; 22:9086–9098.

Kim DH, Fields HL, Barbaro NM. Morphine analgesia and acute physical dependence: rapid onset of two opposing, dose-related processes. *Brain Res* 1990; 516:37–40.

Kirk EJ. Impulses in dorsal spinal nerve rootlets in cats and rabbits arising from dorsal root ganglia isolated from the periphery. *J Comp Neurol* 1974; 155:165–175.

Koetzner L, Hua XY, Lai J, Porreca F, Yaksh T. Nonopioid actions of intrathecal dynorphin evoke spinal excitatory amino acid and prostaglandin E2 release mediated by cyclooxygenase-1 and -2. *J Neurosci* 2004; 24:1451–1458.

Koltzenburg M, Torebjork HE, Wahren LK. Nociceptor modulated central sensitization causes mechanical hyperalgesia in acute chemogenic and chronic neuropathic pain. *Brain* 1994; 117(Pt 3):579–591.

Kovelowski CJ, Ossipov MH, Sun H, et al. Supraspinal cholecystokinin may drive tonic descending facilitation mechanisms to maintain neuropathic pain in the rat. *Pain* 2000; 87:265–273.

Lai J, Ossipov MH, Vanderah TW, Malan TP Jr, Porreca F. Neuropathic pain: the paradox of dynorphin. *Mol Interv* 2001; 1:160–167.

Leem JW, Park ES, Paik KS. Electrophysiological evidence for the antinociceptive effect of transcutaneous electrical stimulation on mechanically evoked responsiveness of dorsal horn neurons in neuropathic rats. *Neurosci Lett* 1995; 192:197–200.

Li J, Simone DA, Larson AA. Windup leads to characteristics of central sensitization. *Pain* 1999a; 79:75–82.

Li WP, Xian C, Rush RA, Zhou XF. Upregulation of brain-derived neurotrophic factor and neuropeptide Y in the dorsal ascending sensory pathway following sciatic nerve injury in rat. *Neurosci Lett* 1999b; 260:49–52.

Li Y, Dorsi MJ, Meyer RA, Belzberg AJ. Mechanical hyperalgesia after an L5 spinal nerve lesion in the rat is not dependent on input from injured nerve fibers. *Pain* 2000; 85:493–502.

Liu CN, Wall PD, Ben-Dor E, et al. Tactile allodynia in the absence of C-fiber activation: altered firing properties of DRG neurons following spinal nerve injury. *Pain* 2000; 85:503–521.

Liu H, Wang H, Sheng M, et al. Evidence for presynaptic N-methyl-D-aspartate autoreceptors in the spinal cord dorsal horn. *Proc Natl Acad Sci USA* 1994; 91:8383–8387.

Liu H, Mantyh PW, Basbaum AI. NMDA-receptor regulation of substance P release from primary afferent nociceptors. *Nature* 1997; 386:721–714.

Liu X, Eschenfelder S, Blenk KH, Jänig W, Habler H. Spontaneous activity of axotomized afferent neurons after L5 spinal nerve injury in rats. *Pain* 2000; 84:309–318.

Ma QP, Woolf CJ. Involvement of neurokinin receptors in the induction but not the maintenance of mechanical allodynia in rat flexor motoneurones. *J Physiol (Lond)* 1995a; 486.769–777.

Ma QP, Woolf CJ. Noxious stimuli induce an *N*-methyl-D-aspartate receptor-dependent hypersensitivity of the flexion withdrawal reflex to touch: implications for the treatment of mechanical allodynia. *Pain* 1995b; 61:383–390.

Ma W, Bisby MA. Increase of calcitonin gene-related peptide immunoreactivity in the axonal fibers of the gracile nuclei of adult and aged rats after complete and partial sciatic nerve injuries. *Exp Neurol* 1998; 152:137–149.

Ma W, Bisby MA. Ultrastructural localization of increased neuropeptide immunoreactivity in the axons and cells of the gracile nucleus following chronic constriction injury of the sciatic nerve. *Neuroscience* 1999; 93:335–348.

Ma W, Eisenach JC. Intraplantar injection of a cyclooxygenase inhibitor ketorolac reduces immunoreactivities of substance P, calcitonin gene-related peptide, and dynorphin in the dorsal horn of rats with nerve injury or inflammation. *Neuroscience* 2003; 121:681–690.

Ma W, Peschanski M, Ralston HJ III. The differential synaptic organization of the spinal and lemniscal projections to the ventrobasal complex of the rat thalamus. Evidence for convergence of the two systems upon single thalamic neurons. *Neuroscience* 1987; 22:925–934.

Malan TP, Ossipov MH, Gardell LR, et al. Extraterritorial neuropathic pain correlates with multisegmental elevation of spinal dynorphin in nerve-injured rats. *Pain* 2000; 86:185–194.

Malcangio M, Ramer MS, Jones MG, McMahon SB. Abnormal substance P release from the spinal cord following injury to primary sensory neurons. *Eur J Neurosci* 2000; 12:397–399.

Malmberg AB, Yaksh TL. Capsaicin-evoked prostaglandin E2 release in spinal cord slices: relative effect of cyclooxygenase inhibitors. *Eur J Pharmacol* 1994; 271:293–299.

Mansikka H, Pertovaara A. Supraspinal influence on hindlimb withdrawal thresholds and mustard oil-induced secondary allodynia in rats. *Brain Res Bull* 1997; 42:359–365.

Mantyh PW, Hunt SP. Evidence for cholecystokinin-like immunoreactive neurons in the rat medulla oblongata which project to the spinal cord. *Brain Res* 1984; 291:49–54.

Mantyh PW, Hunt SP. Setting the tone: superficial dorsal horn projection neurons regulate pain sensitivity. *Trends Neurosci* 2004; 27:582–584.

McGaraughty S, Reinis S, Tsoukatos J. Two distinct unit activity responses to morphine in the rostral ventromedial medulla of awake rats. *Brain Res* 1993; 604:331–333.

McMahon SB, Wall PD. A system of rat spinal cord lamina 1 cells projecting through the contralateral dorsolateral funiculus. *J Comp Neurol* 1983; 214:217–223.

McMahon SB, Wall PD. Descending excitation and inhibition of spinal cord lamina I projection neurons. *J Neurophysiol* 1988; 59:1204–1219.

McNally GP. Pain facilitatory circuits in the mammalian central nervous system: their behavioral significance and role in morphine analgesic tolerance. *Neurosci Biobehav Rev* 1999; 23:1059–1078.

Mendell LM. Physiological properties of unmyelinated fiber projection to the spinal cord. *Exp Neurol* 1966; 16:316–332.

Michaelis M, Liu X, Jänig W. Axotomized and intact muscle afferents but no skin afferents develop ongoing discharges of dorsal root ganglion origin after peripheral nerve lesion. *J Neurosci* 2000; 20:2742–2748.

Miki K, Fukuoka T, Tokunaga A, Noguchi K. Calcitonin gene-related peptide increase in the rat spinal dorsal horn and dorsal column nucleus following peripheral nerve injury: up-regulation in a subpopulation of primary afferent sensory neurons. *Neuroscience* 1998; 82:1243–1252.

Miki K, Iwata K, Tsuboi Y, et al. Dorsal column-thalamic pathway is involved in thalamic hyperexcitability following peripheral nerve injury: a lesion study in rats with experimental mononeuropathy. *Pain* 2000; 85:263–271.

Miquel MC, Emerit MB, Nosjean A, et al. Differential subcellular localization of the 5-HT3-As receptor subunit in the rat central nervous system. *Eur J Neurosci* 2002; 15:449–457.

Molander C, Hongpaisan J, Grant G. Changing pattern of c-FOS expression in spinal cord neurons after electrical stimulation of the chronically injured sciatic nerve in the rat. *Neuroscience* 1992; 50:223–236.

Molander C, Hongpaisan J, Persson JK. Distribution of c-fos expressing dorsal horn neurons after electrical stimulation of low threshold sensory fibers in the chronically injured sciatic nerve. *Brain Res* 1994; 644:74–82.

Molander C, Hongpaisan J, Shortland P. Somatotopic redistribution of c-fos expressing neurons in the superficial dorsal horn after peripheral nerve injury. *Neuroscience* 1998; 84:241–253.

Morgan MM, Fields HL. Pronounced changes in the activity of nociceptive modulatory neurons in the rostral ventromedial medulla in response to prolonged thermal noxious stimuli. *J Neurophysiol* 1994; 72:1161–1170.

Narita M, Ozaki S, Ise Y, Yajima Y, Suzuki T. Change in the expression of c-fos in the rat brain following sciatic nerve ligation. *Neurosci Lett* 2003; 352:231–233.

Nauta HJ, Hewitt E, Westlund KN, Willis WD Jr. Surgical interruption of a midline dorsal column visceral pain pathway. Case report and review of the literature. *J Neurosurg* 1997; 86:538–542.

Nichols ML, Allen BJ, Rogers SD, et al. Transmission of chronic nociception by spinal neurons expressing the substance P receptor. *Science* 1999; 286:1558–1561.

Noguchi K, Kawai Y, Fukuoka T, Senba E, Miki K. Substance P induced by peripheral nerve injury in primary afferent sensory neurons and its effect on dorsal column nucleus neurons. *J Neurosci* 1995; 15:7633–7643.

Nomura H, Ogawa A, Tashiro A, et al. Induction of Fos protein-like immunoreactivity in the trigeminal spinal nucleus caudalis and upper cervical cord following noxious and non-noxious mechanical stimulation of the whisker pad of the rat with an inferior alveolar nerve transection. *Pain* 2002; 95:225–238.

Ohishi H, Nomura S, Ding YQ, et al. Presynaptic localization of a metabotropic glutamate receptor, mGluR7, in the primary afferent neurons: an immunohistochemical study in the rat, *Neurosci Lett* 1995; 202:85–88.

Oku R, Satoh M, Fujii N, et al. Calcitonin gene-related peptide promotes mechanical nociception by potentiating release of substance P from the spinal dorsal horn in rats. *Brain Res* 1987; 403:350–354.

Oliveras JL, Martin G, Montagne J, Vos B. Single unit activity at ventromedial medulla level in the awake, freely moving rat: effects of noxious heat and light tactile stimuli onto convergent neurons. *Brain Res* 1990; 506:19–30.

Ossipov MH, Hong Sun T, Malan P Jr, Lai J, Porreca F. Mediation of spinal nerve injury induced tactile allodynia by descending facilitatory pathways in the dorsolateral funiculus in rats. *Neurosci Lett* 2000a; 290:129–132.

Ossipov MH, Lai J, Malan TP Jr, Porreca F. Spinal and supraspinal mechanisms of neuropathic pain. *Ann NY Acad Sci* 2000b; 909:12–24.

Ossipov MH, Lai J, Malan TP Jr, Vanderah TW, Porreca F. Tonic descending facilitation as a mechanism of neuropathic pain. In: Hansson PT, Fields HL, Hill RG, Marchettini P (Eds). *Neuropathic Pain: Pathophysiology and Treatment,* Progress in Pain Research and Management, Vol. 21. Seattle: IASP Press, 2001, pp 107–124.

Ossipov MH, Zhang ET, Carvajal C, et al. Selective mediation of nerve injury-induced tactile hypersensitivity by neuropeptide Y. *J Neurosci* 2002; 22:9858–9867.

Palecek J, Dougherty PM, Kim SH, et al. Responses of spinothalamic tract neurons to mechanical and thermal stimuli in an experimental model of peripheral neuropathy in primates. *J Neurophysiol* 1992; 68:1951–1966.

Paleckova V, Palecek J, McAdoo DJ, Willis WD. The non-NMDA antagonist CNQX prevents release of amino acids into the rat spinal cord dorsal horn evoked by sciatic nerve stimulation. *Neurosci Lett* 1992; 148:19–22.

Pan ZZ, Williams JT, Osborne PB. Opioid actions on single nucleus raphe magnus neurons from rat and guinea-pig in vitro. *J Physiol* 1990; 427:519–532.

Pan ZZ, Wessendorf MW, Williams JT. Modulation by serotonin of the neurons in rat nucleus raphe magnus in vitro, *Neuroscience* 1993; 54:421–429.

Persson JK, Hongpaisan J, Molander C. c-Fos expression in gracilothalamic tract neurons after electrical stimulation of the injured sciatic nerve in the adult rat. *Somatosens Mot Res* 1993; 10:475–483.

Pertovaara A, Wei H, Hamalainen MM. Lidocaine in the rostroventromedial medulla and the periaqueductal gray attenuates allodynia in neuropathic rats. *Neurosci Lett* 1996; 218:127–130.

Pertovaara A, Kontinen VK, Kalso EA. Chronic spinal nerve ligation induces changes in response characteristics of nociceptive spinal dorsal horn neurons and in their descending regulation originating in the periaqueductal gray in the rat. *Exp Neurol* 1997; 147:428–436.

Polgar E, Puskar Z, Watt C, Matesz C, Todd AJ. Selective innervation of lamina I projection neurones that possess the neurokinin 1 receptor by serotonin-containing axons in the rat spinal cord. *Neuroscience* 2002; 109:799–809.

Porreca F, Burgess SE, Gardell LR, et al. Inhibition of neuropathic pain by selective ablation of brainstem medullary cells expressing the mu-opioid receptor. *J Neurosci* 2001; 21:5281–5288.

Porreca F, Ossipov MH, Gebhart GF. Chronic pain and medullary descending facilitation. *Trends Neurosci* 2002; 25:319–325.

Potrebic SB, Fields HL, Mason P. Serotonin immunoreactivity is contained in one physiological cell class in the rat rostral ventromedial medulla. *J Neurosci* 1994; 14:1655–1665.

Presley RW, Menetrey D, Levine JD, Basbaum AI. Systemic morphine suppresses noxious stimulus-evoked Fos protein-like immunoreactivity in the rat spinal cord. *J Neurosci* 1990; 10:323–335.

Przewlocki R, Przewlocka B. Opioids in chronic pain. *Eur J Pharmacol* 2001; 429:79–91.

Rahman W, Suzuki R, Rygh LJ, Dickenson AH. Descending serotonergic facilitation mediated through rat spinal 5HT3 receptors is unaltered following carrageenan inflammation. *Neurosci Lett* 2004; 361:229–231.

Ren K. Wind-up and the NMDA receptor: from animal studies to humans. *Pain* 1994; 59:157–158.

Robinson D, Calejesan AA, Zhuo M. Long-lasting changes in rostral ventral medulla neuronal activity after inflammation. *J Pain* 2002; 3:292–300.

Rygh LJ, Kontinen VK, Suzuki R, Dickenson AH. Different increase in C-fibre evoked responses after nociceptive conditioning stimulation in sham-operated and neuropathic rats. *Neurosci Lett* 2000; 288:99–102.

Seybold VS, McCarson KE, Mermelstein PG, Groth RD, Abrahams LG. Calcitonin gene-related peptide regulates expression of neurokinin-1 receptors by rat spinal neurons. *J Neurosci* 2003; 23:1816–1824.

Shortland P, Molander C. The time-course of A-beta-evoked c-fos expression in neurons of the dorsal horn and gracile nucleus after peripheral nerve injury. *Brain Res* 1998; 810:288–293.

Skilling SR, Smullin DH, Beitz AJ, Larson AA. Extracellular amino acid concentrations in the dorsal spinal cord of freely moving rats following veratridine and nociceptive stimulation. *J Neurochem* 1988; 51:127–132.

Sluka KA, Westlund KN. Spinal cord amino acid release and content in an arthritis model: the effects of pretreatment with non-NMDA, NMDA, and NK1 receptor antagonists. *Brain Res* 1993; 627:89–103.

Sluka KA, Willis WD. Increased spinal release of excitatory amino acids following intradermal injection of capsaicin is reduced by a protein kinase G inhibitor *Brain Res* 1998; 798:281–286.

Southall MD, Vasko MR. Prostaglandin receptor subtypes, EP3C and EP4, mediate the prostaglandin E2-induced cAMP production and sensitization of sensory neurons. *J Biol Chem* 2001; 276:16083–16091.

Stanfa L, Dickenson A, Xu XJ, Wiesenfeld-Hallin Z. Cholecystokinin and morphine analgesia: variations on a theme. *Trends Pharmacol Sci* 1994; 15:65–66.

Stewart W, Maxwell DJ. Morphological evidence for selective modulation by serotonin of a subpopulation of dorsal horn cells which possess the neurokinin-1 receptor. *Eur J Neurosci* 2000; 12:4583–4588.

Sun H, Ren K, Zhong, CM, et al. Nerve injury-induced tactile allodynia is mediated via ascending spinal dorsal column projections. *Pain* 2001; 90:105–111.

Sun R-Q, Lawand NB, Lin Q, Willis WD. Role of calcitonin gene-related peptide in the sensitization of dorsal horn neurons to mechanical stimulation after intradermal injection of capsaicin. *J Neurophysiol* 2004; 92:320–326.

Sung B, Na HS, Kim YI, et al. Supraspinal involvement in the production of mechanical allodynia by spinal nerve injury in rats. *Neurosci Lett* 1998; 246:117–119.

Suzuki R, Dickenson AH. Neuropathic pain: nerves bursting with excitement. *Neuroreport* 2000; 11:R17–21.

Suzuki R, Morcuende S, Webber M, Hunt SP, Dickenson AH. Superficial NK1-expressing neurons control spinal excitability through activation of descending pathways. *Nat Neurosci* 2002; 5:1319–1326.

Suzuki R, Rahman W, Hunt SP, Dickenson AH. Descending facilitatory control of mechanically evoked responses is enhanced in deep dorsal horn neurones following peripheral nerve injury. *Brain Res* 2004a; 1019:68–76.

Suzuki R, Rygh LJ, Dickenson AH. Bad news from the brain: descending 5-HT pathways that control spinal pain processing. *Trends Pharmacol Sci* 2004b; 25:613–617.

Tal M, Eliav E. Abnormal discharge originates at the site of nerve injury in experimental constriction neuropathy (CCI) in the rat. *Pain* 1996; 64:511–518.

Taylor BK, McCarson KE. Neurokinin-1 receptor gene expression in the mouse dorsal horn increases with neuropathic pain. *J Pain* 2004; 5:71–76.

Todd AJ. Anatomy of primary afferents and projection neurones in the rat spinal dorsal horn with particular emphasis on substance P and the neurokinin 1 receptor. *Exp Physiol* 2002; 87:245–249.

Urban MO, Gebhart GF. Characterization of biphasic modulation of spinal nociceptive transmission by neurotensin in the rat rostral ventromedial medulla. *J Neurophysiol* 1997; 78:1550–1562.

Urban MO, Gebhart GF. Supraspinal contributions to hyperalgesia. *Proc Natl Acad Sci USA* 1999; 96:7687–7692.

Urban MO, Zahn PK, Gebhart GF. Descending facilitatory influences from the rostral medial medulla mediate secondary, but not primary hyperalgesia in the rat. *Neuroscience* 1999; 90:349–352.

Vasko MR. Prostaglandin-induced neuropeptide release from spinal cord. *Prog Brain Res* 1995; 104:367–380.

Wall PD, Gutnick M. Ongoing activity in peripheral nerves: the physiology and pharmacology of impulses originating from a neuroma. *Exp Neurol* 1974a; 43:580–593.

Wall PD, Gutnick M. Properties of afferent nerve impulses originating from a neuroma. *Nature* 1974b; 248:740–743.

Wallin J, Schott E. Substance P release in the spinal dorsal horn following peripheral nerve injury. *Neuropeptides* 2002; 36:252–256.

Wang CC, Willis WD, Westlund KN. Ascending projections from the area around the spinal cord central canal: a *Phaseolus vulgaris* leucoagglutinin study in rats. *J Comp Neurol* 1999; 415:341–367.

Wang YY, Wu SX, Liu XY, Wang W, Li YQ. Effects of c-fos antisense oligodeoxynucleotide on 5-HT-induced upregulation of preprodynorphin, preproenkephalin, and glutamic acid decarboxylase mRNA expression in cultured rat spinal dorsal horn neurons. *Biochem Biophys Res Commun* 2003; 309:631–636.

Wang Z, Gardell LR, Ossipov MH, et al. Pronociceptive actions of dynorphin maintain chronic neuropathic pain. *J Neurosci* 2001; 21:1779–1786.

Wilcox GL, Stone LS, Ossipov MH, Lai J, Porreca F. Pharmacology of pain transmission and modulation. I. Central mechanisms. In: Pappagallo M (Ed). *The Neurologic Basis of Pain*. New York: McGraw-Hill, 2004, pp 31–52.

Willis WD, Coggeshall RE. *Sensory Mechanisms of the Spinal Cord*. New York: Plenum Press, 1991, p 574.

Willis WD, Westlund KN. Neuroanatomy of the pain system and of the pathways that modulate pain. *J Clin Neurophysiol* 1997; 14:2–31.

Woolf CJ. Evidence for a central component of post-injury pain hypersensitivity. *Nature* 1983; 306:686–688.

Woolf CJ. Windup and central sensitization are not equivalent. *Pain* 1996; 66:105–108.

Woolf CJ, Thompson SW. The induction and maintenance of central sensitization is dependent on *N*-methyl-D-aspartic acid receptor activation; implications for the treatment of post-injury pain hypersensitivity states. *Pain* 1991; 44:293–299.

Woolf CJ, Wiesenfeld-Hallin Z. The systemic administration of local anaesthetics produces a selective depression of C-afferent fibre evoked activity in the spinal cord. *Pain* 1985; 23:361–374.

Wu G, Ringkamp M, Hartke TV, et al. Early onset of spontaneous activity in uninjured C-fiber nociceptors after injury to neighboring nerve fibers. *J Neurosci* 2001; RC140:21.

Wu G, Ringkamp M, Murinson BB, et al. Degeneration of myelinated efferent fibers induces spontaneous activity in uninjured C-fiber afferents. *J Neurosci* 2002; 22:7746–7753.

Xie JY, Herman DS, Stiller C-O, et al. Mediation of opioid-induced paradoxical pain and antinociceptive tolerance by cholecystokinin in the rostral ventromedial medulla. *J Neurosci* 2005; 25:409–416.

Zeitz KP, Guy N, Malmberg AB, et al. The 5-HT3 subtype of serotonin receptor contributes to nociceptive processing via a novel subset of myelinated and unmyelinated nociceptors. *J Neurosci* 2002; 22:1010–1019.

Zhuo M, Gebhart GF. Characterization of descending inhibition and facilitation from the nuclei reticularis gigantocellularis and gigantocellularis pars alpha in the rat. *Pain* 1990; 42:337–350.

Zhuo M, Gebhart GF. Spinal serotonin receptors mediate descending facilitation of a nociceptive reflex from the nuclei reticularis gigantocellularis and gigantocellularis pars alpha in the rat. *Brain Res* 1991; 550:35–48.

Zhuo M, Gebhart GF. Characterization of descending facilitation and inhibition of spinal nociceptive transmission from the nuclei reticularis gigantocellularis and gigantocellularis pars alpha in the rat. *J Neurophysiol* 1992; 67:1599–1614.

Zhuo M, Gebhart GF. Biphasic modulation of spinal nociceptive transmission from the medullary raphe nuclei in the rat. *J Neurophysiol* 1997; 78:746–758.

Ziegler EA, Magerl W, Meyer RA, Treede RD. Secondary hyperalgesia to punctate mechanical stimuli. Central sensitization to A-fibre nociceptor input. *Brain* 1999; 122(Pt 12):2245–2257.

Zimmermann M. Pathobiology of neuropathic pain. *Eur J Pharmacol* 2001; 429:23–37.

Correspondence to: Frank Porreca, PhD, Department of Pharmacology, University of Arizona, Tucson, AZ 85724, USA. Fax: 520-626-4182; email: frankp@u.arizona.edu.

Part III

Disease-Specific Targets

Emerging Strategies for the Treatment of Neuropathic Pain, edited by James N. Campbell, Allan I. Basbaum, André Dray, Ronald Dubner, Robert H. Dworkin, and Christine N. Sang, IASP Press, Seattle, © 2006.

11

Disease-Specific Targets: Rapporteur Report

Ralf Baron,[a] John W. Griffin,[b] Robert H. Dworkin,[c] Ahmet Höke,[b] Donald C. Manning,[d] Mitchell B. Max,[e] Karin L. Petersen,[f] Christine Nai-Mei Sang,[g] and William K. Schmidt[h]

[a]Division of Neurological Pain Research and Therapy, Deparment of Neurology, Christian-Albrechts University, Kiel, Germany; [b]Department of Neurology, Johns Hopkins University School of Medicine, Baltimore, Maryland, USA; [c]Department of Anesthesiology, University of Rochester School of Medicine and Dentistry, Rochester, New York, USA; [d]Celgene Corporation, Summit, New Jersey, USA; [e]Pain and Neurosensory Mechanisms Branch, National Institute of Dental and Craniofacial Research, National Institutes of Health, Department of Health and Human Services, Bethesda, Maryland, USA; [f]UCSF Pain Clinical Research, San Francisco, California, USA; [g]Translational Pain Research, Brigham and Women's Hospital, School of Medicine, Harvard University, Boston, Massachusetts, USA; [h]Renovis, Inc., South San Francisco, California, USA

Certain diseases are notorious for producing neuropathic pain. Post-herpetic neuralgia (PHN), diabetic neuropathy, and compression neuropathies are a few examples. The extent to which the pain in these diseases represents distinctive, disease-specific pathology of the nervous system must be determined. It is entirely possible that advances in treatment for neuropathic pain will be based on the development of disease-specific therapies. For example, understanding how diabetes affects nociceptive neurons may lead to new therapies designed to prevent damage to nociceptive afferents and hence reduce or prevent the development of painful diabetic neuropathies. Likewise, the specific impact of other diseases on the nociceptive signaling system needs to be considered.

Regardless of the disease-specific aspects of neuropathic pain, increasing evidence indicates that a multitude of similar mechanisms are operating in many neuropathic pain states. These observations have raised questions regarding whether a new strategy for pain assessment, based on the underlying mechanisms (Jensen and Baron 2003), could provide an alternative approach for examining and classifying patients, with the ultimate aim of improving treatment outcome (Woolf et al. 1998; Dworkin et al. 2003). Our increasing understanding of the mechanisms that underlie chronic pain, together with the discovery of new molecular therapeutic targets, has strengthened the demand for these alternative approaches.

This chapter is based on the consensus of a group colloquium regarding disease-specific targets in neuropathic pain. It highlights three general issues that are of utmost importance in clinical research—novel diagnostic approaches, clinical and proof-of-concept trials, and disease-specific targets. We discuss whether it will be possible to find practical clinical tools to identify one or more pain mechanisms in a particular patient with neuropathic pain and thus treat the pain with agents that target these specific mechanisms. We also consider novel diagnostic approaches that might be helpful in the clinical setting and in future research.

Furthermore, we consider how to improve clinical trial design and outcome measures, given that important information that could improve treatment of neuropathic pain is generally not addressed in industry-funded trials. Examples of potential improvements include combination trials and head-to-head comparisons.

NOVEL DIAGNOSTIC APPROACHES IN NEUROPATHIC PAIN

Extensive preclinical research during the last few years has revealed a variety of potential mechanisms that may play a role in neuropathic pain states. It is likely that several mechanisms may operate in a given patient. The concept of mechanism-based therapy hypothesizes that each mechanism is associated with a certain phenotype (negative and positive somatosensory signs) and that it is possible to design specific therapeutic strategies for each mechanism (Baron 2000).

This concept suggests several questions for future research. Will it be possible to determine individual mechanisms of pain in patients using novel diagnostic procedures? Can we identify subgroups of patients that differ in their phenotype and in the mechanism underlying their pain? Can we use phenotypic differences to identify predictors for the development of neuropathic pain? And can we confirm the mechanisms of neuropathic pain by using therapeutic drugs with a known mechanism of action?

Novel diagnostic tools may help us identify individual mechanisms and should be considered in future mechanistic studies as well as in clinical drug trials. It would be very informative, but also more complex, to incorporate combinations of different diagnostic techniques.

ASSESSMENT OF DISTINCT SENSORY PHENOTYPES

A standardized protocol for quantitative sensory testing (QST) was recently proposed for mechanistic studies and has been applied in PHN patients (Petersen et al. 2000). Besides measuring pain intensity on a visual analogue scale, patients in this study described the specific components of their pain and drew a map of sensory disturbances. Based on these descriptions, precise sensory tests were performed on the PHN-affected side and the unaffected side as well as on a standardized remote body site. Sensory testing included mapping and rating of allodynia intensity and of thresholds for warm and cold detection and heat pain. These measurements were performed in the most painful and second-most painful area of the affected zone. Two different affected sites were included to allow the investigators to assess consistency across the affected dermatome and to reduce variance. Topical capsaicin was applied at a concentration of 0.075% in the most painful area to selectively activate primary afferent nociceptors. During capsaicin stimulation, allodynia mapping and rating were repeated. Finally, skin biopsies were taken just outside the testing site to measure small-fiber density. This approach made it possible to describe subpopulations of PHN patients with distinct somatosensory features and distinct reactions to capsaicin stimulation as well as differences in epidermal nerve fiber densities.

A different approach was established by the German Network on Neuropathic Pain with the introduction of a standardized QST protocol with 13 parameters encompassing thermal and mechanical testing procedures for the analysis of the somatosensory phenotype of patients with neuropathic pain (Rolke et al. 2006). An age- and gender-matched database for absolute and relative QST reference data in healthy human subjects was established as a baseline against which to compare symptoms in patients. This nationwide multicenter trial comprises complete sensory profiles of 180 healthy human subjects and more than 1000 patients with various types of neuropathic pain. Thermal detection and pain thresholds were determined, and tests were included for paradoxical heat sensations, mechanical detection thresholds to von Frey filaments and to a 64-Hz tuning fork, mechanical pain thresholds to pinprick stimuli and blunt pressure, stimulus-response functions for pinprick and dynamic mechanical allodynia (pain evoked by light touch), and pain summation ("wind-up" ratio) using repetitive pinprick stimulation. Data from healthy subjects were analyzed for the influence of body side and region, age, and gender. For most variables, positive and negative signs could be detected on the basis of absolute reference data. The QST data could then be used to create sensory profiles of individual patients or sub-groups of patients to judge impaired somatosensation in patients.

The results of these studies (Rolke et al. 2006) will allow us to characterize the somatosensory profiles of subpopulations of PHN and other neuropathic pain patients. Clinical multicenter drug trials within the German Network are under way using the entire QST protocol in all patients under study to validate the concept of mechanism-based therapy.

Caveats of quantitative sensory testing. Several important caveats regarding QST measures must be taken into account. QST predominantly assesses the phenotype manifested with somatosensory changes in the skin. Changes in the afferent innervation of deep somatic structures that are also affected by the nerve lesion, which may well be involved in the generation of pain, cannot be adequately tested with current QST techniques. Sensory signs that may be indicative of an underlying mechanism can vary among affected skin areas in the same patient, which indicates that multiple mechanisms may be operating in a given patient. Loss of sensory function and denervation have been demonstrated close to areas with preserved sensory function and innervation (Petersen et al. 2000).

Current QST protocols (Rolke et al. 2006), which are much too complicated to be used in large-scale clinical drug trials, must be simplified and made available to primary care physicians. Validation studies are currently being performed to address this issue. Ascertainment bias, which is a systematic distortion in measuring the true frequency of a phenomenon due to the way in which the data are obtained, must be reduced. Other problems with existing protocols include potential interactions with time and the lack of sufficient data to correlate test results with skin biopsies, microneurography and functional imaging.

In summary, by classifying patients according to sensory perception thresholds within the most painful skin area, it is possible to ascertain the predominant sensory profile for each individual. This approach is an important step toward the establishment of a mechanism-based drug therapy for neuropathic pain. If symptoms are closely related to mechanisms, clinical assessment may give an idea of the combination of distinct mechanisms that are relevant for each individual patient. This knowledge may foster optimal polypharmacy with drugs that address the specific combination of mechanisms in each patient.

Recommendations. The following approaches should prove particularly valuable for future research. (1) Standardized QST profiling should be used to detect phenotype subgroups in neuropathic pain patients to help us learn more about pathophysiological mechanisms. (2) Precisely classified phenotype subgroups should be included in proof-of-concept trials. (3) A simplified QST protocol should be defined that can be included in large multicenter trials.

SKIN BIOPSIES

The peripheral nervous system can be directly assessed physiologically and pathologically in mechanistic and disease-modifying studies. Biopsies of nerves such as the sural nerve have been used as outcome measures for clinical trials of aldose reductase inhibitors in diabetes, but this technique has major limitations—it is invasive, it samples only one site, it cannot be done serially (because there is only one sural nerve per leg), and the results are cumbersome and expensive to quantitate, especially for unmyelinated nerve fibers. For these reasons nerve biopsies represent a "last resort" that would be used as an outcome measure only to confirm specific molecular effects.

Multiple assessments of the peripheral nervous system have until recently been restricted to physiological testing, such as EMG and nerve conduction studies. The advent of skin biopsy as a diagnostic and investigative tool has changed the picture; skin biopsies can be done at several sites to establish a spatial profile of nerve fiber involvement and can easily be repeated over time. They have generally met with patient acceptance in neuropathies, even in allodynic states such as PHN. They can be used to assess epidermal nerve fibers, predominantly C-fiber nociceptors, sympathetic fibers innervating the cutaneous sweat glands, and myelinated $A\beta$ and $A\delta$ fibers in the dermis. Detailed anatomical studies using immunochemical markers, including preclinical studies using null mutations and transgenic enhancements, have revealed that fibers presumed to be nociceptive form consistent patterns of cutaneous nerve branches and have similar terminal morphology (Fundin et al. 1997; Rice et al. 1997). Several groups have developed expertise in the identification and quantitation of cutaneous nerve fibers and have refined techniques for the study of cutaneous innervation using skin punch biopsies (Rowbotham et al. 1996; Holland et al. 1997; Oaklander et al. 1998; Petersen et al. 2000; Kennedy 2004; Polydefkis et al. 2004). Several groups have used immunostaining of skin punch biopsies for the panaxonal marker protein gene product 9.5 (PGP9.5), a neuronal ubiquitin hydrolase. This marker is believed to identify axons of all categories of nerve fibers. Initial studies focused on changes in the morphology or density of epidermal nerve fibers or in the innervation of sweat glands (Kennedy and Navarro 1989). Denervation occurs in a length-dependent manner in a variety of neuropathies affecting small-caliber nerve fibers, including diabetes mellitus, HIV-associated sensory neuropathy (Polydefkis et al. 2002), Fabry's disease (Scott et al. 1999), restless legs syndrome, and idiopathic small-fiber sensory neuropathies (Holland et al. 1997). In patients with severe neuropathies, epidermal denervation is found at progressively more rostral levels, with prominent predegenerative axonal swellings or increased branching complexities identified even at asymptomatic sites (Lauria et al. 2003).

Skin punch biopsies have recently been used to examine changes in epidermal innervation over time or after therapeutic interventions in various neuropathic conditions. For example, Nodera et al. (2003) described epidermal reinnervation concomitant with symptomatic improvement in the sensory neuropathy. Impressive increases in the density of epidermal, dermal, and sweat gland innervation have been documented along with improvement in neuropathic status, both spontaneously and after various therapies (Hart et al. 2002). Clinical trials are beginning to incorporate serial determinations of epidermal nerve fiber density as an outcome measure by which to assess therapeutic efficacy (McArthur et al. 2000).

Cutaneous innervation is usually reduced in PHN-affected skin compared to contralateral (mirror-image) skin when assessed with PGP (Rowbotham et al. 1996; Oaklander et al. 1998; Petersen et al. 2000). However, a significant proportion of PHN subjects have similar fiber densities in both PHN and mirror-image skin, suggesting that the symptoms of pain and sensory dysfunction are not due to a mere loss in overall innervation density (Rowbotham et al. 1996; Petersen et al. 2000). Using simple counts of anti-PGP-labeled fibers, Oaklander demonstrated that the average cutaneous fiber density was lower in subjects with established PHN than in those who had recovered from herpes zoster without developing PHN. Furthermore, mirror-image skin had lower fiber densities than skin in other body areas in subjects with established PHN (Oaklander et al. 1998). Linking this information with testing of sensory function has aided in the characterization of phenotypic subtypes in PHN.

Caveats of skin biopsies. Skin biopsies predominantly assess pathology in the skin. Changes in the afferent innervation of deep somatic structures and central changes should also be considered. It remains to be determined whether the pathology shown in a single biopsy is representative of the entire affected area. In PHN, denervation has been demonstrated close to areas with preserved sensory function and innervation (Petersen et al. 2000). In fact, one PHN patient who was treated by removal of a large area of the affected skin showed a variable innervation across the affected dermatome (Petersen et al. 2002). Most groups involved in analysis of human skin biopsies have experienced difficulties using double-labeling immunofluorescence techniques as compared to single-labeling methods. In some cases, antibodies against the same antigen (e.g., TRPV1) have yielded variable results, perhaps because most antibodies are made against nonhuman species and do not bind selectively to human receptors.

Although the skin punch biopsy is a relatively rapid and simple technique, patients with skin that is very delicate, is extremely denervated, or has compromised circulation may not heal quickly. Punch biopsies that are 3 mm in diameter do not need suturing, but some patients will develop a noticeable circular scar at each site. Patients taking anticoagulants or who have a bleeding diathesis are not candidates for skin biopsy.

Recommendations. The information obtained from skin biopsies should greatly improve with validation from double-labeling immunofluorescence techniques using specific molecular markers including sodium and potassium channels, growth factor receptors, and transient receptor potential (TRP) channels such as the capsaicin receptor. Further validation should come from more specific morphological measures that go beyond simple assessment of fiber density to evaluate nerve branching, collateral sprouting, and axonal swellings. Despite being very labor intensive, skin biopsies have the potential to become important outcome measures in trials of disease-modifying agents that affect small nerve fibers.

BIOMARKERS

Biomarkers are specific biochemicals in the body that have a well-defined molecular feature that makes them useful for diagnosing a disease, measuring the progress of a disease, or determining the effect of a treatment. Patterns of protein expression used for diagnostic purposes can reveal subclasses of pathophysiological mechanisms in single patients. Data on the analysis of biomarkers in the pain field are sparse; the available information is reviewed by Urban et al. in this volume.

Measurement of biomarkers is often limited by the invasiveness of obtaining appropriate samples for analysis. Herpes zoster is the condition most amenable for analysis of biomarkers because samples of cerebrospinal fluid are occasionally taken during the acute phase of shingles to assess the severity of spinal inflammation and can be used for the analysis of specific biomarkers. In fact, interleukin (IL)-8 in the cerebrospinal fluid has been described as a predictor for PHN (Kotani et al. 2004), although this study should be replicated to confirm this finding.

In syndromes such as complex regional pain syndrome (CRPS) that are characterized by an inflammatory component within the skin, suction blister fluid analysis can be used to quantify biomarkers. A recent study shows that in CRPS patients, blister fluid contains higher levels of IL-6 and tumor necrosis factor alpha (TNF-α) when taken from the affected limb as compared with the contralateral limb (Huygen et al. 2002).

Cytokines are also involved in common pain comorbidities. IL-6 levels are elevated in sleep and mood disorders as well as in inflammatory central nervous system (CNS) conditions such as transverse myelitis (Irani and Kerr 2000). An interesting question is whether these biomarkers are released to a greater extent if pain is present in addition to these syndromes. Biomarkers might be used to determine a causative relationship between pain and various comorbidities.

The introduction of proteomics to the biomarker field has made possible the analysis of patterns of protein expression (see Urban et al., this volume). Future clinical trials may utilize these new techniques in combination with other measures of somatosensory function such as QST profiling and skin biopsies.

Recommendations. Development of biomarkers for neuropathic pain is desperately needed and would potentially improve clinical trial design and help screen a relatively large number of compounds through early clinical development in a cost-effective manner.

MICRONEUROGRAPHY

Microneurography has been used to assess functional abnormalities in single small fibers. This technique makes it possible to subgroup C nociceptors in healthy controls into a variety of physiologically different classes. The technique requires considerable technical skills from the researcher and is very time-consuming.

It is possible to identify spontaneously active C fibers in patients with conditions such as erythromelalgia (Orstavik et al. 2003). However, results indicating abnormal firing patterns in diabetic neuropathy patients are still inconclusive (H.O. Handwerker, personal communication). One major problem has been that normal aging changes the functional properties of C afferents dramatically. As patient populations with neuropathic conditions are generally older, normative data must be obtained from a cohort of healthy older subjects. Furthermore, since recordings are made from single afferent C fibers and not from whole nerves, it is not possible to obtain reliable quantitative data, and the lack of true quantitation of fibers will limit the use of microneurography in large-scale clinical trials.

Recommendations. Microneurography should be used in research trials only by specialized centers. It does not seem possible to perform this technique in multicenter drug trials.

IMAGING TECHNIQUES

A new magnetic resonance imaging (MRI) technique, magnetic resonance neurography, makes it possible to identify small patches of inflammation in peripheral nerves. This technique might be of value in inflammatory neuropathies, in acute zoster, or in detecting schwannoma and neuroma (Bendszus et al. 2004). One study used MRI in 16 patients with herpes zoster in the cervical and trigeminal distribution (Haanpaa et al. 1998). Of these, nine had lesions in the brainstem and cervical cord that were attributed to the virus. More patients with lesions associated with herpes zoster still had pain 3 months after resolution of the viral infection. No data are available to demonstrate changes that may occur during chronic PHN.

Another technique, diffusion tensor imaging, can also detect degeneration of fibers in the dorsal columns in severe peripheral neuropathies.

AUTOPSIES

Nervous system autopsies are useful for genetic studies and to perform receptor binding autoradiography. Tissue samples from patients who had suffered from PHN (Watson et al. 1988) and chemotherapy-induced neuropathy would be most appropriate for such research. Future studies should include longitudinal observations and should correlate structural MRI data and standardized QST analysis with autopsy data to help us understand the pathophysiology of neuropathic pain states.

DRUG CHALLENGES AS PROBES OF PAIN MECHANISMS

In addition to their role as treatments for pain, selective agonists and antagonists of pain-mediating molecules provide a powerful complement to QST and biopsy studies to distinguish pain mechanisms in patients. Examples include challenges with sympathetic agonists in CRPS (Raja et al. 1991) and PHN (Choi and Rowbotham 1997), topical application of capsaicin or local anesthetics in PHN (Petersen et al. 2000), and two-part clinical studies to enrich the enrollment of diabetic neuropathy patients whose pain is relieved by systemic clonidine (Byas-Smith et al. 1995) or dextromethorphan (Sang et al. 2002). The current and imminent availability of other selective agents such as neurokinin-1 antagonists and TRPV1-receptor antagonists may enlarge the repertoire of strategies useful for making mechanistic distinctions.

CLINICAL TRIALS AND PROOF-OF-CONCEPT TRIALS IN NEUROPATHIC PAIN

IMPROVED CLINICAL TRIAL DESIGN

Participants of the group colloquium regarding disease-specific targets in neuropathic pain, comprising primarily academic and industry clinical pain researchers, reached consensus on many issues regarding clinical trial design.

We agreed that there is "low hanging fruit" to be harvested to improve clinical care and clinical trial methods. The establishment of multi-center academic neuropathic pain clinical trial groups could contribute data that industry generally does not collect, including:

1) Head-to-head comparisons of drugs from different treatment groups. These are a much more reliable guide to comparative efficacy than meta-analyses of studies of single agents compared to placebo. For example, while meta-analyses could not distinguish between the efficacy of opioids, tricyclics, and gabapentin (Dworkin et al. 2003), head-to-head comparisons have shown a trend toward the superiority of opioids over each of the other two classes (Gilron et al. 2005; Raja et al. 2002). European regulatory guidelines encourage the use of comparators in clinical trials, while the U.S. Food and Drug Administration (FDA) does not currently have such recommendations.

2) Combination studies. Data from Gilron et al. (2005) suggest that an opioid-gabapentin combination is superior to either drug alone when titrated to equivalent levels of side effects. This study and others (e.g., C.N. Sang et al., unpublished data) have used a simple two-by-two factorial design, but other designs have been proposed to investigate more complex combinations of three or more drugs (Sveticic et al. 2004).

3) Multi-center cooperative groups can facilitate efficient study of low prevalence neuropathic pain states. These groups can provide a uniform recruitment, testing, and data analysis system.

4) Funding can be sought from governmental and foundation sources similar to the National Cancer Institute's support of the regional cooperative oncology groups. Challenges to this approach would include efficient contract negotiations with individual sites, data ownership, and academic "credit" for investigator participation in individual studies.

A potential barrier to the establishment of multicenter trial groups is the paucity of experienced neuropathic pain researchers, particularly in the United States. A combined approach with more established groups might be workable. Examples are some of the HIV neuropathy pain trials carried out during the 1990s by the neurology section of the AIDS Clinical Trial Group

(Kieburtz et al. 1998; McArthur et al. 2000) and ongoing trials by the German Network on Neuropathic Pain.

When studying analgesic interventions of several weeks to months, we recommend that academic groups consider crossover designs because the greatly increased power of such studies can discern small treatment differences related to drugs or to mechanistic distinctions (Senn 2002). Although some statisticians are reluctant to use these designs, the experience of many single-center groups has shown no systematic carryover effects in neuropathic pain trials.

However, crossover studies are not feasible in studies that alter the natural history of the underlying structural disease (e.g., studies of growth factors in diabetic neuropathy), in studies of the long-term effects of analgesic regimens, in clinical conditions with unstable or rapidly changing pain level, or with drugs with long or uncertain half-life values. Moreover, the effect of expectation should be considered when using a cross-over design.

IMPROVEMENTS IN METHODS OF ANALYZING RESULTS OF RANDOMIZED CONTROLLED TRIALS IN NEUROPATHIC PAIN

Compared to clinical trials in more established fields, analysis methods in chronic analgesic trials have been rather primitive. The recent provision of large data sets by several companies to academic researchers has begun to improve this understanding. For example, Farrar et al. (2001) used pregabalin study results to show that the percentage reduction of pain scores provides a tighter fit to the patient's overall assessment of benefit than do simple differences on the 0–10-point scale during the treatment. We would urge industry and regulatory authorities to find ways of making more of these data available.

The efficiency of clinical trials may be improved by the prerandomization assessment of the subject's ability to interpret assessment scales, so as to determine the subject's readiness to appreciate a change in pain symptoms, similar to what has been proposed before implanting stimulation devices for pain relief. Just as patients have multiple motivations when seeking care from a practitioner, so too may subjects enlisting in a clinical study be driven by different, sometimes confounding, motivations. Knowledge of these sources of variability and strategies to mitigate their effects on therapy assessment may greatly improve the sensitivity of neuropathic clinical trials. It is also apparent that the efficiency of trials can be considerably improved by a study of various prognostic indicators and of the ways in which patients use pain scales in clinical trials.

For example, in many back pain studies, higher education level has predicted a more favorable outcome (Deyo and Diehl 1988). In some types of pain, low catastrophizing scores predict greater reductions in pain (Heinberg et al. 2004). Most clinicians would predict that the number of previous failed treatments for a neuropathic pain condition would correlate negatively with the likelihood of pain improvement, while expectation of pain relief would correlate positively with pain improvement.

We suggest that academic and industry researchers develop tools to assess a number of such possible covariates and perhaps the ways in which patients use pain scales, and test these instruments in academic and industry clinical trials. Reductions in the total variance would translate almost directly into greater power to detect modest treatment differences.

MECHANISM-BASED VERSUS DISEASE-BASED PAIN DIAGNOSIS IN CLINICAL TRIALS

In the early enthusiasm for "mechanism-based diagnosis" (Woolf et al. 1998), traditional disease diagnoses of pain, such as "distal symmetrical diabetic neuropathy," were considered outmoded because they did not specify the pain mechanism. Some investigators proposed enrolling patients for trials based upon inferred pain mechanism, such as patients with mechanical allodynia from a variety of nerve disorders (Wallace et al. 2002; Jensen and Baron 2003; Rolke et al. 2006).

Traditional disease diagnoses retain considerable value because features of the disease pathophysiology tend to create recurring pain-causing lesions and because the similarity of the experience of the patients with these diseases makes it easier to study and correct for other covariates such as environmental influences and demographic variables.

Efforts to establish mechanistic distinctions within disease groups are an important goal. The FDA has stated that it will only accept distinctions made by tests that could be done by a large proportion of clinicians. Such simplification is a feasible second step after extensive laboratory testing has established a mechanistic link. For example, Raja et al. (unpublished data) simplified the extensive zoster sensory testing battery and were able to determine that the finding of a side-to-side difference of 1°C or more in heat pain threshold, suggesting partial denervation, will predict that tricyclics would be more effective than opioids.

USE OF CONCOMITANT ANALGESICS WHILE IN NEUROPATHIC PAIN TRIALS

As knowledge increases about treatment, more and more patients will already be taking one or more analgesics before entering studies. Most group members felt that it is usually impractical to require cessation of other treatments that are not in the same class as the drug to be tested. Institutional review boards may have ethical objections to removing therapies that relieve pain. This issue is usually handled by adding the test drug or placebo to the ongoing regimen, and balancing the randomization for common concomitant treatments such as gabapentin. Patients who are "analgesic naive" can be prospectively collected at the onset of disease, such as in studies of the onset of herpes zoster or acute lumbar root pain.

ISSUES WITH LONG-TERM STUDIES

There are essentially no published studies longer than several months in neuropathic pain. Such studies are urgently needed, particularly for opioids, which are embroiled in controversy about whether they remain effective long-term or are rendered useless by tolerance or hyperalgesia. Placebo controls in studies of 6 months or more are out of the question. However, patients could be randomized to drug regimens at different dose levels (Rowbotham et al. 2003). Further development of innovative study design is needed to address the ethical and practical issues raised by long-term assessment of neuropathic pain therapy.

WHICH APPROACH WILL ESTABLISH PROOF OF CONCEPT FOR NEUROPATHIC PAIN DRUGS?

Experimental surrogate models. The group agreed that there is little evidence that experimental pain models that do not involve nerve damage will predict response in neuropathic pain. However, some secondary phenomena that are present in experimental pain models (i.e., central sensitization or peripheral sensitization) might share common mechanisms.

Pharmacological test study. The best way to quickly get an answer about the analgesic efficacy of a drug is to do a short study in patients with a neuropathic pain condition. Single dose studies with the patient at rest may be misleading because pain may be worst during activity. If pharmacokinetic study makes it safe to rapidly get patients to steady-state drug concentrations, an answer may be forthcoming with a study lasting one to several days. However, animal studies of compounds such as sodium channel blockers and GABA agonists have suggested gradual increase of effect over time. Therefore, a study of at least two weeks duration might avoid many false negatives from such a delayed action.

DISEASE-SPECIFIC TARGETS IN NEUROPATHIC PAIN

It is generally thought that a variety of mechanisms are operating in neuropathic pain, even in any given patient. Furthermore, it is believed that mechanisms are similar across different etiologies. Yet, despite the similarities, some disease-specific mechanisms may be responsible for certain components of pain.

The aim of this section is to identify the etiology- or disease-specific mechanisms of pain generation and to identify targets and therapeutic strategies that may affect these particular mechanisms. We will focus on diabetic neuropathy, PHN, HIV neuropathy, chemotherapy-induced neuropathy, complex regional pain syndrome (CRPS), central neuropathic pain (spinal cord injury pain), and mixed pain syndromes (chronic radiculopathy). We do not specifically address alcohol neuropathy, phantom limb pain, chronic post-surgical neuropathic pain (e.g., mastectomy, thoracotomy, and neuroma pain), trigeminal neuralgia, neuropathic tumor pain, compression neuropathies, post-traumatic neuralgia, radiation-induced pain, central neuropathic pain (poststroke pain), and multiple sclerosis.

DIABETIC NEUROPATHY

Diabetic neuropathy has many attractions as a target. The prevalence is high; over 6% of U.S. residents have diabetes, and another 7% have impaired glucose tolerance. A significant proportion of diabetics have nerve damage, and of these a proportion have pain. The most prevalent form is a distally and sensory predominant neuropathy. Small sensory and autonomic fibers are often involved in the earliest stages; over time, large-caliber sensory and motor fibers become affected. In previous studies, pain in diabetic neuropathy has responded to several agents, including amitriptyline, gabapentin, pregabalin, and duloxetine (Sindrup and Jensen 2000; Dworkin et al. 2003).

Several concerns relate to studies of later stage diabetic neuropathy. It is a heterogeneous disease with many syndromes including some as disparate as diabetic proximal neuropathy, a lumbosacral plexopathy of abrupt onset, and diabetic autonomic neuropathy.

Disease-modification strategies in advanced diabetes are inherently difficult. The relatively slow progression of the disease has mandated long studies to detect possible nerve protection or regeneration. The outcome measures have also been problematic. In the 1980s and 1990s some studies used baseline and endpoint sural nerve biopsies, but this technique is painful and invasive and examines only one site, so it may not be sensitive to more proximal regeneration of nerve fibers.

It is now clear that both early diabetes and impaired glucose tolerance can damage a population of small sensory and autonomic fibers and may be associated with neuropathic pain. Studies of patients with diabetes often have restrictive inclusion criteria, such as range of severity (for example, sural action potential amplitudes within a defined range), and exclusions for specific complications or medication requirements. Recruitment would be simpler for analgesic studies in patients with early diabetes or impaired glucose tolerance, and these patients are also an attractive target for disease modification strategies. Concerns about diabetic complications are less important in these patients, and at early disease stages nerve regeneration is likely to be more robust. Techniques for assessing the rate of regeneration of epidermal nerve fibers after experimental injury have been published, and a prominent defect in diabetics has been documented (Polydefkis et al. 2004). Skin biopsies may provide a relatively simple outcome measure by which to detect protection or regeneration of small sensory fibers. The effect of new regenerative therapies on the rate of regeneration after experimental injury in healthy volunteers can also be assessed prior to larger clinical trials in patients.

POSTHERPETIC NEURALGIA

Many clinical studies have been performed in patients with PHN. The knowledge gained from these studies and from investigations of disease mechanisms in PHN makes this entity especially interesting for future research activities. Furthermore, since neuronal damage is induced by a viral attack, disease-specific and, in particular, virus-specific therapies might emerge.

Histopathological and clinical characteristics. Histopathological studies have demonstrated peripheral and central degenerative changes in many PHN patients, including ganglion cell loss and fibrosis and atrophy of the dorsal horn, dorsal root ganglion, dorsal root, and peripheral nerves (Head and Campbell 1900; Noordenbos 1959; Zacks et al. 1964; Watson et al. 1988, 1991). A more recent study addressed changes after trigeminal PHN that correlated histopathological changes and psychophysical testing (Watson et al. 1999).

Most patients with PHN are able to distinguish four distinct components of their discomfort: (1) a constant deep pain; (2) spontaneous burning pain; (3) a brief, recurrent, shooting, tic-like pain; and (4) pain evoked by very light touch to the skin, which is called dynamic mechanical allodynia. The patient may undergo extraordinary efforts to protect the affected area from innocuous mechanical stimuli, but firm compression of the skin does not usually exacerbate the pain and may even provide relief. Clinical investigations show that negative sensory signs (sensory deficits) and positive ones (mechanical allodynia) may coexist within the affected dermatome. Extreme allodynia to light touch is often restricted to areas surrounding scarred skin or at the border between affected and unaffected dermatomes. In some patients the allodynic area expands far into unaffected adjacent dermatomes, indicating that some CNS mechanisms must be involved in the generation of allodynia. Besides mechanically evoked pain, up to 30% of patients suffer from heat-evoked pain (heat hyperalgesia), whereas pain induced by cold stimuli affects fewer than 10% of patients.

Pathophysiological mechanisms of pain generation. Antiviral drugs used in chronic PHN have failed to relieve pain (Acosta and Balfour 2001). Therefore, a persistent inflammatory reaction due to continuous viral infection or due to immune-cell-mediated inflammation and cytokine release does not seem to be involved in the pathophysiology of PHN in most patients.

Several lines of evidence suggest that distinct pathophysiological changes in the excitability of peripheral and central neurons are involved in pain generation. Standardized QST methods described above can distinguish between three phenotypic subtypes of PHN patients with distinct sensory symptom constellations that may be correlated with different underlying mechanisms.

Type I. Peripheral and central sensitization of nociceptive neurons. Several clinical observations support the concept of sensitized nociceptors and central sensitization in PHN patients. About 30% of patients with PHN show no loss of sensory function in the affected dermatome, indicating that loss of neuronal function is minimal or absent. Accordingly, thermal sensory thresholds in the region of greatest pain are normal or even decreased (indicating heat hyperalgesia) by up to 2–4°C (Pappagallo et al. 2000; Rowbotham and Fields 1996). The decrease of heat pain perception thresholds is a well-known phenomenon of peripheral nociceptor sensitization.

Skin punch biopsy has shown that thermal sensitivity is directly correlated with density of cutaneous innervation in the area of most severe pain (Rowbotham et al. 1996). In addition to their enhanced reactivity to thermal stimuli, sensitized nociceptors also acquire sensitization to chemical stimuli. Another study (Petersen et al. 2000) used capsaicin stimulation to identify "capsaicin responders" characterized by relatively preserved sensory function at baseline compared to nonresponders. In three of the capsaicin responders, the area of allodynia expanded into previously non-allodynic and nonpainful skin that had normal sensory function and cutaneous innervation.

These observations support the hypothesis that allodynia in a subgroup of PHN patients is a form of chronic secondary hyperalgesia maintained by input from intact and possibly "irritable" primary afferent nociceptors to a sensitized CNS (Fields et al. 1998; Petersen et al. 2000). The occurrence of sensitized nociceptors is further supported by observations that topical capsaicin therapy, which is thought to be effective only in patients with sensitized nociceptors, can provide pain relief (Bernstein et al. 1989).

Acute infection of cultured dorsal root ganglion (DRG) neurons with human varicella zoster virus led to an increase in norepinephrine-induced Ca^{2+} influx, indicating adrenergic sensitivity of these neurons. These results suggest that not only a mechanical lesion but also a viral infection may lead to adrenergic sensitivity of afferent neurons (Kress and Fickenscher 2001). Clinical studies support the idea that zoster infection may trigger catecholamine sensitivity in nociceptors. In patients with PHN, intracutaneous injection of epinephrine and phenylephrine increased spontaneous pain and allodynia on the affected side (Choi and Rowbotham 1997). There are also reports that sympathetic blocks, as well as intravenous phentolamine and topical clonidine (Abadir et al. 1996), can transiently relieve pain in the occasional PHN patient.

Type II. Predominant degeneration of nociceptive neurons. In contrast to the patient population with sensitized nociceptors, up to 60% of PHN patients show considerable signs of neuronal degeneration and loss of function within the affected dermatome. Interestingly, many of these patients still suffer from severe dynamic mechanical allodynia, although the function of nociceptors is diminished or absent in the same skin area.

Skin punch biopsies and labeling with the anti-PGP 9.5 antibody were used in PHN patients and zoster patients without pain to quantify epidermal nerve fiber density in the affected and contralateral skin (Rowbotham et al. 1996; Oaklander 1998, 2001). A skin site distant from the shingles involvement was also analyzed. In PHN a severe loss of epidermal nerve fibers could be demonstrated on the affected side. Furthermore, Oaklander (1998) found that mirror-image skin had lower fiber densities than distant control skin in subjects with established PHN. These contralateral changes have not been observed with QST measurements and need to be confirmed in future studies.

Functional studies support the concept of degeneration of cutaneous C-fiber nociceptors. By using these C-fiber axon reflex reactions it is possible to objectively assess cutaneous C-fiber function in the human skin. In some patients, histamine-evoked axon reflex vasodilatation was impaired or abolished and flare size decreased in skin regions with intense dynamic allodynia (Baron and Saguer 1993). Similarly, during capsaicin stimulation, a subgroup did not experience worsening of pain (Petersen et al. 2000). QST has shown that some chronic PHN patients have extremely high thermal thresholds in areas with marked dynamic allodynia (Choi and Rowbotham 1997; Nurmikko and Bowsher 1990; Nurmikko et al. 1994). Thus, there is a subset of PHN patients with pain and *loss* of cutaneous C-nociceptor function in a region that is coextensive with allodynic skin.

Type III. Complete skin deafferentation. Clinically, a third and smaller group of PHN patients can be distinguished. These patients, which account for less than 10% of PHN patients overall, have severe spontaneous pain and profound sensory loss but no evoked sensations (hyperalgesia or allodynia). In association with pain, there is a complete cutaneous deafferentation of the painful area (anesthesia dolorosa). It must be assumed that the DRG cells and the central connections of all afferents are lost in such patients and that their pain must be the result of intrinsic CNS changes.

Three distinct sensory profiles in PHN patients: clinically relevant? The above classification of subtypes of PHN based on nociceptor function and evoked pain types, might be attractive, it should be emphasized that not all patients fit exactly into one category or the other. Furthermore, in a large group of PHN patients many heterogeneous patterns of sensory dysfunction were detected (Pappagallo et al. 2000). In a case study of one PHN patient, detailed testing of sensory function, chemical stimulation, and cutaneous innervation clearly showed areas of relative preservation in close vicinity to areas of impaired thermal sensation, all within the affected dermatome (Petersen et al. 2000). Furthermore, the sensory patterns showed a variation over the time course of PHN. However, by classifying PHN patients according to sensory perception thresholds within the most painful skin area it is possible to detect the predominant individual sensory profile and the most likely underlying mechanism of pain generation.

Animal models. Several animal models of herpes zoster and PHN have been developed. In one model, mice that are inoculated with herpes simplex virus type 1 develop zosteriform skin lesions, exhibit viral DNA in DRG, and manifest allodynia and hyperalgesia beginning approximately 5 days after inoculation (Takasaki et al. 2000). Early treatment with the antiviral agent acyclovir inhibited skin lesions, viral proliferation, allodynia, and hyperalgesia. Gabapentin (Takasaki et al. 2001) and mexiletine (Asano et al. 2003) dose-dependently reduced allodynia and hyperalgesia within 1 week of inoculation. Approximately half of the mice demonstrated persisting allodynia and hyperalgesia, and treatment with morphine, gabapentin, and mexiletine dose-dependently reduced this long-lasting postherpetic pain whereas diclofenac did not (Takasaki et al. 2002). In the most recent study examining this animal model of PHN, when amitriptyline or gabapentin were administered within the first week after inoculation, the highest dose of amitriptyline reduced acute pain and nonsignificantly inhibited persisting pain, whereas gabapentin not only dose-dependently inhibited acute pain but also markedly reduced postherpetic pain, with the highest dose studied completely preventing such pain (Kuraishi et al. 2004). A more recent animal model of herpes zoster and PHN involves inoculation of rats with varicella zoster virus (Dalziel et al. 2004; Fleetwood-Walker et al. 1999). In this model, mechanical allodynia developed within 3 days of inoculation and persisted for 30–60 days.

Research and design of future clinical trials. PHN is clearly responsive to many therapies. Furthermore, it is a well-established model without much heterogeneity. The following approaches are particularly interesting for future research. Since persistent ganglionitis due to continuing viral infection is not likely to occur in the majority of patients, a therapeutic approach aimed at attacking the virus in chronic PHN seems inappropriate. Future studies should include longitudinal observations including standardized QST analysis and imaging and should ideally be correlated with autopsy data to reveal details of pathophysiology. Standardized QST profiling should be used to detect phenotype subgroups to allow us to learn more about pathophysiological mechanisms. Proposed phenotype subgroups should be further validated using pharmacological challenges with agents aimed at specific mechanisms. Precisely classified phenotype subgroups of patients should be included in drug trials. A simplified QST protocol should be developed and validated. PHN is extremely suitable for preventive studies, and preemptive drugs should be explored.

HIV NEUROPATHY

Clinical characteristics and histopathological findings. Patients with neuropathies associated with human immunodeficiency virus present with distal painful paresthesias and mechanical allodynia. They often have spontaneous and evoked shock-like pain, more commonly than is seen in diabetic neuropathy patients. These differences may relate to different underlying pathophysiological mechanisms, but the pattern of involvement (i.e., a distal symmetric stocking-like distribution) is similar to other painful neuropathies, such as idiopathic painful small-fiber sensory neuropathy or painful sensory neuropathy seen in patients with impaired glucose tolerance.

In most patients with HIV-associated neuropathy, nerve damage is often due to a combination of the virus itself and a subset of antiretroviral drugs called nucleoside analogue reverse transcriptase inhibitors. Clinically, these two causes of nerve damage are indistinguishable from each other. Despite the highly active antiretroviral therapy (HAART), the incidence of HIV-associated neuropathy remains high, partly due to toxicity from antiretroviral drugs. Overall incidence is about 15–30% in the HIV population in the current era of HAART.

The initial abnormality in HIV-associated neuropathy is distal intra-epidermal denervation. However, at very early stages of the disease, patients experiencing severe pain may still have "normal" intraepidermal fiber density. However, in later stages of the illness, almost all patients have axonal loss in their sural nerve biopsies. Autopsy series have revealed neuronal atrophy but minimal neuronal loss in the DRG. Unfortunately, the pathology in the dorsal horn is unknown. Dr. Justin McArthur at Johns Hopkins University has a large collection of tissue samples of the spinal cord, peripheral nerves, and DRG from clinically well-characterized patients. These specimens would be useful in future studies to evaluate the mechanisms of unique pain profiles in HIV neuropathy patients.

Research and design of future clinical trials. The neuro-AIDS community is well organized and has completed many clinical trials, including several for HIV-associated neuropathies. There are several well-characterized cohorts, which simplifies patient recruitment. Adherence to drugs is often accomplished by using modern technologies such as personal digital assistants. This issue is especially important in this patient population in which drug adherence is a major concern, due in part to the mild cognitive impairment seen in many patients.

CHEMOTHERAPY-INDUCED NEUROPATHY

Clinical features. Neuropathies induced by cancer chemotherapy are relatively common, and neurotoxicity often limits the dose of the agent used for controlling the cancer. Development of effective neuroprotective or analgesic therapies will allow more effective doses of chemotherapeutic agents to be used. However, these studies will require effective collaborations with oncological groups.

Since the incidence is relatively high and the exact time and dosing of the toxic agent is known, one can easily design trials to ask if a given compound has neuroprotective properties. These trials will need to incorporate a detailed evaluation of "neural health" and can include electrophysiology, skin biopsies, and detailed repeated examinations. One of the advantages of using the chemotherapy-induced neuropathy patient population for neuroprotective treatments is that trials can be accomplished in a relatively short period of time in comparison to other more chronic diseases such as diabetic or HIV neuropathies.

One confounding issue in designing clinical trials involves the possible different mechanisms of neuropathy with different classes of agents. However, it is unknown if the mechanisms underlying neuropathic pain in neuropathies due to different chemotherapeutic agents are unique or are shared among different drug classes.

Animal models. The available literature is limited despite the fact that paclitaxel- and vincristine-induced neuropathy models in rats have been available for many years. Although these models are well studied, many unanswered questions remain, especially those related to disease-specific pain mechanisms. Recent studies examined the role of TRPV4 and integrin/Src tyrosine kinase signaling in paclitaxel-induced neuropathy, and the findings indicate novel therapeutic targets for neuropathic pain in this model (Alessandri-Haber et al. 2004). In another study, inhibition of the calpain activation seen in paclitaxel neuropathy was effective in preventing neuropathy and neuropathic pain behavior in mice (Wang et al. 2004). It remains to be seen whether calpain activation is a common pathway for all chemotherapy-induced neuropathies. In vincristine-induced neuropathy, in contrast to other neuropathies such as diabetic neuropathy, caspase activation seems to play a role, indicating a potential therapeutic role for caspase inhibitors in neuropathic pain in chemotherapy-induced neuropathies. In addition to these animal models, new models are desperately needed, especially those specifically directed to asking mechanistic questions about disease-specific neuropathic pain. One of these areas is oxaliplatin-induced neuropathy, since oxaliplatin use will increase over the next decade due to its recent approval for first-line treatment for colon cancer, a common malignancy.

Research and design of future clinical trials. Chemotherapy-induced neuropathies offer a unique opportunity to test neuroprotective strategies that may also prevent neuropathic pain.

COMPLEX REGIONAL PAIN SYNDROME

Clinical features. CRPS type I patients develop asymmetrical distal extremity pain and swelling in the absence of a demonstrable nerve lesion (Jänig and Baron 2003). These patients often report a burning spontaneous pain in the distal part of the affected extremity. Stimulus-evoked pains are a striking clinical feature; they include mechanical and thermal allodynia and hyperalgesia. These sensory abnormalities are most pronounced distally; they have no consistent spatial relationship to individual nerve territories or to the site of the inciting lesion. Typically pain can be elicited by movement of and pressure on the joints (deep somatic allodynia), even if the joints are not directly affected by the inciting lesion.

Some patients experience generalization of pain to other body areas (spread of hyperalgesia). The underlying mechanism might be generalized descending facilitation. This phenomenon is not seen in other neuropathic pain conditions, at least not in the chronic state. Therefore, it would be worthwhile to look for generalized phenomena acutely after nerve injury so as to be able to analyze the descending facilitation processes.

In a subgroup of patients the pain can be reduced by blocking the efferent sympathetic nerves to the affected extremity; activation of the sympathetic system enhances the pain.

Neuropathic versus inflammatory disorder. In CRPS type II, a nerve lesion is present, which makes the classification of this syndrome as a neuropathic disorder straightforward. In CRPS type I, although no overt nerve lesion is demonstrable, several sensory phenomena are identical to those present in classical painful neuropathies. These close similarities make it likely that the underlying pathophysiological mechanisms are similar to those of neuropathies. However, CRPS patients also demonstrate signs and symptoms of a localized inflammatory process, in particular in the acute stage, which cannot be explained by neuropathic changes alone. To approach this problem, the evaluation of skin biopsies could be helpful. It is noteworthy that CRPS-like symptoms (of the acute type) are common in patients with herpes zoster outbreaks affecting the extremity, particularly if the distal extremity is involved (Berry et al. 2004). Both nerve injury and inflammation during herpes zoster are well documented.

Pathophysiological mechanisms. The generation of pain in CRPS is unknown. It is thought that mechanisms of peripheral and central sensitization are involved. In addition, several studies in CRPS patients address the question as to what extent inflammation mediated by immune cells is involved. Skin biopsies in these patients showed a striking increase in the number of Langerhans cells, which can release immune cell chemoattractants and proinflammatory cytokines. Accordingly, in the fluid of artificially produced skin blisters, significantly higher levels of IL-6 and TNF-α were observed in the involved extremity as compared with the uninvolved extremity (Huygen et al. 2002). The patchy osteoporosis found in more advanced CRPS cases may also be consistent with a regional inflammatory process in deep somatic tissues. Both IL-1 and IL-6 cause proliferation and activation of osteoclasts and suppress the activity of osteoblasts.

Changes in hair growth can also be created by proinflammatory cytokines. TNF and IL-1 directly inhibit hair growth. Keratocyte-derived TNF and IL-6 cause retarded hair growth, signs of fibrosis, and in turn immune infiltration of the dermis, which are all present in CRPS patients.

Sympathetically maintained pain. A pathological interaction between postganglionic sympathetic fibers and afferent fibers is thought to be the underlying cause of sympathetically maintained pain (Baron et al. 2002b). Upregulation of α-adrenoceptors on afferent neurons leading to adrenergic sensitivity seems to be involved. Knowledge about the subtypes of α-adrenoreceptors involved in the sympathetic-afferent coupling following nerve trauma is important for an understanding of the underlying neural mechanism and may be useful in the design of more specific treatment modalities for neuropathic pain conditions involving sympathetic efferent activity.

Central plasticity related to pain generation. Positron emission tomography studies have demonstrated adaptive changes in the thalamus during the course of the disease (Fukumoto et al. 1999). Furthermore, recent magnetoencephalography and functional MRI studies demonstrated a shortened distance between little finger and thumb representations in the primary somatosensory cortex on the painful side (Maihofner et al. 2003; Pleger et al. 2004). This reorganization of the somatosensory cortex was correlated to pain intensity and was reversible after successful treatment. These findings fit into the theoretical concept that decreased lemniscal input to the cortex leads to an increase in nociceptive dominance and therefore to pain.

Animal model. Recently an animal model for CRPS-I was introduced (Coderre et al. 2004). The clinical observation that signs of tissue inflammation and ischemia are present in many CRPS-I patients led to the hypothesis that CRPS-I might depend on an ischemia-reperfusion injury, which may at least in part induce the classical CRPS symptomatology. Consequently, an animal pain model was established that utilizes prolonged hindlimb ischemia for 3 hours, followed by reperfusion, which produces a chronic post-ischemia pain syndrome.

Research and design of future clinical trials. Since the clinical diagnostic criteria for CRPS are in the process of internal and external validation and are now much stricter, it is possible to perform clinical studies in a much less heterogeneous group of patients (Baron and Jänig 2004). Therefore, the time seems ripe for clinical trials in CRPS patients (Baron et al. 2002a).

Integrative research on animal and human models combined with clinical research on CRPS patients is necessary to unravel the mechanisms operating in CRPS and to find the underlying pathophysiological principles that orchestrate the various changes.

The following approaches are particularly interesting for future research. The natural course of fractures should be compared with the development of "real" CRPS. To identify the inflammatory component, the analysis of suction blister fluid or of the effluent of microdialysis devices might be helpful. The inflammatory component in CRPS, as supported by several studies, makes this entity unique from other neuropathic pain states. Therefore, compounds that attack the inflammatory process of the disease are interesting possibilities. Unlike most other neuropathic pain syndromes, CRPS can involve sympathetically maintained pain, and it would be useful to investigate compounds acting on adrenoceptors in patients with this syndrome. CRPS also might be a good model to test therapeutic strategies for cortical reorganization, such as occupational therapy, motor cortex stimulation, and mirror image therapy.

SPINAL CORD INJURY PAIN

Clinical features and taxonomy.   There have been large variations in the reported incidence and prevalence of spinal cord injury (SCI) pain, and until recently, there was little consensus regarding the nature, terminology and definitions of this heterogeneous pain syndrome. This may account for, in part, the large number of negative analgesic trials in this diagnostic group. A proposal for a new taxonomy was put forth in 1997, in which two major divisions can be distinguished (Finnerup and Jensen 2004): (1) nociceptive (musculoskeletal, spastic, and visceral) and (2) neuropathic (above-level and at-level or below-level) pain. At- or below-level neuropathic pain is described in either of two basic anatomical distributions: (a) segmental, in a band-like distribution that is circumferential, and (b) at or below the level of the spinal cord lesion, perceived diffusely in anesthetic regions.

This chapter does not address inflammatory myelopathies, including transverse myelitis and multiple sclerosis, partly because of the acute/subacute nature of these illnesses.

Animal models.   Several recently developed animal models mimic chronic central pain following injury to the spinal cord (Vierck et al. 2000). Lesions of selected spinal pathways have also been used to model SCI pain. In the ischemic model and in a hemisection model of SCI, mechanical allodynia, cold hyperalgesia and allodynia, autotomy, and scratching develop over several days to several weeks. Despite differences in specific lesion type, all rats developed spontaneous and evoked pain behaviors, including allodynia, similar to the human experience in which different etiologies of spinal cord injury may result in similar symptoms.

Research and design of future clinical trials.   Despite the development of animal models whose phenotype and time course are similar to those of patients with SCI pain, the appropriate selection of patients for enrollment into analgesic trials remains the greatest challenge. The extent of cauda equina injury must be considered, and double lesion syndrome, syrinx, and arachnoiditis must be carefully assessed and ruled out. Inadequately controlled central spasticity and other factors that may contribute to a heightened pain state, and perhaps render patients unresponsive to analgesics, need to be addressed prior to admission of SCI patients into clinical trials. Several investigators have suggested that damage to spinothalamic neurons is a necessary, but not sufficient, condition for the development of diffuse neuropathic pain.

The disappointing results across a range of analgesic drug classes is likely to be related in part to methodological issues. Negative trials using chronic oral therapy have been underpowered or lacking in strict entry criteria. Gabapentin has been the exception to date, perhaps because of its antispasmodic effects. The other positive trials have excluded patients with known potential confounders and show both good assay sensitivity, positive responses across a range of drug classes and a low placebo response (C.N. Sang, unpublished data).

MIXED PAIN SYNDROMES: CHRONIC RADICULOPATHY

Pathophysiological mechanisms. In chronic radiculopathy, nociceptive and neuropathic pain components are likely to operate in concert. The nociceptive component stems from activation of intact nociceptors that innervate ligaments, small joints, muscles, and tendons. The neuropathic pain component is caused by mechanical compression of the nerve root (mechanical neuropathic root pain) or by the actions of inflammatory mediators (inflammatory neuropathic pain) originating from the degenerative disk. Cytokines and chemokines have been implicated in the chemical pathomechanism of radicular pain. Increased levels of inflammatory cytokines, such as TNF-α, IL-1, IL-6, and granulocyte-macrophage colony-stimulating factor, have been detected in herniated disk tissue compared with normal, nondegenerated disk tissue. TNF-α, when applied to primary afferent fibers, increases spontaneous discharges. When applied to nerve roots, it can also reproduce the pathological changes observed with nerve root exposure to nucleus pulposus extracts. Finally, in an animal model of radiculopathy induced by intervertebral disk material, inhibitors of TNF-α reversed the radicular pathology. It is unclear whether these mediators are capable of activating intact nerve root fibers even without any mechanical compression, or if the combination of mechanical nerve damage and cytokine attack is the important prerequisite.

Research and design of future clinical trials. Diagnostic procedures must be established that assess the contribution of the neuropathic pain component in patients with mixed radiculopathy. There is evidence that the pathophysiological mechanisms of chronic radiculopathy are different from those of other neuropathic pain syndromes because they involve nociceptive pain, with a combination of compression and cytokine action. Therefore, it seems reasonable that different therapeutic strategies should be tested in clinical trials, such as combinations of nonsteroidal anti-inflammatory drugs, antidepressants, anticonvulsants, and cytokine antagonists.

OVERALL CONCLUSIONS

We need to better understand a broader range of neuropathic pain diseases at a mechanistic level. Individual diseases can have multiple mechanisms. At present, for most purposes, clinical trials are designed around disease-based strategies. Multiple mechanisms can coexist in a disease, and one mechanism may apply to multiple diseases. One drug may have complex downstream consequences. PHN has served as an example of mechanistic analysis.

We encourage broader testing in disease panels when a drug has a novel mechanism. This strategy may require adoption of an experimental medicine approach to early drug development based on proposed pharmacological mechanisms to identify the most appropriate disease conditions. In traditional early-stage development, new compounds are generally tested in only one or a restricted number of specific diseases, which may lead to potentially useful drugs being abandoned prematurely or inappropriately.

We encourage natural history studies to define diseases, study their mechanisms, and identify biomarkers. We also encourage early treatment studies to develop preventive therapies in the case of PHN, diabetes, impaired glucose tolerance, and acute radiculopathy and preemptive therapy in the case of cancer chemotherapy, HIV, and surgery.

We encourage increased opportunities for interdisciplinary interactions to promote new expertise in clinical and basic sciences.

We encourage longer duration trials in phase 4, especially with opioids. Efficacy of opioids is now established in painful diabetic neuropathy and PHN and should be examined in other neuropathic pain states. The role of opioid adjuvants should be established.

We encourage new clinical trial designs, including longer-term, randomized, non-placebo-controlled, add-on, or polypharmacy studies, as well as longitudinal cohort studies. We encourage large-scale head-to-head comparison and combination therapy trials. We encourage registration (http://prsinfo.clinicaltrials.gov) and timely publication of all clinical trials of neuropathic pain for both academic and industry-sponsored trials with either positive or negative findings (De Angelis et al. 2005).

We encourage industry and academic partnerships for post-hoc analysis of neuropathic clinical trial data, and we encourage the establishment of a consortium of academic clinical investigators similar to the German Neuropathic Pain Network and other models of cooperative clinical research and evaluation.

ACKNOWLEDGMENTS

Dr. Baron is supported by the Deutsche Forschungsgemeinschaft (DFG Ba 1921), the German Ministry of Research and Education, the German Research Network on Neuropathic Pain (BMBF, 01EM01/04), and an unrestricted educational grant from Pfizer, Germany.

REFERENCES

Abadir AR, Kraynack BJ, Mayda J II, Gintautas J. Postherpetic neuralgia: response to topical clonidine. *Proc West Pharmacol Soc* 1996; 39:47–48.

Acosta EP, Balfour HH Jr. Acyclovir for treatment of postherpetic neuralgia: efficacy and pharmacokinetics. *Antimicrob Agents Chemother* 2001; 45:2771–2774.

Alessandri-Haber N, Dina OA, Yeh JJ, et al. Transient receptor potential vanilloid 4 is essential in chemotherapy-induced neuropathic pain in the rat. *J Neurosci* 2004; 24:4444–4452.

Asano K, Sameshima T, Shirasawa H, Hisamitsu T. Attenuating effect of mexiletine hydrochloride on herpetic pain in mice infected with herpes simplex virus. *J Pharm Pharmacol* 2003; 55:1365–1370.

Baron R. Peripheral neuropathic pain: from mechanisms to symptoms. *Clin J Pain* 2000; 16:S12–20.

Baron R, Jänig W. Complex regional pain syndromes—how do we escape the diagnostic trap? *Lancet* 2004; 364:1739–1741.

Baron R, Saguer M. Postherpetic neuralgia. Are C-nociceptors involved in signalling and maintenance of tactile allodynia? *Brain* 1993; 116:1477–1496.

Baron R, Fields HL, Jänig W, Kitt C, Levine JD. National Institutes of Health Workshop: reflex sympathetic dystrophy/complex regional pain syndromes—state-of-the-science. *Anesth Analg* 2002a; 95:1812–1816.

Baron R, Schattschneider J, Binder A, Siebrecht D, Wasner G. Relation between sympathetic vasoconstrictor activity and pain and hyperalgesia in complex regional pain syndromes: a case-control study. *Lancet* 2002b; 359:1655–1660.

Bendszus M, Wessig C, Solymosi L, Reiners K, Koltzenburg M. MRI of peripheral nerve degeneration and regeneration: correlation with electrophysiology and histology. *Exp Neurol* 2004; 188:171–177.

Bernstein JE, Korman NJ, Bickers DR, Dahl MV, Millikan LE. Topical capsaicin treatment of chronic postherpetic neuralgia. *J Am Acad Dermatol* 1989; 21:265–270.

Berry JD, Rowbotham MC, Petersen KL. Complex regional pain syndrome-like symptoms during herpes zoster. *Pain* 2004; 110:e1–12.

Byas-Smith MG, Max MB, Muir J, Kingman A. Transdermal clonidine compared to placebo in painful diabetic neuropathy using a two-stage 'enriched enrollment' design. *Pain* 1995; 60:267–274.

Choi B, Rowbotham MC. Effect of adrenergic receptor activation on post-herpetic neuralgia pain and sensory disturbances. *Pain* 1997; 69:55–63.

Coderre TJ, Xanthos DN, Francis L, Bennett GJ. Chronic post-ischemia pain (CPIP): a novel animal model of complex regional pain syndrome-type I (CRPS-I; reflex sympathetic dystrophy) produced by prolonged hindpaw ischemia and reperfusion in the rat. *Pain* 2004; 112:94–105.

Dalziel RG, Bingham S, Sutton D, et al. Allodynia in rats infected with varicella zoster virus— a small animal model for post-herpetic neuralgia. *Brain Res Brain Res Rev* 2004; 46:234–242.

De Angelis CD, Drazen JM, Frizelle FA, et al. Is this clinical trial fully registered? A statement from the International Committee of Medical Journal Editors. *N Engl J Med* 2005; 352:2436–2438.

Deyo RA, Diehl AK. Psychosocial predictors of disability in patients with low back pain. *J Rheumatol* 1988; 15:1557–1564.

Dworkin RH, Backonja M, Rowbotham MC, et al. Advances in neuropathic pain: diagnosis, mechanisms, and treatment recommendations. *Arch Neurol* 2003; 60:1524–1534.

Farrar JT, Young JP Jr, LaMoreaux L, Werth JL, Poole RM. Clinical importance of changes in chronic pain intensity measured on an 11-point numerical pain rating scale. *Pain* 2001; 94:149–158.

Fields HL, Rowbotham M, Baron R. Postherpetic neuralgia: irritable nociceptors and deafferentation. *Neurobiol Dis* 1998; 5:209–227.

Finnerup NB, Jensen TS. Spinal cord injury pain—mechanisms and treatment. *Eur J Neurol* 2004; 11:73–82.

Fleetwood-Walker SM, Quinn JP, Wallace C, et al. Behavioural changes in the rat following infection with varicella-zoster virus. *J Gen Virol* 1999; 80(Pt 9):2433–2436.

Fukumoto M, Ushida T, Zinchuk VS, Yamamoto H, Yoshida S. Contralateral thalamic perfusion in patients with reflex sympathetic dystrophy syndrome. *Lancet* 1999; 354:1790–1791.

Fundin BT, Silos-Santiago I, Ernfors P, et al. Differential dependency of cutaneous mechanoreceptors on neurotrophins, trk receptors, and P75 LNGFR. *Dev Biol* 1997; 190:94–116.

Gilron I, Bailey JM, Tu D, et al. Morphine, gabapentin, or their combination for neuropathic pain. *N Engl J Med* 2005; 352:1324–1334.

Haanpaa M, Dastidar P, Weinberg A, et al. CSF and MRI findings in patients with acute herpes zoster. *Neurology* 1998; 51:1405–1411.

Hart AM, Wiberg M, Youle M, Terenghi G. Systemic acetyl-L-carnitine eliminates sensory neuronal loss after peripheral axotomy: a new clinical approach in the management of peripheral nerve trauma. *Exp Brain Res* 2002; 145:182–189.

Head H, Campbell AW. The pathology of herpes zoster and its bearing on sensory location. *Brain* 1900; 23:353–523.

Heinberg LJ, Fisher BJ, Wesselmann U, Reed J, Haythornthwaite JA. Psychological factors in pelvic/urogenital pain: the influence of site of pain versus sex. *Pain* 2004; 108:88–94.

Holland NR, Stocks A, Hauer P, et al. Intraepidermal nerve fiber density in patients with painful sensory neuropathy. *Neurology* 1997; 48:708–711.

Huygen FJ, De Bruijn AG, De Bruin MT, et al. Evidence for local inflammation in complex regional pain syndrome type 1. *Mediators Inflamm* 2002; 11:47–51.

Irani DN, Kerr DA. 14-3-3 protein in the cerebrospinal fluid of patients with acute transverse myelitis. *Lancet* 2000; 355:901.

Jänig W, Baron R. Complex regional pain syndrome: mystery explained? *Lancet Neurol* 2003; 2:687–697.

Jensen TS, Baron R. Translation of symptoms and signs into mechanisms in neuropathic pain. *Pain* 2003; 102:1–8.

Kennedy WR. Opportunities afforded by the study of unmyelinated nerves in skin and other organs. *Muscle Nerve* 2004; 29:756–767.

Kennedy WR, Navarro X. Sympathetic sudomotor function in diabetic neuropathy. *Arch Neurol* 1989; 46:1182–1186.

Kieburtz K, Simpson D, Yiannoutsos C, et al. A randomized trial of amitriptyline and mexiletine for painful neuropathy in HIV infection. AIDS Clinical Trial Group 242 Protocol Team. *Neurology* 1998; 51:1682–1688.

Kotani N, Kudo R, Sakurai Y, et al. Cerebrospinal fluid interleukin 8 concentrations and the subsequent development of postherpetic neuralgia. *Am J Med* 2004; 116:318–324.

Kress M, Fickenscher H. Infection by human varicella-zoster virus confers norepinephrine sensitivity to sensory neurons from rat dorsal root ganglia. *Faseb J* 2001; 15:1037–1043.

Kuraishi Y, Takasaki I, Nojima H, Shiraki K, Takahata H. Effects of the suppression of acute herpetic pain by gabapentin and amitriptyline on the incidence of delayed postherpetic pain in mice. *Life Sci* 2004; 74:2619–2626.

Lauria G, Morbin M, Lombardi R, et al. Axonal swellings predict the degeneration of epidermal nerve fibers in painful neuropathies. *Neurology* 2003; 61:631–636.

Maihofner C, Handwerker HO, Neundorfer B, Birklein F. Patterns of cortical reorganization in complex regional pain syndrome. *Neurology* 2003; 61:1707–1715.

McArthur JC, Yiannoutsos C, Simpson DM, et al. A phase II trial of nerve growth factor for sensory neuropathy associated with HIV infection. AIDS Clinical Trials Group Team 291. *Neurology* 2000; 54:1080–1088.

Nodera H, Barbano RL, Henderson D, Herrmann DN. Epidermal reinnervation concomitant with symptomatic improvement in a sensory neuropathy. *Muscle Nerve* 2003; 27:507–509.

Noordenbos W. *Pain.* Amsterdam: Elsevier, 1959, pp 68–80.

Nurmikko T, Bowsher D. Somatosensory findings in postherpetic neuralgia. *J Neurol Neurosurg Psychiatry* 1990; 53:135–141.

Nurmikko T, Wells C, Bowsher D. Sensory dysfunction in postherpetic neuralgia. In: Boivie J, Hansson P, Lindblom U (Eds). *Touch, Temperature, and Pain in Health and Disease: Mechanisms and Assessments,* Progress in Pain Research and Management, Vol. 3. Seattle: IASP Press, 1994, pp 133–141.

Oaklander AL. Unilateral postherpetic neuralgia is associated with bilateral sensory neuron damage. *Neurology* 1998; 44:789–795.

Oaklander AL. The density of remaining nerve endings in human skin with and without postherpetic neuralgia after shingles. *Pain* 2001; 92:139–145.

Oaklander AL, Romans K, Horasek S, et al. Unilateral postherpetic neuralgia is associated with bilateral sensory neuron damage. *Ann Neurol* 1998; 44:789–795.

Orstavik K, Weidner C, Schmidt R, et al. Pathological C-fibres in patients with a chronic painful condition. *Brain* 2003; 126:567–578.

Pappagallo M, Oaklander AL, Quatrano-Piacentini AL, Clark MR, Raja SN. Heterogenous patterns of sensory dysfunction in postherpetic neuralgia suggest multiple pathophysiologic mechanisms. *Anesthesiology* 2000; 92:691–698.

Petersen KL, Fields HL, Brennum J, Sandroni P, Rowbotham MC. Capsaicin evoked pain and allodynia in post-herpetic neuralgia. *Pain* 2000; 88:125–133.

Petersen KL, Rice FL, Suess F, Berro M, Rowbotham MC. Relief of post-herpetic neuralgia by surgical removal of painful skin. *Pain* 2002; 98:119–126.

Pleger B, Tegenthoff M, Schwenkreis P, et al. Mean sustained pain levels are linked to hemispherical side-to-side differences of primary somatosensory cortex in the complex regional pain syndrome I. *Exp Brain Res* 2004; 155:115–119.

Polydefkis M, Yiannoutsos CT, Cohen BA, et al. Reduced intraepidermal nerve fiber density in HIV-associated sensory neuropathy. *Neurology* 2002; 58:115–119.

Polydefkis M, Hauer P, Sheth S, et al. The time course of epidermal nerve fibre regeneration: studies in normal controls and in people with diabetes, with and without neuropathy. *Brain* 2004; 127:1606–1615.

Raja SN, Treede RD, Davis KD, Campbell JN. Systemic alpha-adrenergic blockade with phentolamine: a diagnostic test for sympathetically maintained pain. *Anesthesiology* 1991; 74:691–698.

Raja SN, Haythornthwaite JA, Pappagallo M, et al. Opioids versus antidepressants in postherpetic neuralgia: a randomized, placebo-controlled trial. *Neurology* 2002; 59:1015–1021.

Rice FL, Fundin BT, Arvidsson J, Aldskogius H, Johansson O. Comprehensive immunofluorescence and lectin binding analysis of vibrissal follicle sinus complex innervation in the mystacial pad of the rat. *J Comp Neurol* 1997; 385:149–184.

Rolke R, Baron R, Meier C, et al. Quantitative sensory testing in the German Research Network on Neuropathic Pain (DFNS): standardized protocol and reference values. *Pain* 2006; in press.

Rowbotham MC, Fields HL. The relationship of pain, allodynia and thermal sensation in post-herpetic neuralgia. *Brain* 1996; 119:347–354.

Rowbotham MC, Yosipovitch G, Connolly MK, et al. Cutaneous innervation density in the allodynic form of postherpetic neuralgia. *Neurobiol Dis* 1996; 3:205–214.

Rowbotham MC, Twilling L, Davies PS, et al. Oral opioid therapy for chronic peripheral and central neuropathic pain. *N Engl J Med* 2003; 348:1223–1232.

Sang CN, Booher S, Gilron I, Parada S, Max MB. Dextromethorphan and memantine in painful diabetic neuropathy and postherpetic neuralgia: efficacy and dose-response trials. *Anesthesiology* 2002; 96:1053–1061.

Scott LJ, Griffin JW, Luciano C, et al. Quantitative analysis of epidermal innervation in Fabry disease. *Neurology* 1999; 52:1249–1254.

Senn S. *Cross-Over Trials in Clinical Research.* Chichester: John Wiley, 2002.

Sindrup SH, Jensen TS. Pharmacologic treatment of pain in polyneuropathy. *Neurology* 2000; 55:915–920.

Sveticic G, Gentilini A, Eichenberger U, et al. Combinations of bupivacaine, fentanyl, and clonidine for lumbar epidural postoperative analgesia: a novel optimization procedure. *Anesthesiology* 2004; 101:1381–1393.

Takasaki I, Andoh T, Shiraki K, Kuraishi Y. Allodynia and hyperalgesia induced by herpes simplex virus type-1 infection in mice. *Pain* 2000; 86:95–101.

Takasaki I, Andoh T, Nojima H, Shiraki K, Kuraishi Y. Gabapentin antinociception in mice with acute herpetic pain induced by herpes simplex virus infection. *J Pharmacol Exp Ther* 2001; 296:270–275.

Takasaki I, Sasaki A, Andoh T, et al. Effects of analgesics on delayed postherpetic pain in mice. *Anesthesiology* 2002; 96:1168–1174.

Vierck CJ Jr, Siddall P, Yezierski RP. Pain following spinal cord injury: animal models and mechanistic studies. *Pain* 2000; 89:1–5.

Wallace MS, Rowbotham MC, Katz NP, et al. A randomized, double-blind, placebo-controlled trial of a glycine antagonist in neuropathic pain. *Neurology* 2002; 59:1694–1700.

Wang MS, Davis AA, Culver DG, et al. Calpain inhibition protects against Taxol-induced sensory neuropathy. *Brain* 2004; 127:671–679.

Watson CP, Morshead C, Van der Kooy D, Deck J, Evans RJ. Post-herpetic neuralgia: post-mortem analysis of a case. *Pain* 1988; 34:129–138.

Watson CP, Deck JH, Morshead C, Van der Kooy D, Evans RJ. Post-herpetic neuralgia: further post-mortem studies of cases with and without pain. *Pain* 1991; 44:105–117.

Watson CPN, Midha R, Devor M, et al. Trigeminal postherpetic neuralgia postmortem: clinically unilateral, pathologically bilateral. In: Devor M, Rowbotham MC, Wiesenfeld-Hallin Z (Eds). *Proceedings of the 9th World Congress on Pain*, Progress in Pain Management and Research, Vol. 16. Seattle: IASP Press, 1999, pp 733–740.

Woolf CJ, Bennett GJ, Doherty M, et al. Towards a mechanism-based classification of pain? *Pain* 1998; 77:227–229.

Zacks SI, Langfitt RW, Elliott FA. Herpetic neuritis: a light and electron microscopic study. *Neurology* 1964; 14:744–750.

Correspondence to: Prof. Dr. med. Ralf Baron, Division of Neurological Pain Research and Therapy, Department of Neurology, Christian-Albrechts-Universität Kiel, Schittenhelmstr. 10, 24105 Kiel, Germany. Tel: 49-431-597-8504; Fax: 49-431-597-8530; email: r.baron@neurologie.uni-kiel.de.

Emerging Strategies for the Treatment of Neuropathic Pain, edited by James N. Campbell, Allan I. Basbaum, André Dray, Ronald Dubner, Robert H. Dworkin, and Christine N. Sang, IASP Press, Seattle, © 2006.

12

The Roles of Growth Factors in Painful Length-Dependent Axonal Neuropathies

John W. Griffin

Department of Neurology, Johns Hopkins University School of Medicine, Baltimore, Maryland, USA

GROWTH FACTORS AND DISTAL AXONAL DEGENERATION

The final common pathway of axonal degeneration is not fully understood, but we know that it involves energy failure, entry of extracellular calcium, mitochondrial pore formation, and calpain activation, leading to granular degeneration of the cytoskeleton. This sequence can be conceptualized as the equivalent of apoptosis in a "nucleus-free" zone. Axonal degeneration beginning in the distal regions of long axons is the most frequent pathology in peripheral neuropathies. Defects in retrograde transport of growth factors appear to be a common means of triggering this kind of nerve degeneration in neuropathies. The "undertrophed" neuron switches to a regenerative mode in which it abandons stability and maximum caliber for longitudinal growth and plasticity in a search for growth factors.

Axonal length-dependent neuropathies are the most prevalent causes of neuropathic pain. These disorders include diabetic polyneuropathy (Dyck et al. 1987), including the painful neuropathy sometimes seen with impaired glucose tolerance before frank diabetes occurs (Singleton et al. 2001a,b; Sumner et al. 2003). Among patients referred to the Hopkins Peripheral Nerve Clinic for painful neuropathies without previous etiological diagnoses, mild diabetes and impaired glucose tolerance together counted for over 60% of referrals (Sumner et al. 2003). Other frequent causes include the sensory neuropathy of AIDS (So et al. 1990; Cornblath and McArthur 1995; Blum et al. 1996); neuropathies caused by some neurotoxic drugs, including antiretroviral drugs (Cornblath and McArthur 1995) and some cancer chemotherapeutic agents (Chaudhry et al. 1994); and idiopathic painful polyneuropathy, a frequent problem that especially affects elderly individuals (Holland et al. 1998; Periquet et al. 1999).

All of these disorders are characterized by distally predominant axonal degeneration (here termed "distal axonal degeneration" or DAD). The degeneration of the ends of axons in a long-before-short sequence was termed "dying back" by the father of the field, John Cavanagh, at Queens Square in London. It has survived a series of other names, including "central-peripheral distal axonopathy" (Spencer and Schaumburg 1976), and is clinically recognized as "length-dependent axonal degeneration." Implicit in all these terms are the assumptions that: (1) Long axons degenerate before short ones. (2) Degeneration begins in the distalmost region of the axon and proceeds proximally with time. (3) In large-caliber dorsal root ganglion (DRG) neurons with processes ascending the dorsal columns, in general the ends of the peripheral and central processes degenerate roughly synchronously. (4) A fourth element used to be taught—that large-caliber axons degenerate before small-caliber ones (Spencer and Schaumburg 1976, 1977). Recent studies have proved that this concept is often incorrect, because small fibers are involved before or at the same time as large fibers in many neuropathies.

Not all DADs are associated with neuropathic pain; in fact, the majority are painless. Clinical experience would seem to indicate that patients with predominant involvement of "large fibers" are more likely to complain of tingling paresthesias than of spontaneous pain, whereas patients with prominent involvement of small sensory axons are more likely to complain of burning pain in the feet and toes, although no critical series with psychophysical testing and detailed physiological and pathological correlates are available to support or refute this impression. "Large-fiber" involvement is characterized by vibratory and joint position sensibility in the feet and later in the fingers, by loss of tendon reflexes beginning at the ankles, and by weakness beginning in the intrinsic muscles of the feet and the ankles. In contrast, peripheral neurologists have long recognized a group of patients with "small-fiber" neuropathies, characterized by normal strength, normal tendon reflexes, and standard electrophysiological measures, but with spontaneous pain, often including "lightning pains" with or without hyperalgesia, a predilection for painless injuries, and a variable degree of autonomic insufficiency (Holland et al. 1998; Periquet et al. 1999). These "small-fiber" neuropathies typically involve DAD that prominently affects small sensory afferents, including C-fiber nociceptors (Kennedy et al. 1996; Holland et al. 1998).

The prominence of pathology of small sensory fibers in painful neuropathies was revealed by the advent of skin biopsies immunostained for dermal and epidermal nerve fibers (Kennedy and Wendelschafer-Crabb 1993;

McArthur et al. 1994; Hsieh et al. 1996). This approach demonstrated that patients with the severe spontaneous burning in the feet characteristic of these neuropathies usually exhibited *loss* of C-fiber nociceptors from the epidermis of the feet and distal leg (Kennedy et al. 1996; Holland et al. 1998; Periquet et al. 1999).

Distal axonal degeneration as a pathological process. The pathology of "dying back" was recognized in human nerve and spinal cord diseases in the 19th century. The pathology suggested that the nerve cell body was the "alma mater"—the nourishing mother— of a dependent axon, so that the end of the axon was at greatest risk because it was farthest from the cell body. The recognition that the axon utilized special forms of intracytoplasmic transport— the axonal transport systems—suggested that severing an axon might be analogous to interrupting the blood circulation to an organ. In this view the distal axon might be considered the "last field of irrigation," which should degenerate as a result of a passive starvation for essential materials. A corollary was that the basis for DAD might be sought in defects in the cell body.

In the mature nervous system, most of the growth factors derive from the target of innervation. A lesson from the past 10 years is that in most of these models the responsible defects appear to be in axonal transport, especially retrograde transport, or related functions. This finding inverts the "last field of irrigation" concept, suggesting that the target is in fact the "alma mater" and indicating that the cell body receives this trophic support from the periphery via retrograde transport and translates it into the materials that the axon terminals will receive via anterograde transport. The importance of defects in axonal transport have become especially clear in genetic disorders in which molecules involved in axonal transport are responsible for human length-dependent neuropathies. Abnormalities in the retrograde motor system, based on dynein, have been identified, including predominantly motor neuropathies associated with abnormalities in dynamin (Alexander et al. 2000; Delettre et al. 2000) and dynactin (Puls et al. 2003). The importance of mitochondrial renewal is indicated by the fact that one of the most prominent causes of axonal Charcot-Marie-Tooth disease, a dominantly inherited DAD, is a mutation in mitofusin-2, a gene involved in mitochondrial fusion, a process likely to be especially important in axons (Zuchner et al. 2004).

Deficiency in growth factors leads to a reprogramming of perikaryal synthesis and axonal transport. As a simplification, it is useful to think of the growth-factor-deficient neuron as a "lean, mean growing machine." In the peripheral nervous system, separation from the target initiates a series of changes that move the axon away from a state of high radial growth, high stability, and low plasticity to one in which longitudinal growth and plasticity are favored and radial caliber is reduced. The biochemical changes fit with this reprogramming. Neurofilaments, major determinants of axonal caliber, are reduced in both message and protein (Hoffman et al. 1987; Greenberg and Lasek 1988), and the amount of pulse-labeled neurofilament protein undergoing axonal transport is decreased (Hoffman et al. 1984, 1985, 1988). A consequence is centrifugally spreading atrophy of the axon, moving from the perikaryon down the axon. Tubulins and actin, molecules required for longitudinal growth, are increased (Hoffman and Cleveland 1988), as are growth-associated protein-43 (GAP-43) and other axonal growth-cone molecules.

The axotomized peripheral axon can find growth factors "packaged" and presented in the plasmalemma of denervated Schwann cell bands—the Bungner bands. This arrangement provides an ever-changing growth factor gradient that drives the growing axon down individual bands. No comparable longitudinal structural scaffolding or presentation is found in the central nervous system. In order to allow regenerating axons to pass the pia-glial junction of the cord and regenerate intraparenchymally, investigators had to supply higher levels of growth factors (Ramer et al. 2000) or raise perikaryal cyclic AMP (Qiu et al. 2002; Lu et al. 2004).

Axonal degeneration as an active process. Axonal degeneration is now recognized to be an active process, not a passive "starvation" of the axon. The mechanisms of Wallerian degeneration—degeneration of the distal stump following axotomy—appear to be similar to those of DAD. Axonal degeneration represents a neuropathological process comparable in importance to neuronal cell death. Because by definition the neuronal nucleus cannot be involved in Wallerian degeneration (the distal stump is separated from the cell body), cell death mechanisms that do not involve the nucleus may be implicated. However, some of the mechanisms that participate in perikaryal apoptosis, especially those that are mitochondria-based, are likely to operate in axonal degeneration. Axonal degeneration may have elements of what could be termed "apoptosis in a nucleus-free zone."

The pivotal late event in Wallerian degeneration is granular disintegration of the axonal cytoskeleton. It consists of conversion of the normal cytoskeleton to granular and amorphous debris. It is the first morphological change that must be irreversible. The development of granular disintegration appears to be abrupt and explosive. It is an "all or nothing" phenomenon: at any cross-sectional level, partially degenerated axoplasm is rarely seen. The axolemma and some particulate organelles may remain as morphological features for short periods after granular degeneration ensues.

The onset of granular disintegration of the cytoskeleton is triggered by an increase in intra-axonal calcium concentration and by a consequent activation of the calcium-sensitive cysteine proteases, the calpains. The process can be delayed by lowering the temperature (Lunn et al. 2000) and can be prevented by maintaining nerves in low concentrations of calcium (Schlaepfer and Bunge 1973) or by administering membrane-permanent inhibitors of calpains (Schlaepfer and Micko 1979; Glass et al. 1994; George et al. 1995).

The rise in intra-axonal calcium is due, at least in part, to entry of extracellular calcium. This influx of calcium is necessary to activate calpains and results in granular degradation of the axoplasm (Schlaepfer 1974; George et al. 1995). Blockage of entry of calcium or of activation of calpains is sufficient to delay the axonal cytoskeletal degradation (Schlaepfer and Hasler 1979; Mata et al. 1991). Reversal of the sodium-calcium exchanger has been shown to underlie calcium entry in the ischemic optic nerve (Stys et al. 1990, 1991). The Na-Ca exchanger normally moves one molecule of calcium out of the cell for every three molecules of sodium that enter. In conditions of energy deprivation the exchange reverses, so that calcium enters the axon. Some data also suggest that calcium entry may occur via calcium channels, but the status of calcium channels along the axon remains unresolved (George et al. 1995).

There is also evidence for a release of calcium from intracellular stores. Ouardouz and colleagues (2003) showed that in the rat spinal cord dorsal column, ischemia results in axonal injury and in increases intra-axonal calcium levels in the absence of extracellular calcium. This release of calcium from intracellular stores is blocked by ryanodine. At the initial stages of axonal degeneration, local increases in intra-axonal calcium around endoplasmic reticulum profiles lead to dissolution of neurofilaments. Although this process was initiated by ischemia rather than by axonal transection, and therefore might be different from Wallerian degeneration, the resulting rise in intra-axonal calcium and degradation of neurofilaments are very similar to what happens during granular disintegration of the axon.

Axonal breakdown after transection generally moves from the site of transection distally along the nerve with time. Lubinska (1977, 1982) used teased nerve fibers to demonstrate this process in the rat phrenic nerve. Because this nerve by definition remains at core temperature throughout the process, its use eliminates the possibility of a proximal-distal temperature gradient that might slow distal degeneration. Similarly, after lumbar dorsal rhizotomy, degeneration of central projections of DRG sensory neurons begins close to the cell body and spreads rostrally up the dorsal columns (away from the cell body) at a rate of about 3–7 mm/h (Travlos et al. 1990).

The concept that the axon depends from day to day on materials received via axonal transport was implicitly challenged by increasing data that some proteins can be synthesized within the axon, and by observations that axons survive for many days in the face of apparently complete blockade of axonal transport. The most dramatic basis for reconsideration was the identification of profoundly retarded Wallerian degeneration in a substrain of mice called *Wlds* for "Wallerian-like degeneration slow" (Lunn et al. 1989; Perry et al. 1990a,b; Glass et al. 1993). In this spontaneously occurring substrain, degeneration of the transected axons is slowed significantly. In a wild-type animal, transection of the sciatic nerve results in loss of electrical conductivity in the distal portion within a day or two, followed by dissolution of the axoplasm. In contrast, a transected axon in a *Wlds* mouse continues to conduct electricity for up to 2 weeks (Lunn et al. 1989; Tsao et al. 1999).

The *Wlds* mutation in the mouse is an 85-kilobase tandem triplication on the distal arm of the mouse chromosome 4 that contains a translocation. This gene encodes a fusion protein that includes 70 amino acids of the ubiquitin fusion degradation protein 2 (*Ufd2*) and a protein identical to nicotinamide mononucleotide acetyltransferase, expressed in humans by the *NMNAT* gene. Overexpression of this enzyme appears to be responsible for prolonged axonal survival. This synthetic enzyme is involved in the nicotinamide adenine dinucleotide (NAD) salvage pathway. NAD in turn is involved in activation of protein deacetylases within the nucleus. Araki and colleagues (2004) have demonstrated that the NAD-dependent acetylase SIRT1 appears to be the target of the increased NAD; the effect is in the neuronal nucleus. An antibody generated against the N-terminal of the fusion protein gave only a punctate nuclear staining in both the transgenic mouse and the original *Wlds* mouse. There was no accumulation of the fusion protein at the swollen endbulbs of transected axons, suggesting that there was no axonal transport of the protein. Thus the *Wlds* protein, through increased NAD levels, appears to produce deacetylation of transcription factors involved in synthesis of as-yet unknown proteins that promote axonal survival. Importantly, this effect could be achieved by increased NAD levels by exogenous administration in neuronal cultures (Araki et al. 2004).

The challenges in understanding DAD are to imagine how the process of Wallerian degeneration could be compartmentalized into distal axonal segments and to discover how growth factor deficiency could produce this process. An important concept is that growth factors have both obligate perikaryal (nuclear) effects and direct axonal effects. Nerve growth factor (NGF) is a well-studied example. Its high-affinity receptor, the tyrosine kinase A (TrkA) receptor, uses one or more co-receptors, including p75. Binding, dimerization, and internalization of the NGF-TrkA complex with phosphorylation of TrkA forms a signaling endosome that has local effects (Ye et al. 2003) and is also retrogradely transported to the nucleus, where it affects transcriptional and translational events. The multicompartmental Campenot chamber, consisting of axons running through seals between separate compartments, affords a powerful means of testing the regional effects of applied growth factors on the axon. Removal of growth factors from the distalmost compartment can lead to axonal retraction on a local basis (Ye et al. 2003). Conversely, Deckwerth and Johnson (1993) showed that in the *Wlds* mouse, withdrawal of NGF results in degeneration and disappearance of the cell body, whereas the axon survives for days. Pending critically designed experiments, it seems likely that true DAD reflects a perikaryal reordering of synthesis that leads to degeneration of the distal axon. This suggestion is prompted by the fact that simple cessation of fast anterograde axonal transport need not lead to prompt axonal breakdown, yet an "undertrophed" neuron can undergo distal axonal degeneration surprisingly quickly.

GROWTH FACTORS AND NEUROPATHIC PAIN

The NGF system and the glial-cell-line-derived neurotrophic factor (GDNF)/artemin neurotrophic system appear to be counterpoised, so that excessive signaling by NGF through TrkA or deficient signaling by GDNF/ artemin through Ret can each lead to changes in excitability and to spontaneous electrical activity in populations of primary afferent neurons and thereby drive neuropathic pain. Excessive NGF signaling can develop in uninjured C-fiber nociceptors that innervate targets with increased NGF content, such as keratinocytes in the partially denervated skin, or in nociceptors that are ensheathed by "reactive" Remak Schwann cells that make excessive NGF.

Growth factors and primary afferents. Several growth factors are relevant to primary afferent neurons. The large myelinated $A\beta$ afferents include neurons responsive to neurotrophin-3 (NT-3), brain-derived neurotrophic factor (BDNF), and GDNF. C-fiber nociceptors can largely be divided into NGF-responsive neurons, GDNF-responsive nociceptors (Molliver et al. 1997), and a small proportion that are responsive to artemin (Orozco et al. 2001; Gardell et al. 2003).

The NGF-responsive population expresses TrkA, p75, and the peptides calcitonin gene-related peptide (CGRP) and substance P (Molliver et al. 1997). These neurons project to dorsal horn laminae I and II_o. The small sensory neurons responsive to GDNF, a member of the transforming growth factor (TGF)-β family, in general express Ret, GFR-α_1, the $P2X_3$ purinergic receptor, thiamine monophosphatase, and specific Mas-related gene (*Mrg*) products (Dong et al. 2001) and bind the *Griffonia simplicifolia* lectin, isolectin B4 (IB4) (Silverman and Kruger 1988; Molliver et al. 1997). These GDNF-responsive neurons project to lamina II_i. The GDNF-family receptor GFR-α_1 is a coreceptor for the primary signaling receptor, Ret. Artemin,

another TGF-β family member, also uses Ret, but its coreceptor is GFR-α₃
(Orozco et al. 2001; Gardell et al. 2003). Unlike other Ret-positive neurons,
the GFR-α₃-positive neurons may contain CGRP (Gardell et al. 2003). Some
neurons in all of these groups express TRPV1, the capsaicin receptor (Caterina
et al. 1999, 2000). Finally, a population of neurons has mixed phenotypes
(Orozco et al. 2001; Gardell et al. 2003; Kashiba et al. 2003), overlapping the
prototypic NGF-responsive and GDNF-responsive phenotypes outlined above.

Trophic factors are typically taken up at the axon terminal and are
conveyed back to the cell body via retrograde axonal transport. They can be
made by the ensheathing Schwann cells, but in lesser abundance than in the
target. Thus axotomy, by separating the nerve cell body from the axon
terminal, or by impairing retrograde transport, would be expected to reduce
delivery of the appropriate trophic substances to the nerve cell body. Conversely, denervated targets in many systems contain excessive growth factor
protein, which may trigger collateral sprouting from intact axons, so that
they increase their target size and receive greater supplies of growth factors
than normal. Collateral reinnervation is well studied in the neuromuscular
junction (Son and Thompson 1995); it also occurs in the autonomic nervous
system (Voyvodic 1989) and in sensory afferents from the skin (Diamond et
al. 1992a,b; Rajan et al. 2003).

Voyvodic (1989) found that when a portion of the salivary gland was
excised, the sympathetic nerves that innervated it had smaller targets and
underwent atrophy of the axons and cell bodies. Conversely, when the number of innervating axons was reduced surgically, each axon had a larger
target and presumably had access to more NGF; the consequence was that
the axons hypertrophied (increased their diameter). Some segregated into
1:1 relationships with Remak Schwann cells and subsequently myelinated
(Voyvodic 1989). This process was considered to be triggered by excessive
growth factor by Hoke et al. (2003), who found similar changes in the rat
sciatic nerve after administration of high doses of GDNF.

Growth factors and neuropathic pain. It is widely accepted that neuropathic pain can be initiated by sensitization, hyperexcitability, and spontaneous discharge in primary afferent neurons, leading to "central sensitization"
or facilitation. When neuropathic pain of peripheral origin occurs in neuropathies characterized by DAD, are the nerve fibers responsible those that are
dying back (the injured fibers), their intact neighbors, or both? And are large
fibers, small fibers, or both the primary drivers? And where in the afferent
neuron does the spontaneous discharge arise—in the perikaryon, in the degenerating terminal, or in intact terminals? Finally, are the neurons responsible those that are deficient in growth factors or those receiving excessive
growth factors from the periphery?

The following sections review evidence that injured (axotomized) Aβ and Aδ afferents can develop spontaneous activity, arising at least in part in the neuronal perikarya. This last issue can be reformulated to ask whether signaling through the cognate growth factors receptors is normal, increased, or decreased. As a somewhat flippant shorthand, we have come to ask whether the responsible neurons are "undertrophed" or "overtrophed." The discussion below will present evidence that neuropathic pain might be driven by both "undertrophed" afferents (Pattern 1) and "overtrophed" afferents (Pattern 2) (see Table I).

PATTERN 1: THE UNDERTROPHED AFFERENT

A great deal of attention has focused on the role of the injured neuron in hyperalgesia and neuropathic pain. This interest undoubtedly reflects the fact that research on neuropathic pain has been driven in the last 10 years by experimental models of cutaneous hyperalgesia that involve some type of

Table I
Proposed mechanisms of neuropathic pain

	Pattern 1	Pattern 2
Growth factor alteration	*Decreased* signaling of GDNF and/or artemin through Ret	*Increased* signaling of NGF through TrkA
Injured vs. spared neurons	Predominantly injured (axotomized)	Uninjured C-fiber nociceptors in settings of partial nerve injury or inflammation; C-fiber nociceptors with axoterminal degeneration
Proposed ion channel alterations	Increased expression of $Na_v 1.3$	Redistribution into the axon of $Na_v 1.8$
Type of primary afferent neuron affected	Some Aβ and Aδ neurons, C-fiber nociceptors	Some C-fiber nociceptors, some Aδ neurons
Site of origin of spontaneous activity	Cell body of the primary sensory neuron	Peripheral axon terminals
Associated neuronal changes	Decreased neurofilament, with perikaryal/axonal atrophy and reduced TRPV1, IB4, $P2X_3$, SP, and CGRP	Perikaryal/axonal hypertrophy; increased CGRP, SP, TRPV1, ASIC3, bradykinin B2, BDNF
Proposed correction	Increased GDNF or artemin, signaling through Ret	Reduced or blocked NGF signaling through TrkA

Abbreviations: ASIC3 = acid-sensing ion channel 3; BDNF = brain-derived neurotrophic factor; CGRP = calcitonin gene-related peptide; GDNF = glial-cell-line-derived neurotrophic factor; IB4 = isolectin B4; NGF = nerve growth factor; SP = substance P; TrkA = tyrosine kinase A; TRPV1 = transient receptor potential vanilloid 1.

partial nerve injury (Sheen and Chung 1993; Devor and Seltzer 1999; Waxman 1999; Boucher et al. 2000). Most produce a mixture of degenerating and intact fibers in the affected nerves. Especially instructive has been the L5–L6 mixed spinal nerve ligation (SNL) model (Kim and Chung 1992; Liu et al. 2000; Shim et al. 2005). The axotomized primary sensory neurons are in the L5 and L6 DRG, whereas the L4 ganglion contains uninjured intact neurons (Yoon et al. 1996; Fukuoka et al. 2000, 2001; Tsuzuki et al. 2001). In this model the L5 neurons develop oscillating membrane potentials, resulting in spontaneous activity occurring predominantly in the perikarya of the axotomized neurons and at the axotomy site (Liu et al. 2000). Many of these neurons are afferents from muscle; interestingly, cutaneous afferents generally do not become spontaneously active in rodent models (Liu et al. 2000; Michaelis et al. 2000). The axotomized $A\beta$ and $A\delta$ primary afferents implicated in hyperalgesia have increased expression of the tetrodotoxin (TTX)-sensitive sodium channels $Na_V1.3$ (Black et al. 1997; Cummins and Waxman 1997) and $Na_V1.7$. Large afferents that are not normally peptidergic may express substance P (Fukuoka et al. 1998). In contrast to these larger afferents, many of the changes in NGF-responsive C-fiber nociceptors might be regarded as antinociceptive (McMahon et al. 1995; Bennett et al. 1998). The peptides substance P and CGRP are downregulated, as are the receptors TRPV1 (Fukuoka et al. 1999), acid-sensing ion channel 3 (ASIC3) (Mamet et al. 2003), and bradykinin receptor 1 (BR1). These axotomized C-fiber nociceptors develop little spontaneous activity (Liu et al. 2000).

Deficient delivery of GDNF and artemin, both of which signal through Ret, appear to be of special importance in "undertrophing" a population of injured L5–L6 neurons in the SNL model, because both the hyperalgesia and the increased expression of $Na_V1.3$ are reversed by intrathecal administration of GDNF (Boucher et al. 2000; Wang et al. 2003) or by systemic administration of artemin, a related $TGF-\beta$ family growth factor with receptors largely restricted to small sensory neurons (Gardell et al. 2003).

Axotomy or an "undertrophed" state can trigger a number of other changes in the afferent neurons. Various gene products that favor longitudinal growth and regeneration are upregulated, including the growth-associated protein GAP-43 (Jacobson et al. 1986; Skene et al. 1986) and tubulins (Hoffman and Cleveland 1988). These changes may have morphological correlates in abundant collateral sprouting in C fibers (B. Murinson, unpublished data). In contrast, genes associated with radial growth and maintenance of the mature axonal diameter are downregulated, including the neurofilament triplet proteins (Hoffman et al. 1985, 1987). Neurofilaments are important intrinsic regulators of axonal caliber (Hoffman et al. 1985, 1987). Because neurofilament content normally correlates with axonal caliber, after axotomy the axon atrophies, beginning near the cell body and progressing centrifugally (down the peripheral process and up the dorsal root) (Hoffman et al. 1985, 1987).

Pattern I, with "undertrophed" afferents, is an attractive basis for the pain associated with amputation neuromas, in which numerous axons are interrupted and are able to regenerate successfully. Pattern I is also likely to contribute to the neuropathic pain associated with mastectomy and thoracotomy scars. Finally, it may contribute to pain in neuropathies associated with defective retrograde transport.

PATTERN 2: "OVERTROPHED" C-FIBER NOCICEPTORS

C-fiber pathology is prominent in painful human neuropathies. Many painful polyneuropathies prominently or predominantly affect small sensory afferents, including C-fiber nociceptors (Kennedy et al. 1996; Holland et al. 1998). Peripheral neurologists have long recognized a group of patients with "small-fiber" neuropathies, characterized by normal strength, normal tendon reflexes, and normal electrophysiology, but spontaneous pain with or without hyperalgesia, often with autonomic insufficiency and a predilection for painless injuries (Holland et al. 1998; Periquet et al. 1999). In contrast, predominantly large-fiber sensory neuropathies rarely have prominent neuropathic pain. The "small-fiber neuropathies" are now known to include early diabetic neuropathy, often with onset at the stage of impaired glucose tolerance (Low et al. 1975; Singleton et al. 2001a,b; Smith et al. 2001; Sumner et al. 2003). The prominence of pathology of small sensory fibers in painful neuropathies was revealed by the advent of skin biopsies immunostained for dermal and epidermal nerve fibers. This approach (Kennedy and Wendelschafer-Crabb 1993; McArthur et al. 1994; Hsieh et al. 1996) demonstrated that patients with the severe spontaneous burning in the feet characteristic of these neuropathies usually exhibit loss of C-fiber nociceptors from the epidermis of the foot and distal leg (Kennedy et al. 1996; Holland et al. 1998; Periquet et al. 1999).

C-fiber physiology is altered in human and experimental painful neuropathies. In addition to the clinical evidence cited above, some experimental studies in humans have shown that stimulation at C-fiber intensities can produce hyperalgesia (Koppert et al. 2001). Recent microneurographic data suggest increased excitability of C fibers in the painful neuropathic disorder erythromelalgia (Orstavik et al. 2003). Several studies indicate that increased C-fiber excitability can occur in models of hyperalgesia. Koltzenburg et al. (1994) showed increased excitability in C-fiber nociceptors in skin-nerve preparations from animals with the chronic constriction injury (CCI) model.

Sato and Perl (1991) found sensitization of cutaneous afferents after nerve injury and identified adrenergic sensitivity of these afferents. Ali and colleagues (1999) identified spontaneous activity in C-fiber nociceptors in skin-nerve preparations from monkeys with L6 SNL, and again documented adrenergic sensitivity of these nociceptors. Wu and colleagues detected spontaneous activity in cutaneous C fiber nociceptors in rats with L5 SNL (Wu et al. 2001) and L5 ventral rhizotomy (Wu et al. 2002).

Administration of artemin, a growth factor with receptors largely restricted to small sensory neurons, prevents and relieves hyperalgesia in several models of neuropathic pain (Gardell et al. 2003). Ringkamp and others in our group have recently demonstrated that lumbar dorsal root application of resiniferatoxin, a potent analogue of capsaicin that can activate TRPV1 channels and deplete susceptible axons and neurons, prevented hyperalgesia in the L5 SNL model (M. Ringkamp et al., unpublished data). These data provide direct evidence for a role of C-fiber nociceptors in neuropathic pain.

UNINJURED C-FIBER NOCICEPTORS CAN PLAY A ROLE IN THE DEVELOPMENT OF NEUROPATHIC PAIN

A role for uninjured neurons is suggested by work from several laboratories. Li and colleagues (2000) reported that L4, but not L5, dorsal rhizotomy could eliminate hyperalgesia, although this point remains controversial; others have found that L5 dorsal rhizotomy is effective in eliminating hyperalgesia (Yoon et al. 1996; Sukhotinsky et al. 2004). Studies by Koltzenburg (Koltzenburg et al. 1994; Ali et al. 1999) and Wu et al. (2001, 2002) showed increased excitability in C-fiber nociceptors, in which the receptive fields of the neurons could be identified by skin stimulation, indicating that in these models at least some of the excitable nociceptors reached their targets in the skin.

GROWTH FACTORS AND C-FIBER NOCICEPTORS

As noted above, C-fiber nociceptors can largely be divided into NGF-responsive neurons and GDNF-responsive nociceptors. Several lines of evidence suggest that Pattern 2 is based on excessive NGF signaling in TrkA-expressing nociceptors. Access to larger than normal amounts of NGF produces "pronociceptive" biochemical changes, such as an increase in the peptides CGRP and substance P, an increase in the abundance and phosphorylation of the capsaicin receptor TRPV1, and an increased expression of the acid-sensing channel ASIC3 (Mamet et al. 2002, 2003) and the bradykinin B_2 receptor (Lee et al. 2002), all of which may amplify noxious stimuli.

Within the TrkA-positive C-fiber nociceptors, NGF also produces an increase in BDNF synthesis and release at the central synaptic terminals, thereby affecting second-order pain neurons (Thompson et al. 1999; Fukuoka et al. 2001). It is likely that excess NGF can also lead to altered physiology and spontaneous activity in C-fiber nociceptors. These changes may be due to redistribution of the TTX-resistant sodium channel $Na_V1.8$ (Lai et al. 2002; Gardell et al. 2003; Gold et al. 2003), and the spontaneous activity can arise in the peripheral axonal terminals (Wu et al. 2001, 2002).

Strong evidence implicates NGF in pain pathways. NGF injection in humans produces acute local burning pain (Svensson et al. 2003), and in animals it produces hyperalgesia (Lewin and Mendell 1993; Lewin et al. 1993; Kerr et al. 2001). Inflammatory pain due to complete Freund's adjuvant (CFA) injection produces release of NGF from mast cells, and the NGF signals in part through phosphorylation of p38 (Ji et al. 2002) and extracellular signal-regulated kinase (Fukuoka et al. 2000), which can be prevented by administration of anti-NGF. In the L5 SNL model and the CCI models, the Noguchi laboratory in particular has documented prominent changes in the protein expression profiles of the intact, uninjured DRG neurons (Fukuoka et al. 1999, 2001). These changes in the cell bodies of uninjured, non-axotomized neurons (Dai et al. 2002; Obata and Noguchi 2004) include the redistribution of the TTX-resistant sodium channel, $Na_V1.8$, into the axon (Gold et al. 2003).

"Overtrophing" of a population of TrkA-expressing peptidergic C-fiber nociceptors appears to occur after a variety of partial nerve lesions, including the L5 SNL, CCI, and spared nerve models. Fig. 1 speculates on these mechanisms. For C-fiber nociceptors innervating the epidermis, there is solid evidence that NGF is available from basal keratinocytes (Kurihara and Tsukada 1968; Yiangou et al. 2002a; Taherzadeh et al. 2003). Several studies have demonstrated increased NGF protein by immunocytochemistry in basal keratinocytes after denervation (Yiangou et al. 2002b; Li et al. 2003; Taherzadeh et al. 2003). In the center of completely denervated regions, this NGF is not available to any intact axons, but on the margins the epidermal axons respond by a combination of ultraterminal and collateral sprouting (Rajan et al. 2003), so that fibers grow along the basal epidermis. This process has been well documented in humans (Rajan et al. 2003). The implications of alterations in the basal keratinocytes produced by denervation were demonstrated by Taherzadeh and colleagues (2003), who placed dissociated rat DRG neurons on cryostat sections of normal and denervated epidermis. As axons grew toward the epidermis they extended much farther along the dermal-epidermal junction on the denervated skin sections as compared to normal skin. Whether these changes represent alterations in the

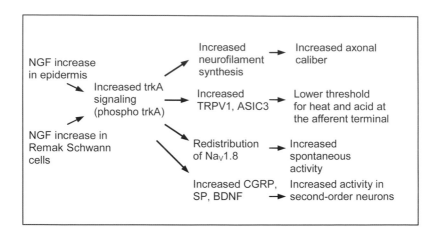

Fig. 1. Overtrophing of a population of TrkA-expressing peptidergic C-fiber nociceptors.

extracellular matrix, increases in growth factor content in the basal keratinocytes, or both, is unresolved.

Remak Schwann cells could also represent a potential source of excessive NGF. Sciatic Remak bundles are innervated by axons from different neurons of different growth factor dependencies and usually from more than one spinal root. In L5 SNL lesions many Remak bundles are partially denervated, and they undergo dramatic reorganization and Schwann cell proliferation (Murinson et al. 2005a,b). These changes can also be stimulated by Wallerian degeneration of neighboring nerve fibers (Murinson et al. 2005a,b). Such "reactive" Remak Schwann cells might produce increased amounts of NGF and GDNF (and other growth factors). Finally, nonneural sources can be important. In CFA-induced inflammation, mast cells and other inflammatory cells release NGF, and anti-NGF strategies ameliorate the inflammatory pain (Woolf et al. 1994; Ji et al. 2002).

Whatever the source of excessive NGF, selective blockers of signaling through TrkA will help place the role of NGF in context. A TrkA-IgG fusion molecule has been used to demonstrate multiple antinociceptive effects (McMahon et al. 1995; Bennett et al. 1998) and to inhibit carrageenan-induced inflammatory pain (McMahon et al. 1995). There is an obvious tension in this approach: if deficient growth factor delivery due to retrograde transport defects is driving the "overtrophing" of as-yet unaffected neighboring axons that are successfully sprouting, an anti-NGF strategy could potentially increase the severity of the neuropathy. More extensive experience in animal models of painful DAD is awaited.

REFERENCES

Alexander C, Votruba M, Pesch UE, et al. OPA1, encoding a dynamin-related GTPase, is mutated in autosomal dominant optic atrophy linked to chromosome 3q28. *Nat Genet* 2000; 26:211–215.

Ali Z, Ringkamp M, Hartke TV, et al. Uninjured C-fiber nociceptors develop spontaneous activity and alpha-adrenergic sensitivity following L6 spinal nerve ligation in monkey. *J Neurophysiol* 1999; 81:455–466.

Araki T, Sasaki Y, Milbrandt J. Increased nuclear NAD biosynthesis and SIRT1 activation prevent axonal degeneration. *Science* 2004; 305:1010–1013.

Bennett DL, Koltzenburg M, Priestley JV, Shelton DL, McMahon SB. Endogenous nerve growth factor regulates the sensitivity of nociceptors in the adult rat. *Eur J Neurosci* 1998; 10:1282–1291.

Black JA, Langworthy K, Hinson AW, Dib-Hajj SD, Waxman SG. NGF has opposing effects on Na+ channel III and SNS gene expression in spinal sensory neurons. *Neuroreport* 1997; 8:2331–2335.

Blum AS, Dal Pan GJ, Feinberg J, et al. Low-dose zalcitabine (ddC)-related toxic neuropathy: frequency, natural history, and risk factors. *Neurology* 1996; 46:999–1003.

Boucher TJ, Okuse K, Bennett DL, et al. Potent analgesic effects of GDNF in neuropathic pain states. *Science* 2000; 290:124–127.

Caterina MJ, Rosen TA, Tominaga M, Brake AJ, Julius D. A capsaicin-receptor homologue with a high threshold for noxious heat. *Nature* 1999; 398:436–441.

Caterina MJ, Leffler A, Malmberg AB, et al. Impaired nociception and pain sensation in mice lacking the capsaicin receptor. *Science* 2000; 288:306–313.

ChaudhryV, Rowinsky EK, Sartorius SE, Donehower RC, Cornblath DR. Peripheral neuropathy from taxol and cisplatin combination chemotherapy: clinical and electrophysiological studies. *Ann Neurol* 1994; 35:304–311.

Cornblath DR, McArthur JC. Peripheral neuropathies in human immunodeficiency virus type 1 infection. In: Asbury AK, Thomas PK (Eds). *Peripheral Nerve Disorders*. Oxford: Butterworth Heinemann, 1995, pp 223–237.

Cummins TR, Waxman SG. Downregulation of tetrodotoxin-resistant sodium currents and upregulation of a rapidly repriming tetrodotoxin-sensitive sodium current in small spinal sensory neurons after nerve injury. *J Neurosci* 1997; 17:3503–3514.

Dai Y, Iwata K, Fukuoka T, et al. Phosphorylation of extracellular signal-regulated kinase in primary afferent neurons by noxious stimuli and its involvement in peripheral sensitization. *J Neurosci* 2002; 22:7737–7745.

Deckwerth TL, Johnson EM Jr. The role of neurite disintegration in trophic factor deprivation-induced programmed neuronal death. *Soc Neurosci Abstracts* 1993; 19:(Pt 1)442.

Delettre C, Lenaers G, Griffoin JM, et al. Nuclear gene OPA1, encoding a mitochondrial dynamin-related protein, is mutated in dominant optic atrophy. *Nat Genet* 2000; 26:207–210.

Devor M, Seltzer Z. Pathophysiology of damaged nerves in relation to chronic pain. In: Wall PD, Melzack R (Eds). *Textbook of Pain*. New York: Churchill Livingstone, 1999, pp 129–164.

Diamond J, Foerester A, Holmes M, Coughlin M. Sensory nerves in adult rats regenerate and restore sensory function to the skin independently of endogenous NGF. *J Neurosci* 1992a; 12:1467–1476.

Diamond J, Holmes M, Coughlin M. Endogenous NGF and nerve impulses regulate the collateral sprouting of sensory axons in the skin of the adult rat. *J Neurosci* 1992b; 12:1454–1466.

Dong X, Han S, Zylka MJ, Simon MI, Anderson DJ. A diverse family of GPCRs expressed in specific subsets of nociceptive sensory neurons. *Cell* 2001; 106:619–632.

Dyck PJ, Thomas PK, Asbury AK, Winegrad AJ, Porte D. *Diabetic Neuropathy*. Philadelphia: WB Saunders, 1987.

Fukuoka T, Tokunaga A, Kondo E, et al. Change in mRNAs for neuropeptides and the GABA (A) receptor in dorsal root ganglion neurons in a rat experimental neuropathic pain model. *Pain* 1998; 78:13–26.

Fukuoka T, Kondo E, Noguchi K. Vanilloid receptor subtype 1 (VR1) messenger RNA expression increases in a subpopulation of L4 dorsal root ganglion (DRG) neurons following L5 spinal nerve ligation; a rat neuropathic pain model. *Abstr Soc Neurosci* 1999; 25:1679.

Fukuoka T, Tokunaga A, Kondo E, Noguchi K. The role of neighboring intact dorsal root ganglion neurons in a rat neuropathic pain model. In: Devor M, Rowbotham R, Wiesenfeld-Hallin Z (Eds). *Proceedings of the 9th World Congress on Pain*, Progress in Pain Research and Management, Vol. 16. Seattle: IASP Press, 2000, pp 137–146.

Fukuoka T, Kondo E, Dai Y, Hashimoto N, Noguchi K. Brain-derived neurotrophic factor increases in the uninjured dorsal root ganglion neurons in selective spinal nerve ligation model. *J Neurosci* 2001; 21:4891–4900.

Gardell LR, Wang R, Ehrenfels C, et al. Multiple actions of systemic artemin in experimental neuropathy. *Nat Med* 2003; 9:1383–1389.

George EB, Glass J, Griffin JW. Axotomy-induced axonal degeneration is mediated by calcium influx through ion-specific channels. *J Neurosci* 1995; 15:6445–6452.

Glass JD, Brushart TM, George EB, Griffin JW. Prolonged survival of transected nerve fibres in C57BL/Ola mice is an intrinsic characteristic of the axon. *J Neurocytol* 1993; 22:311–321.

Glass JD, Schryer BL, Griffin JW. Calcium-mediated degeneration of the axonal cytoskeleton in the Ola mouse. *J Neurochem* 1994; 62:2472–2475.

Gold MS, Weinreich D, Kim CS, et al. Redistribution of Na (V)1.8 in uninjured axons enables neuropathic pain. *J Neurosci* 2003; 23:158–166.

Greenberg SG, Lasek RJ. Neurofilament protein synthesis in DRG neurons decreases more after peripheral axotomy than after central axotomy. *J Neurosci* 1988; 8:1739–1746.

Hoffman PN, Cleveland DW. Neurofilament and tubulin expression recapitulates the developmental program during axonal regeneration: induction of a specific beta tubulin isotype. *Proc Natl Acad Sci USA* 1988; 85:4530–4533.

Hoffman PN, Griffin JW, Price DL. Control of axonal caliber by neurofilament transport. *J Cell Biol* 1984; 99:705–714.

Hoffman PN, Thompson GW, Griffin JW, Price DL. Changes in neurofilament transport coincide temporally with alterations in the caliber of axons in regenerating motor fibers. *J Cell Biol* 1985; 101:1332–1340.

Hoffman PN, Cleveland DW, Griffin JW, et al. Neurofilament gene expression: a major determinant of axonal caliber. *Proc Natl Acad Sci USA* 1987; 84:3472–3476.

Hoffman PN, Koo EH, Muma NA, Griffin JW, Price DL. Role of neurofilaments in the control of axonal caliber in myelinated nerve fibers. In: Lasek RJ, Black MM (Eds). *Intrinsic Determinants of Neuronal Form and Function*. New York: Alan R. Liss, 1988, pp 389–402.

Hoke A, Ho T, Crawford TO, et al. Glial cell line-derived neurotrophic factor alters axon Schwann cell units and promotes myelination in unmyelinated nerve fibers. *J Neurosci* 2003; 23:561–567.

Holland NR, Crawford TO, Hauer P, et al. Small-fiber sensory neuropathies: clinical course and neuropathology of idiopathic cases. *Ann Neurol* 1998; 44:47.

Hsieh S-T, Choi S, Lin W-M, McArthur JC, Griffin JW. Epidermal denervation and its effects on keratinocytes and Langerhans cells. *J Neurocytol* 1996; 25:513–524.

Jacobson RD, Virag I, Skene JHP. A protein associated with axon growth, GAP-43, is widely distributed and developmentally regulated in rat CNS. *J Neurosci* 1986; 6:1843–1855.

Ji RR, Samad TA, Jin SX, Schmoll R, Woolf CJ. p38 MAPK activation by NGF in primary sensory neurons after inflammation increases TRPV1 levels and maintains heat hyperalgesia. *Neuron* 2002; 36:57–68.

Kashiba H, Uchida Y, Senba E. Distribution and colocalization of NGF and GDNF family ligand receptor mRNAs in dorsal root and nodose ganglion neurons of adult rats. *Brain Res Mol Brain Res* 2003; 110:52–62.

Kennedy WR, Wendelschafer-Crabb G. The innervation of human epidermis. *J Neurol Sci* 1993; 115:184–190.

Kennedy WR, Wendelschafer-Crabb G, Johnson T. Quantitation of epidermal nerves in diabetic neuropathy. *Neurology* 1996; 47:1042–1048.

Kerr BJ, Souslova V, McMahon SB, Wood JN. A role for the TTX-resistant sodium channel Na_V 1.8 in NGF-induced hyperalgesia, but not neuropathic pain. *Neuroreport* 2001; 12:3077–3080.

Kim S-H, Chung JM. An experimental model for peripheral neuropathy produced by segmental spinal nerve ligation in the rat. *Pain* 1992; 50:355–363.

Koltzenburg M, Kees S, Budweiser S, Ochs G, Toyka KV. The properties of unmyelinated nociceptive afferents change in a painful chronic constriction neuropathy. In: Gebhart GF, Hammond DL, Jensen TS (Eds). *Proceedings of the 7th World Congress on Pain,* Progress in Pain Research and Management, Vol. 2. Seattle: IASP Press, 1994, pp 511–522.

Koppert W, Dern SK, Sittl R, et al. A new model of electrically evoked pain and hyperalgesia in human skin: the effects of intravenous alfentanil, S+)-ketamine, and lidocaine. *Anesthesiology* 2001; 95:395–402.

Kurihara T, Tsukada Y. 2',3'-cyclic nucleotide 3'-phosphohydrolase in developing chick brain and spinal cord. *J Neurochem* 1968; 15:827–832.

Lai J, Gold MS, Kim CS, et al. Inhibition of neuropathic pain by decreased expression of the tetrodotoxin-resistant sodium channel, $Na_V1.8$. *Pain* 2002; 95:143–152.

Lee YJ, Zachrisson O, Tonge DA, McNaughton PA. Upregulation of bradykinin B2 receptor expression by neurotrophic factors and nerve injury in mouse sensory neurons. *Mol Cell Neurosci* 2002; 19:186–200.

Lewin GR, Mendell LM. Nerve growth factor and nociception. *Trends Neurosci* 1993; 16:353–359.

Lewin GR, Ritter AM, Mendell LM. Nerve growth factor-induced hyperalgesia in the neonatal and adult rat. *J Neurosci* 1993; 13:2136–2148.

Li L, Xian CJ, Zhong JH, Zhou XF. Lumbar 5 ventral root transection-induced upregulation of nerve growth factor in sensory neurons and their target tissues: a mechanism in neuropathic pain. *Mol Cell Neurosci* 2003; 23:232–250.

Li Y, Dorsi MJ, Meyer RA, Belzberg AJ. Mechanical hyperalgesia after an L5 spinal nerve lesion in the rat is not dependent on input from injured nerve fibers. *Pain* 2000; 85:493–502.

Liu CN, Wall PD, Ben Dor E, et al. Tactile allodynia in the absence of C-fiber activation: altered firing properties of DRG neurons following spinal nerve injury. *Pain* 2000; 85:503–521.

Low PA, Walsh JC, Huang CY, et al. The sympathetic nervous system in diabetic neuropathy: a clinical and pathological study. *Brain* 1975; 98:341–356.

Lu P, Yang H, Jones LL, Filbin MT, Tuszynski MH. Combinatorial therapy with neurotrophins and cAMP promotes axonal regeneration beyond sites of spinal cord injury. *J Neurosci* 2004; 24:6402–6409.

Lubinska L. Early course of Wallerian degeneration in myelinated fibers of the rat phrenic nerve. *Brain Res* 1977; 130:47–63.

Lubinska L. Patterns of Wallerian degeneration of myelinated fibres in short and long peripheral stumps and in isolated segments of rat phrenic nerve. Interpretation of the role of axoplasmic flow of the trophic factor. *Brain Res* 1982; 233:227–240.

Lunn ER, Perry VH, Brown MC, Rosen H, Gordon S. Absence of Wallerian degeneration does not hinder regeneration in peripheral nerve. *Eur J Neurosci* 1989; 1:27–33.

Lunn MP, Johnson LA, Fromholt SE, et al. High-affinity anti-ganglioside IgG antibodies raised in complex ganglioside knockout mice: reexamination of GD1a immunolocalization. *J Neurochem* 2000; 75:404–412.

Mamet J, Baron A, Lazdunski M, Voilley N. Proinflammatory mediators, stimulators of sensory neuron excitability via the expression of acid-sensing ion channels. *J Neurosci* 2002; 22:10662–10670.

Mamet J, Lazdunski M, Voilley N. How nerve growth factor drives physiological and inflammatory expressions of acid-sensing ion channel 3 in sensory neurons. *J Biol Chem* 2003; 278:48907–48913.

Mata M, Kupina N, Fink DJ. Calpain II in rat peripheral nerve. *Brain Res* 1991; 564:328–331.

McArthur JC, Hsieh S-T, McCarthy B, et al. Quantitation of intra-epidermal nerves in sensory neuropathies and after nerve transection using punch skin biopsy. *Neurology* 1994; 44(Suppl 2):A275.

McMahon SB, Bennett DL, Priestley JV, Shelton DL. The biological effects of endogenous nerve growth factor on adult sensory neurons revealed by a trkA-IgG fusion molecule. *Nat Med* 1995; 1:774–780.

Michaelis M, Liu X, Janig W. Axotomized and intact muscle afferents but no skin afferents develop ongoing discharges of dorsal root ganglion origin after peripheral nerve lesion. *J Neurosci* 2000; 20:2742–2748.

Molliver DC, Wright DE, Leitner ML, et al. IB4-binding DRG neurons switch from NGF to GDNF dependence in early postnatal life. *Neuron* 1997; 19:849–861.

Murinson BB, Archer DR, Li Y, Griffin JW. Degeneration of myelinated efferent fibers prompt mitosis in Schwann cells of uninjured C-fiber afferents. *J Neurosci* 2005a; 25:1179–1187.

Murinson BB, Hoffman PN, Banihashemi MR, Meyer RA, Griffin JW. C-fiber (Remak) bundles contain both isolectin B4-binding and calcitonin gene-related peptide-positive axons. *J Comp Neurol* 2005b; 484:392–402.

Obata K, Noguchi K. MAPK activation in nociceptive neurons and pain hypersensitivity. *Life Sci* 2004; 74:2643–2653.

Orozco OE, Walus L, Sah DW, Pepinsky RB, Sanicola M. GFRalpha3 is expressed predominantly in nociceptive sensory neurons. *Eur J Neurosci* 2001; 13:2177–2182.

Orstavik K, Weidner C, Schmidt R, et al. Pathological C-fibres in patients with a chronic painful condition. *Brain* 2003; 126:567–578.

Ouardouz M, Nikolaeva MA, Coderre E, et al. Depolarization-induced Ca2+ release in ischemic spinal cord white matter involves L-type Ca^{2+} channel activation of ryanodine receptors. *Neuron* 2003; 40:53–63.

Periquet MI, Novak V, Collins MP, et al. Painful sensory neuropathy: prospective evaluation using skin biopsy. *Neurology* 1999; 53:1641–1647.

Perry VH, Brown MC, Lunn ER, Tree P, Gordon S. Evidence that very slow Wallerian degeneration in C57BL/Ola mice is an intrinsic property of the peripheral nerve. *Eur J Neurosci* 1990a; 2:802–808.

Perry VH, Lunn ER, Brown MC, Cahusac S, Gordon S. Evidence that the rate of Wallerian degeneration is controlled by a single autosomal dominant gene. *Eur J Neurosci* 1990b; 2:408–413.

Puls I, Jonnakuty C, LaMonte BH, et al. Mutant dynactin in motor neuron disease. *Nat Genet* 2003; 33:455–456.

Qiu J, Cai D, Dai H, McAtee M, et al. Spinal axon regeneration induced by elevation of cyclic AMP. *Neuron* 2002; 34:895–903.

Rajan B, Polydefkis M, Hauer P, Griffin JW, McArthur JC. Epidermal innervation after intracutaneous axotomy in man. *J Comp Neurol* 2003; 457:24–36

Ramer MS, Priestley JV, McMahon SB. Functional regeneration of sensory axons into the adult spinal cord. *Nature* 2000; 403:312–316.

Sato J, Perl ER. Adrenergic excitation of cutaneous pain receptors induced by peripheral nerve injury. *Science* 1991; 251:1608–1610.

Schlaepfer WW. Calcium-induced degeneration of axoplasm in isolated segments of rat phrenic nerve. *Brain Res* 1974; 69:203–215.

Schlaepfer WW, Bunge RP. Effects of calcium ion concentration on the degradation of amputated axons in tissue culture. *J Cell Biol* 1973; 59:456–470.

Schlaepfer WW, Hasler MB. Characterization of the calcium-induced disruption of neurofilaments in rat peripheral nerves. *Brain Res* 1979; 168:299–309.

Schlaepfer WW, Micko S. Calcium-dependent alterations of neurofilament proteins of rat peripheral nerve. *J Neurochem* 1979; 32:211–219.

Sheen K, Chung JM. Signs of neuropathic pain depend on signals from injured nerve fibers in a rat model. *Brain Res* 1993; 610:62–68.

Shim B, Kim DW, Kim BH, et al. Mechanical and heat sensitization of cutaneous nociceptors in rats with experimental peripheral neuropathy. *Neuroscience* 2005; 132:193–201.

Silverman JD, Kruger L. Lectin and neuropeptide labeling of separate populations of dorsal root ganglion neurons and associated "nociceptor" thin axons in rat testis and cornea whole-mount preparations. *Somatosens Res* 1988; 5:259–267.

Singleton JR, Smith AG, Bromberg MB. Increased prevalence of impaired glucose tolerance in patients with painful sensory neuropathy. *Diabetes Care* 2001a; 24:1448–1453.

Singleton JR, Smith AG, Bromberg MB. Painful sensory polyneuropathy associated with impaired glucose tolerance. *Muscle Nerve* 2001b; 24:1225–1228.

Skene JHP, Jacobson RD, Snipes GJ, et al. A protein induced during nerve growth (GAP-43) is a major component of growth-cone membranes. *Science* 1986; 233:783–786.

Smith AG, Ramachandran P, Tripp S, Singleton JR. Epidermal nerve innervation in impaired glucose tolerance and diabetes- associated neuropathy. *Neurology* 2001; 57:1701–1704.

So YT, Engstrom JW, Olney RK. The spectrum of electrodiagnostic abnormalities in patients with human immunodeficiency virus infection. *Muscle Nerve* 1990; 13:855.

Son Y-J, Thompson WJ. Nerve sprouting in muscle is induced and guided by processes extended by Schwann cells. *Neuron* 1995; 14:133–141.

Spencer PS, Schaumburg HH. Central-peripheral distal axonopathy—the pathogenesis of dying-back polyneuropathies. In: Zimmerman H (Ed). *Progress in Neuropathology,* Vol. 3. New York: Grune and Stratton, 1976, pp 253–295.

Spencer PS, Schaumburg HH. Ultrastructural studies of the dying back process. III. The evolution of experimental peripheral giant axonal degeneration. *J Neuropathol Exp Neurol* 1977; 36:276–299.

Stys PK, Ransom BR, Waxman SG. Effects of polyvalent cations and dihydropyridine calcium channel blockers on recovery of CNS white matter from anoxia. *Neurosci Lett* 1990; 115:293–299.

Stys PK, Waxman SG, Ransom BR. Na^+-Ca^{2+} exchanger mediates Ca^{2+} influx during anoxia in mammalian central nervous system white matter. *Ann Neurol* 1991; 30:375–380.

Sukhotinsky I, Ben Dor E, Raber P, Devor M. Key role of the dorsal root ganglion in neuropathic tactile hypersensitivity. *Eur J Pain* 2004; 8:135–143.

Sumner CJ, Sheth S, Griffin JW, Cornblath DR, Polydefkis M. The spectrum of neuropathy in diabetes and impaired glucose tolerance. *Neurology* 2003; 60:108–111.

Svensson P, Cairns BE, Wang K, Arendt-Nielsen L. Injection of nerve growth factor into human masseter muscle evokes long-lasting mechanical allodynia and hyperalgesia. *Pain* 2003; 104:241–247.

Taherzadeh O, Otto WR, Anand U, Nanchahal J, Anand P. Influence of human skin injury on regeneration of sensory neurons. *Cell Tissue Res* 2003; 312:275–280.

Thompson SW, Bennett DL, Kerr BJ, Bradbury EJ, McMahon SB. Brain-derived neurotrophic factor is an endogenous modulator of nociceptive responses in the spinal cord. *Proc Natl Acad Sci USA* 1999; 96:7714–7718.

Travlos J, Goldberg I, Boome RS. Brachial plexus lesions associated with dislocated shoulders. *J Bone Joint Surg Br* 1990; 72B:68–71.

Tsao JW, George EB, Griffin JW. Temperature modulation reveals three distinct stages of Wallerian degeneration. *J Neurosci* 1999; 19:4718–4726.

Tsuzuki K, Kondo E, Fukuoka T, et al. Differential regulation of P2X(3) mRNA expression by peripheral nerve injury in intact and injured neurons in the rat sensory ganglia. *Pain* 2001; 91:351–360.

Voyvodic JT. Target size regulates calibre and myelination of sympathetic axons. *Nature* 1989; 342:430–433.

Wang R, Guo W, Ossipov MH, et al. Glial cell line-derived neurotrophic factor normalizes neurochemical changes in injured dorsal root ganglion neurons and prevents the expression of experimental neuropathic pain. *Neuroscience* 2003; 121:815–824.

Waxman SG. The molecular pathophysiology of pain: abnormal expression of sodium channel genes and its contributions to hyperexcitability of primary sensory neurons. *Pain* 1999; (Suppl 6):S133–S140.

Woolf CJ, Safieh-Garabedian B, Ma QP, Crilly P, Winter J. Nerve growth factor contributes to the generation of inflammatory sensory hypersensitivity. *Neuroscience* 1994; 62:327–331.

Wu G, Ringkamp M, Hartke TV, et al. Early onset of spontaneous activity in uninjured C-fiber nociceptors after injury to neighboring nerve fibers. *J Neurosci* 2001; 21:RC140.

Wu G, Ringkamp M, Murinson BB, et al. Degeneration of myelinated efferent fibers induces spontaneous activity in uninjured C-fiber afferents. *J Neurosci* 2002; 22:7746–7753.

Ye H, Kuruvilla R, Zweifel LS, Ginty DD. Evidence in support of signaling endosome-based retrograde survival of sympathetic neurons. *Neuron* 2003; 39:57–68.

Yiangou Y, Facer P, Sinicropi DV, et al. Molecular forms of NGF in human and rat neuropathic tissues: decreased NGF precursor-like immunoreactivity in human diabetic skin. *J Peripher Nerv Syst* 2002a; 7:190–197.

Yiangou Y, Facer P, Sinicropi DV, et al. Molecular forms of NGF in human and rat neuropathic tissues: decreased NGF precursor-like immunoreactivity in human diabetic skin. *J Peripher Nerv Syst* 2002b; 7:190–197.

Yoon YW, Na HS, Chung JM. Contributions of injured and intact afferents to neuropathic pain in an experimental rat model. *Pain* 1996; 64:27–36.

Zuchner S, Mersiyanova IV, Muglia M, et al. Mutations in the mitochondrial GTPase mitofusin 2 cause Charcot-Marie-Tooth neuropathy type 2A. *Nat Genet* 2004; 36:449–451.

Correspondence to: John W. Griffin, MD, Department of Neurology, Johns Hopkins University School of Medicine, 600 N. Wolfe Street, Meyer 6-113, Baltimore, MD 21287-7613, USA. Tel: 410-955-5103; Fax: 410-955-0672; email: jgriffi@jhmi.edu.

Emerging Strategies for the Treatment of Neuropathic Pain, edited by James N. Campbell, Allan I. Basbaum, André Dray, Ronald Dubner, Robert H. Dworkin, and Christine N. Sang, IASP Press, Seattle, © 2006.

13

Pain Related to Inflammatory, Infectious, and Toxic Neuropathies: Mechanisms and Perspectives on Treatment

Ahmet Höke

Departments of Neurology and Neuroscience, Johns Hopkins University, School of Medicine, Baltimore, Maryland, USA

Painful peripheral neuropathies are common complications of cancer chemotherapies and human immunodeficiency virus-1 (HIV-1) infection. They often affect the quality of life of the patients and limit their therapeutic options. The exact mechanisms of sensory neuronal and axonal damage are not fully known, but a growing body of evidence points to the role of immune mediators in the pathogenesis of neuropathic pain in these conditions. In HIV infection, there is minimal, if any, direct infection of neurons or glial cells; however, cytokines and other inflammatory mediators released by invading infected macrophages seem to play an important role in the development of neuropathic pain. The sites of action of these inflammatory mediators are unknown, but they are likely to contribute to both peripheral and central mechanisms of neuropathic pain. The mechanism of neuropathic pain in chemotherapy-induced peripheral neuropathies may differ from those seen in inflammatory diseases such as HIV-induced neuropathy. However, it may share common pathways with other metabolic or toxic neuropathies in which pain may be a prominent feature. This chapter will critically review the available literature on pathophysiological mechanisms of HIV- and chemotherapy-associated neuropathies and offer novel avenues of research.

HIV-ASSOCIATED NEUROPATHIES

Since the introduction of highly active antiretroviral therapy (HAART) in 1996 (Autran et al. 1997; Mouton et al. 1997), central nervous system

(CNS) complications of HIV-1 infection have declined dramatically. However, the incidence and prevalence of peripheral nervous system (PNS) complications of HIV infection remain high (Sacktor 2002) and, in fact, may be increasing. Many types of peripheral neuropathies are seen in HIV patients, but only a few appear to be HIV-specific, i.e., not seen in other patient populations. Starting with early observations, it appeared that there was a link between the type of neuropathy and the stage of HIV infection and that certain non-HIV-specific neuropathies may be overrepresented in HIV-infected patients. Additionally, while the first PNS complications of HIV were described in 1985 (Levy et al. 1985; Lipkin et al. 1985), the pathogenesis of most peripheral neuropathies in HIV-infected patients remains unknown.

One of the most striking features of the neuropathies that occur in the HIV-infected population is the relative specificity of the individual neuropathic syndromes for each stage of HIV infection (Cornblath et al. 1987; Cornblath and McArthur 1988; Miller et al. 1988; Leger et al. 1989). This disease-stage specificity is likely to reflect different pathogenetic mechanisms of the various syndromes. For example, the inflammatory demyelinating polyneuropathies, both acute (Guillain-Barré syndrome) and chronic (chronic inflammatory demyelinating polyneuropathy), occur mainly during the early phases of HIV-1 infection, often when individuals are otherwise asymptomatic. These disorders are likely to be immunopathogenic. During the early stages of infection, the immune system is relatively competent, but it is stimulated and has altered responsiveness. This may provide the setting for development of autoimmune disorders, including the inflammatory demyelinating polyneuropathies. A vasculitic syndrome occurs mainly during the early symptomatic phase of HIV-1 infection and has been hypothesized to be due to circulating immune complexes of HIV-1 antibody and antigen that are deposited in vessel walls (Gherardi et al. 1989; Mahadevan et al. 2001). Distal symmetric polyneuropathy (DSP) occurs mainly in the late phase of HIV-1 infection (i.e., acquired immunodeficiency syndrome, AIDS), when there is severe immunoincompetence. At this stage, the proposed mechanisms include productive infection of neural tissue with HIV-1 (Ho et al. 1985) or cytomegalovirus (CMV) (Grafe and Wiley 1989; Wiley 1989; Miller et al. 1990), but these explanations have not been supported by subsequent studies. More recently proposed explanations include indirect neurotoxicity by secreted HIV envelope proteins and inflammatory mediators released by infected macrophages infiltrating the nervous system (Tan and Guiloff 1998; Wulff et al. 2000; Pardo et al. 2001; Keswani et al. 2002, 2003b; Höke and Cornblath 2005). In addition to DSP, another painful sensory neuropathy that is commonly seen in HIV patients is caused by the neurotoxicity of a subclass of antiretroviral agents, a condition known as antiretroviral toxic neuropathy (ATN). This chapter will concentrate on the mechanisms underlying the neuropathic pain in the most common forms of HIV-associated neuropathies, namely DSP and ATN.

CLINICAL FEATURES

The clinical presentations of the predominantly sensory polyneuropathies DSP and ATN are very similar (Bailey et al. 1988; Cornblath and McArthur 1988; Lange et al. 1988; Miller et al. 1988; Parry 1988; Yarchoan et al. 1988; Leger et al. 1989; LeLacheur and Simon 1991; Berger and Levy 1993; Simpson and Tagliati 1995; Schifitto et al. 2002). In both DSP and ATN, the initial symptoms are distal dysesthesias, which start in the toes and slowly progress up the lower extremities. They often involve the ankles by the time the patients seek medical attention. These dysesthesias are often painful and have a burning quality. In a recent study, severity of pain was related to HIV viral load (Simpson et al. 2002). Patients may develop allodynia, in some cases so severe that walking or even the weight of bedsheets at night is unbearable. As the disease progresses, dysesthesias may reach up to the knees. Rarely, they may involve the hands. At later stages, patients complain of numbness. The distal loss of sensory function is corroborated on examination. Sensory thresholds are raised to all modalities, especially to those testing small-fiber functions. The ankle reflex is almost universally lost. The deep tendon reflexes at the knees are often normal but may be brisk. In such instances the diagnosis of concomitant myelopathy should be considered. Although patients may complain of weakness, weakness is rarely found on examination, and when present it is rarely due to neuropathy. The only clinical feature that may help differentiate between DSP and ATN is a recent history of using nucleoside reverse transcriptase inhibitor (NRTI). In patients without symptoms before using NRTI, ATN may start soon after beginning NRTI therapy, often within weeks, but sometimes after a delay of several months. Even if the drug is discontinued, most patients experience worsening of their symptoms for a month or two as a result of a phenomenon known as "coasting." Later, most patients will see an improvement in their symptoms, but often they never return to an asymptomatic state. This observation has raised the hypothesis that use of NRTI "unmasks" DSP in susceptible patients, although a failure to completely return to normal is a feature of many toxic axonal polyneuropathies (Schaumberg et al. 1983).

MECHANISMS OF PAIN IN DISTAL
SYMMETRIC POLYNEUROPATHY

The exact pathogenic mechanisms responsible for the development of neuropathic pains such as DSP in HIV-infected individuals are unknown. Over the years various hypotheses have been put forward, but recent data suggest that multiple mechanisms are likely to play a role in neuronal or axonal injury and for the development of neuropathic pain observed in DSP.

Prior to antiretroviral therapy, patients with HIV infection often died of AIDS with multiple opportunistic infections. It was not clear whether DSP was due to co-infection with other viruses or to the HIV itself. In fact, as a result of the high association of CMV and HIV co-infection in other organs, Fuller and coworkers (1989) postulated that CMV infection of the sensory ganglia was responsible for DSP. However, other studies did not find an increased incidence of CMV in the dorsal root ganglia (DRG) or the peripheral nerves (Grafe and Wiley 1989). Since these early clinical observations, most of the experimental studies on the neuropathogenesis of HIV have focused on the CNS complications. Very few experimental studies have looked at the role of HIV in causing degeneration of sensory neurons. Clinical observations and autopsy findings suggest a length-dependent neuropathy with "dying-back axonopathy" features (reviewed by Pardo et al. 2001).

Neuronal infection by HIV occurs rarely (Yoshioka et al. 1994), if at all. Thus, in a search for other mechanisms, attention fell on the HIV-1 envelope glycoprotein gp120. It has been hypothesized that neurotoxicity from gp120 plays a role in the pathogenesis of HIV-associated DSP via binding to chemokine receptors on glial cells and neurons. Two studies showed that recombinant gp120 could bind to DRG sensory neurons (Apostolski et al. 1993) and cause complement-mediated cytotoxicity in vitro (Apostolski et al. 1994). Although there is experimental evidence of complement activation leading to neuropathic pain behavior in rats (Twining et al. 2004), complement activation has not been seen in biopsy specimens of HIV neuropathy patients (Rizzuto et al. 1995). Therefore, it is unclear whether potential complement activation by gp120 plays any role in the development of neuropathic pain in HIV patients with neuropathy.

Furthermore, the concentration of gp120 used in these studies was higher than is likely to occur in the sensory ganglia. More recent studies have failed to show significant levels of circulating gp120 in the DRG (Smith et al. 2000). However, brief exposure to gp120 may initiate a cascade of pathological processes that might lead to neuropathic pain. In a recent study, Herzberg and Sagen (2001) applied topical gp120 to the epineuria of sciatic nerve in rats using oxidized cellulose as a delivery method. Animals that received gp120 developed tactile allodynia, mechanical hyperalgesia, cold allodynia, and thermal hyperalgesia. These behavioral changes correlated with intense astrocytic and microglial activation in the spinal cord and an increase in tumor necrosis factor alpha (TNF-α) at the site of gp120 application in the sciatic nerve.

Further insights into the role of spinal astrocytic and microglial activation in neuropathic pain were reported by Watkins and colleagues in a recent series of papers (Milligan et al. 2000, 2001a,b; Holguin et al. 2004; Spataro et al. 2004). These investigators used intrathecal administration of gp120 to induce spinal and microglial activation in rats and demonstrated the development of thermal hyperalgesia and mechanical allodynia (Milligan et al. 2000). Intrathecal gp120 caused elevated levels of TNF-α and interleukin-1 (IL-1) in the lumbar spinal cord and cerebrospinal fluid (CSF). Furthermore, antagonists of TNF-α and IL-1 as well as fluorocitrate, a glial metabolic inhibitor, blocked the gp120-induced neuropathic state (Milligan et al. 2001b). These findings suggested that activated glia in the dorsal spinal cord can create exaggerated pain states via the release of proinflammatory cytokines. In a separate set of experiments, Watkins and colleagues examined the effects of CNI-1493, a p38 mitogen-activated protein kinase (MAPK) inhibitor, on gp120-induced glial activation in the spinal cord, as well as its effects on neuropathic state. Systemic administration of CNI-1493 prevented the development of neuropathic pain behaviors in rats receiving intrathecal gp120, but it did not prevent glial activation or release of TNF-α and IL-1 (Milligan et al. 2001a). These findings strongly suggest that activation of p38 MAPK occurs downstream from glial activation and release of proinflammatory cytokines. Nevertheless, CNI-1493 or similar inhibitors of p38 MAPK may have a potential use in centrally mediated neuropathic pain.

In contrast to these central effects of gp120, we recently examined the complex interplay between the sensory neuron and the supporting glial cells within the DRG (Keswani et al. 2003b). In this in vitro study, gp120-induced neurotoxicity did not occur directly on the sensory neuron but was mediated by the chemokine receptors on the Schwann cells. Binding of the gp120 to the CXCR4 chemokine receptor on Schwann cells caused release of a CCR5 ligand, RANTES (regulated upon activation, normal T-cell expressed and secreted), which in turn bound to the CCR5 receptors on the sensory neurons and induced a TNF-α-mediated axonal degeneration and apoptotic cell death. The investigators studied the interaction between the sensory neuron and the surrounding Schwann cells, omitting the role of the infiltrating macrophages. Often there is an increase in the number of activated macrophages in the DRG of patients with HIV, and these macrophages immunostain with markers of HIV such as p24 (Pardo et al. 2001). Because there is little evidence for direct infection of the sensory neuron or the Schwann cell by HIV, the infiltrating infected macrophages may serve to create a reservoir of secreted viral proteins such as gp120.

In addition to this indirect neurotoxicity, it has been shown that gp120 can directly bind to chemokine receptors on sensory neurons and induce intracellular calcium fluxes (Oh et al. 2001). The gp120-responsive subset of neurons also expressed the capsaicin receptor, TRPV-1. When their paws were injected with gp120, rats developed neuropathic pain behavior.

At this stage, it is difficult to determine what role direct versus indirect neurotoxicity plays in HIV-associated DSP and in neuropathic pain in these patients. Further in vivo studies are needed to corroborate the in vitro studies. What is needed is a reliable animal model of HIV infection that also shows PNS neurotoxicity. In recent years, an accelerated version of simian immunodeficiency virus infection in macaques has been used successfully as a model of HIV encephalitis (Mankowski et al. 2002; Zink and Clements 2002). The pathology of the PNS in these macaques is largely unknown. However, recent unpublished studies demonstrate large numbers of infiltrating activated macrophages in the DRG (C.A. Pardo, personal communication, 2004). Skin biopsies in the footpads of these animals, however, failed to show a reduction in intraepidermal nerve fiber density (J.C. McArthur, unpublished data, 2000). Therefore, it is unclear whether these animals will serve as a good model of HIV neuropathy.

Another potentially useful animal model of HIV neuropathy is the development of neuropathy in newborn cats infected with the feline immunodeficiency virus (FIV) (Kennedy et al. 2004). FIV-infected cats developed a lower density of intraepidermal nerve fibers and had fewer myelinated fibers in their sural nerves compared to control littermates. Furthermore, there was evidence of macrophage infiltration in their peripheral nerves and DRG (Kennedy et al. 2004). It is not clear whether this animal can be a model for adult-onset DSP, because these cats were infected with the FIV at a time when they were developing. The model may be more applicable to HIV infection in children. Nevertheless, FIV may be a useful model to study DSP, but further studies are needed, especially behavioral studies to examine whether these animals develop neuropathic pain behavior.

A promising new development in the field has been the creation of a transgenic rat that expresses human CD4 and CCR5 (Keppler et al. 2002). These animals can be infected with HIV and show evidence of immune deficiency. The nervous system pathology has not been examined in detail. However, if these animals develop pathology in the PNS, they will serve as a very useful rodent model to study mechanisms of neuronal injury and neuropathic pain in HIV infection.

MECHANISMS OF PAIN IN ANTIRETROVIRAL TOXIC NEUROPATHY

The literature on the mechanisms of pain in ATN is less developed. Initial cases of ATN were reported in AIDS patients receiving ddC (dideoxycytidine, also called zalcitabine) (Dubinsky et al. 1988, 1989; Yarchoan et al. 1988; Merigan et al. 1989). As the newer NRTIs came to market, it was clear that some of them, namely ddC, ddI (dideoxyinosine, also called didanosine), and d4T (didehydrodeoxythymidine, also called stavudine) also caused a predominantly sensory painful neuropathy (Cooley et al. 1990; Lambert et al. 1990, 1993; Murray et al. 1995; Skowron 1995). Moore and coworkers (2000) found a greater incidence of neuropathy when two or more neurotoxic agents were used together or when two such agents were used with hydroxyurea. While the exact etiology of this neurotoxic neuropathy remains unclear, inhibition of mitochondrial DNA polymerase-gamma is thought to play an important role (Starnes and Cheng 1987; Chen et al. 1991; Keilbaugh et al. 1991). Theoretically, inhibition of mitochondrial DNA polymerase-gamma could result in reduced numbers of mitochondria and subsequent mitochondrial failure, causing axonal/neural degeneration. This line of argument has been promoted over the years (Carey 2000; Simpson 2002; Rossero et al. 2003), albeit with little evidence that inhibition of DNA polymerase-gamma is the cause of neurotoxicity. In fact, although the mitochondrial DNA content in the subcutaneous fat tissue correlates well with NRTI use, there is no correlation of reduced mitochondrial content with the incidence of neuropathy (Cherry et al. 2002). Furthermore, although all of the NRTIs inhibit mitochondrial DNA polymerase-gamma in vitro, only some cause neuropathy. Of the six NRTIs in clinical use, only ddC, ddI, and d4T have been associated with clinical neuropathy. There are no clinical reports of AZT (azidothymidine, also known as zidovudine), 3TC (deoxythiacytidine, also known as lamivudine), or abacavir causing neuropathy (Bozzette et al. 1991; French et al. 2002).

Recent in vitro studies also argue against the inhibition of mitochondrial DNA-polymerase-gamma as the main cause of neurotoxicity. In a study by Cui and coworkers (1997), although ddI and ddC toxicity on PC-12 rat pheochromocytoma cells correlated with inhibition of mitochondrial DNA synthesis, no change in mitochondrial DNA content was observed with d4T at doses that caused toxic effects on neurites (Cui et al. 1997). Furthermore, AZT inhibited the mitochondrial DNA polymerase-gamma and caused a reduction in DNA content in PC-12 cells but did not cause degeneration of neurites. This finding suggests that NRTI mitochondrial toxicity may be mediated by mechanisms other than mitochondrial DNA depletion.

In a recent report, investigators studied the mechanism of neurotoxicity of NRTIs using primary DRG neurons (Keswani et al. 2003a). In this study, neurotoxicity exhibited by ddC, ddI, and d4T correlated with the incidence of neuropathy in clinical experience (ddC > ddI > d4T); AZT, which does not cause neuropathy, was not toxic to DRG neurons even at very high doses. The neurotoxicity of these NRTIs was mediated by mitochondrial toxicity and by energy failure from loss of the electrical potential differential that exists across the inner mitochondrial membrane. The loss of electrical potential differential was not due to inhibition of mitochondrial DNA polymerase-gamma, given that the effect was very rapid and there was no such effect with AZT, even at very high doses.

Another study arguing against the inhibition of mitochondrial DNA polymerase-gamma hypothesis is the toxicity of ddC on cardiac myocytes. Skuta and colleagues (1999) noted that ddC induced rapid cardiotoxicity in rats, which was associated with decreased activity of respiratory complexes, but not with mitochondrial DNA depletion.

Despite the studies that argue against a pivotal role for inhibition of mitochondrial DNA polymerase-gamma in mediating the NRTI neurotoxicity, recent clinical-pathological data do suggest that abnormal mitochondria are a feature of ATN. Dalakas and coworkers (2001) demonstrated structural abnormalities in mitochondria in axons and Schwann cells in the sural nerve biopsies of HIV neuropathy patients exposed to ddC as compared to HIV neuropathy patients who were not exposed to ddC or non-HIV-infected patients with neuropathy (Dalakas et al. 2001). While a larger study would be helpful in confirming this observation, detailed mechanistic studies are also needed to assess the primary abnormality or abnormalities.

Studies on the mechanism of NRTI-induced neurotoxicity have also suffered from lack of a reliable in vivo model. In animal studies, ddC was shown to cause a neuropathy in rabbits after 16 weeks of exposure (Anderson et al. 1992; Feldman et al. 1992). However, this neuropathy was characterized by prominent changes in Schwann cells in the proximal segments of the sciatic nerves and in the ventral roots, with demyelination and remyelination (Anderson et al. 1994). Primary demyelination is not a characteristic pathological feature of NRTI-induced neuropathy in patients. Therefore, it is unclear if the ddC-induced neuropathy in rabbits is a model of human ATN.

Based on patient studies, two other hypotheses have been put forward to explain ATN. A recent prospective study compared the serum lactate levels in 20 patients with ATN due to d4T, 10 patients with DSP, 20 patients without neuropathy who were taking d4T, and 23 HIV patients who were not taking d4T and did not have neuropathy (Brew et al. 2003). Elevated serum lactate levels discriminated between d4T-induced ATN and DSP.

Before elevated serum lactate levels can be considered as a unifying pathogenic marker for all cases of ATN, this study needs confirmation by a larger study that should include patients who develop ATN due to ddC or ddI

Another study raised the possibility of low carnitine levels in ATN patients (Famularo et al. 1997). In this small study with 12 ATN patients on dideoxynucleoside analogues, serum acetyl-carnitine level was lower in comparison with HIV-infected patients on dideoxynucleosides without neuropathy. However, a subsequent study with a larger cohort failed to show any association between serum carnitine levels and incidence of neuropathy (Simpson et al. 2001).

What do all of these studies tell us about the mechanism of neuropathic pain in HIV-positive patients with ATN? Unfortunately, these studies were directed toward understanding the mechanisms and pathways underlying neuronal and/or axonal injury in ATN and not toward elucidating specific mechanisms of neuropathic pain in this condition. In a recent study, Joseph and colleagues (2004) brought some answers to this question by giving rats either daily oral doses of ddC or a single intravenous dose of ddI, ddC, or d4T. Animals in all groups exhibited neuropathic pain as evidenced by mechanical hypersensitivity and allodynia. Peripheral administration of inhibitors of protein kinase A, protein kinase C, protein kinase G, extracellular regulated kinase 1/2, or nitric oxide synthase, which had antihyperalgesic effects in other models of neuropathic pain in rats, did not reverse ddC-induced hyperalgesia, suggesting that the neuropathic pain induced by NRTIs may not involve these pathways. However, intradermal or spinal injection of intracellular calcium modulators significantly attenuated ddC-induced hyperalgesia. Furthermore, C-fiber recording in ddC-treated animals showed alterations in the pattern of firing. Taken together, these studies suggest a calcium-mediated mechanism of pain induced by the NRTIs. This calcium-mediated mechanism of neuropathic pain may be seen in other toxic neuropathies, such as suramin (Joseph et al. 2004). The authors conclude that alterations in calcium homeostasis due to mitochondrial dysfunction cause ddC to lead to abnormal activity of calcium-activated potassium channels SK-1 and IK-1, which in turn have been implicated in neuropathic pain in patients with painful neuropathies (Boettger et al. 2002).

CHEMOTHERAPY-INDUCED NEUROPATHIES AND NEUROPATHIC PAIN

Peripheral neuropathies are common complications of chemotherapies. Depending on the mechanism of action, various chemotherapeutic agents cause peripheral neuropathies that affect different populations of sensory or motor neurons (reviewed in Hilkens and ven den Bent 1997; Windebank 1999; Quasthoff and Hartung 2002; Visovsky 2003). In general, platinum compounds such as cisplatin, oxaliplatin, and carboplatin cause a sensory predominant, painful polyneuropathy, whereas taxanes (paclitaxel, docetaxel), vinca alkaloids (vincristine), and suramin cause a sensory-motor polyneuropathy with or without the involvement of the autonomic system. Peripheral neurotoxicity is often dependent on the cumulative dose, but in susceptible patients even a single dose can cause peripheral neuropathy. Pre-existing neuropathies due to diabetes, overconsumption of alcohol, or genetic factors increase the risk of developing chemotherapy-induced peripheral neuropathies. After the cessation of chemotherapy, recovery is often incomplete, and even a partial improvement takes a long time.

Several animal and in vitro models have been developed to examine the mechanisms underlying the neurotoxicity of chemotherapeutic agents and the manifestation of neuropathic pain. The best models are of the paclitaxel and cisplatin-induced neuropathies, with studies dedicated to the mechanisms of neuropathic pain.

PACLITAXEL-INDUCED NEUROPATHY AND NEUROPATHIC PAIN

Paclitaxel-induced neuropathy models in rats have been available for almost 20 years (Roytta et al. 1984; Roytta and Raine 1985, 1986). However, researchers have only recently begun to explore the potential mechanisms of neuropathic pain in paclitaxel-induced peripheral neuropathy (Dina et al. 2001; Polomano et al. 2001; Alessandri-Haber et al. 2004; Flatters and Bennett 2004; Wang et al. 2004). Similar to the role of protein kinase A (PKA) and protein kinase C (PKC) in neuropathic pain in inflammatory conditions, intradermal application of PKA and PKC antagonists abolished paclitaxel-induced hypersensitivity in rats (Dina et al. 2001). Since paclitaxel alters microtubule function, which may affect many cellular pathways, it is unclear how specific the role of PKA and PKC might be in mediating paclitaxel-induced neuropathic pain.

A more promising line of study from the same laboratory examined the role of transient receptor potential vanilloid 4 (TRPV4) in paclitaxel-induced neuropathic pain (Alessandri-Haber et al. 2004). In this study, intraspinal administration of antisense oligonucleotides to TRPV4 reduced the expression of TRPV4 in the sensory nerve and dramatically reduced mechanical hyperalgesia in paclitaxel-treated rats. In DRG sensory neurons isolated from paclitaxel-treated rats, enhanced osmotransduction was noted, which was dependent on integrin/Src tyrosine kinase signaling. Even though

these novel findings open up new avenues of research for potential therapeutic targets, further studies are needed to examine the specificity of TRPV4
and integrin/Src kinase signaling for paclitaxel-induced neuropathic pain.

In another important recent study, Wang and colleagues (2004) examined the role of calpains in paclitaxel-induced neuropathy and neuropathic
pain. Calpains are calcium-activated proteases that are important in limited
cleavage of target proteins in a variety of cellular processes including axonal
degeneration. Paclitaxel-induced axonal degeneration involves activation of
calpains, similar to that seen with Wallerian degeneration. AK295, a specific
calpain inhibitor, blocked axonal degeneration and development of neuropathic pain behavior in paclitaxel-treated animals, but did not interfere with
paclitaxel's antimitotic effects. These findings suggest that inhibition of
calpain activation may be a useful neuroprotective therapy for chemotherapy-
induced peripheral neuropathies.

VINCRISTINE-INDUCED PERIPHERAL NEUROPATHY

Neuropathy caused by vinca alkaloids has been recognized for almost
40 years (Gottschalk et al. 1968). Even though animal models were developed early on (Gottschalk et al. 1968; Sahenk et al. 1987), only recently
have researchers focused on neuropathic pain in vincristine-induced neuropathy (Aley et al. 1996; Tanner et al. 1998; Authier et al. 1999, 2003;
Nozaki-Taguchi et al. 2001; Higuera and Luo 2004). Unfortunately, most of
these recent studies have failed to shed any significant light onto the potential mechanism of neuropathic pain in vincristine-induced peripheral neuropathy. One exception is a study examining C-fiber responsiveness in vivo
(Tanner et al. 1998). In animals treated with vincristine, single-fiber recordings revealed that 41% of C fibers were hyperresponsive to suprathreshold
mechanical stimuli and that a subset of these neurons were also hyperresponsive to heat stimuli. However, there were no differences in the percentage of spontaneously active C fibers in vincristine-treated and control-
treated animals. These findings indicate a specific effect of vincristine on
suprathreshold mechanical stimuli rather than a nonspecific impairment of
C-fiber function. The effect of vincristine in sensory neurons may involve
activation of caspases (aspartate-specific cysteinyl proteases involved in mediating cell death pathways including apoptosis), because administration of
caspase inhibitors prevented neuropathic pain behavior in vincristine-treated
rats, but not in rats with diabetic neuropathy induced by streptozotocin
(Joseph and Levine 2004). Many questions remain as to how specific these
findings may be. Can caspase inhibition be developed as a therapeutic tool
for neuropathic pain?

CONCLUSION

Mechanisms of neuropathic pain in painful neuropathies may share some common pathways, but there is ample evidence to suggest that specific pathways are also activated in inflammatory and toxic neuropathies. Treatments directed at elucidating common pathways may lead to development of therapeutic targets that can be used in multiple diseases. However, as with many therapeutic interventions targeting common pathways, there is the potential of more widespread side effects. In contrast, drugs targeting specific pathways in inflammatory and toxic neuropathies may lead to more specific treatments that are likely to be better tolerated.

ACKNOWLEDGMENTS

This work is supported by NINDS (NS-43911, NS-46262) and NIMH (MH-70056).

REFERENCES

Alessandri-Haber N, Dina OA, Yeh JJ, et al. Transient receptor potential vanilloid 4 is essential in chemotherapy-induced neuropathic pain in the rat. *J Neurosci* 2004; 24:4444–4452.

Aley KO, Reichling DB, Levine JD. Vincristine hyperalgesia in the rat: a model of painful vincristine neuropathy in humans. *Neuroscience* 1996; 73:259–265.

Anderson TD, Davidovich A, Arceo R, et al. Peripheral neuropathy induced by 2',3'-dideoxycytidine. A rabbit model of 2',3'-dideoxycytidine neurotoxicity. *Lab Invest* 1992; 66:63–74.

Anderson TD, Davidovich A, Feldman DH, et al. Mitochondrial schwannopathy and peripheral myelinopathy in a rabbit model of dideoxycytidine neurotoxicity. *Lab Invest* 1994; 70:724–739.

Apostolski S, McAlarney T, Quattrini A, et al. The gp120 glycoprotein of human immunodeficiency virus type 1 binds to sensory ganglion neurons. *Ann Neurol* 1993; 34:855–863.

Apostolski S, McAlarney T, Hays AP, Latov N. Complement dependent cytotoxicity of sensory ganglion neurons mediated by the gp120 glycoprotein of HIV-1. *Immunol Invest* 1994; 23:47–52.

Authier N, Coudore F, Eschalier A, Fialip J. Pain related behaviour during vincristine-induced neuropathy in rats. *Neuroreport* 1999; 10:965–968.

Authier N, Gillet JP, Fialip J, Eschalier A, Coudore F. A new animal model of vincristine-induced nociceptive peripheral neuropathy. *Neurotoxicology* 2003; 24:797–805.

Autran B, Carcelain G, Li TS, et al. Positive effects of combined antiretroviral therapy on CD4+ T-cell homeostasis and function in advanced HIV disease. *Science* 1997; 277:112–116.

Bailey RO, Baltch AL, Venkatesh R, Singh JK, Bishop MB. Sensory motor neuropathy associated with AIDS. *Neurology* 1988; 38:886–891.

Berger JR, Levy RM. The neurologic complications of human immunodeficiency virus infection. *Med Clin North Am* 1993; 77:1–23.

Boettger MK, Till S, Chen MX, et al. Calcium-activated potassium channel SK1- and IK1-like immunoreactivity in injured human sensory neurones and its regulation by neurotrophic factors. *Brain* 2002;125:252–263.

Bozzette SA, Santangelo J, Villasana D, et al. Peripheral nerve function in persons with asymptomatic or minimally symptomatic HIV disease: absence of zidovudine neurotoxicity. *J Acquir Immune Defic Syndr* 1991; 4:851–855.

Brew BJ, Tisch S, Law M. Lactate concentrations distinguish between nucleoside neuropathy and HIV neuropathy. *AIDS* 2003; 17:1094–1096.

Carey P. Peripheral neuropathy: zalcitabine reassessed. *Int J STD AIDS* 2000; 11:417–423.

Chen CH, Vazquez-Padua M, Cheng YC. Effect of anti-human immunodeficiency virus nucleoside analogs on mitochondrial DNA and its implication for delayed toxicity. *Mol Pharmacol* 1991; 39:625–628.

Cherry CL, Gahan ME, McArthur JC, et al. Exposure to dideoxynucleosides is reflected in lowered mitochondrial DNA in subcutaneous fat. *J Acquir Immune Defic Syndr* 2002; 30:271–277.

Cooley TP, Kunches LM, Saunders CA, et al. Once-daily administration of 2',3'-dideoxyinosine (ddI) in patients with the acquired immunodeficiency syndrome or AIDS-related complex. Results of a Phase I trial. *N Engl J Med* 1990; 322:1340–1345.

Cornblath DR, McArthur JC. Predominantly sensory neuropathy in patients with AIDS and AIDS-related complex. *Neurology* 1988; 38:794–796.

Cornblath DR, McArthur JC, Kennedy PG, Witte AS, Griffin JW. Inflammatory demyelinating peripheral neuropathies associated with human T-cell lymphotropic virus type III infection. *Ann Neurol* 1987; 21:32–40.

Cui L, Locatelli L, Xie MY, Sommadossi JP. Effect of nucleoside analogs on neurite regeneration and mitochondrial DNA synthesis in PC-12 cells. *J Pharmacol Exp Ther* 1997; 280:1228–1234.

Dalakas MC, Semino-Mora C, Leon-Monzon M. Mitochondrial alterations with mitochondrial DNA depletion in the nerves of AIDS patients with peripheral neuropathy induced by 2',3'-dideoxycytidine (ddC). *Lab Invest* 2001; 81:1537–1544.

Dina OA, Chen X, Reichling D, Levine JD. Role of protein kinase C-epsilon and protein kinase A in a model of paclitaxel-induced painful peripheral neuropathy in the rat. *Neuroscience* 2001; 108:507–515.

Dubinsky RM, Dalakas M, Yarchoan R, Broder S. Follow-up of neuropathy from 2',3'-dideoxycytidine. *Lancet* 1988; 1:832.

Dubinsky RM, Yarchoan R, Dalakas M, Broder S. Reversible axonal neuropathy from the treatment of AIDS and related disorders with 2',3'-dideoxycytidine (ddC). *Muscle Nerve* 1989; 12:856–860.

Famularo G, Moretti S, Marcellini S, et al. Acetyl-carnitine deficiency in AIDS patients with neurotoxicity on treatment with antiretroviral nucleoside analogues. *AIDS* 1997; 11:185–190.

Feldman D, Brosnan C, Anderson TD. Ultrastructure of peripheral neuropathy induced in rabbits by 2',3'-dideoxycytidine. *Lab Invest* 1992; 66:75–85.

Flatters SJ, Bennett GJ. Ethosuximide reverses paclitaxel- and vincristine-induced painful peripheral neuropathy. *Pain* 2004;109:150–161.

French M, Amin J, Roth N, et al. Randomized, open-label, comparative trial to evaluate the efficacy and safety of three antiretroviral drug combinations including two nucleoside analogues and nevirapine for previously untreated HIV-1 Infection: the OzCombo 2 study. *HIV Clin Trials* 2002; 3:177–185.

Fuller GN, Jacobs JM, Guiloff RJ. Association of painful peripheral neuropathy in AIDS with cytomegalovirus infection. *Lancet* 1989; 2:937–941.

Gherardi R, Lebargy F, Gaulard P, et al. Necrotizing vasculitis and HIV replication in peripheral nerves. *N Engl J Med* 1989; 321:685–686.

Gottschalk PG, Dyck PJ, Kiely JM. Vinca alkaloid neuropathy: nerve biopsy studies in rats and in man. *Neurology* 1968; 18:875–882.

Grafe MR, Wiley CA. Spinal cord and peripheral nerve pathology in AIDS: the roles of cytomegalovirus and human immunodeficiency virus. *Ann Neurol* 1989; 25:561–566.

Herzberg U, Sagen J. Peripheral nerve exposure to HIV viral envelope protein gp120 induces neuropathic pain and spinal gliosis. *J Neuroimmunol* 2001; 116:29–39.

Higuera ES, Luo ZD. A rat pain model of vincristine-induced neuropathy. *Methods Mol Med* 2004; 99:91–98.

Hilkens PH, ven den Bent MJ. Chemotherapy-induced peripheral neuropathy. *J Peripher Nerv Syst* 1997; 2:350–361.

Ho DD, Rota TR, Schooley RT, et al. Isolation of HTLV-III from cerebrospinal fluid and neural tissues of patients with neurologic syndromes related to the acquired immunodeficiency syndrome. *N Engl J Med* 1985;313:1493–1497.

Hoke A, Cornblath DR. Peripheral neuropathies in human immunodeficiency virus infection. In: Dyck PJB, Thomas PK (Eds). *Peripheral Neuropathy*, 4th ed. Philadelphia: Saunders, 2005.

Holguin A, O'Connor KA, Biedenkapp J, et al. HIV-1 gp120 stimulates proinflammatory cytokine-mediated pain facilitation via activation of nitric oxide synthase-I (nNOS). *Pain* 2004; 110:517–530.

Joseph EK, Levine JD. Caspase signalling in neuropathic and inflammatory pain in the rat. *Eur J Neurosci* 2004; 20:2896–2902.

Joseph EK, Chen X, Khasar SG, Levine JD. Novel mechanism of enhanced nociception in a model of AIDS therapy-induced painful peripheral neuropathy in the rat. *Pain* 2004; 107:147–158.

Keilbaugh SA, Prusoff WH, Simpson MV. The PC12 cell as a model for studies of the mechanism of induction of peripheral neuropathy by anti-HIV-1 dideoxynucleoside analogs. *Biochem Pharmacol* 1991; 42:R5–8.

Kennedy JM, Hoke A, Zhu Y, et al. Peripheral neuropathy in lentivirus infection: evidence of inflammation and axonal injury. *AIDS* 2004;18:1241–1250.

Keppler OT, Welte FJ, Ngo TA, et al. Progress toward a human CD4/CCR5 transgenic rat model for de novo infection by human immunodeficiency virus type 1. *J Exp Med* 2002;195:719–736.

Keswani SC, Pardo CA, Cherry CL, Hoke A, McArthur JC. HIV-associated sensory neuropathies. *AIDS* 2002;16:2105–2117.

Keswani SC, Chander B, Hasan C, et al. AFK506 is neuroprotective in a model of antiretroviral toxic neuropathy. *Ann Neurol* 2003a; 53:57–64.

Keswani SC, Polley M, Pardo CA, et al. Schwann cell chemokine receptors mediate HIV-1 gp120 toxicity to sensory neurons. *Ann Neurol* 2003b; 54:287–296.

Lambert JS, Seidlin M, Reichman RC, et al. 2',3'-dideoxyinosine (ddI) in patients with the acquired immunodeficiency syndrome or AIDS-related complex. A phase I trial. *N Engl J Med* 1990; 322:1333–1340.

Lambert JS, Seidlin M, Valentine FT, Reichman RC, Dolin R. Didanosine: long-term follow-up of patients in a phase 1 study. *Clin Infect Dis* 1993; 16(Suppl 1):S40–45.

Lange DJ, Britton CB, Younger DS, Hays AP. The neuromuscular manifestations of human immunodeficiency virus infections. *Arch Neurol* 1988; 45:1084–1088.

Leger JM, Bouche P, Bolgert F, et al. The spectrum of polyneuropathies in patients infected with HIV. *J Neurol Neurosurg Psychiatry* 1989; 52:1369–1374.

LcLacheur SF, Simon GL. Exacerbation of dideoxycytidine-induced neuropathy with dideoxyinosine. *J Acquir Immune Defic Syndr* 1991; 4:538–539.

Levy RM, Bredesen DE, Rosenblum ML. Neurological manifestations of the acquired immunodeficiency syndrome (AIDS): experience at UCSF and review of the literature. *J Neurosurg* 1985; 62:475–495.

Lipkin WI, Parry G, Kiprov D, Abrams D. Inflammatory neuropathy in homosexual men with lymphadenopathy. *Neurology* 1985; 35:1479–1483.

Mahadevan A, Gayathri N, Taly AB, et al. Vasculitic neuropathy in HIV infection: a clinico-pathological study. *Neurol India* 2001; 49:277–283.

Mankowski JL, Clements JE, Zink MC. Searching for clues: tracking the pathogenesis of human immunodeficiency virus central nervous system disease by use of an accelerated, consistent simian immunodeficiency virus macaque model. *J Infect Dis* 2002;186(Suppl 2):S199–208.

Merigan TC, Skowron G, Bozzette SA, et al. Circulating p24 antigen levels and responses to dideoxycytidine in human immunodeficiency virus (HIV) infections. A phase I and II study. *Ann Intern Med* 1989;110:189–194.

Miller RG, Parry GJ, Pfaeffl W, et al. The spectrum of peripheral neuropathy associated with ARC and AIDS. *Muscle Nerve* 1988; 11:857–863.

Miller RG, Storey JR, Greco CM. Ganciclovir in the treatment of progressive AIDS-related polyradiculopathy. *Neurology* 1990; 40:569–574.

Milligan ED, Mehmert KK, Hinde JL, et al. Thermal hyperalgesia and mechanical allodynia produced by intrathecal administration of the human immunodeficiency virus-1 (HIV-1) envelope glycoprotein, gp120. *Brain Res* 2000; 861:105–116.

Milligan ED, O'Connor KA, Armstrong CB, et al. Systemic administration of CNI-1493, a p38 mitogen-activated protein kinase inhibitor, blocks intrathecal human immunodeficiency virus-1 gp120-induced enhanced pain states in rats. *J Pain* 2001a; 2:326–333.

Milligan ED, O'Connor KA, Nguyen KT, et al. Intrathecal HIV-1 envelope glycoprotein gp120 induces enhanced pain states mediated by spinal cord proinflammatory cytokines. *J Neurosci* 2001b; 21:2808–2819.

Moore RD, Wong WM, Keruly JC, McArthur JC. Incidence of neuropathy in HIV-infected patients on monotherapy versus those on combination therapy with didanosine, stavudine and hydroxyurea. *AIDS* 2000; 14:273–278.

Mouton Y, Alfandari S, Valette M, et al. Impact of protease inhibitors on AIDS-defining events and hospitalizations in 10 French AIDS reference centres. Federation National des Centres de Lutte contre le SIDA. *AIDS* 1997; 11:F101–105.

Murray HW, Squires KE, Weiss W, et al. Stavudine in patients with AIDS and AIDS-related complex: AIDS clinical trials group 089. *J Infect Dis* 1995; 171(Suppl 2):S123–130.

Nozaki-Taguchi N, Chaplan SR, Higuera ES, Ajakwe RC, Yaksh TL. Vincristine-induced allodynia in the rat. *Pain* 2001; 93:69–76.

Oh SB, Tran PB, Gillard SE, et al. Chemokines and glycoprotein 120 produce pain hypersensitivity by directly exciting primary nociceptive neurons. *J Neurosci* 2001; 21:5027–5035.

Pardo CA, McArthur JC, Griffin JW. HIV neuropathy: insights in the pathology of HIV peripheral nerve disease. *J Peripher Nerv Syst* 2001; 6:21–27.

Parry GJ. Peripheral neuropathies associated with human immunodeficiency virus infection. *Ann Neurol* 1988; 23 Suppl:S49–53.

Polomano RC, Mannes AJ, Clark US, Bennett GJ. A painful peripheral neuropathy in the rat produced by the chemotherapeutic drug, paclitaxel. *Pain* 2001; 94:293–304.

Quasthoff S, Hartung HP. Chemotherapy-induced peripheral neuropathy. *J Neurol* 2002; 249:9–17.

Rizzuto N, Cavallaro T, Monaco S, et al. Role of HIV in the pathogenesis of distal symmetrical peripheral neuropathy. *Acta Neuropathol (Berl)* 1995; 90:244–250.

Rossero R, Asmuth DM, Grady JJ, et al. Hydroxyurea in combination with didanosine and stavudine in antiretroviral-experienced HIV-infected subjects with a review of the literature. *Int J STD AIDS* 2003; 14:350–355.

Roytta M, Raine CS. Taxol-induced neuropathy: further ultrastructural studies of nerve fibre changes in situ. *J Neurocytol* 1985; 14:157–175.

Roytta M, Raine CS. Taxol-induced neuropathy: chronic effects of local injection. *J Neurocytol* 1986;15:483–496.

Roytta M, Horwitz SB, Raine CS. Taxol-induced neuropathy: short-term effects of local injection. *J Neurocytol* 1984; 13:685–701.

Sacktor N. The epidemiology of human immunodeficiency virus-associated neurological disease in the era of highly active antiretroviral therapy. *J Neurovirol* 2002; 8(Suppl 2):115–121.

Sahenk Z, Brady ST, Mendell JR. Studies on the pathogenesis of vincristine-induced neuropathy. *Muscle Nerve* 1987; 10:80–84.

Schaumberg HH, Spencer PS, Thomas PK. *Disorders of Peripheral Nerves*. Philadelphia: Davis, 1983.

Schifitto G, McDermott MP, McArthur JC, et al. Incidence of and risk factors for HIV-associated distal sensory polyneuropathy. *Neurology* 2002; 58:1764–1768.

Simpson DM. Selected peripheral neuropathies associated with human immunodeficiency virus infection and antiretroviral therapy. *J Neurovirol* 2002; 8(Suppl 2):33–41.

Simpson DM, Tagliati M. Nucleoside analogue-associated peripheral neuropathy in human immunodeficiency virus infection. *J Acquir Immune Defic Syndr Hum Retrovirol* 1995; 9:153–161.

Simpson DM, Katzenstein D, Haidich B, et al. Plasma carnitine in HIV-associated neuropathy. *AIDS* 2001; 15:2207–2208.

Simpson DM, Haidich AB, Schifitto G, et al. Severity of HIV-associated neuropathy is associated with plasma HIV-1 RNA levels. *AIDS* 2002; 16:407–412.

Skowron G. Biologic effects and safety of stavudine: overview of phase I and II clinical trials. *J Infect Dis* 1995; 171(Suppl 2):S113–117.

Skuta G, Fischer GM, Janaky T, et al. Molecular mechanism of the short-term cardiotoxicity caused by 2',3'-dideoxycytidine (ddC): modulation of reactive oxygen species levels and ADP-ribosylation reactions. *Biochem Pharmacol* 1999; 58:1915–1925.

Smith KM, Crandall KA, Kneissl ML, Navia BA. PCR detection of host and HIV-1 sequences from archival brain tissue. *J Neurovirol* 2000; 6:164–171.

Spataro LE, Sloane EM, Milligan ED, et al. Spinal gap junctions: potential involvement in pain facilitation. *J Pain* 2004; 5:392–405.

Starnes MC, Cheng YC. Cellular metabolism of 2',3'-dideoxycytidine, a compound active against human immunodeficiency virus in vitro. *J Biol Chem* 1987; 262:988–991.

Tan SV, Guiloff RJ. Hypothesis on the pathogenesis of vacuolar myelopathy, dementia, and peripheral neuropathy in AIDS. *J Neurol Neurosurg Psychiatry* 1998; 65:23–28.

Tanner KD, Reichling DB, Levine JD. Nociceptor hyper-responsiveness during vincristine-induced painful peripheral neuropathy in the rat. *J Neurosci* 1998; 18:6480–6491.

Twining CM, Sloane EM, Milligan ED, et al. Peri-sciatic proinflammatory cytokines, reactive oxygen species, and complement induce mirror-image neuropathic pain in rats. *Pain* 2004; 110:299–309.

Visovsky C. Chemotherapy-induced peripheral neuropathy. *Cancer Invest* 2003; 21:439–451.

Wang MS, Davis AA, Culver DG, et al. Calpain inhibition protects against Taxol-induced sensory neuropathy. *Brain* 2004; 127:671–679.

Wiley CA. Neuromuscular diseases of AIDS. *FASEB J* 1989; 3:2503–2511.

Windebank AJ. Chemotherapeutic neuropathy. *Curr Opin Neurol* 1999; 12:565–571.

Wulff EA, Wang AK, Simpson DM. HIV-associated peripheral neuropathy: epidemiology, pathophysiology and treatment. *Drugs* 2000; 59:1251–1260.

Yarchoan R, Perno CF, Thomas RV, et al. Phase I studies of 2',3'-dideoxycytidine in severe human immunodeficiency virus infection as a single agent and alternating with zidovudine (AZT). *Lancet* 1988; 1:76–81.

Yoshioka M, Shapshak P, Srivastava AK, et al. Expression of HIV-1 and interleukin-6 in lumbosacral dorsal root ganglia of patients with AIDS. *Neurology* 1994; 44:1120–1130.

Zink MC, Clements JE. A novel simian immunodeficiency virus model that provides insight into mechanisms of human immunodeficiency virus central nervous system disease. *J Neurovirol* 2002; 8(Suppl 2):42–48.

Correspondence to: Ahmet Höke, MD, PhD, FRCPC, Johns Hopkins Hospital, Department of Neurology, 600 N. Wolfe Street, Path 509, Baltimore, MD 21287, USA. Tel: 410-614-1196; Fax: 410-614-1008; email: ahoke@jhmi.edu.

Emerging Strategies for the Treatment of Neuropathic Pain, edited by James N. Campbell, Allan I. Basbaum, André Dray, Ronald Dubner, Robert H. Dworkin, and Christine N. Sang, IASP Press, Seattle, © 2006.

14

The Depression-Pain Complex: Overlap between the Two Problems and Implications for Neuropathic Pain

M. Dolores Ferrer-Garcia,[a] Joachim F. Wernicke,[b]
Michael J. Detke,[b,c,d] and Smriti Iyengar[b]

aDepartment of Anesthesiology, Reanimation and Pain Control, IMAS Hospitals of Barcelona, Barcelona, Spain; bLilly Research Laboratories, Eli Lilly and Company, Indianapolis, Indiana, USA; cIndiana University School of Medicine, Indianapolis, Indiana, USA; dMcLean Hospital and Harvard Medical School, Belmont, Massachusetts, USA

Chronic pain is a disease state intimately related to many pathological conditions. One such condition is major depressive disorder (MDD). Patients with MDD frequently express pain as one of the manifestations of the disorder or as a comorbidity. To be diagnosed with MDD, patients must experience a cluster of defined symptoms almost every day for at least 2 weeks and must have significantly impaired functioning in one or more domains, such as work and personal life. Symptoms include depressed mood (or irritability, particularly in children) and anhedonia (a reduced ability to experience pleasure in things such as friends, work, and hobbies that normally give pleasure). In addition, patients may display several other symptoms. Some are emotional or cognitive, such as excessive or ruminative guilt, impaired concentration, and thoughts of suicide. Other symptoms are more physical, such as increases in psychomotor activity (restlessness and fidgeting) or reduced activity; altered sleep patterns, including insomnia at the beginning, middle, or end of the sleep cycle, or a mixture, or hypersomnia; reduced energy; and either reduced or increased appetite, occasionally with specific cravings for certain types of food such as carbohydrates (American Psychiatric Association 2004). In the latest version of the *Diagnostic and Statistical Manual* of the American Psychiatric Association (2004), many important additional symptoms are listed as being associated with MDD.

These symptoms include anxiety, which is quite common, and complaints of pain, including headaches, joint pain, and abdominal pain.

Several extensive literature reviews have studied the association between pain and depression (Brodaty 1993; De Wester 1996; Evans et al. 1999; O'Malley et al. 1999; Bair et al. 2003; Briley 2003; Greden 2003; Kroenke 2003). Patients with depression, particularly those seen by primary care physicians, may report somatic symptoms such as headache, constipation, and back pain (Kirmayer et al. 1993; Kroenke et al. 1997; Simon et al. 1999; Fava 2002) or fatigue and insomnia (Kirmayer et al. 1993; Kroenke et al. 1994), all of which are grouped within the common denomination of physical illness (Detke et al. 2002a).

This chapter reviews the link between pain and depression and clarifies the contribution of the neurotransmitters 5-hydroxytryptamine (5HT) and norepinephrine (NE) to the pathophysiology of these related conditions. We examine treatment options that target these neurotransmitter systems that affect both depression and pain.

RELATIONSHIP BETWEEN PAIN AND DEPRESSION

The relationship between chronic pain and depression is complex and incompletely understood. Either condition can be associated with or may aggravate the other, as has been demonstrated with biopsychosocial models (Ong and Keng 2003). Pain and psychological illness are viewed as having reciprocal psychological and behavioral effects (Von Korff and Simon 1996). Clearly, in some cases pain precedes depression and is only one of the associated phenomena (Katon 1984; Magni 1984, 1986; Atkinson et al. 1988; Von Korff et al. 1988, 1993; Magni et al. 1990; Ruoff 1996; Fishbain et al. 1997; Katon et al. 2001; Kroenke et al. 2001). In other cases, the causal relationship is plainly the opposite (Von Knorring et al. 1983; Leino and Magni 1993). However, a significant number of patients present with a depression-pain complex in which it is difficult to elucidate the relative contribution of each of the components. In this case, the clinician needs a combined approach that can address both aspects.

EPIDEMIOLOGICAL DATA

In the United States and Europe, MDD has a lifetime prevalence of approximately 17% (Katon and Schulberg 1992; Kessler et al. 1994; Lepine et al. 1997). The prevalence of "minor" depression is approximately twice that of major depression (Crum et al. 1994; Beck and Koenig 1996; Pincus et al. 1999). Depression is a leading cause of disability (Murray and Lopez 1997); in the United States, it involves costs of approximately $83 billion annually (Greenberg et al. 2003; Stewart et al. 2003).

Pain is a common and disabling condition in the U.S. workforce. The mean prevalence of chronic pain is about 35% for the adult population, with prevalence estimates ranging from 11% to 55% (Andersson et al. 1993; Bair et al. 2003). Most pain results in lost productive time and reduced performance at work (Stewart et al. 2003). Headache is the most common pain condition to result in lost productive time, accounting for 5.4% of lost productivity, followed by back pain (3.2%), arthritis pain (2.0%), and other musculoskeletal pain. Lost productive time from common pain conditions among active workers costs an estimated $61.2 billion per year in the United States (Stewart et al. 2003). Chronic pain often occurs as a physical manifestation of a primary affective disorder. Physical symptoms are the presenting complaint in 69% of MDD patients (Simon et al. 1999) and in 76% of patients with mood or anxiety disorders (Kirmayer et al. 1993). Approximately 60% of these physical symptoms are related to pain (Kroenke and Price 1993). The presence of these symptoms indicates a reduced likelihood of remission from MDD, whereas antidepressants that are also effective for the treatment of painful physical symptoms may yield higher remission rates from depression (Fava 2003). The number of physical symptoms correlates highly with the severity of depression (Kroenke et al. 1994) and with the risk of relapse (Greden 2003). Depressed patients are more likely than healthy, nondepressed persons to develop chest pain, headache, and other types of pain (Von Korff et al. 1993). A concomitant sleep disorder may indicate the likelihood of higher pain intensity and a higher level of psychosocial disability (Aigner et al. 2003).

Among physical symptoms, gastrointestinal problems, sleep disturbances, headaches, appetite changes, and diffuse aches and pains have a strong association with psychiatric disorders. The presence of any of these symptoms may increase the likelihood of a mood or anxiety disorder by two- to threefold. Persons with depression and concomitant pain consume significantly more health resources (Bao et al. 2003), and their pain is less responsive to treatment (Fishbain 2000; Gureje et al. 2001). Given the additional disease burden caused by physical symptoms in depression, effective treatment of the physical symptoms and chronic pain associated with depression would certainly be of value (Bailey 2003; Bair et al. 2004) and could help avoid treatment failure (Linton 2000).

Depression prevalence rates in patients with persistent pain range from 30% to 54% (Banks and Kerns 1996). The intensity, frequency, and duration of pain are associated with depression, as is the occurrence of back pain and migraine (Bair et al. 2003). Approximately 43% of patients with MDD also have a chronic painful physical condition; the odds are four times higher for MDD patients than for persons without MDD to have chronic pain (Ohayon and Schatzberg 2003). Therefore, patients seeking consultation for chronic pain should be systematically evaluated for depression, and those with depression should be systematically evaluated for chronic pain. Specialists involved in the treatment of the emotional symptoms of depression frequently do not recognize and treat the painful physical symptoms, and vice versa (Williams et al. 2003).

THE CONTRIBUTION OF SEROTONIN AND NOREPINEPHRINE IN PAIN AND DEPRESSION

The monoamine hypothesis of depression has provided an important organizing paradigm for the treatment of MDD and has spurred the development of antidepressant therapies. This hypothesis proposes that depression is due to a deficit of synaptic monoamines, especially 5HT and NE. Depressed patients also have significantly reduced 5HT in blood platelets (Coppen and Wood 1979) and reduced levels of NE in the cerebrospinal fluid (Delgado and Moreno 2000).

Considerable evidence shows that most currently available antidepressants act primarily by increasing serotonergic, noradrenergic, and/or dopaminergic neurotransmission, presumably at key synapses within critical pathways. At least three distinct, but not necessarily mutually exclusive, mechanisms may accomplish this action: first, blockade of monoamine reuptake at the presynaptic terminal; second, blockade of monoamine binding to autoreceptors; and third, inhibition of monoamine oxidase, a key enzyme involved in monoamine catabolism (Delgado and Moreno 1999). Given that serotonergic and noradrenergic neurons are widespread throughout the nervous system, the effects of antidepressants may occur at several sites (Drevets 2001). Neuroanatomical and functional neuroimaging studies support the idea that several relatively discrete areas of the central nervous system may be malfunctioning in patients with depression (Drevets 2001), possibly resulting in specific subsets of symptoms (Delgado and Moreno 1999). It follows that the most effective therapies may be those that alter neurotransmission signaling by more than one type of monoaminergic neuron to "normalize" multiple inputs, resulting in improved mood and possibly ameliorating various affective symptoms.

Both neurotransmitters also exert analgesic effects via descending modulatory pain pathways and therefore play a key modulating role in pain (reviewed by Fields and Basbaum 1994). Noradrenergic neurons of the brainstem's locus ceruleus provide the major spinal catecholaminergic projection relevant to the descending control of "pain" transmission (reviewed by Fields and Basbaum 1994). Serotonergic neurons from the rostroventral medulla and noradrenergic neurons from the dorsolateral pontine tegmentum directly modulate dorsal horn neurons in the spinal cord. 5HT modulates both the descending inhibitory and descending facilitatory arms of the descending pain-modulatory system; it can thus exert both an antinociceptive and a pronociceptive effect, presumably acting via several receptor subtypes (Suzuki et al. 2004). NE typically acts in an antinociceptive fashion centrally (Jones 1991; Fields and Basbaum 1994). The facilitatory component of the descending pain-modulatory system may contribute to maintenance of normal pain sensitivity important for survival, while the descending inhibitory components help to achieve a balance of nociception and antinociception in the dorsal horn of the spinal cord in normal physiological states. A change in this balance could lead to persistent pain states (reviewed by Millan 2002; Ren and Dubner 2002; Ren et al. 2000; Suzuki et al. 2004). Monoaminergic drugs have thus been of interest both in treating depression as well as pain. This chapter will primarily focus on clinical observations and studies pertaining to pain and depression.

CLINICAL STUDIES FOCUSING ON PAIN ASSOCIATED WITH DEPRESSION

Numerous clinical studies have assessed the problem of pain associated with depression. The characteristics that most strongly predict depression are diffuseness of pain and the extent to which pain interferes with activities (Von Korff and Simon 1996). Impairment of daily activities (as indicated by occupational role disability) was the strongest predictor for the onset of both persistent pain and psychological disorders (Gureje et al. 2001). Back pain, headaches, chronic sinusitis, and joint pain are the most frequent pain conditions (Gureje et al. 2001; Patten 2001). Depression is a strong and independent predictor for the onset of intense or disabling neck and low back pain, with four-fold increased risk in those with high depression scores (Carroll et al. 2004). Major depression correlates in a linear fashion with pain severity, and the combination of chronic back pain and major depression is associated with greater disability than either condition alone (Currie and Wang 2004). Data from a trial designed to test the effectiveness of a collaborative care intervention on major depression or dysthymia showed that more than 50% of elderly patients with affective illnesses suffered from chronic pain with functional impairment, predominantly due to osteoarthritis (Unutzer et al. 2001).

Clinical experience and clinical trials have documented the beneficial role of antidepressants in a variety of persistent pain conditions, both in depressed and nondepressed patients (Panerai et al. 1990; Magni 1991; Max et al. 1992; Onghena and Van Houdenhove 1992; Von Korff and Simon 1996; Vrethem et al. 1997; Atkinson et al. 1999; Sindrup and Jensen 1999; Fishbain 2000; Fishbain et al. 2000; Ehrnrooth et al. 2001; Kroenke 2001; Maina et al. 2002; Salerno et al. 2002; Drossman et al. 2003; Kirwin and Goren 2005). These agents have proven useful in managing both depressed mood and associated painful physical symptoms in depressed patients (Detke et al. 2002a,b). One meta-analysis examined 94 trials including more than 6,500 patients with six symptom syndromes (headache, fibromyalgia, functional gastrointestinal syndromes, idiopathic pain, tinnitus, and chronic fatigue syndrome) treated with antidepressants, placebos, or alternative drugs (O'Malley et al. 2000). The meta-analysis concluded that in patients with medically unexplained physical symptoms or syndromes, antidepressants are effective for improving outcomes, including symptoms and disability; it excluded patients with neuropathic pain, cancer pain, or degenerative joint pain (O'Malley et al. 2000).

SEROTONIN AND NOREPINEPHRINE ANTIDEPRESSANTS

The selective serotonin reuptake inhibitors (SSRIs) are better tolerated than older antidepressants such as tricyclics and monoamine oxidase inhibitors and have shown efficacy in depression (O'Malley et al. 2000). However, SSRIs have shown limited efficacy in pain conditions (McQuay et al. 1996; Sindrup and Jensen 1999, 2000). Agents with primarily NE or mixed monoamine reuptake inhibition are more effective as analgesics (Max et al. 1992; Onghena and Van Houdenhove 1992). Moreover, the concentration-response effect is suggested to be more consistent in these compounds than in SSRIs (Sindrup et al. 1991). Consistent with these data are observations that the efficacy of antidepressants in pain is greater with tricyclic antidepressants having dual 5HT/NE actions than with the SSRIs in both depressed and nondepressed patients (Max et al. 1992; Sindrup and Jensen 1999, 2000; Collins et al. 2000). A review of 22 trials of tricyclic antidepressants for the treatment of back pain found no benefit in pain relief or functional status with antidepressants that do not inhibit NE reuptake as well (Salerno et al. 2002). Nontricyclic selective NE reuptake inhibitors such as reboxetine have not been systematically studied.

TRICYCLIC ANTIDEPRESSANTS

Tricyclic antidepressants (TCAs) are noted to be effective in various pain conditions and are associated with fewer dropouts from side effects at lower doses (Furukawa et al. 2002). However, they show poor tolerability at higher doses. The analgesic effect of TCAs has been confirmed by meta-analyses in chronic nonmalignant pain (Onghena and Van Houdenhove 1992), psychogenic pain and somatoform pain disorder (Fishbain et al. 1998), unexplained symptoms and symptom syndromes (O'Malley et al. 1999), neuropathic pain (McQuay et al. 1996; Collins et al. 2000; Sindrup and Jensen 2000), chronic headache (Tomkins et al. 2001), and fibromyalgia (Rossy et al. 1999; Arnold et al. 2000; O'Malley et al. 2000). Low back pain (Atkinson et al. 1999), chronic back pain (Salerno et al. 2002), and functional gastrointestinal disorders (Jackson et al. 2000) also may be responsive to treatment with TCAs, although the findings are less conclusive. Tricyclic and tetracyclic antidepressants reduce symptoms moderately in patients with chronic low back pain; the benefit appears to be independent of depression status (Staiger et al. 2003).

TCAs have an independent analgesic effect in chronic pain, and this effect may result from several pharmacological actions (Sawynok et al. 2001). These drugs inhibit presynaptic reuptake of NE and (in some cases) 5HT, but they also have an antagonistic effect on N-methyl D-aspartate (NMDA) receptors (Reynolds and Miller 1988) and block sodium channels in neuronal tissue (Deffois et al. 1996; Pancrazio et al. 1998). Other actions include blockade of calcium channels (Lavoie 1990) and of α-adrenergic, H_1 histaminergic, and muscarinic receptors, as well as interactions with opioid receptors with a quinidine-like effect; all of these receptors could also influence the antinociceptive effects of TCAs (Pancrazio et al. 1998; Schreiber et al. 2002) but also contribute to their limiting side effects.

SELECTIVE SEROTONIN-NOREPINEPHRINE (DUAL) REUPTAKE INHIBITORS

In recent years, dual reuptake inhibitor therapy has emerged as an attractive option for treating depression and pain comorbidity. Antidepressant agents have been developed that selectively incorporate both 5HT and NE reuptake inhibition, but do not have the multiple receptor affinities of the TCAs. Several trials with selective SNRIs such as venlafaxine, milnacipran, and duloxetine suggest their efficacy in pain, either associated with or in the absence of depression (Mattia et al. 2002; Briley 2003), and have also shown relief of painful physical symptoms in depression (Detke et al. 2002a,b; Bailey 2003). Furthermore, dual reuptake inhibitors such as venlafaxine or duloxetine may hasten the onset of antidepressant activity or may have greater antidepressant efficacy compared to compounds that act on only one monoamine pathway (Thase et al. 2001; Tran et al. 2003).

With regard to painful physical symptoms in depression, duloxetine is an interesting example of agents in this class because it has been studied the most in controlled trials of pain disorders, as well as in controlled trials of MDD that systematically assessed pain symptoms. Duloxetine is a potent and relatively balanced dual reuptake inhibitor of both 5HT and NE, as demonstrated in preclinical studies (Bymaster et al. 2001). A clinical study at a dose of 80–120 mg a day showed a decrease in the urinary excretion of NE metabolites in a similar magnitude to 100 mg desipramine, indicating NE uptake inhibition in vivo (Chalon et al. 2003). At a dose of 60 mg/day, duloxetine inhibits platelet 5HT (Turcotte et al. 2001). Controlled studies in depression have demonstrated the drug's efficacy, tolerability, and safety (Detke et al. 2002a,b; Goldstein et al. 2002).

The specific outcome of painful physical symptoms associated with depression was analyzed based on the results of three large randomized, double-blind, placebo-controlled studies in major depression (Detke et al. 2002a,b; Goldstein et al. 2002). Patients treated with duloxetine had a significant reduction in the depression scale as well as in painful physical symptoms. The results showed that duloxetine significantly reduced pain severity as compared with placebo. The response pattern showed improvement as early as after the first week of therapy on some pain items. Other studies with duloxetine have confirmed its significant benefit in the treatment of the painful physical symptoms associated with depression (Nemeroff et al. 2002; Fava et al. 2004; McIntyre and Konarski 2005). However, the improvement in pain was probably underestimated in the clinical context of the trials because the primary outcome of these studies was depression and because the patients did not have high levels of pain at baseline (Goldstein et al. 2004).

ANTIDEPRESSANTS IN DIFFERENT PAIN CONDITIONS

NEUROPATHIC PAIN

TCAs have demonstrated efficacy in different painful conditions such as painful neuropathy (Sindrup et al. 2003) and diabetic neuropathy (Max et al. 1992). In a 6-week randomized, double-blind crossover trial, 20 patients received 12.5 to 250 mg/day of desipramine, a selective inhibitor of NE reuptake transporter, as compared with active placebo (Max et al. 1991). Patients were required to have signs and symptoms of daily neuropathic pain for at least 3 months prior to randomization and were required to have diabetes and normal cognition. Patients recorded their pain in a diary once a day, choosing from a list of 13 verbal descriptors of pain intensity. Patients receiving desipramine had statistically significant pain relief as compared with patients taking the placebo (Max et al. 1991).

Max et al. (1992) conducted two comparative trials in patients with pain from peripheral diabetic neuropathy. In the first trial, 38 patients received the SNRI amitriptyline and desipramine in a double-blind crossover study; in the companion trial, 46 patients received fluoxetine and placebo. The dose ranges were 12.5–150 mg/day for desipramine and amitriptyline and 20–40 mg/day for fluoxetine. The duration of treatment in both studies was 6 weeks, during which time the patients recorded pain intensity in a daily diary by selecting from a list of 13 descriptors. Desipramine and amitriptyline both relieved pain with similar efficacy, but pain relief in patients treated with fluoxetine, an SSRI, did not differ from that recorded in the placebo group (Max et al. 1992).

Clomipramine, a selective inhibitor of 5HT reuptake transporter, was examined in a clinical trial in comparison with desipramine and placebo (Sindrup et al. 1990). Twenty-six patients were randomized to receive clomipramine for 2 weeks followed by a 2-week treatment with desipramine and a 2-week treatment with placebo. The patients had neurological signs of peripheral neuropathy prior to randomization. Doses were 75 mg/day for clomipramine and 200 mg/day for desipramine. Patients recorded their pain intensity in diaries using a six-item neuropathy observer scale. Both clomipramine and desipramine were more effective than placebo in relieving peripheral diabetic neuropathic pain. Clomipramine was more effective than both desipramine and placebo in relieving the pain (Sindrup et al. 1990).

Sindrup et al. (2005) reviewed data from several clinical trials covering pain of different origin, including central post-stroke pain, spinal cord injury pain, postherpetic neuralgia, painful neuropathy, postmastectomy pain, HIV neuropathy, and pain of mixed types. They concluded that TCAs with affinity for 5HT and NE reuptake transporter, along with SNRIs, were more effective in relieving pain in patients with peripheral neuropathy as compared to other classes of drugs such as SSRIs (Sindrup et al. 2005).

Meta-analysis (McQuay et al. 1996; Collins et al. 2000; Sindrup and Jensen 2000) firmly supports the beneficial effects of this group of drugs in neuropathy as well as in postherpetic neuralgia (Collins et al. 2000; Ahmad and Goucke 2002), and a randomized controlled trial (Raja et al. 2002) comparing opioids versus antidepressants in postherpetic neuralgia also supports the use of TCAs in this condition. The selective SNRI venlafaxine has been studied at two doses (75 and 150–225 mg/day) for efficacy in diabetic neuropathic pain in a double-blind, placebo-controlled, parallel-group study (Rowbotham et al. 2004). While the lower dose was numerically superior, only the higher dose (which is more likely to inhibit reuptake of both 5HT and NE) was significantly superior to placebo in this 6-week study. In this multicenter study, which included 244 adult patients, the primary efficacy measures were scores on daily 100-mm visual analogue scales of pain intensity (VAS-PI) and pain relief (VAS-PR). At week 6, the percentage reduction from baseline on the VAS-PI scale was 50% in the 150–225-mg group, 32% in the 75-mg group, and 27% in the placebo group.

The SNRI duloxetine has also been studied in pain disorders. The results have shown an analgesic effect independent of the drug's antidepressant efficacy, at the same doses (i.e., 60–120 mg/day) used in depression studies. Three double-blind, placebo-controlled, parallel-group studies (Wernicke et al. 2004; Goldstein et al. 2005; Raskin et al. 2005) were performed in patients with diabetic peripheral neuropathic pain. In these studies, about 90% of the patients had type II diabetes, about 60% were male, and the average age was approximately 60 years. Patients had on average had diabetes for 11 years and neuropathic pain for 4 years. They were required to have a baseline pain score of at least 4 out of 10 on a 10-point Likert scale as measured by a daily diary, and the average baseline score was approximately 6. The first study (Goldstein et al. 2005) compared the pain-relieving effects of duloxetine at doses of 20 mg once daily, 60 mg once daily, and 60 mg twice daily. The latter two doses provided relief that was significantly superior to placebo at each time point (weeks 1–12). The two active doses of duloxetine (60 and 120 mg/day) reduced pain by roughly 50% on average. They also produced improvements in a variety of secondary pain measures (e.g., pain at night) and functional outcomes. The second study (Raskin et al. 2005) included only three conditions: placebo, 60 mg duloxetine once daily, and 60 mg duloxetine twice daily. This study replicated the above findings. The third study was similar to the second in design and results (Wernicke et al. 2004). Patients with major depression were specifically excluded from these studies in order to ensure that the analgesic effect seen was independent of any effect on depression. Thus, these studies on venlafaxine and duloxetine provide very strong clinical evidence for the efficacy of nontricyclic SNRIs in diabetic peripheral neuropathic pain.

An interesting new area of research is the preemptive use of antidepressants to avoid the development of chronic pain conditions. A controlled trial showed that a low dose of amitriptyline during the acute phase of herpes zoster may reduce the risk of developing postherpetic neuralgia (Bowsher 1997). Antidepressants are also an essential part of the treatment of patients with the difficult clinical problem of postsurgical neuropathic pain (Power and Barratt 1999). Venlafaxine was studied perioperatively for possible efficacy in the prevention of postmastectomy pain syndrome. Patients received 75 mg of venlafaxine or placebo for 2 weeks prior to surgery, and VAS pain scores were recorded 1 day, 1 month, and 6 months after surgery. Scores of pain with movement were lower at 6 months in the patients treated with venlafaxine as compared to patients treated with placebo; a significant decrease in the incidence of pain in the chest wall, axilla, and arm was also observed (Bulut et al. 2004).

FIBROMYALGIA

Patients with fibromyalgia suffer from musculoskeletal pain, neuroendocrine disorders, and often psychological distress, including anxiety and depression. Depression is more common in patients with fibromyalgia than in controls or patients with rheumatoid arthritis (Hudson and Pope 1994). Approximately 25% of patients with fibromyalgia have current major depression, and 50% have a lifetime history of depression. In addition, many of the symptoms of depression and fibromyalgia are identical. However, the primary symptoms of fibromyalgia include pain and specific "tender points" (Wolfe 1990; Wolfe et al. 1990).

SSRIs have shown mixed results in fibromyalgia, whereas TCAs have shown evidence of efficacy (Arnold et al. 2000). Of the SNRIs, duloxetine has been studied in two double-blind, placebo-controlled, parallel-group trials of fibromyalgia syndrome. In the first study (Arnold et al. 2004), patients were predominantly female (about 90%), with an average age of approximately 50 years, and all met the American College of Rheumatology criteria for fibromyalgia. Patients were treated either with placebo or with 60 mg duloxetine twice daily, and the latter group had significantly greater reduction in average pain intensity and tender points and in a variety of secondary pain and overall function measures. The second study (Arnold et al. 2005) showed similar results except that only females were enrolled, and there were three arms: placebo, 60 mg duloxetine once daily, and 60 mg duloxetine twice daily. Duloxetine significantly improved pain and function in both active treatment arms (Arnold et al. 2005). Because of the relatively high comorbidity between fibromyalgia and MDD, both studies included patients with MDD, who made up about one-third of the population. The effects of duloxetine on pain were similar in patients with and without MDD.

Milnacipran, another SNRI, was also recently studied in fibromyalgia patients (Gendreau et al. 2005). One hundred and twenty-five patients with fibromyalgia were randomly assigned in a 3:3:2 ratio to receive milnacipran twice daily, milnacipran once daily, or placebo for 3 months in a double-blind dose escalation trial. In this study, 92% of the twice-daily and 81% of the once-daily participants achieved dose escalation to 200 mg. Both the once-daily and twice-daily groups showed statistically significant improvements in pain. Improvements were also noted in global well-being, fatigue, and other domains. Response rates were similar in patients with or without depression, but placebo response rates were considerably higher in depressed patients, leading to a significantly greater overall efficacy of the drug in the nondepressed group. Milnacipran was reported to be well tolerated in this study (Gendreau et al. 2005).

MIGRAINE AND IRRITABLE BOWEL SYNDROME

Major depression increases the risk for migraine, and migraine increases the risk for major depression (Breslau 2003). Meta-analysis supports the efficacy of antidepressants in migraine (Jackson et al. 2000; O'Malley et al. 2000; Tomkins et al. 2001). Recently, a double-blind crossover trial of venlafaxine and amitriptyline has shown the utility of these agents in prophylactic migraine treatment (Reuben et al. 2004). Only one randomized, double-blind, placebo-controlled study has shown efficacy of TCAs in functional bowel disorders (Drossman et al. 2003).

LOW BACK PAIN

Atkinson and colleagues (1998) found a modest reduction in pain intensity in a randomized controlled trial of TCAs in patients with low back pain, excluding patients with depression. The authors suggested that physicians should carefully weigh the risks and benefits of nortriptyline in chronic back pain without depression. Salerno and colleagues (2002), using meta-analyses, concluded that before antidepressants can be routinely recommended as therapy for back pain in patients with depression, larger, well-designed, randomized, controlled trials are needed to weigh the benefits and adverse effects of antidepressant therapy. In general, the use of TCAs or selective SNRIs for treatment of chronic low back pain has not been well studied.

RHEUMATOID ARTHRITIS AND OSTEOARTHRITIS

Few studies have systematically studied antidepressants in arthritis or other joint-related pain disorders. In persons with rheumatoid arthritis, cognitive-behavioral approaches to the management of depression were not found to be additive to antidepressant medication alone, but antidepressant intervention was superior to no treatment (Parker et al. 2003).

In a randomized controlled trial of 1,801 depressed older adults with joint pain (mostly osteoarthritis), which was performed at 18 primary care clinics within eight health care organizations, Lin et al. (2003) concluded that improved depression care extended beyond reduced depressive symptoms and included decreased pain as well as improved functional status and better quality of life.

FUTURE PERSPECTIVES FOR TREATMENT OF PAIN SYNDROMES

Because depression and pain are often comorbid, appropriate treatment of both emotional and painful symptoms may be most beneficial overall in patients with depression or chronic pain. It is important to note the growing consensus among the psychiatric community that the treatment goal for patients with MDD should be not merely symptomatic improvement but rather remission, or virtually complete symptom resolution. Treatment to remission prevents a host of bad outcomes, such as a higher risk of relapse into another episode of MDD, impairment of physical and social functioning, increased risk of suicide and substance abuse, and worsened prognosis for comorbid medical illnesses (Hirschfeld et al. 1997; Doraiswamy et al. 2001; Thase et al. 2001). It stands to reason that treating a broad spectrum of MDD symptoms, including painful physical symptoms, is likely to help a greater proportion of patients achieve remission.

In contrast, resolution of mood symptoms in chronic pain patients has received less attention and should be the focus of future treatment paradigms. Currently, in the United States, about 25 compounds have been approved by the Food and Drug Administration as antidepressants. To date, the pharmacological and clinical studies suggest that 5HT/NE reuptake inhibitors are indeed promising therapeutic options. The use of these compounds in persistent pain needs to be explored further in well-designed trials with pain relief as the primary outcome. Non-monoaminergic antidepressant treatment options need to be developed as well and their potential utility evaluated in managing depression, painful physical symptoms, and pain disorders.

ACKNOWLEDGMENTS

Supported in part by a grant of the Fondo de Investigaciones Sanitarias (FIS BA03/00042). Dr. Ferrer was a Visiting Fellow at Eli Lilly and Company from 2002 to 2004. The authors thank Dr. Durisala Desaiah for his assistance with manuscript preparation.

REFERENCES

Ahmad M, Goucke CR. Management of strategies for the treatment of neuropathic pain in the elderly. *Drugs Aging* 2002; 19:929–945.

Aigner M, Graf A, Freidl M, et al. Sleep disturbances in somatoform pain disorder. *Psychopathology* 2003; 36:324–328.

American Psychiatric Association. *Diagnostic and Statistical Manual of Mental Disorders,* 4th ed. Primary Care Version. Washington, DC: American Psychiatric Association Press, 2004.

Andersson HI, Ejlertsson G, Leden I, Rosenberg C. Chronic pain in a geographically defined general population: studies of differences in age, gender, social class, and pain localization. *Clin J Pain* 1993; 9:174–182.

Arnold LM, Keck PE Jr, Welge JA. Antidepressant treatment of fibromyalgia. A meta-analysis and review. *Psychosomatics* 2000; 41:104–113.

Arnold LM, Lu Y, Crofford LJ, et al. Duloxetine Fibromyalgia Trial Group. A double-blind, multicenter trial comparing duloxetine with placebo in the treatment of fibromyalgia patients with or without major depressive disorder. *Arthritis Rheum* 2004; 50:2974–2984.

Arnold LM, Rosen AS, Pritchett YL, et al. A randomized, double-blind, placebo-controlled trial of duloxetine in the treatment of women with fibromyalgia with or without major depressive disorder. *Pain* 2005; 119:5–15

Atkinson JH, Slater MA, Grant I, Patterson TL, Garfin SR. Depressed mood in chronic low back pain: relationship with stressful life events. *Pain* 1988; 35:47–55.

Atkinson JH, Slater MA, Williams RA, et al. A placebo-controlled randomized clinical trial of nortriptyline for chronic low back pain. *Pain* 1998; 76:287–296.

Atkinson JH, Slater MA, Wahlgren DR, et al. Effects of noradrenergic and serotonergic antidepressants on chronic low back pain intensity. *Pain* 1999; 77:137–145.

Bailey KP. Physical symptoms comorbid with depression and the new antidepressant duloxetine. *J Psychosoc Nurs Ment Health Serv* 2003; 41:13–18.

Bair MJ, Robinson RL, Katon W, Kroenke K. Depression and pain comorbidity: a literature review. *Arch Intern Med* 2003; 163:2433–2445.

Bair MJ, Robinson RL, Eckert GJ, et al. Impact of pain on depression treatment response in primary care. *Psychosom Med* 2004; 66:17–22.

Banks S, Kerns R. Explaining high rates of depression in chronic pain. A diathesis-stress framework. *Psychol Bull* 1996; 119:95–110.

Bao Y, Sturm R, Croghan TW. A national study of the effect of chronic pain on the use of health care by depressed persons. *Psychiatr Serv* 2003; 54:693–697.

Beck DA, Koenig HG. Minor depression: a review of the literature. *Int J Psychiatry Med* 1996; 26:177–209.

Bowsher D. The effects of pre-emptive treatment of postherpetic neuralgia with amitriptyline: a randomized, double-blind, placebo-controlled trial. *J Pain Symptom Manage* 1997; 13:327–331.

Breslau N, Lipton RB, Stewart WF, Schultz LR, Welch KM. Comorbidity of migraine and depression: investigating potential etiology and prognosis. *Neurology* 2003; 60:1308–1312.

Briley M. New hope in the treatment of painful symptoms in depression. *Curr Opin Investig Drugs* 2003; 4:42–45.

Brodaty H. Think of depression: atypical presentations in the elderly. *Aust Fam Physician* 1993; 22:1195–203.

Bulut S, Berilgen MS, Baran A, et al. Venlafaxine versus amitriptyline in the prophylactic treatment of migraine: randomized, double-blind, crossover study. *Clin Neurol Neurosurg* 2004; 107:44–48.

Bymaster FP, Dreshfield-Ahmad LJ, Threlkeld PG, et al. Comparative affinity of duloxetine and venlafaxine for serotonin and norepinephrine transporters in vitro and in vivo, human serotonin receptor subtypes, and other neuronal receptors. *Neuropsychopharmacology* 2001; 25:871–880.

Carroll LJ, Cassidy JD, Cote P. Depression as a risk factor for onset of an episode of troublesome neck and low back pain. *Pain* 2004; 107:134–139.

Chalon SA, Granier LA, Vandenhende FR, et al. Duloxetine increases serotonin and norepinephrine availability in healthy subjects: a double-blind, controlled study. *Neuropsychopharmacology* 2003; 28:1685–1693.

Collins SL, Moore RA, McQuay HJ, Wiffen P. Antidepressants and anticonvulsants for diabetic neuropathy and post-herpetic neuralgia: a quantitative systematic review. *J Pain Symptom Manage* 2000; 20:449–458.

Coppen A, Wood K. Adrenergic and serotonergic mechanisms in depression and their response to amitriptyline. *Ciba Found Symp* 1979; 74:157–166.

Crum RM, Cooper-Patrick L, Ford DE. Depressive symptoms among general medical patients: prevalence and one-year outcome. *Psychosom Med* 1994; 56:109–117.

Currie SR, Wang J. Chronic back pain and major depression in the general Canadian population. *Pain* 2004; 107:54–60.

Deffois A, Fage D, Carter C. Inhibition of synaptosomal veratridine-induced sodium influx by antidepressants and neuroleptics used in chronic pain. *Neurosci Lett* 1996; 220:117–120.

Delgado PL, Moreno FA. Antidepressants and the brain. *Int Clin Psychopharmacol* 1999; 14:S9–S16.

Delgado PL, Moreno FA. Role of norepinephrine in depression. *J Clin Psychiatry* 2000; 61:S5–S12.

Detke MJ, Lu Y, Goldstein DJ, Hayes JR, Demitrack MA. Duloxetine, 60 mg once daily, for major depressive disorder: a randomized double-blind placebo-controlled trial. *J Clin Psychiatry* 2002a; 63:308–315.

Detke MJ, Lu Y, Goldstein DJ, McNamara RK, Demitrack MA. Duloxetine 60 mg once daily dosing versus placebo in the acute treatment of major depression. *J Psychiatr Res* 2002b; 36:383–390.

De Wester JN. Recognizing and treating the patient with somatic manifestations of depression. *J Fam Pract* 1996; 43:S3–S15.

Doraiswamy PM, Khan ZM, Donahue RM, Richard NE. Quality of life in geriatric depression: a comparison of remitters, partial responders, and nonresponders. *Am J Geriatr Psychiatry* 2001; 9:423–428.

Drevets WC. Neuroimaging and neuropathological studies of depression: implications for the cognitive-emotional features of mood disorders. *Curr Opin Neurobiol* 2001; 11:240–249.

Drossman DA, Toner BB, Whitehead WE, et al. Cognitive-behavioral therapy versus education and desipramine versus placebo for moderate to severe functional bowel disorders. *Gastroenterology* 2003; 125:19–31.

Ehrnrooth E, Grau C, Zachariae R, Andersen J. Randomized trial of opioids versus tricyclic antidepressants for radiation-induced mucositis pain in head and neck cancer. *Acta Oncol* 2001; 40:745–750.

Evans DL, Staab JP, Petitto JM, et al. Depression in the medical setting: biopsychological interactions and treatment considerations. *J Clin Psychiatry* 1999; 60:S40–S55.

Fava M. Somatic symptoms, depression, and antidepressant treatment. *J Clin Psychiatry* 2002; 63:305–357.

Fava M. The role of the serotonergic and noradrenergic neurotransmitter systems in the treatment of psychological and physical symptoms of depression. *J Clin Psychiatry* 2003; 64:S26–S29.

Fava M, Mallincrodt CH, Detke MJ, Watkin JG, Wohlreich MM. The effect of duloxetine on painful physical symptoms in depressed patients: do improvements in these symptoms result in higher remission rate. *J Clin Psychiatry* 2004; 65:521–530.

Fields HL, Basbaum AI. Central nervous system mechanisms of pain modulation. In: Wall P, Melzack R (Eds). *Textbook of Pain*. New York: Churchill Livingstone, 1994, pp 243–257.

Fishbain DA. Evidence-based data on pain relief with antidepressants. *Ann Med* 2000; 32:305–316.

Fishbain DA, Cutler R, Rosomoff HL, Rosomoff RS. Chronic pain-associated depression: antecedent or consequence of chronic pain? A review. *Clin J Pain* 1997; 13:116–137.

Fishbain DA, Cutler RB, Rosomoff HL, Rosomoff RS. Do antidepressants have an analgesic effect in psychogenic pain and somatoform pain disorder? A meta-analysis. *Psychosom Med* 1998; 60:503–509.

Fishbain DA, Cutler R, Rosomoff HL, et al. Evidence-based data from animal to experimental studies on pain relief with antidepressants: a structural review. *Pain Med* 2000; 1:310–316.

Furukawa TA, McGuire H, Barbui C. Meta-analysis of effects and side effects of low dosage tricyclic antidepressants in depression: systematic review. *BMJ* 2002; 325:991–999.

Gendreau RM, Thorn MD, Gendreau JF, et al. Efficacy of milnacipran in patients with fibromyalgia. *J Rheumatol* 2005; 32:1975–1985.

Goldstein DJ, Mallinckrodt C, Lu Y, Demitrack MA. Duloxetine in the treatment of major depressive disorder: a double-blind clinical trial. *J Clin Psychiatry* 2002; 63:225–231.

Goldstein DJ, Lu Y, Detke MJ, et al. Effects of duloxetine on painful physical symptoms associated with depression. *Psychosomatics* 2004; 45:17–28.

Goldstein DJ, Lu Y, Detke MJ, Lee TC, Iyengar S. Duloxetine vs. placebo in patients with painful diabetic neuropathy. *Pain* 2005; 116:109–118.

Greden JF. Physical symptoms of depression: unmet needs. *J Clin Psychiatry* 2003; 64:S5–S11.

Greenberg PE, Leong SA, Birnbaum HG, Robinson RL. The economic burden of depression with painful symptoms. *J Clin Psychiatry* 2003; 64:S17–S23.

Gureje O, Simon GE, Von Korff M. A cross-national study of the course of persistent pain in primary care. *Pain* 2001; 92:195–200.

Hirschfeld RM, Keller MB, Panico S, et al. The National Depressive and Manic-Depressive Association consensus statement on the undertreatment of depression. *JAMA* 1997; 277:333–340.

Hudson JL, Pope HG. The concept of affective disorder: relationship to fibromyalgia and other symptoms of chronic muscle pain. *Baillieres Clin Rheumatol* 1994; 8:839–856.

Jackson JL, O'Malley PG, Tomkins G, et al. Treatment of functional gastrointestinal disorders with antidepressant medications: a meta-analysis. *Am J Med* 2000; 108:65–72.

Jones SL. Descending noradrenergic influences on pain. *Prog Brain Res* 1991; 88:381–394.

Katon W. Panic disorder and somatization. Review of 55 cases. *Am J Med* 1984; 77:101–106.

Katon W, Schulberg H. Epidemiology of depression in primary care. *Gen Hosp Psychiatry* 1992; 14:237–247.

Katon W, Sullivan M, Walker E. Medical symptoms without identified pathology: relationship to psychiatric disorders, childhood and adult trauma, and personality traits. *Ann Intern Med* 2001; 134:917–925.

Kessler RC, McGonagle KA, Zhao S, et al. Lifetime and 12-month prevalence of DSM-III-R psychiatric disorders in the United States. Results from the National Comorbidity Survey. *Arch Gen Psychiatry* 1994; 51:8–19

Kirmayer LJ, Robbins JM, Dworkin M, Yaffe MJ. Somatization and the recognition of depression and anxiety in primary care. *Am J Psychiatry* 1993; 150:734–741.

Kirwin JL, Goren JL. Duloxetine: a dual serotonin-norepinephrine reuptake inhibitor for treatment of major depressive disorder. *Pharmacotherapy* 2005; 25:396–410.

Kroenke K. Studying symptoms: sampling and measurement issues. *Ann Intern Med* 2001; 134:844–853.

Kroenke K. Patients presenting with somatic complaints: epidemiology, psychiatric comorbidity and management. *Int J Methods Psychiatr Res* 2003; 12:34–43.

Kroenke K, Price RK. Symptoms in the community. Prevalence, classification, and psychiatric comorbidity. *Arch Intern Med* 1993; 153:2474–2480.

Kroenke K, Spitzer RL, Williams JB, et al. Physical symptoms in primary care. Predictors of psychiatric disorders and functional impairment. *Arch Fam Med* 1994; 3:774–779.

Kroenke K, Jackson JL, Chamberlin J. Depressive and anxiety disorders in patients presenting with physical complaints: clinical predictors and outcome. *Am J Med* 1997; 103:339–347.

Kroenke K, West SL, Swindle R, et al. Similar effectiveness of paroxetine, fluoxetine, and sertraline in primary care: a randomized trial. *JAMA* 2001; 286:2947–2955.

Lavoie PA, Beauchamp G, Elie R. Tricyclic antidepressants inhibit voltage-dependent calcium channels and Na^+-Ca^{2+} exchange in rat brain cortex synaptosomes. *Can J Physiol Pharmacol* 1990; 68:1414–1418.

Leino P, Magni G. Depressive and distress symptoms as predictors of low back pain, neck-shoulder pain, and other musculoskeletal morbidity: a 10-year follow-up of metal industry employees. *Pain* 1993; 53:89–94.

Lepine JP, Gastpar M, Mendlewicz J, Tylee A. Depression in the community: the first pan-European study DEPRES (Depression Research in European Society). *Int Clin Psychopharmacol* 1997; 12:19–29.

Lin EHB, Katon W, Von Korff M, et al. IMPACT Investigators. Effect of improving depression care on pain and functional outcomes among older adults with arthritis: a randomized controlled trial. *JAMA* 2003; 290:2428–2434.

Linton SJ. A review of psychological risk factors in back and neck pain. *Spine* 2000; 25:1148–1156.

Magni G. Chronic low-back pain and depression: an epidemiological survey. *Acta Psychiatr Scand* 1984; 70:614–617.

Magni G. Chronic pain and depression. *Can J Psychiatry* 1986; 31:878–879.

Magni G. The use of antidepressants in the treatment of chronic pain. A review of the current evidence. *Drugs* 1991; 42:730–748.

Magni G, Caldieron C, Rigatti-Luchini S, Merskey H. Chronic musculoskeletal pain and depressive symptoms in the general population. An analysis of the 1st National Health and Nutrition Examination Survey data. *Pain* 1990; 43:299–307.

Maina G, Vitalucci A, Gandolfo S, Bogetto F. Comparative efficacy of SSRIs and amisulpride in burning mouth syndrome: a single-blind study. *J Clin Psychiatry* 2002; 63:38–43.

Mattia C, Paoletti F, Coluzzi F, Boanelli A. New antidepressants in the treatment of neuro-pathic pain. A review. *Minerva Anestesiol* 2002; 68:105–114.

McQuay HJ, Tramèr M, Nye BA, et al. A systematic review of antidepressants in neuropathic pain. *Pain* 1996; 68:217–227.

Max MB, Kishore-Kumar R, Schafer SC, et al. Efficacy of desipramine in painful diabetic neuropathy: a placebo-controlled trial. *Pain* 1991; 45:3–9.

Max MB, Lynch SA, Muir J, et al. Effects of desipramine, amitriptyline, and fluoxetine on pain in diabetic neuropathy. *N Engl J Med* 1992; 326:1250–1256.

McIntyre RS, Konarski JZ. Duloxetine: pharmacoeconomic implications of an antidepressant that alleviates painful physical symptoms. *Expert Opin Pharmacother* 2005; 6:707–713.

Millan MJ. Descending control of pain. *Prog Neurobiol* 2002; 66:355–474

Murray CJ, Lopez AD. Alternative projections of mortality and disability by cause 1990–2020: Global Burden of Disease Study. *Lancet* 1997; 349:1498–1504.

Nemeroff CB, Schatzberg AF, Goldstein DJ, et al. Duloxetine for the treatment of major depressive disorder. *Psychopharmacol Bull* 2002; 36:106–132.

Ohayon MM, Schatzberg AF. Using chronic pain to predict depressive morbidity in the general population. *Arch Gen Psychiatry* 2003; 60:39–47.

O'Malley PG, Jackson JL, Santoro J, et al. Antidepressant therapy for unexplained symptoms and symptom syndromes. *J Fam Pract* 1999; 48:980–990.

O'Malley PG, Balden E, Tomkins G, et al. Treatment of fibromyalgia with antidepressants: a meta-analysis. *J Gen Intern Med* 2000; 15:659–666.

Ong KS, Keng SB. The biological, social, and psychological relationship between depression and chronic pain. *Cranio* 2003; 21:286–294.

Onghena P, Van Houdenhove B. Antidepressant-induced analgesia in chronic non-malignant pain: a meta-analysis of 39 placebo-controlled studies. *Pain* 1992; 49:205–219.

Pancrazio JJ, Kamatchi GL, Roscoe AK, Lynch C III. Inhibition of neuronal Na$^+$ channels by antidepressant drugs. *J Pharmacol Exp Ther* 1998; 284:208–214.

Panerai AE, Monza G, Movilia P, et al. A randomized, within-patient, cross-over, placebo-controlled trial on the efficacy and tolerability of the tricyclic antidepressants chlorimipramine and nortriptyline in central pain. *Acta Neurol Scand* 1990; 82:34–38.

Parker JC, Smarr KL, Slaughter JR, et al. Management of depression in rheumatoid arthritis: a combined pharmacologic and cognitive-behavioral approach. *Arthritis Rheum* 2003; 49:766–277.

Patten SB. Long-term medical conditions and major depression in a Canadian population study at waves 1 and 2. *J Affect Disord* 2001; 63:35–41.

Pincus HA, Davis WW, McQueen LE. 'Subthreshold' mental disorders. A review and synthesis of studies on minor depression and other 'brand names'. *Br J Psychiatry* 1999; 174:288–296.

Power I, Barratt S. Analgesic agents for the postoperative period. Nonopioids. *Surg Clin North Am* 1999; 79:275–295.

Raja SN, Haythornthwaite JA, Pappagallo M, et al. Opioids versus antidepressants in postherpetic neuralgia: a randomized, placebo-controlled trial. *Neurology* 2002; 59:1015–1021.

Raskin J, Pritchett YL, Wang F, et al. A double-blind, randomized multicenter trial comparing duloxetine with placebo in the management of diabetic peripheral neuropathic pain. *Pain Med* 2005; 6:346–356.

Ren K, Dubner R. Descending modulation in persistent pain: an update. *Pain* 2002; 1001–1006.

Ren K, Zhuo M, Willis WD. Multiplicity and plasticity of descending modulation of nociception: implications for persistent pain. In: Devor M, Rowbotham MC, Wiesenfeld-Hallin Z (Eds). *Proceedings of the 9th World Congress on Pain,* Progress in Pain Research and Management, Vol. 16. Seattle: IASP Press, 2000, pp 371–386.

Reuben SS, Makari-Judson G, Lurie SD. Evaluation of efficacy of the perioperative administration of venlafaxine XR in the prevention of postmastectomy pain syndrome. *J Pain Symptom Manage* 2004; 27:133–139.

Reynolds IJ, Miller RJ. Tricyclic antidepressants block *N*-methyl-D-aspartate receptors: similarities to the action of zinc. *Br J Pharmacol* 1988; 95:102.

Ruoff GE. Depression in the patient with chronic pain. *J Fam Pract* 1996; 43:S25–S33.

Rowbotham MC, Goli V, Kunz NR, Lei D. Venlafaxine extended release in the treatment of painful diabetic neuropathy: a double-blind, placebo-controlled study. *Pain* 2004; 110(3):697–706.

Salerno SM, Browning R, Jackson JL. The effect of antidepressant treatment on chronic back pain: a meta-analysis. *Arch Intern Med* 2002; 15:19–24.

Sawynok J, Esser MJ, Reid AR. Antidepressants as analgesics: an overview of central and peripheral mechanisms of action. *J Psychiatry Neurosci* 2001; 26:21–29.

Schreiber S, Bleich A, Pick CG. Venlafaxine and mirtazapine: different mechanisms of antidepressant action, common opioid-mediated antinociceptive effects—a possible opioid involvement in severe depression? *J Mol Neurosci* 2002; 18:143–149.

Simon GE, Von Korff M, Piccinelli M, Fullerton C, Ormel J. An international study of the relation between somatic symptoms and depression. *N Engl J Med* 1999; 341:1329–1335.

Sindrup SH, Jensen TS. Efficacy of pharmacological treatments of neuropathic pain: an update and effect related to mechanism of drug action. *Pain* 1999; 83:389–400.

Sindrup SH, Jensen TS. Pharmacologic treatment of pain in polyneuropathy. *Neurology* 2000; 55:915–920.

Sindrup SH, Gram LF, Skjold T, et al. Clomipramine vs desipramine vs placebo in the treatment of diabetic neuropathy symptoms. A double-blind cross-over study. *Br J Clin Pharm* 1990; 30:683–691.

Sindrup SH, Grodum E, Gram LF, Beck-Nielsen H. Concentration-response relationship in paroxetine treatment of diabetic neuropathy symptoms: a patient-blinded dose-escalation study. *Ther Drug Monit* 1991; 13:408–414.

Sindrup SH, Bach FW, Madsen C, Gram LF, Jensen TS. Venlafaxine versus imipramine in painful polyneuropathy: a randomized, controlled trial. *Neurology* 2003; 60(8):1284–1289.

Sindrup SH, Otto M, Flinnerup NB, Jensen TS. Antidepressants in the treatment of neuropathic pain. *Basic Clin Pharmacol Toxicol* 2005; 96:399–409.

Staiger TO, Gaster B, Sullivan MD, Deyo RA. Systematic review of antidepressants in the treatment of chronic low back pain. *Spine* 2003; 28:2540–2545.

Stewart WF, Ricci JA, Chee E, Hahn SR, Morganstein D. Cost of lost productive work time among US workers with depression. *JAMA* 2003; 289:3135–3144.

Suzuki R, Rygh L, Dickenson A. Bad news from the brain: descending 5-HT pathways that control spinal pain processing. *Trends Pharmacol Sci* 2004; 25:613–617.

Thase ME, Entsuah AR, Rudolph RL. Remission rates during treatment with venlafaxine or selective serotonin reuptake inhibitors. *Br J Psychiatry* 2001; 178:234–241.

Tomkins GE, Jackson JL, O'Malley PG, Balden E, Santoro JE. Treatment of chronic headache with antidepressants: a meta-analysis. *Am J Med* 2001; 111:54–63.

Tran PV, Bymaster FP, McNamara RK, Potter WZ. Dual monoamine modulation for improved treatment of major depressive disorder. *J Clin Psychopharmacol* 2003; 23:78–86.

Turcotte JE, Delsonnel G, de Montigny C, Herbert C, Blier P. Assessment of the serotonin and norepinephrine reuptake blocking properties of duloxetine in healthy subjects. *Neuropsychopharmacology* 2001; 24:511–521.

Unutzer J, Katon W, Williams JW Jr, et al. Improving primary care for depression in late life: the design of a multicenter randomized trial. *Med Care* 2001; 39:785–799.

von Knorring L, Perris C, Eisemann M, Eriksson U, Perris H. Pain as a symptom in depressive disorders. II. Relationship to personality traits as assessed by means of KSP. *Pain* 1983; 17(4):377–384.

Von Korff M, Simon G. The relationship between pain and depression. *Br J Psychiatry* 1996; 30(Suppl):101–108.

Von Korff M, Dworkin SF, Le Resche L, Kruger A. An epidemiologic comparison of pain complaints. *Pain* 1988; 32:173–183.

Von Korff M, Le Resche L, Dworkin SF. First onset of common pain symptoms: a prospective study of depression as a risk factor. *Pain* 1993; 55:251–258.

Vrethem M, Boivie J, Arnqvist H, et al. A comparison amitriptyline and maprotiline in the treatment of painful polyneuropathy in diabetics and nondiabetics. *Clin J Pain* 1997; 13:313–323.

Wernicke J, Lu Y, D'Souza D, et al. Duloxetine at doses of 60mg QD and 60mg BID is effective in treatment of diabetic neuropathic pain (DNP). *J Pain* 2004; 5(S1):S48.

Williams LS, Jones WJ, Shen J, et al. Prevalence and impact of depression and pain in neurology outpatients. *J Neurol Neurosurg Psychiatry* 2003; 74:1587–1589.

Wolfe F. Fibromyalgia. *Rheum Dis Clin North Am* 1990; 16:681–698.

Wolfe F, Smythe HA, Unus MB, et al. The American College of Rheumatology 1990. Criteria for the classification of fibromyalgia. Report of the Multicenter Criteria Committee. *Arthritis Rheum* 1990; 33:160–172.

Correspondence to: Smriti Iyengar, PhD, Lilly Research Laboratories, Drop Code 0510, Eli Lilly and Company, Indianapolis, IN 46285, USA. Tel: 317-276-2479; Fax: 317-276-5546; email: iyengar@lilly.com.

Emerging Strategies for the Treatment of Neuropathic Pain, edited by James N. Campbell, Allan I. Basbaum, André Dray, Ronald Dubner, Robert H. Dworkin, and Christine N. Sang, IASP Press, Seattle, © 2006.

15

Dissecting Molecular Causes of the Components of Chronic Neuropathic Pain Syndromes

Mitchell B. Max and Beata Buzas

Pain and Neurosensory Mechanisms Branch, National Institute of Dental and Craniofacial Research, National Institutes of Health, Department of Health and Human Services, Bethesda, Maryland, USA

Over the years I have referred to chronic pain as a "disease state"—a position that provoked criticism by those who insist that pain is a *symptom* of disease. Fortunately, beginning in the late 1960's … Merskey and Spear, Sternbach, Fordyce, and Pilowsky [began to develop a detailed account of chronic pain as a disease]. John J. Bonica (1990)

The many pain researchers who have echoed Bonica's characterization of "pain as a disease" often mean different things. Some just mean it as a marketing slogan: "pain is important, pain kills, pain needs more research money, pain needs its own national funding institute," and so on. The clinicians whom Bonica cited above focused on making clinical assessment and care as comprehensive for pain patients as for those with other serious psychiatric or medical diseases.

However, as a superb anatomist and pioneer of modern pain research, Bonica also must have been describing a research approach. For a clinical scientist trained in the 1940s, a research understanding of pain as a disease would resemble the understanding of syphilis or systemic lupus or breast cancer as a disease—a temporal sequence of clinical manifestations and underlying structural changes in organs, whose causes can be inferred by correlating the two.

What clinical aspects of neuropathic pain are essential mediating features of this "disease"? Patients with chronic pain have a high prevalence of anxiety and depression, sleep impairment, and substance abuse (Von Korff and Simon 1996; Casarett et al. 2001; Bair et al. 2003; Smith and

Haythornthwaite 2004; Sullivan et al. 2005). All of these conditions are easy to correlate with fundamental brain processes and appear to be reasonable targets for molecular dissection. Apkarian et al. (2004) have suggested that chronic pain may also cause brain atrophy and cognitive dysfunction, which would be an ominous complication indeed, but these results await replication. At the moment I will not discuss some higher-order phenomena such as the patient's functional status, psychological coping strategies, or assessments of meaning and dignity, but these are also important clinical dimensions, and molecular contributions to these constructs may be found.

Although pain neurobiologists have made great progress in defining pain-related short-term structural changes in the nervous system, we have barely begun to unravel the causal relations between pain and these other mediating clinical features. We will offer examples of the types of studies that allow us to optimize our ability to define the molecular basis and treatment of these clinical manifestations.

POTENTIAL CAUSAL LINKS BETWEEN PAIN AND MOOD, SLEEP, AND SUBSTANCE ABUSE DISORDERS

Why should pain researchers study the mechanisms of mood, sleep, or substance abuse disorders in pain patients rather than relying upon the ongoing research on these entities in patients without pain? Perhaps depression in pain is triggered and reinforced by the same complex cortical assessment pathways that are activated by reverses in one's career or in one's intimate relationships. Perhaps the same antidepressants or sleeping pills developed for patients with primary psychiatric illness are adequate.

However, I would make two arguments for studying mood, sleep, and substance abuse disorders specifically in the context of pain. First, perhaps the neural pathways and neurochemistry initiating and maintaining these other entities is somewhat unique in the pain patient. Second, we will gain statistical power in looking for molecular causes of pain by analyzing and extracting from the error term the variance caused by intervening variables such as mood, sleep, and substance abuse. This increase in statistical efficiency is essential if we are to be able to test many variables for their link with pain outcome, whether these variables are gene polymorphisms, cerebrospinal fluid proteins, functional brain imaging patterns, sensory testing results, or the results of drug challenges.

Fig. 1 (Burstein 1996) illustrates pathways that may provide a unique neurochemistry underlying pain-mediated disorders of mood, sleep, reward, or other vegetative functions. In the 1980s, several laboratories (Cechetto et

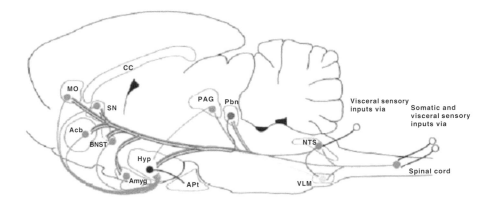

Fig. 1. Schematic illustration shows neural pathways conveying somatosensory and visceral information to the hypothalamus and other limbic structures mediating mood, sleep, and endocrine and cardiovascular function. Line drawing represents sagittal view of the rat's brain. Sites of origin (large circles) and of neural pathways are indicated. Acute pain alters many of these functions in humans, but a better understanding of the mechanisms and consequences of chronic pain for these functions might decrease the morbidity of painful illnesses. Abbreviations: Acb, nucleus accumbens; Amyg, amygdala; APt, anterior pituitary gland; BNST, bed nucleus stria terminals; cc, corpus callosum; Hyp, hypothalamus; MO, medial orbita cortex; NTS, nucleus tractus solitarius; PAG, periaqueductal gray; Pbn, parabrachial nuclei; SN, septa nucleus; VLM, ventrolateral medulla. (Reprinted from Burstein [1996], with permission from Elsevier.)

al. 1985; Burstein et al. 1987; Bernard et al. 1989; Hylden et al. 1989) described powerful spinal, trigeminal, and solitary tract pathways by which nociceptive inputs are multiplied by several orders of magnitude at synapses in the parabrachial and solitary tract nuclei and then synapse in the hypothalamus, amygdala, nucleus accumbens, septal nuclei, and medial orbital cortex. These are structures that mediate most of the manifestations of chronic pain seen in the clinic—dysfunctions of mood, sleep, appetite, reward from activities or drugs, sexual activity, and endocrine regulation.

It is plausible that pain might adversely affect mood through the direct synapses from spinal pathways to the limbic brain structures shown in Fig. 1 (Neugebauer et al. 2004). Although the neurotransmitters, receptors, and intracellular signaling pathways involved have not yet been described, they may differ in many cases from those on pathways through which other life stresses give rise to mood change (Charney and Manji 2004). Therefore, it is possible that treatments optimally suited to prevent or lessen pain-related dysphoria might differ from the usual antidepressants and anti-anxiety agents. Consistent with this suggestion is the report by Bair et al. (2004) from a large randomized trial of three selective serotonin reuptake-inhibiting antidepressants in depressed patients in primary care settings. Patients who also had pain disorders were less likely to have improvement in mood, and the severity of pain was correlated with treatment resistance. I would offer a similar neuroanatomical argument for the possibility of a unique neuro-chemical contribution of pain to insomnia, drug addiction, or other vegeta-tive disorders. Possible therapeutic leads could be uncovered by anatomical studies in animal pain models or by clinical studies of the effects on pain-related mood and vegetative disorders by polymorphisms of neurotransmit-ters or signaling molecules.

In order to interpret these relationships, we need to understand the di-rection of causative links among these phenomena. We know from cross-sectional studies that pain, mood and sleep disorders, and substance abuse coexist, but such designs tell us little about long-term processes or the direction of causation. For example, dozens of studies have reported that a large proportion of pain clinic patients have major depressive or anxiety disorders. The discussion sections of these papers almost uniformly give three equally weighted explanations: pain may cause mood disorder, mood disorder may amplify pain complaint, or similar biochemical substrates or environmental stresses may predispose to both.

The most powerful way to infer causation is through a longitudinal cohort study, but there are only a few longitudinal studies of pain and mood (Von Korff and Simon 1996). Does mood before lumbar diskectomy for sciatica predict surgical relief of pain? Very little; Carragee's (2001) review of his own preliminary data and the literature concludes that baseline mood is only weakly predictive of long-term outcome. The strongest predictor is the size of the herniated disk fragment observed with MRI and with surgical exploration. Patients with larger herniated disk fragments are more likely to improve. We have tentatively observed the same independence of surgical outcome from baseline mood in the Maine Lumbar Spine Study interverte-bral disk herniation cohort (Atlas et al. 1996; R.R. Edwards et al., unpub-lished data).

Our knowledge of the causal interactions between pain and insomnia is similar to that for the pain-mood nexus: pain and insomnia coexist in cross-sectional studies, but few longitudinal studies dissect the causal links and inform us about how to best intervene (Smith and Haythornthwaite 2004; Smith et al. 2005). Several studies have suggested that experimental inter-ruption of sleep may decrease experimental pain thresholds, or that experi-mental pain given during sleep causes microarousal and diminishes the amount of slow-wave sleep. A few longitudinal studies in fibromyalgia and rheuma-toid arthritis suggest bidirectional influences; e.g., insomnia worsens later pain, while pain worsens later insomnia. Several other studies stress that the most important link is between insomnia and depression. Recent industry studies of gabapentin and pregabalin in neuropathic pain (Sabatowsky et al. 2004) show that these drugs significantly improve pain, sleep, and mood, but causal inferences are difficult because these drugs are acutely sedative, and the time sequence of these changes was not teased out.

Smith and colleagues (2005) suggest that future longitudinal studies of the effect of cognitive behavioral therapy for insomnia, which is quite effective in a range of conditions, may be particularly useful in chronic pain patients. Such studies may both evaluate the causal contribution of insomnia to chronic pain and determine whether these safe interventions should be added to, or substitute for, the multiple drug treatments commonly used. Of the two available studies in patients with chronic pain of mixed etiologies, both showed significant improvements in sleep (Morin et al. 1989; Currie et al. 2000), and one showed a trend toward later pain improvement (Currie et al. 2000).

The U.S. National Institutes of Health funds a broad range of basic and clinical sleep studies (the funding for 2002 was $162 million, according to the American Academy of Sleep Medicine), but we pain researchers rarely invite these scientists to our meetings. Both fields might benefit from symposia to develop a research agenda to explore the neurobiological links between pain and sleep processing and their clinical implications.

Longitudinal data on the relationship between pain, mood, and abuse of alcohol, opioids, and other substances is even sparser than data on sleep or mood. Controlled trials or cohort studies of opioid treatment rarely exceed 6 weeks in duration. The bitter and unsatisfying controversies about the indications for opioid treatment in chronic pain directly result from this lack of data with which to infer cause. University of Washington clinical epidemiologists have begun to examine these relationships with a cross-sectional study of more than 14,000 patients in a population-based sample (Sullivan et al. 2005). They report that 435 cancer-free patients took an opioid at least several times a week for a month or more, and that these patients were 3–4 times more likely than non-opioid users to meet DSM-IV criteria (American Psychiatric Association 2000) for major depression, dysthymia, generalized anxiety disorder, or panic disorder. Possible interpretations are that pain leads to both opioid treatment and mood disorder, that patients with mood disorder are more likely to complain of enough pain to get an opioid prescription, or that chronic opioids worsen mood. Here again, longitudinal studies are needed to shed more light on the causal relationships.

COMPLEMENTARY APPROACHES TO CHARACTERIZING
THE CAUSES OF POSTHERPETIC NEURALGIA

Communities of scientists have laid the groundwork for many break-through discoveries by adopting model organisms or disease states in which hundreds of studies have characterized many sources of variation in the system's behavior. Such an approach to neuropathic pain conditions might accelerate our progress. Herpes zoster and postherpetic neuralgia has already had enough study to show the potential advantages of such concerted research efforts.

Dworkin and colleagues have conducted many large longitudinal cohort studies. In one recent study (Jung et al. 2004), they examined baseline and 4-month follow-up data from 965 patients with acute herpes zoster enrolled within 72 hours of rash onset into two clinical trials of famciclovir. They found that older age, female sex, presence of a prodrome, greater rash severity, and greater acute pain severity made independent contributions to identifying which patients would have persistent postherpetic neuralgia (PHN). These factors were able to explain 29% of the variance in the likelihood of developing PHN.

Because the sample size in any clinical trial or epidemiological study is proportional to the unexplained variance in the primary outcome, the ability to explain and then extract much of the variance from the error variance means that future researchers will be able to enroll almost one-third fewer patients, compared to the time prior to the knowledge of these covariates. This increase in power will be available whether the investigator is examining the effect of a new molecular, psychological, or sociological variable upon outcome.

A final point is that Jung, Dworkin, and colleagues were more interested in pain mechanisms than in antiviral drug development, but they lacked the resources to enroll almost a thousand patients in their own pain study. As in the case of the Maine Lumbar Spine Study, pain researchers of modest means expanded their resources by piggybacking on the large studies of established internal medicine researchers.

The longitudinal multicenter cohort approach necessary to detect and explain modest portions of the variance in pain patient outcomes stands in contrast to the norm in academic pain research, the intensive single-center bedside sensory physiology study. We seek to emulate at the bedside the successful approach of the bench neurobiologists, most of whom started out as sensory neurophysiologists trained by Patrick Wall or his students. Other fields, such as cardiology, began with bedside physiology studies, but many of the recent advances in understanding the mechanism, prevention, and treatment of cardiac disease have depended upon longitudinal cohort studies. Several decades of quantitative sensory testing (QST) have yielded relatively few practical advances in the treatment of neuropathic pain, and "mechanism-based treatment" guided by sensory examination remains a slogan. Although the standard recommendation for new pain fellows in many universities is to get a QST machine and examine a few dozen patients, I think that more can be gained by sending them for a degree in clinical epidemiology and setting them to work on vast prospective medical or surgical data sets.

Nevertheless, the intensive clinicopathological study of small patient groups will remain a crucial component of pain research and can synergize with the large cohort approach. We would all agree that the University of California San Francisco (UCSF) group's delineation of several distinct anatomical and mechanistic subsets in PHN (Petersen et al. 2000) has advanced our understanding. But QST takes many hours and costly equipment. One can only stimulate intact nerve endings, and it is hard to infer how things are working deeper than the skin. We have argued (Woolf and Max 2001) that drug treatments may be a far more powerful way to infer mechanisms in individual patients than sensory testing, because one can target thousands of distinct receptor sites anywhere in the body.

For example, consider a repeated-dose crossover trial of morphine, nortriptyline, and placebo in 76 PHN patients (Raja et al. 2002). Fig. 2 plots

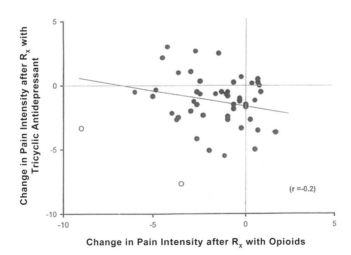

Change in Pain Intensity after R$_x$ with Opioids

Fig. 2. Relationship between pain reduction in postherpetic neuralgia in individual patients treated with chronic tricyclic antidepressants vs. opioids. Each filled circle represents one patient in the crossover study by Raja et al. (2002). Response to the two classes of drugs appears to be independent, suggesting that the drugs reduce neuropathic pain by different mechanisms.

pain reduction with morphine vs. nortriptyline, where each filled circle represents a patient. The complete independence of these responses to the two drugs in individual patients may indicate that they target different pain mechanisms. One might suspect from this data that a tricyclic-opioid combination might be superior to each drug alone, but this hypothesis has not been adequately tested.

In the same study, Raja and colleagues used QST (unpublished data) to subdivide the patients into the UCSF categories of "intact peripheral afferents" versus "partial denervation" by using a cut point for denervation of an elevation of the heat pain threshold of 1°C or more on the PHN-affected side. They hypothesized that the loss of primary nociceptive afferents, whose central synapses bear inhibitory presynaptic opioid receptors, would reduce the efficacy of opioids. As predicted, morphine was not as effective as nortriptyline in this subset. In contrast, morphine far surpassed nortriptyline in the patients without any hypoalgesia, who presumably had ample presynaptic opioid receptors as targets for the drug. These data suggest that for large multicenter studies, the extensive sensory testing battery of the UCSF group might be reduced to a single thermal threshold measurement.

Skin biopsy studies by Oaklander (2001) and the few precious autopsy studies of PHN (Oaklander 1999) are also providing essential information. The advanced age of PHN patients makes PHN the most likely common neuropathic pain condition to be readily studied at autopsy, given more concerted efforts at enrollment. The discriminating power of these small analyses can be enhanced by analyses of simpler endpoints from the large cohort studies discussed above. For example, correlations of peripheral nerve fiber counts with pain outcome in PHN might be sharpened by considering the variance in pain produced by the prognostic variables reported by Jung et al. (2004), to the degree that these variables affect pain by mechanisms independent from the death of peripheral afferents.

MOLECULAR EPIDEMIOLOGY OF CHRONIC NEUROPATHIC PAIN

Pain researchers have identified very few Mendelian disorders of pain processing among the patients in their waiting rooms. Hereditary sensory and autonomic neuropathy, type IV, caused by a mutation in the tyrosine kinase A (TrkA) receptor, is a rare exception. A genetic variant must increase the relative risk of a disorder by at least 50-fold in order for a large family pedigree chart to show an obvious pattern. It is quite possible, however, that chronic neuropathic pain syndromes are "complex genetic disorders," in which common polymorphisms often confer relative risks of between 1.25 and 4 (Mogil and Max 2005).

If we are lucky, there will be variants whose discovery will revolutionize clinical neuropathic pain research. Alzheimer's and Crohn's disease researchers recently had such luck. Inheriting two copies of high-risk alleles such as *APOEε4* in Alzheimer's, and *NOD2* in Crohn's, will increase the risk of disease 4-fold and 17-fold, respectively (Economou et al. 2004; Bird 2005). Common alleles with an effect of this strength can account for one-half or more of the disease burden in the general population. The ability to select high-risk patients by genotyping for these alleles has reduced the needed sample size of natural history or prevention studies by factors almost as high as these relative risks. Even if we are as unlucky as psychiatric geneticists (and I think we can define our cases better), current results in schizophrenia and mood disorders suggest that we would still find multiple candidate genes, each of which might contribute a few percentage points to the variance in pain outcome—and every bit of explained variance helps. Within several years, it will be feasible to assay 500,000 to 1 million single nucleotide polymorphisms (SNPs) to examine every common genetic variant in the human genome for associations with one's disease of interest. If there are common polymorphisms that confer a relative risk of at least 1.5 and we systematically study other prognostic variables, it should be possible to search all human genes with adequate power with sample sizes of several thousand patients or fewer (Fig. 3; Belfer et al. 2004).

PRELIMINARY EVIDENCE THAT CHRONIC
PAIN IS PARTLY HERITABLE

When a researcher applies for funding to carry out candidate gene studies, the first thing the reviewers want to know is whether there is evidence that the disorder is heritable. Some diseases have very low heritability, either because environmental issues predominate or because genes that favor their development reduce the bearer's likelihood of having offspring and are reduced by negative selection.

The finding by Mogil and colleagues (1999) that all 22 different pain phenotypes they studied in inbred mice, including pain behaviors in the Chung and autotomy nerve injury model, have heritabilities of 40–60% demonstrates that common polymorphisms affecting pain behavior did not impair the ability of their ancestor mice to live a good life in the wild. Humans are unlikely to have the same specific polymorphisms as mice, because most human genetic variability arose from a small number of "founder

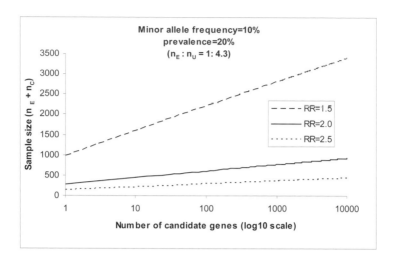

Fig. 3. Merely linear increases in sample size allow *exponential* increases in the numbers of independent genetic loci one can test simultaneously, providing a major incentive to collect large cohorts of patients in genetic association studies. Sample size is plotted against the number of independent polymorphisms tested in a scan of up to 10,000 loci. The injury or disease is assumed to produce an incidence of chronic pain of 20% in patients exposed to at least one copy of the minor allele (i.e., a dominant model; see Belfer et al. [2004] for calculations for co-dominant and recessive models). The three curves in each panel correspond to relative risk (RR) of 1.5, 2.0, and 2.5, and the population frequency of the minor allele is 10%. n_E = number exposed; n_U = number unexposed. The same principle holds for other types of exploratory analyses—whether one wishes to do multiple tests of hypotheses about chemical or psychosocial measures. (Figure provided by courtesy of Dr. Tianxia Wu; reprinted from Max 2004.)

individuals" during recent human population bottlenecks. However, the mouse findings make it plausible that pain-modulating variants might also be present in humans.

Unfortunately, skeptical grant reviewers usually insist on human evidence for heritability, commonly provided by dizygotic vs. monozygotic twin studies. Very few of these have been done in the young field of clinical pain research. Moreover, twin studies are ill-suited to studying specific neuropathic pain conditions. The main question of neuropathic pain researchers is "Why does pain expression vary in patients with the same nerve injury or disease?" It is rare that twins will have the same nerve injury, and even when they do, they develop it at different times, making comparative pain assessment largely retrospective and therefore imprecise.

An alternative to twin studies is examination of candidate polymorphisms. If one can convincingly replicate an association between a common polymorphism and a trait or disease phenotype, the study will support the concept that the trait is somewhat heritable, and that nature does not select against genetic heterogeneity for the trait.

Evidence of such associations is starting to appear for chronic pain. Solovieva et al. (2004a,b) showed that the *3954T* allele of the inflammatory cytokine interleukin 1-β is associated with the prevalence of low back pain, sciatica, and intervertebral disk degeneration in a cohort of Finnish workers. The allele was previously reported to be associated with greater IL-1β expression in vitro.

Several groups have recently replicated associations of another candidate gene with pain and negative affect. Zubieta et al. (2003) showed that a polymorphism in the catechol-*O*-methyl transferase (*COMT*) gene, which reduces the function of this enzyme in breaking down norepinephrine, epinephrine, and dopamine, is associated with higher pain and sensations of unpleasantness and with altered brain enkephalin secretion after infusion of hypertonic saline into the masseter of normal subjects. Diatchenko et al. (2005) have extended this result to show that the hypofunctional *COMT* haplotype is associated with both amplification of experimental pain at baseline and development of temporomandibular muscle pain syndrome during a 3-year follow-up in a cohort of 200 normal young women.

These positive findings, together with the inbred mouse studies, have strengthened the case that genetic variation may account for much of the variation in chronic pain phenotypes. Genetic association studies often leave the investigator with the unanswered question of how the associated polymorphism alters gene function. A demonstration of a plausible effect makes the result far more convincing. But while the Human Genome and HapMap projects have provided a treasure trove of information about gene sequence and common variants, lack of functional data about the variants remains the great missing piece. In the Appendix, we describe the time-intensive methods by which a molecular biologist can explore whether a polymorphism affects protein structure or gene regulation, and raise some questions about whether this can be an ad hoc activity or whether pain neuroscientists should take a more organized approach to elucidating functional consequences of gene variants.

OTHER PHENOTYPE MEASURES

Quantitative sensory testing. Apart from thermal sensation in PHN, QST has thus far provided few clues to central nervous system structural changes or choice of treatment (Rasmussen et al. 2004). A generalized amplification of experimental pain is the hallmark of multisomatoform pain disorders, but it is not obvious that QST responses in body regions free of neural damage provides insight into chronic neuropathic pain. Edwards (2005) reviews recent data suggesting that QST responses can predict postsurgical pain, and speculates that standard tests of pain amplification and inhibition may predict chronic pain outcomes in patients with clear-cut anatomical lesions of nerve or somatic tissues and in those with generalized unexplained pain. Most patients with neuropathic pain are available for study only after the initial injury, so most experimental designs will not have a pain-free baseline. One could study the patients before and after treatment, such as chronic drug administration or surgical release of nerve entrapment.

Measurements of neurotransmitters and proteins in blood, cerebrospinal fluid, and neural tissue. It is likely that there are potential biochemical measurements that could explain some of the variance in the course and features of chronic neuropathic pain. These measurements might be limited to a single chemical entity or a pattern of many molecules, as has been used to diagnose ovarian cancer. Sample size considerations that we have discussed for "fishing" among 25,000 genes can also apply to a search among 100,000 or more proteins. It is surprising that so little work has been done with cerebrospinal fluid chemical measurements, which might reflect chemical processes in the lamina I nociceptive neurons within a millimeter of the interface with pia and cerebrospinal fluid. Provocative experimental pain testing in lumbosacral segments or clinical nociceptive events such as surgery or childbirth might enhance this chemical signal (Mannes et al. 2003; Eisenach et al. 2004).

Brain imaging. Although functional brain imaging has produced novel findings about acute pain processing, we have been disappointed with the limited insights thus far about the pathophysiology of chronic pain. Perhaps this failure to meet expectations is due to the emphasis on techniques that measure brain blood flow. Other methods will be more useful, such as structural magnetic resonance imaging (Apkarian et al. 2004), deoxyglucose uptake, magnetic resonance spectroscopy, or positron emission tomography and single photon emission computed tomography assessment of neurotransmitter physiology.

ENVIRONMENTAL INFLUENCES ON CHRONIC NEUROPATHIC PAIN

The current red-hot topic in the psychiatric genetics literature is gene-environment interactions. It has been difficult to show significant associations between genetic polymorphisms and behavioral disorders, but Caspi and Moffit and their coworkers (Moffit et al. 2005) have shown that several such associations become significant when they rigorously measured a key environmental variable and included it in the genetic analysis. These variables included multiple stressful life events in the effect of the serotonin transporter gene on depression (Caspi et al. 2003), child abuse in the effect of monoamine oxidase A on antisocial personality and adult crime (Caspi 2002), and cannabis use in the effect of *COMT* on adult psychosis.

In a certain sense, we are already reaping the advantages Moffit illustrates for gene by environment analyses when we do genetic studies of chronic neuropathic pain syndromes. Postherpetic pain or chronic lumbar radiculopathy represent a relatively uncommon event triggered by a stereotyped and relatively measurable lesion. From the perspective of central nervous system processing of pain, an inflammatory or compressive lesion of nerve is part of the "environment."

Michael Feuerstein, a pain psychologist who has spent two decades quantifying physical and psychosocial stresses in the workplace and assessing their impact in producing chronic pain (Huang et al. 2003), has observed that pain researchers have virtually ignored the environment. The accessibility of the nerve and the established methods for evaluating upper-extremity mechanics might make carpal tunnel syndrome a good model for mechanistic dissection, but there are few large cohort studies (Manktelow et al. 2004). Significant favorable environmental factors that have been noted in cohort studies include higher educational level as well as timing of surgical diskectomy for lumbar radiculopathy before prolonged disability has occurred (Carragee 2001); surgical sparing of major nerve trunks in breast surgery (Jung et al. 2003); and better glycemic control in diabetic neuropathy (Gooch and Podwall 2004). Childhood physical and sexual abuse is associated with later development of multisomatoform disorders (Katon et al. 2001), but we are not aware of data pertaining to neuropathic pain.

CONCLUSIONS

To better understand and treat the "disease" of a neuropathic pain condition, we must use large prospective studies to determine the causal relationships among pain, mood, sleep, and substance abuse disorders. We must take into account the contributions of covariates that may include demographic variables, coping style, work environment, and genetic polymorphisms. The study of each variable in this web reduces unexplained error variance in the clinical outcome and makes it easier to detect the effects of other biological or psychosocial variables.

Preliminary evidence suggests that the risk of chronic pain in the human as well as the mouse may be partly determined by common genetic variants. Because of the expense of large cohort studies, pain researchers may need to piggyback their questions into studies funded by more established medical researchers. Advances may be more rapid if pain researchers focus on several common neuropathic pain conditions such as PHN, carpal tunnel syndrome, or lumbar radiculopathy.

To assess the clinical domains discussed in large longitudinal cohort studies, we may need briefer measures of variables such as sleep, mood, or substance abuse suited to molecular epidemiology studies. Clinical epidemiology is the most critical underrepresented skill among pain researchers and should be a priority in fellowship programs.

REFERENCES

American Psychiatric Association. *Diagnostic and Statistical Manual of Mental Disorders*, 4th ed. Washington, DC: American Psychiatric Association, 2000.

Apkarian AV, Sosa Y, Sonty S, et al. Chronic back pain is associated with decreased prefrontal and thalamic gray matter density. *J Neurosci* 2004; 24:10410–10415.

Atlas SJ, Deyo RA, Keller RB, et al. The Maine Lumbar Spine Study. Part II. 1-year outcomes of surgical and nonsurgical management of sciatica. *Spine* 1996; 21:1777–1786.

Bair MJ, Robinson RL, Katon W, Kroenke K. Depression and pain comorbidity: a literature review. *Arch Intern Med* 2003; 163:2433–2445.

Bair MJ, Robinson RL, Eckert GJ, et al. Impact of pain on depression treatment response in primary care. *Psychosom Med* 2004; 66:17–22.

Belfer I, Wu T, Kingman A, et al. Candidate gene studies of human pain mechanisms: a method for optimizing choice of polymorphisms and sample size. *Anesthesiology* 2004; 100:1562–1572.

Bernard JF, Peschanski M, Besson JM. A possible spino (trigemino)-ponto-amygdaloid pathway for pain. *Neurosci Lett* 1989; 100:83–88.

Bird TD. Genetic factors in Alzheimer's disease. *N Engl J Med* 2005; 352:862–864.

Bonica JJ. *The Management of Pain,* 2nd ed. Philadelphia: Lea & Febiger, 1990.

Botstein D, Risch N. Discovering genotypes underlying human phenotypes: past successes for Mendelian disease, future approaches for complex disease. *Nat Genet* 2003; 33:228–237.

Burstein R. Somatosensory and visceral input to the hypothalamus and limbic system. *Prog Brain Res* 1996; 107:257–267.

Burstein, Cliffer KD, Giesler GJ Jr. Direct somatosensory projections from the spinal cord to the hypothalamus and telencephalon. *J Neurosci* 1987; 7:4159–4164.

Carragee EJ. Psychological screening in the surgical treatment of lumbar disc herniation. *Clin J Pain* 2001; 7:215–219.

Casarett D, Karlawish, Sankar P, Hirschman K, Asch DA. Designing pain research from the patient's perspective: what trial end points are important to patients with chronic pain. *Pain Med* 2001; 2:309–316.

Caspi A, McClay J, Moffitt TE, et al. Role of genotype in the cycle of violence in maltreated children. *Science* 2002; 297:851–853.

Caspi A, Sugden K, Moffitt TE, et al. Influence of life stress on depression: moderation by a polymorphism in the 5-HTT gene. *Science* 2003; 301:386–389.

Cechetto DF, Standaert DB, Saper CB. Spinal and trigeminal dorsal horn projections to the parabrachial nucleus in the rat. *J Comp Neurol* 1985; 240:153–160.

Charney DS, Manji HK. Life stress, genes, and depression: multiple pathways lead to increased risk and new opportunities for intervention. *Sci STKE* 2004; 225:re5.

Currie SR, Wison KG, Pontefract AJ, deLaplante L. Cognitive-behavioral treatment of insomnia secondary to chronic pain. *J Consult Clin Psychol* 2000; 68:407–416.

Diatchenko L, Slade GD, Bhalang K, et al. Genetic basis for individual variations in pain perception and the development of a chronic pain condition. *Hum Mol Genet* 2005; 14:135–143.

Economou M, Trikalinos TA, Loizou KT, Tsianos EV, Ioannidis JP. Differential effects of NOD2 variants on Crohn's disease risk and phenotype in diverse populations: a meta-analysis. *Am J Gastroenterol* 2004; 99:2393–2404.

Edwards RR. Hypothesis: individual differences in endogenous pain modulation as a risk factor for chronic pain. *Neurology* 2005; 65:437–443.

Eisenach JC, Thomas JA, Rauck RL, Curry R, Li X. Cystatin C in cerebrospinal fluid is not a diagnostic test for pain in humans. *Pain* 2004; 107:207–212.

Gooch C, Podwall D. The diabetic neuropathies. *Neurologist* 2004; 10:311–322.

Huang GD, Feuerstein M, Kop WJ, Schor K, Arroyo F. Individual and combined impacts of biomechanical and work organization factors in work-related musculoskeletal symptoms. *Am J Ind Med* 2003; 43:495–506.

Hylden JL, Anton F, Nahin RL. Spinal lamina I projection neurons in the rat: collateral innervation of parabrachial area and thalamus. *Neuroscience* 1989; 28:27–37.

Jung BF, Ahrendt GM, Oaklander AL, Dworkin RH. Neuropathic pain following breast cancer surgery: proposed classification and research update. *Pain* 2003; 104:1–13.

Jung BF, Johnson RW, Griffin DRJ, Dworkin RH. Risk factors for postherpetic neuralgia in patients with herpes zoster. *Neurology* 2004; 62:1545–1551.

Katon W, Sullivan M, Walker E. Medical symptoms without identified pathology: relationship to psychiatric disorders, childhood and adult trauma, and personality traits. *Ann Intern Med* 2001; 134(9, pt 2):917–925.

Knight JC, Keating BJ, Rockett KA, Kwiatkowski DP. In vivo characterization of regulatory polymorphisms by allele-specific quantification of RNA polymerase loading. *Nat Genet* 2003; 33:469–475.

Manktelow RT, Binhammer P, Tomat LR, Bril V, Szalai JP. Carpal tunnel syndrome: cross-sectional and outcome study in Ontario workers. *J Hand Surg* 2004; 29A:307–317.

Mannes AJ, Martin BM, Yang HY, et al. Cystatin C as a cerebrospinal fluid biomarker for pain in humans. *Pain* 2003; 102:251–256.

Max MB. Assessing pain candidate gene studies. *Pain* 2004; 109:1–3.

Morin CM, Kowatch RA, Wade JB. Behavioral management of sleep disturbances secondary to chronic pain. *J Behav Ther Exp Psychiatry* 1989; 20:295–302.

Moffitt TE, Caspi A, Rutter M. Strategy for investigating interactions between measured genes and measured environments. *Arch Gen Psychiatry* 2005; 62:473–481.

Mogil JS, Max MB. The genetics of pain. In: Koltzenburg M, McMahon SB (Eds.) *Wall and Melzack's Textbook of Pain,* 5th ed. London: Elsevier, 2005, pp 159–174.

Mogil JS, Wilson SG, Bon K, et al. Heritability of nociception I: responses of 11 inbred mouse strains on 12 measures of nociception. *Pain* 1999; 80:67–82.

Neugebauer V, Li W, Bird GC, Han JS. The amygdale and persistent pain. *Neuroscientist* 2004; 10:221–234.

Oaklander AL. The pathology of shingles: Head and Campbell's 1900 monograph. *Arch Neurol* 1999; 56:1292–1294.

Oaklander AL. The density of remaining nerve endings in human skin with and without postherpetic neuralgia after shingles. *Pain* 2001; 92:139–145.

Petersen KL, Fields HL, Brennum J, Sandroni P, Rowbotham MC. Capsaicin evoked pain and allodynia in post-herpetic neuralgia. *Pain* 2000; 88:125–133.

Rasmussen PV, Sindrup SH, Jensen TS, Bach FW. Therapeutic outcome in neuropathic pain: relationship to evidence of nervous system lesion. *Eur J Neurol* 2004; 11:545–553.

Raja SN, Haythornthwaite JA, Pappagallo M, et al. A placebo-controlled trial comparing the analgesic and cognitive effects of opioids and tricyclic antidepressants in postherpetic neuralgia. *Neurology* 2002; 59:1015–1021.

Sabatowsky R, Galvez R, Cherry DA, et al. Pregabalin reduces pain and improves sleep and mood disturbances in patients with post-herpetic neuralgia: results of a randomised, placebo-controlled clinical trial. *Pain* 2004; 109:26–35.

Smith MT, Haythornthwaite JA. How do sleep disturbance and chronic pain inter-relate? Insights from the longitudinal and cognitive-behavioral clinical trials literature. *Sleep Med Rev* 2004; 8:119–132.

Smith MT, Huang MI, Manber R. Cognitive behavior therapy for chronic insomnia occurring within the context of medical and psychiatric disorders. *Clin Psychol Rev* 2005; 25:559–592.

Solovieva S, Leino-Arjas P, Saarela J, et al. Possible association of interleukin 1 gene locus polymorphisms with low back pain. *Pain* 2004a; 109:8–19.

Solovieva S, Kouhia S, Leino-Arjas P, et al. Interleukin 1 polymorphisms and intervertebral disc degeneration. *Epidemiology* 2004b; 15:626–633.

Sullivan M, Edlund M, Steffic D, Unutzer J. Regular use of prescribed opioids: association with common psychiatric disorders in a population-based sample. *Abstracts: Annual Meeting of the American Pain Society.* Glenview, IL: American Pain Society, 2005.

Von Korff M, Simon G. The relationship between pain and depression. *Br J Psychiatry* 1996; 168(Suppl 30):101–108.

Woolf CJ, Max MB. Mechanism-based pain diagnosis: issues for analgesic drug development. *Anesthesiology* 2001; 95:241–249.

Zubieta JK, Heitzeg MM, Smith YR, et al. *COMT val158met* genotype affects mu-opioid neurotransmitter responses to a pain stressor. *Science* 2003; 299:1240–1243.

Correspondence to: Mitchell Max, MD, NIH, Building 10, 3C-405, Bethesda, MD 20892-1258, USA. Tel: 301-594-3630; Fax: 301-402-4347; email: mm77k@nih.gov.

Appendix

SO YOU HAVE A SIGNIFICANT CLINICAL ASSOCIATION WITH A SNP: DO YOU NEED A MOLECULAR BIOLOGIST?

A common result of clinical candidate gene studies is that one finds a statistically significant association of a single nucleotide polymorphism (SNP) or combination of SNPs (haplotype) with the primary clinical outcome, but it is not obvious how the polymorphisms alter the function of the gene or resulting mRNA or protein. For example, a SNP in a coding region may be "synonymous," that is, specifying the same amino acid in both of its alleles. The majority of the associations initially reported in the literature have not been replicated and are probably chance findings. Obviously, the finding should be replicated in a second clinical cohort, but if one cannot find colleagues with similar data sets, this task may take years. In the meantime, one cannot publish such a result in a high-impact journal or convince skeptics that the findings are real without a better understanding of the functional mechanism.

Perhaps the common polymorphism that was tested has no effect by itself, but owes its statistical power to another rarer genetic variant at a nearby locus in linkage disequilibrium that alters an amino acid in a critical part of the protein. Botstein and Risch (2003) have suggested that such important variants may be missed if one relies on the standard haplotype approach using genotype data and inference of haplotypes from the International HapMap Project. Many of the genetic variants in this project were identified in a sample of 20 individual chromosomes or less, an approach that often misses variants of 5–10% population frequency. We are not aware of a comprehensive database of resequencing data, so one must search the published literature to see if others have resequenced the gene of interest in 50–100 individuals. If so, one can do additional genotyping for uncommon SNPs of interest, and if not, any genetics laboratory can resequence the gene for interesting individuals with extreme clinical results, or with the high-risk haplotype.

Unfortunately, one may still be left with an associated SNP without clear functional effect. In the next few pages we will describe some of the studies that might be used to delineate functional ramifications of the presence of a given genetic variant.

As part of the long-term strategy for neuropathic pain research, particularly pain genetics, we want to summarize how pain neurobiologists in the coming years may address this dearth of functional data.

BIOINFORMATIC TOOLS

Ninety-eight percent of the human genome does not encode proteins. The noncoding sequences contain regulatory regions in which polymorphisms may alter gene expression, as well as noncoding and nonfunctional sequences. These two functionally different types of sequences are difficult to distinguish. Comparative sequence analysis of phylogenetically different organisms is the most powerful tool to identify sequences that are conserved between species and may harbor functionally important regulatory sequences. These phylogenetic footprints are regions that change much less during evolution than adjacent nonfunctional sequences due to stabilizing selection. With the completion of several vertebrate genome sequencing efforts (in rat, mouse, cow, dog, chicken, and fish species), sequence comparison of ortholog genes and adjacent (±E 10 kb) regions from several species is feasible, as well as the less computationally intensive alignment of human-mouse ortholog sequences. A SNP that shows association with a phenotype and is located in a phylogenetically conserved region is more likely to possess functional significance than SNPs situated in phylogenetically divergent, thus presumably nonfunctional, regions. The GenomeBrowser of the University of California at Santa Cruz (http://genome.ucsc.edu/) displays the alignment of these phylogenetically conserved regions among several species, and SNPs can be also displayed in this context. In silico analysis may also indicate if a SNP is in a putative transcription factor-binding site and might interrupt or alter binding of a transcription factor to its cognate element. However, in silico prediction of transcription factor binding should be taken only as a helpful hint; it should not be relied on without further in vitro or in vivo investigation.

EXPERIMENTAL APPROACHES TO DEFINING THE FUNCTION OF NONCODING POLYMORPHISMS

Single nucleotide polymorphisms that are identified in putative regulatory regions may be further analyzed to show that they indeed alter the transcription of the gene in question. Messenger RNA levels for the gene can be measured in individuals homozygous for the two alleles. Tissue-specificity is a major concern in these experiments, since many regulatory elements influence cell- or tissue-specific gene expression. As a result, a SNP that influences gene expression in the heart or vasculature may not have any effect on expression in other tissues. Access to some cells in humans is relatively easy (different blood cells or cells from routinely performed tissue biopsies); however, it is difficult to assess many tissues. Postmortem tissue samples in large enough numbers (particularly for rare variants) are hard to find, and additional significant variability comes from age, sex, medications, disease states, environmental factors, and postmortem interval. In addition, these individuals differ not only in the SNP in question, but also in millions of other loci. These confounding factors make it very difficult, if not impossible, to detect whether a polymorphism has a modest effect on transcription.

In vitro methods offer an alternative in which one can keep constant all other factors besides the SNP in question. Regulation of gene expression most commonly happens through DNA protein interaction, whereas transcription factors regulate transcription following their binding to specific short sequences in the promoter region. There are several in vitro methods to assay these DNA-protein interactions.

ELECTROPHORETIC MOBILITY SHIFT ASSAYS

If the SNP appears to be located in a transcription factor binding site, electrophoretic mobility shift assays (EMSA) are the technically easiest to perform to evaluate whether a sequence polymorphism results in altered DNA-protein interaction. In EMSA, short DNA sequences are synthesized for both SNP alleles. After annealing and radiolabeling, these probes are incubated with nuclear protein extracts, which are prepared from cells where the gene is expressed. The DNA/protein complexes are then resolved on non-denaturing polyacrylamide gels. Both free and protein-bound probes are detected by autoradiography, and the intensity of the bound probe reflects the extent of binding to transcription factors in the nuclear extracts. Comparison of the intensity of the protein-DNA complexes of two SNP alleles can reveal whether the SNP alters transcription factor binding to the DNA element. Further information regarding the identity of the transcription factor forming a complex with the probe can be obtained in "supershift" experiments, which use specific antibodies against transcription factors. Addition of these antibodies to the DNA-protein complexes either specifically disrupts the interaction, leading to diminished amounts of protein-DNA complexes detected, or may result in a complex with higher molecular mass that is further retained in the gel, as a result "supershifting" the complex.

DNA FOOTPRINTING

The limitations of the EMSA technique are that it requires prior knowledge of putative transcription factor-binding element in the region surrounding the SNP and that it is amenable only for analysis of a short sequence (about 20 bp). In promoter regions where more than one SNP may be present and may show association with a phenotype, DNA footprinting may offer a better alternative. In these experiments, the DNA may be several hundred base pairs in length and may contain several SNP alleles that reflect the haplotypes in which they occur. The DNA is labeled on one end and is either chemically or enzymatically cleaved in such a way that each molecule is cleaved only once and at a random site. The DNA is then resolved by denaturing polyacrylamide gel electrophoresis. The resulting ladder-like DNA fragments are visualized by autoradiography. When the DNA is cleaved following incubation with nuclear extracts, protein binding to specific DNA regions protects the DNA from cleavage. The autoradiogram then reveals gaps in the DNA ladder corresponding to the footprint of the protecting proteins. When a sequencing reaction is run side by side with the DNA footprinting, the exact sequence of the footprints can be determined. Comparison of the footprints (if they are present) on the DNA probes containing different SNP alleles may indicate functional differences between the two alleles.

REPORTER GENE ASSAYS

Differential binding of transcription factors to DNA sequences containing each SNP allele suggests that the particular SNP may be functional. Nevertheless, to show that the SNP alleles indeed regulate transcription differentially, further experiments are needed. The assay most commonly used to investigate the functional effects of polymorphic sites, deletions, or mutations on transcriptional activity involves reporter gene constructs transiently transfected into cell lines. This approach involves creating a plasmid vector in which a reporter gene (most commonly luciferase) is linked to the regulatory regions differing in the SNP alleles. In a promoterless vector, expression of the reporter gene is fully driven by the regulatory region being inserted. Alternatively, vectors may contain a constituently active promoter, and the putative regulatory element inserted upstream from the promoter may influence transcription driven by the promoter. In any case, the reporter plasmid is introduced into an appropriate cell line by transient transfection, and the activity of the reporter gene, which reflects its level of expression, is measured. Since efficiency of transient transfection varies considerably between samples, an additional reporter plasmid, which contains a different reporter, is usually co-transfected and used for normalization. It is essential to use a cell line for the transfections that is close to the cell types physiologically expressing the gene from which the regulatory element is derived, because transcription factors that bind to the given regulatory element may not be ubiquitously expressed in all cells. In addition to cell specificity, one also needs to consider inducibility. If the regulatory sequence is responsible for inducible, and not constitutive, expression, then reporter activity following appropriate activation should be monitored at multiple time points. Reporter constructs in transient transfection assays provide valuable information regarding the potential influence of sequence variation in regulatory regions on the rate of transcription. However, these assays often yield different and sometimes conflicting results in the context of different cell types, method of transfection, level of reporter vector, and mode of induction.

GENOMIC FOOTPRINTING

Assays described above are particularly suited for the analysis of regulatory elements and their polymorphisms in isolation, but the functional effects of sequence variations may also depend upon the haplotype on which they occur and could be influenced by interactions with other polymorphisms on the same haplotype. All the in vitro experiments described above use "naked" DNA segments isolated from their natural context on the chromosome. In reality, transcription occurs on chromatin templates, which have an intricate interaction between modified DNA and histone molecules. In vivo protein-DNA interaction may also be investigated, but it is much more challenging technically. In vivo genomic DNA footprinting involves treatment of living cells with dimethylsulfate, which penetrates the cells and causes the modification of accessible guanine residues of the DNA, which are not protected by a bound protein. The modified DNA is then cleaved, and the fragments are amplified by ligation-mediated polymerase chain reaction (PCR). Although this method can be used for identifying in vivo DNA-protein interaction, its inherent variability so far has not allowed the demonstration that SNP alleles differentially influence in vivo protein-DNA interaction. When the factor binding to the regulatory sequence is known, chromatin immunoprecipitation may also be used. In these assays, DNA is covalently crosslinked with interacting proteins using formaldehyde, and then sheared to yield fragments of certain size. The DNA-protein complexes are then immunoprecipitated using antibodies specific to different transcription factors. Afterwards, the crosslink is reversed, and the DNA fragments are purified. Level of DNA-protein interaction can be assessed by real-time PCR to measure the amount of specific sequences in the immunoprecipitated DNA.

HAPLOCHIP ASSAYS

In recognition of the importance of studying the effect of a sequence variation in vivo in the context of naturally occurring transcription machinery and chromatin landscape, Knight et al. (2003) developed a new method called HaploChip. The method uses chromatin immunoprecipitation and mass spectrometry to measure how alleles of "regulatory" SNPs influence transcription by monitoring the amount of phosphorylated polymerase II enzyme associated with DNA strands containing each SNP allele.

REGULATION OF GLOBAL GENE EXPRESSION

Global gene expression profiles may also be considered molecular phenotypes that are dependent on functional genetic polymorphism. Microarray analysis of tissue-specific gene expression in individuals or cells carrying different SNP alleles may identify gene networks and complex adaptive changes in response to different alleles of regulatory SNPs, particularly if the SNP is in the promoter of a gene involved in the regulation of numerous targets, such as transcription factors and intracellular signaling molecules. However, the cost and technical difficulties associated with this technique make it less amenable for large-scale analysis of regulatory SNPs.

DIFFERENTIAL ALLELIC EXPRESSION

The effect of SNPs that do not encode non-synonymous changes but are located in the region transcribed to mRNA may be assessed by measuring differential allelic expression. Studying heterozygous individuals, so the SNP alleles share the same cellular environment, can eliminate confounding factors mentioned previously. Differential allelic expression can be measured by real-time reverse transcription PCR using primers specific for the alleles. It is important in these experiments to consider cell- and tissue-specific expression, since the effect of regulatory polymorphisms in tissue-specific regulatory regions may not be evident in all tissues.

ANALYSIS OF PROTEIN LEVELS

The previous paragraphs described how to assess whether SNPs in regulatory regions affect transcription. However, gene expression and protein levels often correlate poorly. When a polymorphism does not alter the primary protein sequence, it needs to alter expression levels in order to be considered functional. Therefore, the most direct way to assess functionality of a SNP may be to measure protein levels in certain tissues and correlate them with SNP alleles. This approach would give the ultimate answer as to whether the SNP alleles indeed correspond to different amounts of the protein encoded by the gene within whose regulatory region the SNP is located. The method for assaying protein levels may vary according to the tissue or cell type one wishes to analyze, and according to the type of protein. In general, antibodies against the protein are used in Western blot or ELISA assays.

Enzyme-linked immunosorbent Assays (ELISAs) are designed for detection and quantification of substances such as peptides, proteins, and hormones and are particularly useful to assay serum, plasma, or cerebrospinal fluid. In an ELISA, an antigen is immobilized to a solid surface. The antigen is then complexed with an antibody that is linked to an enzyme. Detection is accomplished by incubating this enzyme complex with a substrate that produces a detectable and quantifiable product. ELISA assays are relatively high throughput, which can be performed in 96-well (or 384-well) plates. The ability to wash away nonspecifically bound materials makes ELISA a powerful tool for measuring specific proteins within a crude preparation.

In Western blot experiments, aliquots of tissue or cell extracts are loaded onto sodium dodecyl sulfate polyacrylamide gels, and the proteins are separated by molecular mass. The separated proteins are then blotted to nylon, nitrocellulose, or polyvinylidene difluoride (PVDF) membranes. After blocking nonspecific binding, it is possible to detect specific proteins by incubation with an antibody or polyclonal antiserum. A detection enzyme may be linked directly to the primary antibody or introduced through a secondary antibody that recognizes the primary antibody and then linked to an enzyme, most commonly to horseradish peroxidase or alkaline phosphatase. A large selection of substrates is available for performing quantitative analysis with these conjugates.

Although analysis of protein levels may seem to be an ideal way to assess the functionality of a regulatory SNP, there are disadvantages to this approach. Obtaining tissue samples from humans is difficult, and finding homozygotes for a rare allele in particular may also be problematic. Other confounding factors, including genetic differences at other loci, age, gender, disease states, medications, and environmental differences, may hamper interpretation of the data.

The techniques listed above range from simple and straightforward to difficult, time-consuming, and expensive. The extent to which each SNP is analyzed may depend on several factors, such as the strength of association or successful replication in an independent data set. However, the best approach may be the combination of several experimental assays following an initial bioinformatics analysis.

Emerging Strategies for the Treatment of Neuropathic Pain, edited by James N. Campbell, Allan I. Basbaum, André Dray, Ronald Dubner, Robert H. Dworkin, and Christine N. Sang, IASP Press, Seattle, © 2006.

16

Tailoring Pharmacotherapy to Diagnostic Subgroups in the Treatment of Neuropathic Pain

William K. Schmidt and Randall W. Moreadith

Renovis, Inc., South San Francisco, California, USA

Neuropathic pain represents a group of heterologous acute and chronic disorders of sensory perception characterized by mild, moderate, or severe pain that may vary in sensory quality from burning, tingling, shooting, stabbing, or "electric" shock pain, to abnormal evoked pain responses occurring during routine daily activities, or to persistent spontaneous pain (continuous or intermittent) throughout the day (Dworkin 2002). Some patients may have further "negative" changes in sensory perception that are not necessarily painful by themselves (paresthesias, dysesthesias), but which may lead to changes in sensitivities to other sensory stimuli including pinprick, touch, pressure, cold, heat, and vibration (Dworkin 2002; Herr 2004).

Neuropathic pain syndromes share certain key features including hyperalgesia (exaggerated perception of pain or shifts in stimulation thresholds to noxious stimuli) and allodynia (perception of pain to non-noxious stimuli) that help to distinguish them from inflammatory, visceral, or somatic pain. Some types of neuropathic pain may be characterized as "mixed pain" and may share features with, and yet still be identifiably different from, inflammatory pain or musculoskeletal pain (Baron and Binder 2004). For example, lumbar radiculopathy pain (sciatica) may occur in patients with lower back pain, but the neuropathic pain component may have further external or internal characteristics suggestive of chronic nerve damage. Other types of neuropathic pain may be caused by chronic nerve injury with no obvious inflammation or target organ dysfunction other than distortions of sensory perception, such as central post-stroke pain. For most patients with neuropathic pain, the altered sensory qualities of sensory perception represent only part of the total "pain experience," which may include changes in physical, emotional, and spiritual health, the ability to work, and changes in family and social relationships (Arnstein 2004).

Neuropathic pain syndromes that are most often studied in controlled clinical trials of novel pharmaceutical agents include postherpetic neuralgia (PHN), painful diabetic neuropathy (PDN), lumbar radiculopathy, HIV neuropathies, persistent lower back pain, trigeminal neuralgia, and cancer pain (Backonja and Serra 2004a). Other types of neuropathic pain that are less often evaluated in drug registration trials, but which remain of considerable interest for the study of mechanisms of action, include phantom limb pain, complex regional pain syndrome (CRPS), central post-stroke pain (CPSP), spinal cord injury (SCI) pain, chemotherapy-induced neuropathies, alcohol-induced neuropathy, postmastectomy and post-thoracotomy neuropathies, post-traumatic neuralgia, and chronic postsurgical neuropathic pain (Backonja and Serra 2004b; Finnerup and Jensen 2004).

Patients may differ substantially in their perception of or resistance to neuropathic pain, and not everyone experiencing the same initial insult will experience similar changes in sensory perception, if indeed any at all. For instance, it is estimated that 25–50% of normal healthy patients with acute herpes zoster may develop postherpetic neuralgia, defined as persistent pain 3 months after the onset of the initial rash (Schmader 2002); the incidence of persistent pain is lower in those who receive antiviral therapy within days after presentation of the initial herpes zoster rash. Risk factors for a higher incidence of PHN include advanced age, female sex, greater severity of acute pain, greater rash severity, greater sensory impairment, psychological distress, and a painful prodrome (Schmader 2002; Jung et al. 2004). Patients with certain leukemias or lymphomas, HIV infection, or compromised immune function following transplantation and treatment with immunosuppressive drugs may have a greater incidence of both herpes zoster and PHN (Lojeski and Stevens 2000; Herrero et al. 2004).

Large systematic reviews of neuropathic pain treatment have shown that only one-third to one-half of patients achieve moderate or better levels of pain relief, regardless of diagnostic category (McQuay et al. 1996; Sindrup and Jensen 1999; Collins et al. 2000). Intolerable side effects often limit the ability to achieve adequate pain control with a single agent, leading either to discontinuation of specific agents or to progressive treatment strategies to optimize pain control for individual patients (Namaka et al. 2004).

CURRENT TREATMENT OPTIONS

Even within the same disease, responses to neuropathic pain treatment may vary from patient to patient, and few patients obtain complete pain relief. Most patients receive multiple agents with divergent mechanisms of action that collectively work to diminish the peripheral and central manifestations of pain. For more intense pain, opioids and nonsteroidal anti-inflammatory drugs (NSAIDs) are often used in conjunction with gabapentin or amitriptyline for treating PHN pain; other treatment options include antidepressants, anticonvulsants, and topical analgesics. Table I provides a list of currently available medications with indications for specific neuropathic pain syndromes approved by the U.S. Food and Drug Administration (FDA). Table II lists additional medications that are FDA-approved for other diseases (most often epilepsy) that are being evaluated for specific neuropathic pain conditions (Backonja 2004; Schmidt 2004). Older, generically available compounds (e.g., amitriptyline, nortriptyline, carbamazepine, and dextromethorphan) that are indicated for treatment of depression or epilepsy are frequently used to treat neuropathic pain symptoms based on a combination of empirical and rational evidence-based medical approaches.

TOWARD A MORE RATIONAL PHARMACOTHERAPY: USE OF DIAGNOSTIC SUBGROUPS

Evaluation of mechanisms responsible for the initiation or maintenance of neuropathic pain may offer treatments with greater efficacy and selectivity with fewer side effects. Woolf and others (Sindrup and Jensen 1999; Jensen and Baron 2003; Woolf 2004) have emphasized the rationale for using treatments directed toward specific symptoms or mechanisms of neuropathic pain rather than at traditional disease classifications. For example, treatment strategies may be more successful if they focus on specific

Table I
Medications for neuropathic pain that are approved in the United States

Generic Name	Trade Name	Sponsor	Indication(s)	Approval Date
Carbamazepine	Tegretol®	Novartis	Epilepsy, trigeminal neuralgia	1968
Lidocaine patch	Lidoderm®	Endo	PHN	1999
Gabapentin	Neurontin®	Pfizer	Epilepsy, PHN	2002
Duloxetine	Cymbalta®	Eli Lilly	Depression, PDN	2004
Ziconotide	Prialt™	Elan	Morphine-resistant severe pain	2004
Pregabalin	Lyrica®†	Pfizer	Epilepsy, PHN, PDN	2004

Abbreviations: PDN = peripheral diabetic neuropathy; PHN = postherpetic neuralgia.
†Launched in the United States in September 2005.

Table II
Investigational compounds for neuropathic pain
with approvals for other diseases

Generic Name	Trade Name	Sponsor	Approved Indication(s)	Clinical Status for Neuropathic Pain
Memantine	Namenda™	Forest	Alzheimer's	Phase III
Oxcarbazepine	Trileptal®	Novartis	Epilepsy	Phase III
Lamotrigine	Lamictal®	GSK	Epilepsy	Phase III
Topiramate	Topamax®	Johnson & Johnson	Epilepsy, migraine	Phase III
Tiagabine	Gabitril®	Cephalon	Epilepsy	Phase II
Levetiracetam	Keppra®	UCB	Epilepsy	Phase II
Zonisamide	Zonegran®	Eisai	Epilepsy	Phase I

Source: Data from Pharmaprojects (July 2005).

neuropathic pain phenomena such as pain paroxysms (possibly due to excessive ion channel stimulation in the dorsal root ganglion or dorsal horn), C-fiber hyperalgesia (possibly due to overexpression of TRPV1 or other ligand-gated ion channels in the dermis), touch-evoked allodynia (Aβ-fiber-recruited central sensitization), or sympathetic hyperactivity. Current treatment strategies might then be directed toward reducing touch-evoked pain using compounds that work locally on ion channels or using compounds with known actions on central hyperexcitability, much as we use anti-inflammatory agents to reduce inflammation-driven traumatic or musculoskeletal pain.

Simple diagnostic techniques may be used to assess the presence of negative symptoms including reduced sensitivity to touch, pinprick, cold or warm sensations, or vibration, and positive symptoms such as ongoing spontaneous pains (paresthesias, paroxysms, superficial burning pain, or deep pain), touch-evoked allodynia, cold-induced hyperalgesia, or sympathetically-maintained pain. These positive symptoms may point either to specific neurological deficits or to ectopic hyperexcitability, suggesting a basis for specific pharmacological interventions (Jensen and Baron 2003; Woolf 2004).

Multiple mechanisms coexisting within a given patient may provide the basis for rational combinations of pharmacotherapies to treat specific symptoms. Over time, there may be an evolution from one or more early drivers of pain to others, as aberrant nociceptors shift to deafferentation or central sensitization begins to dominate. While this evolution may demand a periodic change in treatment strategies, it also demands attention to earlier, more comprehensive strategies directed toward *preventing* the onset of more insidious drivers of pain that are progressively more difficult to treat.

This strategy may become increasingly important as newer treatments are developed based on the presumed biological mechanisms that underlie the pain. A recent survey identified at least 14 targeted strategies in current clinical development that may be used to reduce specific drivers of ongoing neuropathic pain (Table III; Schmidt 2004). Other strategies that may be considered for future clinical development include methods to target mechanisms responsible for alterations in the density, distribution, phenotype, or kinetics of ion channels that maintain ectopic excitability, or methods to block alterations in the transcription, post-translational changes, and trafficking of ion channels after nerve injury. Other potential strategies might target central nervous system mechanisms responsible for the neuroplasticity involved in changing receptive fields or that maintain perceptions of pain even in the absence of intact peripheral nociceptors or spinothalamic processes that carry the signals to the brain (Devor 2004; Woolf 2004). Novel strategies may also be used to reduce the activation of glial cells, interfere with the recruitment of monocytes or macrophages that attack neurons or Schwann cells, or inhibit the release and action of pro-inflammatory cytokines that influence the development or maintenance of neuropathic pain (Manning 2004).

PRACTICAL CONSIDERATIONS FOR FUTURE DRUG DEVELOPMENT

As indicated above, current and future clinical trials are likely to involve both antinociceptive and disease-modifying approaches for the treatment of

Table III
Newer approaches to the treatment of neuropathic pain

Neuronal Na^+ channel blockers ($Na_v1.8$, $Na_v1.9$)
Neuronal Ca^{2+} channel blockers ($Ca_v2.2$)
Neuronal K^+ channel antagonists (KCNQ)
Neuronal nicotinic agonists ($\alpha_4\beta_2$)
Nerve growth factor antagonists
NMDA antagonists (glycine site, NR2B site, PCP site)
AMPA/kainite antagonists (GluR5 site)
Adenosine (A1a) agonists/receptor modulators
N-acetylated α-linked acidic dipeptidase (NAALADase) inhibitors
Superoxide dismutase (SOD) mimetics
Cytokine antagonists: tumor necrosis factor-α, interleukin (IL)-1, IL-6
Lipoxygenase or leukotriene inhibitors (5-LO, LTB4)
Cannabinoid agonists (CB-1, CB-2)
Vanilloid TRPV1 agonists/antagonists

specific neuropathic pain *symptoms*. Where there are commonalities in the underlying pathology, compounds may work in multiple types of neuropathic pain syndromes; for example, postherpetic neuralgia and diabetic neuropathy may both benefit from drugs which reduce ectopic hyperexcitability. Thus, novel agents developed to treat specific neuropathic pain syndromes may have application in other types of inflammatory or nociceptive pain. Hence, *mechanistic distinctions* and knowledge about the presence or absence of specific receptors, ion channels, nociceptive transmitters, or trophic factors that initiate or support the maintenance of neuropathic pain may be key to understanding the generalizability of drugs from one type of pain syndrome to another or between neuropathic pain and other neurological or psychiatric diseases.

CONCOMITANT MEDICATIONS/DRUG COMBINATION TRIALS

For patients with existing pain, most will have been treated with commercially available medications that may have failed to provide adequate pain relief, hence their motivation for seeking more effective treatments or treatments with fewer side effects. Nevertheless, most will continue to receive concomitant medications during the trial period that may either facilitate or reduce the effectiveness of drug responses. This consideration is especially important for P450 enzyme inducers or inhibitors if the test medication or any concomitant medications are subject to oxidative metabolism. For trials in PHN in particular, many patients will have received gabapentin prior to enrollment; strategies must be addressed in advance to include or exclude such patients from the clinical trial or to prospectively analyze those who use specific medications.

In a recent 5-week, four-period, crossover clinical trial, Gilron et al. (2005) found that a combination of controlled-release morphine with gabapentin was more effective at lower doses than either drug alone. Such therapies should be explored in greater detail where there is a rational basis to target drug combinations to reduce pain or other symptoms in neuropathic pain trials.

PLACEBO RESPONSE/SPONTANEOUS RESOLUTION

In some neuropathic pain syndromes such as PHN, patients may have spontaneous resolution of pain over a period of months to years. There are no current strategies to evaluate *who* might have spontaneous recovery or *what mechanisms* drive this response. Strategies that are targeted toward disease modification to prevent onset of symptoms where there is a predictable onset time or that hasten the resolution of symptoms would be highly desirable. However, spontaneous resolution of symptoms is too often attributed to "placebo response" without a systematic evaluation of the causes of pain relief. While most studies report the mean or median and variance in placebo versus test group responses over time, few studies have reported individual responses over time.

For acute pain studies, Farrar et al. (2003) have shown that changes of 2.0 or greater (33%) in pain intensity difference on a 0–10-point numeric rating scale are associated with a clinically meaningful response. Similar validation is urgently required to determine "clinically meaningful" response rates in specific neuropathic pain *syndromes*, or for specific *symptoms* irrespective of clinical diagnosis.

CONCLUSIONS

Diagnostic subgroups that attempt to identify *mechanisms* responsible for the initiation or maintenance of neuropathic pain are clearly important in evaluating changes in specific *symptoms* of neuropathic pain over time. Neurophysiological and molecular data indicate that there may be similarities in certain drivers for allodynia in PHN, diabetic neuropathy, and other neuropathic pain states. These similarities suggest commonalities in pharmacological approaches for treating those specific symptoms. Individual neuropathic pain diseases may have multiple drivers of pain responses, particularly over time, which produce multiple symptoms that are important in the expression and interpretation of the pain state. Current drugs often produce multiple effects on receptors, ion channels, and transmitter systems, whereas newer drugs are likely to have more narrowly targeted pharmacological effects. A better understanding of the molecular mechanisms driving specific neuropathic pain syndromes may lead to more rational therapies across multiple neuropathic pain syndromes. Highly targeted pharmacotherapies that inhibit the drivers of specific pain states, used in combination with existing therapies, may improve the treatment of specific neuropathic pain diseases.

REFERENCES

Arnstein P. Chronic neuropathic pain: issues in patient education. *Pain Manag Nurs* 2004; 5(4 Suppl 1):34–41.
Backonja M. Neuromodulating drugs for the symptomatic treatment of neuropathic pain. *Curr Pain Headache Rep* 2004; 8:212–216.
Backonja MM, Serra J. Pharmacologic management part 1: better-studied neuropathic pain diseases. *Pain Med* 2004a; 5(Suppl 1):S28–47.

Backonja MM, Serra J. Pharmacologic management part 2: lesser-studied neuropathic pain diseases. *Pain Med* 2004b; 5(Suppl 1):S48–59.

Baron R, Binder A. [How neuropathic is sciatica? The mixed pain concept]. *Orthopade* 2004; 33:568–575.

Collins SL, Moore RA, McQuay HJ, Wiffen P. Antidepressants and anticonvulsants for diabetic neuropathy and postherpetic neuralgia: a quantitative systematic review. *J Pain Symptom Manage* 2000; 20:449–458.

Devor M. Strategies for finding new pharmacological targets for neuropathic pain. *Curr Pain Headache Rep* 2004; 8:187–191.

Dworkin RH. An overview of neuropathic pain: syndromes, symptoms, signs, and several mechanisms. *Clin J Pain* 2002; 18:343–349.

Farrar JT, Berlin JA, Strom BL. Clinically important changes in acute pain outcome measures: a validation study. *J Pain Symptom Manage* 2003; 25:406–411.

Finnerup NB, Jensen TS. Spinal cord injury pain—mechanisms and treatment. *Eur J Neurol* 2004; 11:73–82.

Gilron I, Bailey JM, Tu D, et al. Morphine, gabapentin, or their combination for neuropathic pain. *N Engl J Med* 2005; 352:1324–1334.

Herr K. Neuropathic pain: a guide to comprehensive assessment. *Pain Manag Nurs* 2004; 5(4 Suppl 1):9–18.

Herrero JI, Quiroga J, Sangro B, et al. Herpes zoster after liver transplantation: incidence, risk factors, and complications. *Liver Transpl* 2004; 10:1140–1143.

Jensen TS, Baron R. Translation of symptoms and signs into mechanisms in neuropathic pain. *Pain* 2003; 102:1–8.

Jung BF, Johnson RW, Griffin DR, Dworkin RH. Risk factors for postherpetic neuralgia in patients with herpes zoster. *Neurology* 2004; 62:1545–1551.

Lojeski E, Stevens RA. Postherpetic neuralgia in the cancer patient. *Curr Rev Pain* 2000; 4:219–226.

McQuay HJ, Tramer M, Nye BA, et al. A systematic review of antidepressants in neuropathic pain. *Pain* 1996; 68:217–227.

Manning DC. New and emerging pharmacological targets for neuropathic pain. *Curr Pain Headache Rep* 2004; 8:192–198.

Namaka M, Gramlich CR, Ruhlen D, et al. A treatment algorithm for neuropathic pain. *Clin Ther* 2004; 26:951–979.

Schmader KE. Epidemiology and impact on quality of life of postherpetic neuralgia and painful diabetic neuropathy. *Clin J Pain* 2002; 18:350–354.

Schmidt WK. What drugs are in the neuropathic pain pipeline? Paper presented at: 7th International Conference on the Mechanisms and Treatment of Neuropathic Pain, University of Rochester School of Medicine & Dentistry, Southampton, Bermuda, November 4–6, 2004.

Sindrup SH, Jensen TS. Efficacy of pharmacological treatments of neuropathic pain: an update and effect related to mechanism of drug action. *Pain* 1999; 83:389–400.

Woolf CJ. Dissecting out mechanisms responsible for peripheral neuropathic pain: implications for diagnosis and therapy. *Life Sci* 2004; 74:2605–2610.

Correspondence to: William K. Schmidt, PhD, President, NorthStar Consulting, LLC, 1337 Marina Circle, Davis, CA 95616, USA. Tel: 650-438-3018; Fax: 866-410-8835; email: schmidtwk@sbcglobal.net.

Part IV

Measurement and New Technologies

Emerging Strategies for the Treatment of Neuropathic
Pain, edited by James N. Campbell, Allan I. Basbaum,
André Dray, Ronald Dubner, Robert H. Dworkin, and
Christine N. Sang, IASP Press, Seattle, © 2006.

17

Measurement and New Technologies: Rapporteur Report

Allan I. Basbaum,[a] M. Catherine Bushnell,[b] James N.
Campbell,[c] Sandra R. Chaplan,[d] Patrick W. Mantyh,[e]
Frank Porreca,[f] Donald D. Price,[g] Laszlo Urban,[h]
Charles J. Vierck,[i] and Jon-Kar Zubieta[j]

*[a]Department of Anatomy, University of California San Francisco, San
Francisco, California, USA; [b]Department of Anesthesia, Faculty of Medicine,
and Faculty of Dentistry, McGill University, Montreal, Quebec, Canada;
[c]Department of Neurosurgery, Johns Hopkins Hospital, Baltimore, Maryland,
USA; [d]Johnson & Johnson Pharmaceutical Research & Development, LLC, San
Diego, California, USA; [e]Neurosystems Laboratory, University of Minnesota,
Minneapolis, Minnesota, USA; [f]Department of Pharmacology, College of
Medicine, University of Arizona, Tucson, Arizona, USA; [g]Departments of Oral
and Maxillofacial Surgery, College of Dentistry, University of Florida,
Gainesville, Florida, USA; [h]Preclinical Compound Profiling, Lead Discovery
Center, Discovery Technologies, Novartis Institutes for BioMedical Research,
Inc., Cambridge, Massachusetts, USA; [i]Department of Neuroscience and
McKnight Brain Institute, University of Florida College of Medicine,
Gainesville, Florida, USA; [j]Mental Health Research Institute, University
of Michigan, Ann Arbor, Michigan, USA*

This chapter is based on a group colloquium regarding the measurement
of pain and the use of technology to understand, diagnose, and treat neuropathic pain. A consensus was that many new biopharmaceutical developments are held back because of limitations in these areas. Specifically, although numerous targets have been identified, their validation has been
difficult to achieve. Members of the group expressed concern that many
molecules may be inappropriately rejected based on animal testing, while
other molecules that appear efficacious in animal testing may not be effective in the clinic.

In some sense, development of drugs to treat pain has many advantages over the development of drugs to treat other neurological conditions. The generation of painful stimuli is easy and can be done in a reproducible fashion. The proof of principle as to the utility of the stimulus conditions comes from extensive studies of morphine, which reliably produces analgesia to noxious stimuli. These paradigms work in models of acute and postoperative pain. With neuropathic pain, however, ongoing pain is frequently the major problem, and drugs that are useful in treating neuropathic pain do not necessarily have conventional analgesic effects. In contrast to the modeling of exogenous stimuli, ongoing stimulus-independent pain is a major clinical problem. Modeling such pain in animals remains problematic.

WHAT IS NEUROPATHIC PAIN, AND HOW SHOULD IT BE ADDRESSED?

Our group felt compelled to discuss fundamental issues of definition. We know that neuropathic pain can arise from diseases that affect the peripheral nervous system, the spinal cord, and the brain. A rule that appears to apply uniformly to these diverse sources of pain is that the lesion must involve the nociceptive signaling system (Boivie et al. 1989). Thus, lesions of the medial lemniscal pathway, for example, are not expected to cause pain. The question of why injury to the pain-signaling system should be associated with pain (a negative event leading to positive symptoms) represents a longstanding, yet fascinating paradox. A reasonable answer to this paradox is that injury to pain-signaling pathways in fact results in *increased* signaling. Indeed, after nerve injury, pain can result from increased activity in (1) nociceptive fibers of the injured nerve (neuroma), (2) the dorsal root ganglion (DRG), (3) nociceptors that innervate the partly denervated peripheral tissue, or (4) nociceptive dorsal horn cells (Campbell 2001). Logically, then, this abnormal activity becomes the most important focus of treatment. Multiple mechanisms account for this abnormal activity, and thus the physiology becomes quite complicated. Moreover, these mechanisms may vary not only among different diseases but also between patients with a given disease. Indeed, a frustrating aspect of clinical treatment is that for the same disease, a given treatment typically works well in only a minority of patients.

NEURONAL INJURY AND PAIN

Many of the prototypic neuropathic pain conditions involve neuronal injury, whether in the form of an axotomy or an injury to the cell body. Painful diabetic neuropathy involves loss of nociceptor innervation of the skin. Similar evidence of neuronal injury is seen in postherpetic neuralgia. We now appreciate that our concepts of "neuropathic" must be broadened. Erythromelalgia, a rare disorder characterized by striking heat hyperalgesia so severe that patients are known to keep their feet in ice buckets, appears to be a sodium channelopathy (Waxman and Dib-Hajj 2005). A familial form of this condition has been traced to a single gene mutation of *SCN9a* ($Na_V1.7$) in sensory and sympathetic neurons. Conceivably, other channel disorders are a major source of pain. In the case of erythromelalgia, we might presume that gene therapy that downregulates *SCN9a* can solve the problem without the use of traditional analgesics. This strategy is a disease modification approach to treating the pain condition. It remains to be seen to what extent it might be of value to target the $Na_V1.7$ channel in order to address other types of pain, such as inflammatory pain, even if the inciting pathology is upstream. In other words, expression of *SCN9a* may not even be abnormal in some pain conditions, but regulating *SCN9a* expression may nevertheless hold significant promise as a pain therapy.

PRIMARY AFFERENTS

Uninjured primary afferents. We now recognize that the nociceptors that survive injury and that innervate partially innervated tissues (such as the skin) acquire abnormal properties that are relevant to the problem of neuropathic pain. Spontaneous activity and sensitization to natural stimuli and catecholamines have been documented in primates and rats (Ali et al. 1999). This finding has led to speculation that targeting the partly denervated skin may provide a means to treat neuropathic pain. Hence, capsaicin applied to the abnormal skin in patients with nerve injury (e.g., postherpetic neuralgia) may reduce pain by reducing the spontaneous activity and sensitization of the uninjured nociceptors (Rowbotham and Fields 1996). An intriguing explanation for the abnormalities in these intact nociceptors is that the target tissue overexpresses growth factors that in turn sensitize the remaining nociceptors. For example, overexpression of nerve growth factor in mice results in increased numbers of nociceptors (Goodness et al. 1997), although the extent to which these changes produce hypersensitivity is not clear (Molliver et al. 2005). Interestingly, even when the expression is increased in skin, there is a hypertrophy of sympathetic efferents and greater sympathetic innervation of DRG (Davis et al. 1996). Regarding the concept that neuropathic pain may exist without axotomy, pain could result from abnormalities in the expression of any of a variety of growth factors. We predict that such abnormalities will be discovered to be a novel mechanism for the generation of neuropathic pain—the only missing element is data.

Injured afferents. The opposite may also be true. Thus, nerve injury can result in reduced transport of growth factors to DRG neurons, which can produce a host of injury-associated biochemical changes that may contribute to the neuropathic pain condition (Boucher and McMahon 2001). Some of these problems, including the neuropathic pain state produced by nerve injury, may be remedied by administration of exogenous growth factors (Boucher et al. 2000; Averill et al. 2004). A particularly comprehensive example comes from studies of the effects of the neurotrophic factor artemin in animals that underwent the Chung model procedure (Gardell et al. 2003). Artemin targets the c-ret neurotrophin receptor, which is expressed by the so-called nonpeptide population of primary afferent nociceptors (Snider and McMahon 1998). Artemin not only reliably prevented and reversed the pain behaviors (tactile allodynia) that develop in the Chung model, but it also reversed all of the neurochemical consequences of the injury, which are manifest in the DRG and dorsal horn. For this reason, the authors argued that artemin therapy provides a disease-modifying approach, rather than merely being a pain therapy.

The dorsal horn. Treating the primary afferent pathology may not suffice. For example, some laboratories report that peripheral nerve injury can induce a loss of interneurons in the superficial dorsal horn (Sugimoto et al. 1990; Moore et al. 2002). Thus, some investigators have reported the appearance of "dark neurons" in the substantia gelatinosa after peripheral nerve injury, proposing that they were remnants of GABAergic inhibitory interneurons (Sugimoto et al. 1990). Whether or not these dark neurons represent dying neurons is disputed, and one laboratory was unable to find any evidence for loss of interneurons (Polgar et al. 2004). A recent study presented evidence of a 20% loss of neurons in lamina II in peripheral nerve pain models and demonstrated that inhibitors of apoptosis (via inhibition of caspase) attenuated hyperalgesia and blocked cell death (Scholz et al. 2005). Once again there is lack of agreement in the literature, and the utility and reliability of the traditional markers of apoptosis have been questioned. Clearly, additional neuroanatomical studies documenting large numbers of neurons may address this important controversy. However, the death of a neuron might not be essential for it to be nonfunctional.

Another controversy concerns the issue of whether there are enduring anatomical changes (neuronal sprouting) such that tactile afferents acquire the capacity to activate central pain-signaling neurons. There is evidence both for and against this hypothesis (Woolf et al. 1995; Bennett et al. 1996; Hughes et al. 2003). Part of the controversy results from the fact that cell bodies of injured peripheral nerves have significantly altered phenotypes, making it difficult to distinguish myelinated from unmyelinated axons in transneuronal tracing experiments. The evidence for sprouting may in fact reflect altered expression of these markers, rather than sprouting (Tong et al. 1999).

Regardless of the above controversy, there is wide agreement that the phenotype of injured afferents (and of the afferents that share the innervation territory of the injured axons) is drastically altered (Wiesenfeld-Hallin and Xu 1996). Following peripheral nerve injury, there are, in fact, unequivocal and profound biochemical changes such as upregulation of galanin and neuropeptide Y expression in DRG neurons (Landry et al. 2000) as well as de novo expression of substance P in large-diameter neurons (Noguchi et al. 1995). To what extent any one change contributes to the neuropathic pain condition is not known, but clearly this is a fruitful area of investigation. Moreover, the neurochemical reorganization that occurs in the primary afferents and in the spinal cord almost certainly will lead to changes at other levels of the neuraxis. In other words, there will be profound changes in circuits throughout the nervous system, any of which could contribute to the maladaptive plasticity that is presumed to underlie the development of neuropathic pain. There was broad consensus in our group that further studies should address the extent to which manipulating (indeed reversing) these central changes can ameliorate pain.

PAIN AFTER SPINAL CORD INJURY

Studies of neuropathic pain in animals tend to emphasize peripheral nerve disease or injury. In humans, however, there is a very high incidence of pain after spinal cord injury (Ravenscroft et al. 2000). With complete transection pain can occur not only at the border zone of innervation but also in the distal, deafferented lower extremities and sacral regions. In humans, pain and hyperalgesia in this border zone of innervation and deafferentation correlates with distal pain (Finnerup et al. 2003).

A variety of animal models have been developed to mimic central neuropathic pain associated with spinal cord injury- (Yezierski 2005). These include injection of quisqualic acid into the spinal cord gray matter (Yezierski 2005), photochemical destruction of dorsal gray and white matter (Xu et al. 1992), and contusion injury of the core region of the spinal cord (Siddall et al. 1995). Below-level pain (referred to segments well below the level of the injury) can be attributed to combined white and gray matter injury, producing a combination of rostral deafferentation (especially from interruption of the spinothalamic tract) and diffuse rostral propagation of abnormal activity from gray matter that is located rostral to the lesion (Vierck and Light 2000). In humans, distal pain (in essence phantom pain in the case of complete spinal cord transection) correlates with at-level hyperalgesia. Therefore, tests of hyperalgesia in dermatomes that correspond to the level of injury may provide a surrogate measure of distal pain and may be useful ways to assess the efficacy of treatments designed to treat central neuropathic pain.

SHOULD WE TARGET THE DISEASE OR THE PAIN?

Given that axotomy by itself can induce pain, the question therapeutically becomes an issue of whether the treatment should be directed to the disease that causes the axotomy or to the generic issue of axotomy-induced pain. In other words, should we treat the underlying specific disease or the pain? Or, is pain itself the disease? Max suggested that the concept of pain as a disease is overly simplistic. Pain may be considered a neurological disease, but its characterization as a disease is largely based on animal studies, where changes are observed over a very short period of time. He challenged the group to provide evidence that there are human correlates that can be considered hallmarks of a "disease of pain." What are the clinical changes that occur in the course of the disease of pain? He suggested that a consideration of the complexity of depression, which may be complicated by other somatic disorders, might be instructive. Although the predominant focus in depression is on the cognitive or psychiatric component of the disease, complex changes in other systems may, for example, lead to osteoporosis and cardiovascular problems. There are also complex endocrine changes that should also be considered part of the disease. He argued that proper characterization of a disease must take into account and identify all of the associated features, which must be assessed in a longitudinal fashion as the disease progresses.

Other members of the group pointed to a contrary example. Specifically, although patients with epilepsy may have concurrent, complex non-neurological changes, the latter features are not something that the neurologist commonly considers in the evaluation and treatment of a patient with seizures. The focus is on the neurological component of the disease, and thus a selective focus on the neurological features of the proposed "disease of pain" may be reasonable.

Having one's clinical problem of interest labeled a disease has obvious sociopolitical value because treatment of diseases, rather than of symptoms, is the goal of medically oriented philanthropic organizations. This view was not considered to be the driving force for defining neuropathic pain as a disease, as there appear to be many strong examples of pathophysiological changes in the nervous system that are intimately linked to the development of the persistent pain condition. Apkarian and colleagues (2004b) reported a particularly dramatic example of central nervous system reorganization. They found a remarkable loss of gray matter density in the prefrontal cortex in patients with lumbar root pain. That this pathology is also profoundly functional was demonstrated by their observation that these same patients have a deficit in performing an emotional decision-making task (Apkarian et al. 2004a), which presumably reflects cognitive abnormalities generated by the cortical pathology.

If there is significant reorganization of the nervous system (at the molecular and circuit level), perhaps treatment could be directed at reversing the neuroanatomical and biochemical changes. In this regard the recent studies of Flor and colleagues are relevant. These authors reported that providing coherent input to the cortex with a myoelectric prosthesis could significantly alleviate phantom limb pain, and perhaps more interestingly, reduce the cortical reorganization that normally occurs following limb amputation (Lotze et al. 1999). These examples are illustrative of a pathophysiological plasticity of the cortex that can contribute to a persistent pain condition, one that perhaps can be prevented by addressing the neurological disease process that appears to contribute to, or certainly correlate with, the development of the pain condition.

The principle has been elegantly demonstrated in another set of recent experiments that examined cortical reorganization and pain. Merzenich reported that repetitive movements intensively performed over time induce peripheral inflammation, as well as a reorganization of the topographic map in the somatosensory cortex, and that these changes parallel those observed in patients with focal dystonia (Byl et al. 2002). Importantly, his laboratory demonstrated that a structured regimen of a different form of exercise not only may resolve the peripheral inflammation, but also may normalize the somatosensory map structure. This demonstration of activity-dependent neuroplasticity may have considerable relevance to the development of approaches to the resolution of chronic pain after peripheral or central neural injury. In particular, because partial deafferentation is common to many forms of neuropathic pain, one should consider the use of a training regimen designed to appropriately influence the deafferentation-induced neuroplastic changes that inevitably occur at all levels of the neuroaxis.

Another important influence on neural plasticity, which might be relevant to the treatment of neuropathic pain, comes from preclinical models of Alzheimer's disease. Animal studies show that enriched environments decrease markers for Alzheimer's disease, namely transcripts that are specifically associated with cortical function (Lazarov et al. 2005). Furthermore, epidemiological studies of Alzheimer patients have identified education and occupation as environmental factors that help determine the risk of developing the disease (Moceri et al. 2001). In a somewhat related vein, psychologists point to coping styles as issues germane to the question of pain and suffering. Passive behaviors (passive versus active coping) appear to correlate with more pain (Mercado et al. 2005). The animal work with enriched environments at least raises the possibility that these psychological influences could have morphological and neurophysiological underpinnings. Future research in this area could have very important implications.

MEASUREMENT, PAIN MODELS, AND PSYCHOPHYSICS

WHAT CAN PSYCHOPHYSICAL STUDIES TELL US ABOUT MECHANISMS?

Languages are rich with adjectives that describe pain, and some descriptors regularly emerge with regard to neuropathic pain. For example, the pain in the feet that accompanies painful diabetic neuropathy is often described as "burning." In principle, this characteristic should say something about mechanism. Heat stimuli evoke a burning sensation, and this sensation appears to be signaled by activity in polymodal C-fiber nociceptors (LaMotte and Campbell 1978; Torebjork et al. 1984). Thus, the burning pain in painful diabetic neuropathy may be signaled by the activity in this class of nociceptors. Touch-evoked pain (allodynia) arises in particular with stroking stimuli (Ochoa and Yarnitsky 1993), and we now know that this phenomenon results from central sensitization to the inputs carried by tactile afferents (Campbell et al. 1988). That stroking is more bothersome than static pressure suggests that the quickly adapting mechanoreceptors (Aδ guard fibers and Meissner fibers) are the culprit, but a role for low-threshold, slowly adapting mechanoreceptors has not been excluded. Of course, there are other types of mechanical hyperalgesia. Punctate hyperalgesia (LaMotte et al. 1991) has now been shown to be due to central sensitization to the inputs carried by TRPV1-negative Aδ mechano-(only)-nociceptors (Magerl et al. 2001). This we know purely from psychophysics, a point that effectively illustrates how psychophysics can point to mechanism.

Different forms of neuropathic pain present with different patterns of hyperalgesia. Traumatic neuropathies in humans are associated with prominent cooling hyperalgesia (Frost et al. 1988; Treede et al. 1992). By contrast, in painful diabetic neuropathy, cooling may be soothing and heat hyperalgesia may predominate. These observations beg for mechanistic explanations. Heat hyperalgesia may be mediated by heat sensitization of nociceptors in the skin. Cooling hyperalgesia is also evident in many cases of traumatic nerve injury, perhaps due to abnormal expression of channels sensitive to cooling stimuli, such as TRPM8 or even TRPA1 (McKemy et al. 2002; Obata et al. 2005). Finally, psychophysics may also predict response to drug therapy. For example, patients with postherpetic neuralgia who have preserved innervation of the skin respond better to opioids than do patients with denervation (Raja et al. 2002). For response to tricyclics, this variable does not appear to predict efficacy.

We still are in the early stages of studying the psychophysics of pain. Our group felt that pain psychophysics might augment the understanding of pain in a way similar to how vision physiology has been furthered by psychophysical studies.

ANIMAL MODELS

The group, not surprisingly, spent considerable time on the topic of animal testing. The focus of the discussion centered on the following three questions:

1) Do drug studies in animal models of neuropathic pain predict efficacy in humans?

2) Are withdrawal reflexes a valid measure of pain, in particular in animal models of neuropathic pain?

3) What is the role of operant tests, and does operant testing provide an efficient means to evaluate analgesics?

Consideration of these issues evoked some of the sharpest differences of opinion. Preclinical evaluation of putative analgesics eventually involves behavioral testing of animals. This pivotal stage in drug development determines which drugs get selected for clinical testing. There is no question that a major breakthrough in the preclinical analysis of neuropathic pain followed from the development of animal models that mimic, at least to some extent, the pains associated with various nerve-injury-induced (neuropathic) conditions. The Chung model (Kim and Chung 1992) appears to be the one most commonly used, particularly in the pharmaceutical setting. Yet how valid are the conclusions drawn when the endpoint in the Chung and other neuropathic pain models is a withdrawal reflex?

The group voiced two immediate concerns. First, in these animal models we depend on tests of stimulus-evoked pain. It is possible, however, that the dominant clinical problem experienced by patients is ongoing pain, not allodynia or hyperalgesia. The bottom-line question, therefore, is: To what extent do we model human neuropathic pain when our behavioral screen relies principally on increased responses to natural stimuli?

The predominant animal pain model involves measurement of when and how often the paw is withdrawn to a mechanical or heat stimulus. These measures involve segmental spinal reflexes. Licking and guarding are more complex behaviors that most likely involve spino-bulbar reflexes, but they are still reflexive in nature. Of course, these tests offer significant advantages, and in a retrospective sense they have to some extent been validated. That is, drugs that are effective for neuropathic pain in the clinic are generally effective in the animal models. On the other hand, what these tests measure are generally threshold changes for withdrawal responses, not pain, and certainly not stimulus-independent pain. To address this limitation, Vierck advocated the use of behavioral tests that involve an operant paradigm, one in which the animal learns how to avoid a painful stimulus (see the chapter by Vierck in this volume).

ANOMALIES AND DISCREPANCIES: COMPARING REFLEX AND OPERANT MODELS

Vierck described results using operant tests that are very different from those observed when reflex tests are used (Vierck et al. 2002). For example, the dose of morphine required to suppress behavior in an operant task is much lower than is required to block paw-withdrawal responses. In fact, a low dose of morphine (0.5 mg/kg) is antinociceptive in an operant test of pain behavior, but it actually enhances "behavior" in reflex tests of pain (Vierck et al. 2002). Furthermore, in a stress situation, Vierck finds hyperalgesia, not analgesia, which is typical in the reflex tests (King et al. 2003). He argues that results using the operant test are more meaningful because stress-induced enhancement of pain is likely to be more common in the clinic than stress-induced analgesia.

Vierck also pointed out other potential weaknesses of reflex testing, particularly when it comes to the partial nerve injury models. Following unilateral chronic constriction injury (CCI) of the sciatic nerve, reflex responses to mechanical, cold, and heat stimulation are typically enhanced, for 40 days. In contrast, bilateral CCI enhances operant escape responses to cold, but not heat, for more than 100 days (Vierck et al. 2005). Importantly, humans with nerve injury show a robust cooling hyperalgesia, but much less pronounced heat hyperalgesia. In this respect, the operant behavioral response, which is free from the asymmetrical motor consequences of unilateral CCI, is more consistent with clinical findings in humans with nerve-injury-induced pain.

VALIDATION OF THE OPERANT MODELS

Although there was general interest in the utility of operant models, the importance of validation was emphasized strongly by members of the group who represented the pharmaceutical industry. Other concerns were raised, including the relative difficulty of performing operant compared to reflex tests. The latter is particularly important because of the requirement of high throughput, so that large numbers of candidate drugs can be quickly assessed. On the other hand, the operant tests can be performed automatically, so that some scale-up may be possible. The "n" required to power the testing adequately is dependent on variability (noise). The noise level in reflexive versus operant tasks is simply unknown. Thus, we really cannot determine at present the relative merits of operant conditioning, despite the enormous importance of this issue. Finally, it was pointed out that operant measures are particularly important if the target of therapy is supraspinal, given that operant tests tap into elements of suffering and motivation. The lesser relevance of these features in reflex testing may therefore be a limitation of reflex tests, not an advantage. Then again, these concerns may vary with the mechanism of action of a given drug (e.g., spinal vs. supraspinal). In other words, the value of the screens in behavioral testing may vary according to how the drug affects pain.

There was general agreement that studying mechanical hyperalgesia in a neuropathic pain model, using operant testing, is a critical next step to validating the utility of operant approaches. In addition, it is essential that a detailed analysis of different drug effects be performed to establish the validity of the operant tests. These should be performed for drugs already shown to have utility in the clinic and also to show that drugs that do not work in the clinic do not work in the operant model. Neurokinin-1 receptor antagonists were offered as an example of a drug that should be evaluated. Thus, although they are reportedly effective in some preclinical models of persistent pain, such drugs are generally ineffective in reflex tests of neuropathic pain (Cumberbatch et al. 1998) and have not yet proven effective for the treatment of neuropathic pain in patients.

Of course, in the mind of all participants was a key unanswered question. Has reliance on reflex tests resulted in misses of candidate molecules (i.e., Type II error)? If this is true, then the operant approach may in the long run have greater utility, despite the many difficulties that were pointed out. A study reported just after our meeting upheld the value of operant conditioning in a neuropathic pain model (Baliki et al. 2005). This study suggested a 10-fold improvement in sensitivity in the operant model.

HOW CAN WE EVALUATE SPONTANEOUS PAIN?

Whereas the testing for allodynia and hyperalgesia offers good opportunities to screen treatments for neuropathic pain, a variety of "spontaneous" behavioral responses of animals have been used to infer the presence of ongoing pain. For example, following unilateral CCI or spinal nerve ligation (SNL), rats elevate the affected hindpaw for a period of approximately 40 days. Although it looks as if the guarding responses represent attempts to avoid tactile or pressure stimulation of the paw, Vierck pointed out that there is a flexor bias for the affected paw, because of the reciprocal nature of spinal reflex control and due to an ipsilateral motor deficit that is produced by the lesion. He added that guarding responses are not observed following bilateral CCI, i.e., where there is no postural asymmetry (Vierck et al. 2005). These observations indicate that elevation of a paw after CCI does not necessarily reflect the presence of ongoing pain or avoidance of tactile and pressure stimulation. Similar experiments have not been conducted to determine whether paw elevation after SNL is similarly related to postural asymmetry. In this model, analgesic treatment can normalize weight bearing by the affected limb.

Several other potentially important approaches to the production and evaluation of spontaneous pain were mentioned. Local DRG compression appears to induce clinically relevant persistent pain behavior (Song et al. 1999) and should be evaluated further. Eisenach reported that self-administration of analgesic compounds by animals can be an effective tool to monitor spontaneous pain. Self-administration to attenuate prolonged noxious stimulation (e.g., cold) should clearly be compared with self-administration after CCI and SNL and in other models of neuropathic pain.

Vocalization may be another useful measure of spontaneous pain in the laboratory. Interestingly, vocalizations induced by noxious stimuli are suppressed by low doses of systemic morphine, much lower than are typically required to suppress reflex behaviors. This finding suggests that vocalization may indeed be a measure of spontaneous pain. On the other hand, a recent study reported that ultrasonic vocalizations in rodents correlate poorly with other measures of pain behavior (Wallace et al. 2005). Furthermore, vocalizations of monkeys that occur while they perform operant responses for food reinforcement in the absence of pain are also suppressed by low doses of morphine (Cooper and Vierck 1986). Similarly, vocalizations that occur when monkeys or rats are performing an operant escape task are not evoked reliably by intensities of stimulation that are escaped. Taken together, these data indicate that our anthropomorphic assumptions of the significance of vocalization in the setting of injury or intense stimulation may be incorrect.

Measures of self-injurious behaviors, such as autotomy (Wallace et al. 2005), were not discussed in detail, but the longstanding controversy as to their relevance to spontaneous pain behavior was mentioned. The potential utility of central recording of neural activity during expression of spontaneous behaviors was also touched on, but no consensus was reached as to whether this is practical. Dubner and colleagues did pioneering studies of this type in monkeys (Bushnell et al. 1984), but this work is very time intensive and difficult. Food intake and sleep patterns were also proposed as surrogate measures of ongoing pain, but it was pointed out that these measures can be greatly influenced by motivational factors. For example, in certain models, such as diabetic neuropathy, there could be several reasons for abnormal behaviors that are not directly related to the magnitude of the pain that is being assessed.

CHRONICITY OF NEUROPATHIC PAIN
AND OPIOID SENSITIVITY

The issue of the time dependency of the neuropathic pain phenotype was raised. Because the typical duration of "pain" behavior in animals with partial nerve injury nerve is short (less than 2 months), it is difficult to be certain that it is modeling the normal evolution of pain that develops in neuropathic pain conditions in humans. Hyperalgesia in the SNL model extends beyond 100 days. Prior work has also shown that the duration of abnormal behavior depends on whether the lesion is favorable to regeneration (Lancelotta et al. 2003). If recovery from the injury occurs, the neuropathic pain behavior tends to go away. This recovery may vary with modality of stimulation; for example, cooling hyperalgesia is more durable.

The group also addressed the important and longstanding question of the efficacy of opioids in the treatment of neuropathic pain. There was considerable agreement among the clinicians in the group that opioids can be effective for the treatment of many patients. Nevertheless, it was also agreed that many patients do not respond (Raja et al. 2002). An interesting unanswered question is whether the patient with neuropathic pain who does not respond to opioids has decreased sensitivity to opioids for treatment of other types of pain. Of the many mechanisms that could account for individual differences in efficacy of opioids, the group discussed polymorphisms in the opioid receptor, differences in levels of expression of receptors in target regions, and differences in second messenger coupling. It has not yet been determined whether morphine can be more or less effective at different times during the evolution of a neuropathic pain condition, and whether nonresponsive patients ever become responsive at a different time point. Several members of the group expressed the opinion that any given patient who is opioid responsive will continue to respond for a long period of time, but this contention has not been studied systematically. Dissecting out the genetics and the fascinating biochemistry of opioid responsiveness (for example, see Waldhoer et al. 2004) will almost certainly be a promising area of research in the future.

PLACEBO EFFECTS

Although considerable evidence indicates that placebo effects operate in the context of pain treatment (Hrobjartsson and Gotzsche 2001), there is little information about the magnitude of placebo effects in patients with neuropathic pain. Future research should be directed at determining whether there are unique placebo mechanisms that operate in patients with neuropathic pain and at revealing the magnitude of these effects among various neuropathic pain conditions.

There was much discussion of the body of work performed by Benedetti and colleagues (2005) that has provided insights into the complex pharmacological underpinnings of the placebo response. Using several pain models in healthy volunteers, these authors confirmed a prior observation (Levine et al. 1978) that placebo analgesia created by expectation is blocked by naloxone, and thus is presumed to be endorphin-mediated. However, placebo analgesia created through classical conditioning may or may not be endorphin-mediated, depending on whether or not the conditioning involved opioid-related treatments. In contrast to the findings of the Benedetti group, Price and colleagues suggested that antihyperalgesic expectation-related placebo effects in irritable bowel syndrome are not endorphin-mediated (Vase et al. 2005). These data indicate that the placebo for pain control is not a unitary phenomenon, and thus it would be worthwhile to study to what extent it operates in the setting of neuropathic pain, and indeed which form of placebo analgesia might operate.

Is there any evidence that patients with chronic pain in general, or neuropathic pain in particular, have exaggerated or reduced placebo responses? Brain-imaging evidence (Wager et al. 2004) shows that when healthy subjects experience placebo analgesia, there is activation in the dorsolateral prefrontal cortex (DLPFC), which correlates with expectation-related placebo analgesia. Interestingly, this region is where Apkarian and colleagues (2004b) found a reduced volume of gray matter in patients with chronic low back pain. If the DLPFC is important in the generation and maintenance of placebo analgesia, then it is possible that chronic pain patients, including neuropathic pain patients, have a reduced placebo analgesic response. The fact that the typical chronic pain patient has experienced a multitude of failed treatments should further reduce expectation of treatment success. Studies need to be performed to address these possibilities. Of course, placebo is not the only psychological manipulation that can alter pain perception and change neural functioning. There is substantial psychophysical and brain-imaging evidence that psychological factors, including attentional state and emotions, alter pain perception and pain-related cortical activation (Villemure et al. 2003).

OTHER TECHNOLOGIES

FUNCTIONAL BRAIN IMAGING

There was general agreement that functional brain imaging has tremendous value in the analysis of normal and pathological pain conditions. Whether imaging can serve as an alternative measure of pain in humans is not at all clear. Finding activation patterns in animals that are similar to those observed in humans who are experiencing pain might provide important support for the assumption that animals submitted to various injury models are, in fact, experiencing pain. Functional brain imaging in humans has also been proposed as a way to validate verbal reports of patients (Borsook and Becerra 2005). Of great interest is the use of imaging to reveal some of the circuitry that underlies both pharmacologically and psychologically produced changes in pain perception. For example, as described above, the approach is now commonly used to examine functional connectivity in the brain, as well as anatomical changes that occur in patients with chronic pain. The use of imaging to test novel analgesic agents also has a bright future.

DNA ARRAYS, GENE SCREENS, AND PROTEOMICS

Characterization of olfactory transduction mechanisms has revealed that large numbers of receptors in combinatorial associations confer specificity to the sense of smell. The murine odorant G-protein-coupled receptor repertoire is estimated at 1% of the genome, or 1000 genes (Mombaerts 1999).

What can this finding teach us about the molecular basis of specificity in the somatosensory system? The idea of a similar complexity underlying the specificity of somatosensation is daunting. Certainly, the neurochemical complexity of the nociceptor is remarkable, and we are only beginning to appreciate how this diversity relates to nociception.

The ability to leverage technology to address questions of this scale has obvious appeal. One example that is already reasonably well implemented in pain research is the DNA microarray. In theory, this technology lends itself well to the urge to compare, contrast, and catalogue large numbers of previously undefined variables. There, in fact, is an ongoing effort to catalogue the composition of the normal DRG. Several microarray studies of the rat DRG are already under way, as are attempts to identify the molecular makeup of individual DRG neurons. To this end, large numbers of individual neurons are randomly captured, mRNA extracted, amplified, and characterized. Chaplin reported on a preliminary analysis of 100 DRG neurons using this approach. She and her colleagues found that 12 clusters of genes predominated. Of course, depending on the definition of the minimum degree of difference necessary to define a distinct neuronal type, the number of groups may be larger or smaller. Association of each defined group with one or more gene markers should provide a highly useful tool to other investigators in the field. Finally, while it is tempting to leap into a similar experiment that compares the normal and injured DRG, the inherent difficulty of this experiment was emphasized. We already know that injury brings out considerable changes in the gene expression profile in DRG neurons. However, the functional significance of the few major changes that have been identified is still unclear.

Not surprisingly, it is the large pharmaceutical companies with pain programs that have performed microarray studies in nerve injury models. These studies generally use homogenized whole DRG, and to date, they do not appear to be yielding the hoped-for gold mine of novel targets. Limits in resolution along with the overwhelming amount of information make for slow progress. Clearly, different changes will be expected to occur in different classes of DRG cells. Sampling of individual cells may be required to make sense of the changes in gene expression. Many changes are seen in "mystery genes," rather than in the traditionally "preferred" drug targets, namely G-protein-coupled receptors and enzymes, and it is not known whether to interpret upregulation as an event contributing to hyperalgesia, or as a homeostatic attempt to reach a compensatory state (toward resolution of the injury-induced changes). Similarly, downregulation could represent a deficiency of the target leading to pain, or an effort to counterbalance some other influence toward normalcy.

Similar studies of neurons in the spinal cord dorsal horn have proven to be even more difficult. An earlier study that attempted to correlate morphology with gene expression profile ran into difficulty because of the need to discriminate intrinsic and projection neurons (Kamme et al 2004). The projection neurons were identified by a retrograde tracer approach. Unfortunately, the shape and relatively flat nature of those neurons required that they be captured in the coronal plane, which significantly reduced the sample that could be captured. A comprehensive analysis would probably require far more animals than a comparable analysis of DRG neurons. The value of these studies is not questioned, but technological hurdles must still be crossed. An obvious and important technological improvement for these studies would be the use of whole, living neurons that are characterized either electrophysiologically or pharmacologically, prior to amplification and hybridization. Despite the problem of damage that is introduced during dissociation of the neurons in culture, the functional information that this approach offers is clearly important. Moreover, far more mRNA can be extracted from each neuron using this approach.

Other uses of microarrays should be considered as well. Profiling an injury in the presence and absence of an effective analgesic could give important information on the molecular contrast between the two states. Using microarray technology to try to discern the molecular targets of drugs with unknown mechanisms of action may also be productive.

SUMMARY

There are no shortages of new technologies or of new targets for pain treatment. Having valid, reliable, capital-efficient measurement techniques to test these innovations is of extraordinary importance. Perhaps the most pressing need is for the development of new behavioral screening tests that meet these standards. The fact that these do not yet exist increases the likelihood that many candidate molecules are being routinely and inappropriately discarded. And even more disappointing is the likelihood that other drug candidates are brought into later phase testing because inappropriate decisions were made based on preclinical analyses. Present data indicate that over 80% of centrally acting drug candidates that reach phase III ultimately fail. This high rate of failure makes drug development very expensive and erects a barrier to the discovery of new treatments. Because the cost of drug development from animal studies up to phase II is relatively small compared to the cost of phase III trials, it is obvious that the screening methods in preclinical analyses are critical. To promote new treatments it will be important to combine the great progress in basic science with better screening techniques in animals and in early phase human trials.

REFERENCES

Ali Z, Ringkamp M, Hartke TV, et al. Uninjured C-fiber nociceptors develop spontaneous activity and alpha-adrenergic sensitivity following L6 spinal nerve ligation in monkey. *J Neurophysiol* 1999; 81:455–466.

Apkarian AV, Sosa Y, Krauss BR, et al. Chronic pain patients are impaired on an emotional decision-making task. *Pain* 2004a; 108:129–136.

Apkarian AV, Sosa Y, Sonty S, et al. Chronic back pain is associated with decreased prefrontal and thalamic gray matter density. *J Neurosci* 2004b; 24:10410–10415.

Averill S, Michael GJ, Shortland PJ, et al. NGF and GDNF ameliorate the increase in ATF3 expression which occurs in dorsal root ganglion cells in response to peripheral nerve injury. *Eur J Neurosci* 2004; 19:1437–1445.

Baliki M, Calvo O, Chialvo DR, Apkarian AV. Spared nerve injury rats exhibit thermal hyperalgesia on an automated operant dynamic thermal escape task. *Mol Pain* 2005; 1:18.

Benedetti F, Mayberg HS, Wager TD, Stohler CS, Zubieta JK. Neurobiological mechanisms of the placebo effect. *J Neurosci* 2005; 25:10390–10402.

Bennett DL, French J, Priestley JV, McMahon SB. NGF but not NT-3 or BDNF prevents the A fiber sprouting into lamina II of the spinal cord that occurs following axotomy. *Mol Cell Neurosci* 1996; 8:211–220.

Boivie J, Leijon G, Johansson I. Central post-stroke pain—a study of the mechanisms through analyses of the sensory abnormalities. *Pain* 1989; 37:173–185.

Borsook D, Becerra L. Functional imaging of pain and analgesia—a valid diagnostic tool? *Pain* 2005; 117:247–250.

Boucher TJ, McMahon SB. Neurotrophic factors and neuropathic pain. *Curr Opin Pharmacol* 2001; 1:66–72.

Boucher TJ, Okuse K, Bennett DL, et al. Potent analgesic effects of GDNF in neuropathic pain states. *Science* 2000; 290:124–127.

Bushnell MC, Duncan GH, Dubner R, He LF. Activity of trigeminothalamic neurons in medullary dorsal horn of awake monkeys trained in a thermal discrimination task. *J Neurophysiol* 1984; 52:170–187.

Byl NN, Nagarajan SS, Merzenich MM, Roberts T, McKenzie A. Correlation of clinical neuromusculoskeletal and central somatosensory performance: variability in controls and patients with severe and mild focal hand dystonia. *Neural Plast* 2002; 9:177–203.

Campbell JN. Nerve lesions and the generation of pain. *Muscle Nerve* 2001; 24:1261–1273.

Campbell JN, Raja SN, Meyer RA, Mackinnon SE. Myelinated afferents signal the hyperalgesia associated with nerve injury. *Pain* 1988; 32:89–94.

Cooper BY, Vierck CJ Jr. Vocalizations as measures of pain in monkeys. *Pain* 1986; 26:393–407.

Cumberbatch MJ, Carlson E, Wyatt A, et al. Reversal of behavioural and electrophysiological correlates of experimental peripheral neuropathy by the NK1 receptor antagonist GR205171 in rats. *Neuropharmacology* 1998; 37:1535–1543.

Davis BM, Wang HS, Albers KM, et al. Effects of NGF overexpression on anatomical and physiological properties of sympathetic postganglionic neurons. *Brain Res* 1996; 724:47–54.

Finnerup NB, Johannesen IL, Fuglsang-Frederiksen A, Bach FW, Jensen TS. Sensory function in spinal cord injury patients with and without central pain. *Brain* 2003; 126:57–70.

Frost SA, Raja SN, Campbell JN, Meyer RA, Khan AA. Does hyperalgesia to cooling stimuli characterize patients with sympathetically-maintained pain (reflex sympathetic dystrophy)? In: Dubner R, Gebhart GF, Bond MR (Eds). *Proceedings of the Vth World Congress on Pain*. Amsterdam: Elsevier Science, 1988, pp 151–156.

Gardell LR, Wang R, Ehrenfels C, et al. Multiple actions of systemic artemin in experimental neuropathy. *Nat Med* 2003; 9:1383–1389.

Goodness TP, Albers KM, Davis FE, Davis BM. Overexpression of nerve growth factor in skin increases sensory neuron size and modulates Trk receptor expression. *Eur J Neurosci* 1997; 9:1574–1585.

Hrobjartsson A, Gotzsche PC. Is the placebo powerless? An analysis of clinical trials comparing placebo with no treatment. *N Engl J Med* 2001; 344:1594–1602.

Hughes DI, Scott DT, Todd AJ, Riddell JS. Lack of evidence for sprouting of A-beta afferents into the superficial laminas of the spinal cord dorsal horn after nerve section. *J Neurosci* 2003; 23:9491–9499.

Kamme F, Zhu J, Luo L, et al. Single-cell laser-capture microdissection and RNA amplification. *Methods Mol Med* 2004; 99:215–223.

Kim SH, Chung JM. An experimental model for peripheral neuropathy produced by segmental spinal nerve ligation in the rat. *Pain* 1992; 50:355–363.

King CD, Devine DP, Vierck CJ, Rodgers J, Yezierski RP. Differential effects of stress on escape and reflex responses to nociceptive thermal stimuli in the rat. *Brain Res* 2003; 987:214–222.

LaMotte RH, Campbell JN. Comparison of responses of warm and nociceptive C-fiber afferents in monkey with human judgments of thermal pain. *J Neurophysiol* 1978; 41:509–528.

LaMotte RH, Shain CN, Simone DA, Tsai EF. Neurogenic hyperalgesia: psychophysical studies of underlying mechanisms. *J Neurophysiol* 1991; 66:190–211.

Lancelotta MP, Sheth RN, Meyer RA, et al. Severity and duration of hyperalgesia in rat varies with type of nerve lesion. *Neurosurgery* 2003; 53:1200–1208; discussion 1208–1209.

Landry M, Holmberg K, Zhang X, Hokfelt T. Effect of axotomy on expression of NPY, galanin, and NPY Y1 and Y2 receptors in dorsal root ganglia and the superior cervical ganglion studied with double-labeling in situ hybridization and immunohistochemistry. *Exp Neurol* 2000; 162:361–384.

Lazarov O, Robinson J, Tang YP, et al. Environmental enrichment reduces A-beta levels and amyloid deposition in transgenic mice. *Cell* 2005; 120:701–713.

Levine JD, Gordon NC, Fields HL. The mechanism of placebo analgesia. *Lancet* 1978; 2:654–657.

Lotze M, Grodd W, Birbaumer N, et al. Does use of a myoelectric prosthesis prevent cortical reorganization and phantom limb pain? *Nat Neurosci* 1999; 2:501–502.

Magerl W, Fuchs PN, Meyer RA, Treede RD. Roles of capsaicin-insensitive nociceptors in cutaneous pain and secondary hyperalgesia. *Brain* 2001; 124:1754–1764.

McKemy DD, Neuhausser WM, Julius D. Identification of a cold receptor reveals a general role for TRP channels in thermosensation. *Nature* 2002; 416:52–58.

Mercado AC, Carroll LJ, Cassidy JD, Cote P. Passive coping is a risk factor for disabling neck or low back pain. *Pain* 2005; 117:51–57.

Moceri VM, Kukull WA, Emanual I, et al. Using census data and birth certificates to reconstruct the early-life socioeconomic environment and the relation to the development of Alzheimer's disease. *Epidemiology* 2001; 12:383–389.

Molliver DC, Lindsay J, Albers KM, Davis BM. Overexpression of NGF or GDNF alters transcriptional plasticity evoked by inflammation. *Pain* 2005; 113:277–284.

Mombaerts P. Seven-transmembrane proteins as odorant and chemosensory receptors. *Science* 1999; 286:707–711.

Moore KA, Kohno T, Karchewski LA, et al. Partial peripheral nerve injury promotes a selective loss of GABAergic inhibition in the superficial dorsal horn of the spinal cord. *J Neurosci* 2002; 22:6724–3671.

Noguchi K, Kawai Y, Fukuoka T, Senba E, Miki K. Substance P induced by peripheral nerve injury in primary afferent sensory neurons and its effect on dorsal column nucleus neurons. *J Neurosci* 1995; 15:7633–7643.

Obata K, Katsura H, Mizushima T, et al. TRPA1 induced in sensory neurons contributes to cold hyperalgesia after inflammation and nerve injury. *J Clin Invest* 2005; 115:2393–2401.

Ochoa JL, Yarnitsky D. Mechanical hyperalgesias in neuropathic pain patients: dynamic and static subtypes. *Ann Neurol* 1993; 33:465–472.

Polgar E, Gray S, Riddell JS, Todd AJ. Lack of evidence for significant neuronal loss in laminae I-III of the spinal dorsal horn of the rat in the chronic constriction injury model. *Pain* 2004; 111:144–150.

Raja SN, Haythornthwaite JA, Pappagallo M, et al. Opioids versus antidepressants in postherpetic neuralgia: a randomized, placebo-controlled trial. *Neurology* 2002; 59:1015–1021.

Ravenscroft A, Ahmed YS, Burnside IG. Chronic pain after SCI. A patient survey. *Spinal Cord* 2000; 38:611–614.

Rowbotham MC, Fields HL. The relationship of pain, allodynia and thermal sensation in post-herpetic neuralgia. *Brain* 1996; 119(Pt 2):347–354.

Scholz J, Broom DC, Youn DH, et al. Blocking caspase activity prevents transsynaptic neuronal apoptosis and the loss of inhibition in lamina II of the dorsal horn after peripheral nerve injury. *J Neurosci* 2005; 25:7317–7323.

Siddall P, Xu CL, Cousins M. Allodynia following traumatic spinal cord injury in the rat. *Neuroreport* 1995; 6:1241–1244.

Snider WD, McMahon SB. Tackling pain at the source: new ideas about nociceptors. *Neuron* 1998; 20:629–632.

Song XJ, Hu SJ, Greenquist KW, Zhang JM, LaMotte RH. Mechanical and thermal hyperalgesia and ectopic neuronal discharge after chronic compression of dorsal root ganglia. *J Neurophysiol* 1999; 82:3347–3358.

Sugimoto T, Bennett GJ, Kajander KC. Transsynaptic degeneration in the superficial dorsal horn after sciatic nerve injury: effects of a chronic constriction injury, transection, and strychnine. *Pain* 1990; 42:205–213.

Tong YG, Wang HF, Ju G, et al. Increased uptake and transport of cholera toxin B-subunit in dorsal root ganglion neurons after peripheral axotomy: possible implications for sensory sprouting. *J Comp Neurol* 1999; 404:143–158.

Torebjork HE, LaMotte RH, Robinson CJ. Peripheral neural correlates of magnitude of cutaneous pain and hyperalgesia: simultaneous recordings in humans of sensory judgments of pain and evoked responses in nociceptors with C-fibers. *J Neurophysiol* 1984; 51:325–339.

Treede RD, Davis KD, Campbell JN, Raja SN. The plasticity of cutaneous hyperalgesia during sympathetic ganglion blockade in patients with neuropathic pain. *Brain* 1992; 115:(Pt 2):607–621.

Vase L, Robinson ME, Verne GN, Price DD. Increased placebo analgesia over time in irritable bowel syndrome (IBS) patients is associated with desire and expectation but not endogenous opioid mechanisms. *Pain* 2005; 115:338–347.

Vierck CJ Jr, Light AR. Allodynia and hyperalgesia within dermatomes caudal to a spinal cord injury in primates and rodents. *Prog Brain Res* 2000; 129:411–428.

Vierck CJ, Acosta-Rua A, Nelligan R, Tester N, Mauderli A. Low dose systemic morphine attenuates operant escape but facilitates innate reflex responses to thermal stimulation. *J Pain* 2002; 3:309–319.

Vierck CJ, Acosta-Rua AJ, Johnson RD. Bilateral chronic constriction of the sciatic nerve: a model of long-term cold hyperalgesia. *J Pain* 2005; 6:507–517.

Villemure C, Slotnick BM, Bushnell MC. Effects of odors on pain perception: deciphering the roles of emotion and attention. *Pain* 2003; 106:101–108.

Wager TD, Rilling JK, Smith EE, et al. Placebo-induced changes in FMRI in the anticipation and experience of pain. *Science* 2004; 303:1162–1167.

Waldhoer M, Bartlett SE, Whistler JL. Opioid receptors. *Annu Rev Biochem* 2004; 73:953–990.

Wallace VC, Norbury TA, Rice AS. Ultrasound vocalisation by rodents does not correlate with behavioural measures of persistent pain. *Eur J Pain* 2005; 9:445–452.

Waxman SG, Dib-Hajj SD. Erythromelalgia: a hereditary pain syndrome enters the molecular era. *Ann Neurol* 2005; 57:785–788.

Wiesenfeld-Hallin Z, Xu XJ. Plasticity of messenger function in primary afferents following nerve injury: implications for neuropathic pain. *Prog Brain Res* 1996; 110:113–124.

Woolf CJ, Shortland P, Reynolds M, et al. Reorganization of central terminals of myelinated primary afferents in the rat dorsal horn following peripheral axotomy. *J Comp Neurol* 1995; 360:121–134.

Xu XJ, Hao JX, Aldskogius H, Seiger A, Wiesenfeld-Hallin Z. Chronic pain-related syndrome in rats after ischemic spinal cord lesion: a possible animal model for pain in patients with spinal cord injury. *Pain* 1992; 48:279–290.

Yezierski RP. Spinal cord injury: a model of central neuropathic pain. *Neurosignals* 2005; 14:182–193.

Correspondence to: Allan I. Basbaum, PhD, Department of Anatomy, University of California San Francisco, Box 2722, 1550 4th Street, San Francisco, CA 94143-2722, USA. Email: allan.basbaum@ucsf.edu.

Emerging Strategies for the Treatment of Neuropathic Pain, edited by James N. Campbell, Allan I. Basbaum, André Dray, Ronald Dubner, Robert H. Dworkin, and Christine N. Sang, IASP Press, Seattle, © 2006.

18

Brain Imaging as a Surrogate Measure of Pain: Human and Animal Studies

M. Catherine Bushnell

Department of Anesthesia, Faculty of Medicine, and Faculty of Dentistry, McGill University, Montreal, Quebec, Canada

Most neuropathic conditions are dominated by ongoing pain. Our major means of assessing clinical pain is to communicate with language. This chapter will consider whether it is feasible to use brain and spinal cord imaging to measure nociceptive processing and, by implication, pain in animals and humans. Measurement of ongoing pain in animals may afford an impetus to development of new treatments.

The health care industry has much at stake in the question as to whether we can use brain imaging as a surrogate measure of pain. Insurance companies want to know if brain imaging can tell them whether a person on disability really has low back pain or is just malingering. Pharmaceutical companies want to know if brain imaging can provide objective evidence of their drugs' effectiveness. Can it provide a more sensitive and reliable measure than self-report in patients? Marketing executives want to show pictures to consumers and say: "This is pain in your brain before and after taking our drug." As brain imaging evolves, many of these questions can be answered in the affirmative. Nevertheless, as will be discussed below, brain-imaging data must always be interpreted with caution.

BRAIN IMAGING TO MEASURE NOCICEPTIVE PROCESSES

The use of brain imaging in humans to study nociceptive processes dates back to the 1970s, when Lassen and colleagues (1978) injected the radioisotope Xenon[133] into human volunteers and produced the first images of cerebral hemodynamic changes related to pain. Although this technique provided only crude spatial resolution and no temporal resolution, the results suggested that presentation of a noxious stimulus led to increased blood flow to the frontal lobes. Although these were exciting results, researchers using these techniques did not continue to study pain, partly because of the prolonged stimulation periods that were required. Nevertheless, when new radiotracers with short half-lives were developed in the late 1980s, imaging of pain in the human brain came into its own. Today, there are numerous imaging techniques for studying pain in the human brain, including positron emission tomography (PET), single photon emission computed tomography (SPECT), functional magnetic resonance imaging (fMRI), electroencephalographic (EEG) dipole source analysis, and magnetoencephalographic analysis (MEG). Each technique has advantages and disadvantages in terms of spatial and temporal resolution, sensitivity, and cost. However, all of these techniques provide measures that can be used as indirect indices of neural activity, and some can be used as measures of neurochemical activity. This chapter will concentrate on data obtained using PET and MRI methodology, which provide better spatial information than other techniques and thus are particularly important for determining pain pathways and pain-modulatory systems.

There have now been scores of brain-imaging studies of pain processing, using both PET and fMRI (see (Apkarian et al. 2004 for an in-depth review]. Although there are many differences in activation patterns across studies, a consistent cortical and subcortical network has emerged that includes sensory, limbic, associative, and motor areas. The most commonly activated brain regions include parts of the primary and secondary somatosensory cortices (S1 and S2), the anterior cingulate cortex (ACC), insular cortex (IC), prefrontal cortex (PFC), thalamus (Th), and cerebellum (CB).

BRAIN IMAGING TO MEASURE PAIN PERCEPTION

The earliest human brain-imaging studies used a block design in which stimuli were turned on and off, and hemodynamic measures were compared during different stimulus conditions. For example, Talbot et al. (1991) measured regional cerebral blood flow (rCBF) when painful heat stimuli as compared to nonpainful warm stimuli were applied to the arm. Similar techniques were used by many investigators in both PET and fMRI scanning protocols. Although the investigators usually confirmed that the subjects were or were not experiencing pain, depending on the condition, they did not factor the intensity of pain into the analysis. Analytical techniques now allow us to correlate the imaging signal with the individual's perception. Different aspects of perception, such as perceived pain intensity and pain

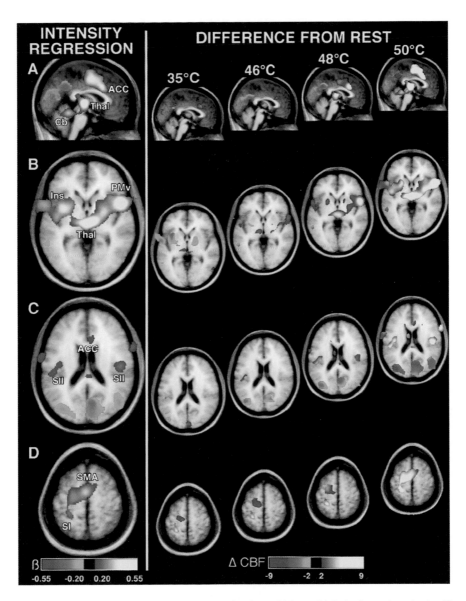

Fig. 1. Regression analysis showing that activation within multiple brain regions is significantly related to subjects' perceptions of pain intensity. Left panel: regression coefficients (β) are color coded such that red-yellow shows positive correlations with pain intensity and blue-violet shows a negative correlation with pain intensity ($P < 0.001$). The right panel shows differences in cerebral blood flow (CBF) between application of heat stimuli at each temperature and rest. Functional data are displayed on the averaged structural magnetic resonance imaging (MRI) data of all subjects. The left side of the image corresponds to the subjects' left. ACC, anterior cingulate cortex; Thal, thalamus; Cb, cerebellum; Ins, insula; PMv, ventral premotor cortex; SII, secondary somatosensory cortex; SI, primary somatosensory cortex; SMA, supplementary motor area. (From Coghill et al. 1999, Fig. 2.)

unpleasantness, can be correlated with the same imaging data to determine which regional activations are best correlated with different aspects of perception. Using PET blood flow imaging, both Rainville et al. (1997) and Tölle et al. (1999) were able to show that pain-evoked activity in the ACC correlated better with subjects' ratings of pain unpleasantness than with their ratings of pain intensity. Coghill et al. (1999) used correlational techniques and PET to show that pain-evoked activity in S1, S2, IC, and ACC significantly correlated with pain perception, whereas that in the dorsolateral prefrontal cortex did not (Fig. 1). Correlating perceptual features with the imaging signal is now being applied to fMRI blood-oxygen-level-dependent (BOLD) techniques. This application incurs some complications not encountered using PET blood flow imaging. Using PET H_2O^{15} blood flow imaging, stimuli are presented during periods of about 1 minute, and scans are separated by 10–12 minutes. During the inter-scan rest periods, subjects can provide ratings of the stimuli in the previous stimulation period. Using fMRI BOLD techniques, subjects are scanned during longer periods (usually 5–10 minutes), with multiple types of stimuli presented during each trial, since the best sensitivity for comparing conditions is obtained within a trial. Having the subjects give perceptual ratings of each stimulus would be ideal, except that providing the rating produces both motor and cognitive confounds. In order to obtain subjective perceptual responses on a stimulus-by-stimulus basis, Koyama et al. (2003) developed a "single-epoch" design, in which a single stimulation period was presented between two baseline periods. The subjects gave ratings during the baseline periods, thus allowing subjective ratings to be acquired after each stimulus, while minimizing rating-induced confounds. Using these techniques, Coghill et al. (2003) showed that highly pain-sensitive subjects showed larger pain-evoked cortical activations than did subjects who gave lower perceptual ratings to the same physical stimulus.

CONNECTIVITY ANALYSIS

Using fMRI, researchers are now performing cross-correlations between activation in different brain regions. Such analyses can shed light both on networks that are activated by pain and on networks that are involved in different types of analgesic manipulations. For example, Lorenz and colleagues (2002, 2003) used network analyses to examine the role of subregions of the frontal cortex in pain processing. The authors compared brain activity evoked during capsaicin-produced heat allodynia and normal heat pain of equal intensities and found that allodynia led to more activity in multiple frontal regions, as well as the medial thalamus, nucleus accumbens, and midbrain. A cross-correlation analysis of this activity demonstrated that dorsal frontal and orbital frontal cortical activities showed a negative correlation, whereas the orbital frontal cortical activation was positively correlated with that in the medial thalamus and nucleus accumbens. These correlations led the authors to hypothesize that a orbital frontal-accumbens-medial thalamus network is engaged in affective perception of pain, while the dorsal frontal cortex acts as a "top-down" controller that modulates pain and thus limits the extent of suffering.

Valet et al. (2004) have applied similar covariation analyses to the study of attentional modulation of pain (Fig. 2). These authors used fMRI to examine activations elicited by painful heat stimuli while subjects were focusing on the pain and when they were distracted by performing a visual incongruent color-word Stroop task. The distraction task increased the activation of the orbitofrontal and perigenual ACC, as well as the periaqueductal gray (PAG) and the posterior thalamus. The covariation analysis revealed a functional interaction between these structures during pain stimulation and distraction, but not during pain stimulation alone, leading the authors to conclude that pain suppression during distraction may be related to top-down influences of the cingulofrontal cortex on the PAG and posterior thalamus.

IMAGING ABNORMAL PAIN PROCESSING

A number of studies have now been performed imaging abnormal pain processing, including peripheral neuropathic pain (Hsieh et al. 1995, 1999a; Iadarola et al. 1995; Duncan et al. 1998; Petrovic et al. 1999; Apkarian et al. 2001b), central pain (Willoch et al. 2000; Olausson et al. 2001), low back pain (Grachev et al. 2000; Apkarian et al. 2004), fibromyalgia (Wik et al. 1999; Gracely et al. 2002), irritable bowel syndrome (Silverman et al. 1997; Mertz et al. 2000; Naliboff et al. 2001; Bernstein et al. 2002), and vulvovestibulitis (Pukall et al. 2005). Because both PET and fMRI analytical techniques are based on signal changes in response to a stimulus, it is difficult to image ongoing tonic pain. Thus, most of the PET and fMRI studies of abnormal pain processing image allodynia related to the clinical condition. For example, in studying peripheral or central neuropathic pain, experimenters often stimulate the subject with a soft brush or a warm or cool stimulus, which produces pain in patients but not in healthy control subjects. Such studies have found that during allodynia, at least some cortical pain-related regions are activated (Peyron et al. 1998, 2000; Hsieh et al. 1999a; Olausson et al. 2001) and concluded that such activation most likely underlies

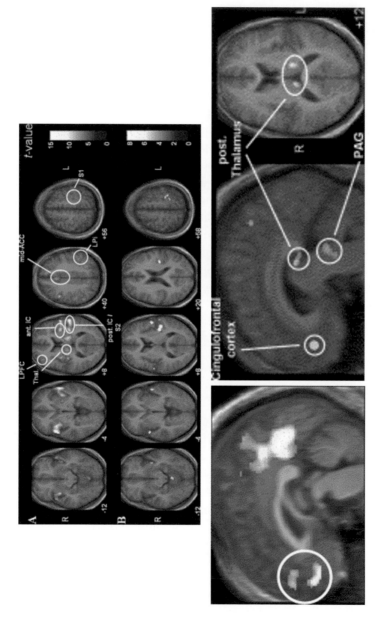

the pain experience. Similarly, in syndromes such as fibromyalgia, irritable bowel syndrome, or vulvovestibulitis, patients are abnormally sensitive to pressure stimuli, and imaging studies show enhanced activation to normally nonpainful stimuli. For example, Gracely et al. (2002) showed a pattern of cortical pain-related activity in response to mild pressure stimuli in fibromyalgia patients. The experimenters equated stimulus intensities and perception intensities between patients and normal subjects and found that weaker stimuli were needed in fibromyalgia patients to produce the same pain as in normal control subjects. When perceived stimulus intensity was equated, similar regions were activated for patients and controls, but when the physical stimulus intensity was equated, fibromyalgia patients showed greater activation in pain-related brain regions.

Nevertheless, the results of other studies suggest that unique aspects of forebrain functioning may be associated with pathological pain states. One example is the evidence of a decrease in thalamic activity in patients with aberrant pain states (Iadarola et al. 1995; Fukumoto et al. 1999). Not only is there less activity in the thalamus contralateral to the pain, but in some cases there is a positive relationship between the duration of the chronic pain and the reduction in activity (Fukumoto et al. 1999).

The imaging of spontaneous pain during chronic conditions has presented a problem to researchers. Nevertheless, one can take advantage of natural fluctuations in spontaneous pain, using real-time pain measures during fMRI scanning to correlate ongoing pain with the BOLD signal. Although this technique can be both powerful and sensitive, the on-line pain measurements require both motor activity (finger or hand movement) and cognitive processing, both of which must be taken into account when interpreting the

---

← **Fig. 2.** Top figure: fMRI BOLD response to painful stimuli (A) without distraction and (B) during the Stroop distraction task. The images represent pain-specific activation effects ($P < 0.05$ corr.) that are corrected for temperature-related activation effects. Without distraction, noxious stimulation (A) evokes significant activation of S1 and S2 sensory cortices, the anterior cingulate cortex (ACC), the anterior and posterior insular cortex (IC), and the thalamus. During distraction (B) induced by the Stroop task, the same noxious stimulation fails to significantly activate these regions. Activation maps are superimposed on the mean normalized anatomical images of the subjects. The right side of the image corresponds to the left side of the brain. Bottom left figure: Pain-specific regions that show a higher activation level during distraction than without distraction ($P < 0.05$ corr.). Activation is observed in the cingulofrontal cortex, including the perigenual ACC (BA 32) and orbitofrontal cortex (BA 10/11), and a part of the occipital transition zone. Bottom right figure: Covariation analysis with the BOLD signal pattern of the cingulofrontal cortex (blue area). Covariation with the periaqueductal gray (PAG) and the posterior thalamus were only observed during noxious stimulation with distraction ($P < 0.001$ uncorr.). No covariation between these structures was detected during any of the other conditions. (From Valet et al. 2004, Figs. 2, 3, 4.)

data. Researchers are beginning to apply such techniques to the study of chronic and acute pain (Apkarian et al. 2001a). As these techniques are new, a consensus of findings remains to be determined.

ANATOMICAL IMAGING—VOXEL-BASED MORPHOMETRY

The study of regional anatomical changes in the human brain related to disease is an important new area of investigation. Voxel-based morphometry (VBM) is a method used to compare local concentrations of gray matter between groups of individuals. The technique includes first spatially normalizing high-resolution anatomical MRI images from all the subjects in the study into the same stereotactic space. Next, the gray matter of the normalized brains is segmented into distinct regions. Finally, the density of gray matter in each region is compared between groups. A number of studies have used this technique to examine anatomical differences between patients with various psychiatric disorders and control subjects (Lyoo et al. 2004; Moorhead et al. 2004; Wilke et al. 2004). Apkarian and colleagues (2004) have now applied this technique to the study of chronic pain (Fig. 3). They found that patients with long-term low back pain have reduced gray matter density in the bilateral dorsolateral PFC and right thalamus, compared to matched control subjects. Further, there was a negative correlation between the duration of the back pain and the amount of gray matter in these regions. Thus, although less gray matter in the dorsolateral PFC and thalamus could be a predisposing factor for pain to become chronic, the negative correlation with duration of pain suggests that the reduced gray matter may in fact be a result of the long-term pain.

IMAGING NEUROPHARMACOLOGICAL PROCESSES RELATED TO PAIN AND ANALGESIA

Neuropharmacological processes related to pain and analgesia have been studied in humans using several methods. One important technique involves imaging of radio-labeled chemical substances in the brain. The distribution of different types of receptors in the brain can be imaged, using exogenously administered radiolabeled substances that bind to specific receptor types. Several studies have examined the distribution of opioid receptors in the normal human brain (Frost et al. 1990; Villemagne et al. 1994; Zubieta et al. 1999; Bencherif et al. 2002), finding receptors in the thalamus, striatum, and cortical areas involved in pain processing, such as the cingulate cortex.

A technique that has great potential for increasing our understanding of the neuropharmacology of pain transmission and pain modulation is the competitive binding technique. This technique allows one to examine differences in binding of an exogenously applied radiolabeled substance in the presence and absence of pain. This technique has been used to study the role of forebrain opioid receptors in pain. The hypothesis is that when a painful stimulus is applied, endogenous opioids will be released in regions important for analgesia. If an exogenous radiolabeled opiate is administered at the same time as the pain, its uptake will be reduced in regions important for analgesia, since the receptors will be occupied by the endogenously released opioids. In opioid-rich regions not important for analgesia, there should be no difference in uptake of the exogenous opiate in the presence or absence of pain. Studies using this approach and the radiolabeled μ-opioid receptor agonist [^{11}C]-carfentanil have found dynamic changes in the activity of μ-opioid receptors (Zubieta et al. 2001, 2003; Bencherif et al. 2002). Reductions in the in vivo availability of μ-opioid receptors, reflecting the activation of this neurotransmitter system, were observed in the ACC, PFC, IC, thalamus, basal ganglia, amygdala, and PAG, thus suggesting that opioid receptors in these regions are involved in the production of analgesia (Fig. 4).

Another neurotransmitter system that has been implicated in pain is dopamine. Using radiolabeled raclopride, an agonist of the D2 and D3 dopamine receptors, and PET imaging in healthy human volunteers, Hagelberg et al. (2002) found an inverse correlation between subjects' cold pain threshold and tolerance and striatal and extrastriatal D2/D3 binding potential, suggesting that low pain sensitivity is related to high basal dopamine tone.

Hagelberg et al. (2002) also found a positive correlation between the magnitude of pain-evoked analgesia (diffuse noxious inhibitory control) and striatal D2/D3-binding potential, suggesting the possibility that at least one endogenous pain inhibitory system in the brain involves dopamine (Fig. 5). Other data from the same group suggest that in chronic pain patients, low levels of endogenous dopamine may contribute to the pain syndrome. A PET study of patients with burning mouth syndrome showed a consistent reduction of 6-[^{18}F]-fluoro-L-DOPA uptake in the striatum compared with healthy controls (Jaaskelainen et al. 2001). Another study found higher [^{11}C]-raclopride binding in the striatum of these patients compared to healthy volunteers (Hagelberg et al. 2003). Together, these findings suggest reduced endogenous dopamine in some chronic pain patients.

Another method of examining modulatory systems activated during analgesia is to study brain metabolic function in response to pharmacological agents. Using this approach, several investigators have tested the effect of μ-opioid agonists on regional CBF responses to painful stimuli (Casey et al.

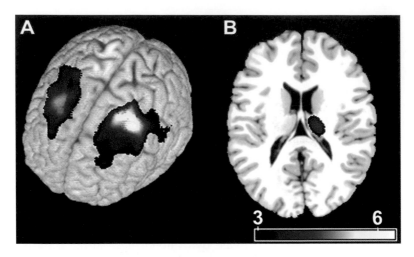

Fig. 3. Regional gray matter density decreases in subjects with chronic back pain. A nonparametric comparison of voxel-based morphometry between back pain and control subjects is shown. (A) Gray matter density is bilaterally reduced in the dorsolateral prefrontal cortex. Pseudocolor highly positive values indicate regions where gray matter density was reduced in back pain subjects (controls minus subjects). (B) A nonparametric comparison spatially limited to the thalami revealed a significant decrease in gray matter density in the right anterior thalamus. A slice at the peak of decreased thalamic gray matter is shown. Pseudo-*t* values are color coded in a range of 3–6. (From Apkarian et al. 2004, Fig. 2.)

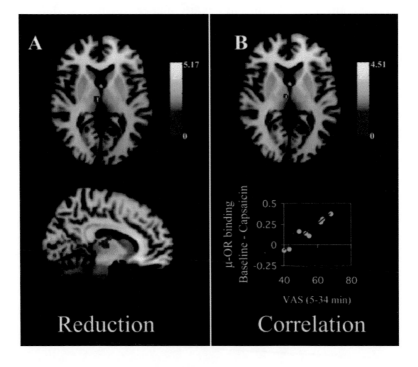

2000; Petrovic et al. 2002; Wise et al. 2004). These studies showed that pain-evoked activation in the ACC and IC, areas rich in opioid receptors, is reduced during opiate analgesia (Fig. 6).

IMAGING NONPHARMACOLOGICAL ANALGESIA

The mechanisms underlying psychological or behavioral modulation of pain are difficult to address in animal studies. On the other hand, complex psychological variables and their effect on pain processing can be readily addressed using human brain-imaging methods. A number of investigators have conducted human imaging studies examining the effects of attention and distraction on pain, and in general these show that distraction leads to a reduction of pain-evoked activity in the thalamus and in several cortical regions, including the S1 cortex, ACC, and IC (Bushnell et al. 1999; Longe et al. 2001; Bantick et al. 2002). Other regions, including the PAG, parts of the ACC, and the PFC are activated when subjects are distracted from pain, suggesting that these regions may be involved in the modulatory circuitry related to attention (Petrovic et al. 2000; Frankenstein et al. 2001; Tracey et al. 2002; Valet et al. 2004).

Other studies have shown that hypnosis and hypnotic suggestions alter pain-evoked activity. Further, the regions showing modulation depend on the nature of the suggestions (Rainville et al. 1997; Faymonville et al. 2000; Hofbauer et al. 2001). When subjects receive suggestions to interpret a burning sensation as extremely unpleasant in one condition and as not at all unpleasant in another condition, pain-evoked activity in the ACC differs between conditions, even though the physical stimulus is the same (Rainville et al. 1997). On the other hand, when subjects are given suggestions leading them to feel the burning sensation as more or less intense, the most prominent modulation is in the S1 cortex (Hofbauer et al. 2001). These findings not only show that hypnotic suggests have a clear modulatory effect on pain processing, but they also suggest that the nature of the modulation is dependent on the nature of the suggestions. Since subjects are required to attend to the

---

← **Fig. 4.** Reduction in regional brain μ-opioid receptor (OR) binding during capsaicin-induced pain to the left hand and regional correlation with pain ratings. Statistical *t* maps after fusion on coregistered MRI show a unique cluster of decreased μ-OR binding in the right thalamus during the capsaicin PET session compared to the baseline PET session. Positive correlation between decrease in μ-OR binding and average VAS pain rating 5–34 minutes after administration of [^{11}C]-carfentanil was also seen in the region showing an absolute decrease in μ-OR binding. Higher pain ratings during the capsaicin PET session were associated with a greater reduction in μ-OR binding compared to the baseline PET session in the right thalamus. (From Bencherif et al., Fig. 2.)

pain stimulus in all conditions, it is likely that hypnotic suggestions invoke modulatory systems other than those involved in selective attention, and these systems most likely involve frontal cortical areas (Rainville et al. 1999).

Other studies have examined the effect of anticipation on pain-evoked activity in the brain. Regions such as the S1 cortex, ACC, PAG, IC, PFC, and cerebellum are all activated during periods of expectation, before the painful stimulus is presented (Hsieh et al. 1999b; Ploghaus et al. 1999; Sawamoto et al. 2000; Porro et al. 2002).

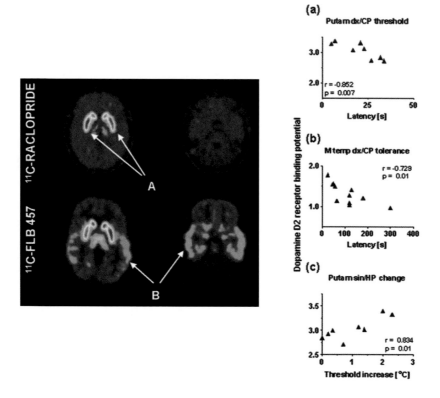

Fig. 5. Left panel: Examples of a [¹¹C]-raclopride scan of striatal dopamine D2 receptors (upper graphs) and an [¹¹C]-FLB 457 scan of extrastriatal D2 receptors (lower graphs) in two healthy subjects. The graphs show axial slices at the striatal (left) and cerebellar (right) level. The arrow A indicates the head of the putamen. The arrow B indicates the temporal cortex. Right panel: Associations of dopamine D2-receptor-binding potentials in selected brain regions of interest with sensory responses. (a) The right putamen and cold pain (CP) threshold. (b) The right medial temporal cortex and cold pain tolerance. (c) The left putamen and the elevation of heat pain (HP) threshold by conditioning stimulation. In panel (b), the radioligand was [¹¹C]-FLB 457, and in other graphs it was [¹¹C]-raclopride. The Pearson coefficient of correlation and the significance of correlation are given in each graph. Putam dx, the right putamen; Putam sin, the left putamen; M temp dx, the right medial temporal cortex. (From Hagelberg et al. 2002, Figs. 1 and 2).

Investigators have now begun to explore the neural basis of placebo analgesia, which can involve expectation, attention, and conditioning (Petrovic et al. 2002; Wager et al. 2004). Wager and colleagues (2004) performed fMRI experiments involving two types of experimental pain (evoked by heat and electrical stimuli) and expectation-induced placebo analgesia. They found that placebo analgesia was related to decreased brain activity in pain-sensitive brain regions, including the thalamus, IC, and ACC. Furthermore, the placebo analgesia was associated with increased activity in the prefrontal cortex. Thus, it appears that endogenous modulatory circuits that are activated during placebo analgesia reduce pain transmission to cortical pain-processing areas.

SPINAL CORD IMAGING IN HUMANS

Since the advent of fMRI, pain researchers have asked "Can we image the spinal cord in humans?" Despite the intense interest in applying this method to the spinal cord, there have been few reports of such imaging,

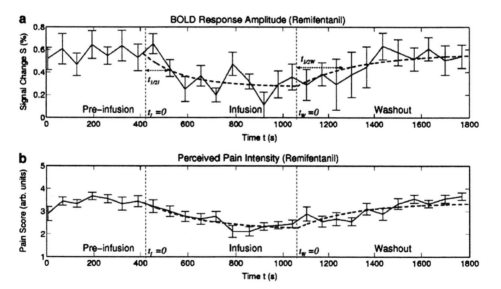

Fig. 6. Time-course of fMRI in the insular cortex and perceived pain intensity. Mean amplitude of the BOLD response to pain (solid line, a) and mean perceived pain intensity scores (solid line, b) during the course of sessions in which subjects received the opioid agonist remifentanil. Each point represents the response to one stimulus. Error bars indicate the standard error of the mean across subjects. $t_I = 0$ and $t_W = 0$ indicate the onset and cessation of remifentanil infusion, respectively. The heavy broken lines indicate the fitted exponential models from which the onset equilibration half-life ($t_{1/2I}$) and the washout half-life of drug activity ($t_{1/2W}$) were estimated. (From Wise et al. 2004, Fig. 5).

because of the unique problems associated with it. First, a resolution of no more than 1 mm is necessary to obtain any relevant information. In imaging of the brain, the spatial resolution is typically 2–5 mm. Other problems include poor field homogeneity caused by the bone surrounding the spinal cord and pulsations of the cerebrospinal fluid. For the cervical spinal cord, additional problems include respiratory motion and the effects of changing lung volumes on the local field homogeneity (Stroman et al. 1999). Yoshizawa et al. (1996) were the first to investigate the potential use of fMRI to study spinal cord activity. These investigators reported changes in signal intensity in BOLD-sensitive MRI of the human cervical spinal cord between periods of rest and hand exercise. This initial study, however, lacked the spatial resolution and sensitivity necessary to demonstrate specific areas of activation. Later, Stroman et al. (1999) used a 3-Tesla (T) MRI and BOLD imaging in the human cervical spinal cord to examine the signal produced by hand exercise alternated with rest. They found regions of activation between the levels of the sixth cervical and first thoracic spinal cord segments, with the activation being predominantly ipsilateral to the moving hand. This study produced somewhat more regional specificity and sensitivity than the Yoshizawa study and demonstrated that spinal fMRI is feasible. The same group then went on to examine contrast changes in fMRI of the human spinal cord using a 1.5-T scanner, a type that is readily available in clinical settings, using both spin-echo and gradient-echo echo-planer imaging (Stroman and Ryner 2001). Their analyses suggested a non-BOLD contribution to the signal changes observed in spinal fMRI and hypothesized that this contribution is a local proton density increase due to increased water exudation from capillaries with increased blood flow during neuronal activation, termed SEEP (signal enhancement by extravascular protons). Stroman and colleagues have published several papers showing both sensory and motor activation in the human cervical and lumbar spinal cord using SEEP fMRI (Stroman et al. 2002, 2004; Kornelsen and Stroman 2004) (Fig. 7). These investigators feel that the SEEP methodology more accurately and sensitively represents spinal cord neural activity. Nevertheless, the technique is controversial and has recently been criticized by Jochimsen et al. (2005), who suggest that the use of a low threshold to identify activated voxels may generate an artificial offset in functional contrast due to the inclusion of false-positives in the analysis. Thus, spinal cord imaging in humans is an evolving technique. To date, it has produced only crude images that would do little to tell us about subtle physiological changes related to nerve damage or chronic pain conditions. However, with improvements both in scanners and analytical techniques, it seems likely that this method will soon yield a sensitivity that will be useful for pain researchers.

MAGNETIC RESONANCE IMAGING IN ANIMALS

High-resolution fMRI of the animal brain began more than a decade ago, but it has received little application in terms of pain. When pain researchers consider using animal MRI to examine brain and spinal cord nociceptive mechanisms, the first question that usually arises is "What is the resolution?" The temporal and spatial resolution in any given study depends on many factors, including magnet strength and the type of response being measured. Imaging the metabolic change (e.g., by 2-deoxyglucose autoradiography) yields high spatial specificity, since increased metabolism will occur at the activated tissue. Given that the magnitude of CBF change is well correlated with that of glucose consumption change, CBF mapping can identify the most active regions of neural activity. In contrast, the most commonly used gradient-echo BOLD technique is sensitive to paramagnetic deoxyhemoglobin changes occurring at both the capillaries and the draining venous system, with the latter reducing the spatial specificity of the conventional gradient-echo BOLD signal. Thus, among the available hemodynamic fMRI approaches, the CBF-based signal is expected to be the most specific to sites of neuronal activity, since most of the signal originates from tissue and capillaries. Tissue-specific BOLD signals that are obtained using spin-echo, instead of gradient-echo, techniques will have less contribution from large vessels and thus will yield better spatial specificity. However, the spin-echo BOLD technique can be used only when ultrahigh fields (such as 9.4 T) are available. Nevertheless, with such techniques, spatial resolution of 100 μm can be achieved (Kim and Ugurbil 2003). Temporal resolution is more of a problem, because the hemodynamic response is sluggish, usually beginning 1–2 seconds after the onset of neuronal activity, with the peak of activity occurring 5–8 seconds after neuronal activity begins. Furthermore, the timing of the vascular response varies in different brain tissue. Nevertheless, by using an approach with multiple experiments with different stimulus conditions, temporal resolution can be improved to approximately 100 ms (Kim and Ugurbil 2003).

Effects of anesthesia on animal MRI. It is usually necessary to anesthetize animals when performing fMRI, and the effect of anesthesia on the signal is an important issue. Austin et al. (2005) used a rat model of direct cortical stimulation to investigate the effects of anesthesia in rodent fMRI. Using halothane, the investigators found no significant differences in the amplitude of the BOLD response at different halothane doses, despite electroencephalography recordings indicating a dose-dependent reduction in neuronal activity with increasing halothane levels. When anesthesia was changed to chloralose, there was an immediate reduction in the spatial extent of

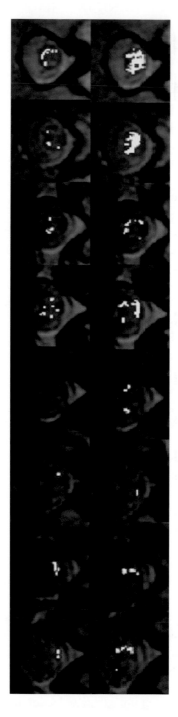

Fig. 7. Combined activity map of the lumbar spinal cord of normal human subjects while they were engaged in passive pedaling or active pedaling, using an MRI-compatible pedaling device that was attached to their feet in the scanner. During passive pedaling (top row) there was motor and reflex activity, and during active pedaling (bottom row) there was bilateral motor activity and sensory activity. Images are axial and in radiological orientation, with the right side of the body to the left of the image; dorsal is toward the bottom. Eight image slices are shown, spanning from the 3rd sacral spinal cord segment (S3) on the left, moving rostrally along the spinal cord, reaching the 1st lumbar spinal cord segment (L1) on the right. (From Kornelsen and Stroman 2004, Fig. 2.)

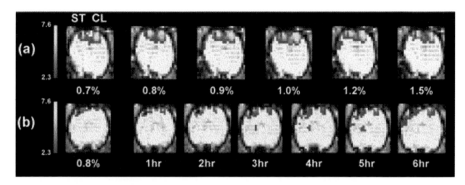

Fig. 8. fMRI responses to direct cortical stimulation of the left hindpaw motor cortex under halothane and α-chloralose anesthesia in two representative animals. Z-score activation maps (thresholded at $P = 0.01$) are overlaid on the gradient-echo images under (a) different levels of halothane anesthesia and (b) under 0.8% halothane and at hourly intervals following transfer to α-chloralose anesthesia. ST and CL indicate the stimulated and contralateral cortices, respectively. (From Austin et al. 2005, Fig. 1.)

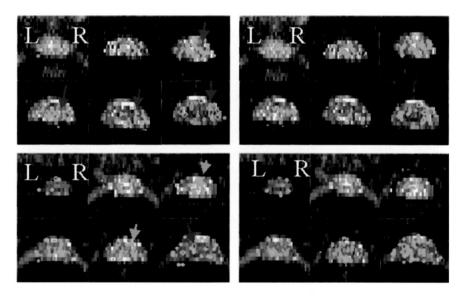

Fig. 9. Combined activation map showing activations (left) and deactivations (right) of six slices of the lumbar spinal cord from L2 to T13 of the vertebral column (spinal cord segments S2–L3) after application of a light touch stimulus without (top) and with (bottom) physiotherapy manipulation, 3 hours after capsaicin injection into the right ankle. Dorsal is toward the top and ventral toward the bottom of the images. Red illustrates the greatest amount of overlap in activations or deactivations between animals, followed by blue, then green. The arrows point to the greatest amount of overlap of interest. Individual data sets were analyzed using direct correlation to the paradigm with $R = 0.312$ ($P \geq 0.05$). The final overlay map was obtained with a cut-off value of 0.33 and 3×3 kernal smoothing. (From Malizsa et al. 2003, Fig. 3.)

the BOLD response, followed several hours later by a significant increase in both the spatial extent and peak height of the BOLD signal (Fig. 8). These results suggest a substantial variation in the effect of anesthetic agents on the BOLD response, which could introduce considerable variability into studies.

Animal fMRI to study nociceptive mechanisms in the brain. Although several studies have used fMRI to examine dynamic changes in the rat brain during forepaw electrical stimulation (Hyder et al. 1994; Mandeville et al. 1998; Marota et al. 1999), few studies have used the technique to examine the effect of noxious stimuli on brain activity. However, a recent study used correlational analyses in animal fMRI studies to examine possible nociceptive connectivity. Shyu et al. (2004) examined connectivity between the medial thalamus and ACC in rats using electrical microstimulation and fMRI. These authors implanted glass-coated carbon fiber microelectrodes in the left medial thalamus of anesthetized rats, and obtained T2*-weighted gradient-echo images on a 4.7-T MRI scanner. A series of two-slice images were acquired during electrical stimulation of the medial thalamus, and a cross-correlation analysis was used to show that the signal intensities of activated areas in the ipsilateral ACC were significantly increased during thalamic stimulation.

Animal fMRI in the spinal cord. There have been several recent reports of fMRI in the rat spinal cord (Malisza and Stroman 2002; Malisza et al. 2003a; Lawrence et al. 2004), using high field imaging (7 T or 9.4 T). Malisza and Stroman (2002) used fMRI to examine the rat cervical spinal cord during two types of painful stimulation—capsaicin injection and electrical stimulation of the forepaw. The investigators observed activation in the dorsal horn of the spinal cord using both types of stimulation, and they were able to reproduce the nociceptive response several times in each animal. They concluded that spinal fMRI can be a useful tool in animal models of pain and injury. The same group reproduced the capsaicin findings in the rat lumbar spinal cord (Malisza et al. 2003b), using injections into the hindpaw and ankle joint. Further, they observed activation in response to light touch after the capsaicin injection (corresponding to allodynia), although this response was less reliable (Fig. 9). Finally, following ankle joint manipulation resembling that used in physiotherapy they found a trend toward a decreased area of activation during the allodynia. These results suggest that fMRI of the spinal cord in rats may provide enough sensitivity to examine analgesic manipulations.

POSITRON EMISSION TOMOGRAPHY IN ANIMALS

The development of small-animal PET scanners has taken place during the last decade (see Chatziioannou 2002 for review). The first PET system developed specifically for rodent imaging was the RAT-PET scanner (Bloomfield et al. 1995, 1997), developed by Hammersmith Hospital in collaboration with the manufacturer. This system, the first to demonstrate the potential utility of a dedicated small-animal PET scanner, has been used for neuroreceptor work on the rat brain (Hume et al. 1995). Since then several other institutions have developed small-animal PET scanners, and commercial small-animal PET systems are now available. As these systems develop, it appears that the resolution limit for small-animal PET investigations lies below 1 mm. The PET technology in small animals allows researchers to transform in vitro biology into the in vivo setting of animal models. This development is of particular interest to pharmaceutical companies, since the technology provides the ability to quickly perform in vivo pharmacokinetic and pharmacodynamic investigations for many different compounds across multiple species. The combined use of small-animal PET and gene-manipulated animal models holds great potential for accelerating the drug discovery process. The application of small-animal PET to the study of nociceptive processes has received limited attention to date, but as scanners become more readily available and the spatial resolution improves, there is great potential for the application of this technology to pain research in rats and mice.

CONCLUSION

Brain imaging in humans and animals has the potential to reveal much about normal and abnormal nociceptive processes. It can be used as a tool to examine sites of action of new pharmaceutical agents and to provide an overview of brain areas ultimately affected by an analgesic manipulation. Nevertheless, the spatial and temporal resolution is still limited, and the statistical nature of the data analysis makes the interpretation of negative results problematic. A lack of an observed effect with either fMRI or PET technologies does not mean that a clinically important effect does not exist. The sensitivity for detecting what could be a physiologically important signal is limited. However, the technology is advancing at a great rate, so that the spatial and temporal resolution, as well as the sensitivity, of the techniques will continue to improve.

REFERENCES

Apkarian AV, Krauss BR, Fredrickson BE, Szeverenyi NM. Imaging the pain of low back pain: functional magnetic resonance imaging in combination with monitoring subjective pain perception allows the study of clinical pain states. *Neurosci Lett* 2001a; 299:57–60.

Apkarian AV, Thomas PS, Krauss BR, Szeverenyi NM. Prefrontal cortical hyperactivity in patients with sympathetically mediated chronic pain. *Neurosci Lett* 2001b; 311:193–197.

Apkarian AV, Sosa Y, Sonty S, et al. Chronic back pain is associated with decreased prefrontal and thalamic gray matter density. *J Neurosci* 2004; 24:10410–10415.

Austin VC, Blamire AM, Allers KA, et al. Confounding effects of anesthesia on functional activation in rodent brain: a study of halothane and alpha-chloralose anesthesia. *Neuroimage* 2005; 24:92–100.

Bantick SJ, Wise RG, Ploghaus A, et al. Imaging how attention modulates pain in humans using functional MRI. *Brain* 2002; 125:310–319.

Bencherif B, Fuchs PN, Sheth R, et al. Pain activation of human supraspinal opioid pathways as demonstrated by [¹¹C]-carfentanil and positron emission tomography (PET). *Pain* 2002; 99:589–598.

Bernstein CN, Frankenstein UN, Rawsthorne P, et al. Cortical mapping of visceral pain in patients with GI disorders using functional magnetic resonance imaging. *Am J Gastroenterol* 2002; 97:319–327.

Bloomfield PM, Rajeswaran S, Spinks TJ, et al. The design and physical characteristics of a small animal positron emission tomograph. *Phys Med Biol* 1995; 40:1105–1126.

Bloomfield PM, Myers R, Hume SP, et al. Three-dimensional performance of a small-diameter positron emission tomograph. *Phys Med Biol* 1997; 42:389–400.

Bushnell MC, Duncan GH, Hofbauer RK, et al. Pain perception: is there a role for primary somatosensory cortex? *Proc Natl Acad Sci USA* 1999; 96:7705–7709.

Casey KL, Svensson P, Morrow TJ, et al. Selective opiate modulation of nociceptive processing in the human brain. *J Neurophysiol* 2000; 84:525–533.

Chatziioannou AF. Molecular imaging of small animals with dedicated PET tomographs. *Eur J Nucl Med Mol Imaging* 2002; 29:98–114.

Coghill RC, Sang CN, Maisog JM, Iadarola MJ. Pain intensity processing within the human brain: a bilateral, distributed mechanism. *J Neurophysiol* 1999; 82:1934–1943.

Coghill RC, McHaffie JG, Yen YF. Neural correlates of interindividual differences in the subjective experience of pain. *Proc Natl Acad Sci USA* 2003; 100:8538–8542.

Duncan GH, Kupers RC, Marchand S, et al. Stimulation of human thalamus for pain relief: possible modulatory circuits revealed by positron emission tomography. *J Neurophysiol* 1998; 80:3326–3330.

Faymonville ME, Laureys S, Degueldre C, et al. Neural mechanisms of antinociceptive effects of hypnosis. *Anesthesiology* 2000; 92:1257–1267.

Frankenstein UN, Richter W, McIntyre MC, Remy F. Distraction modulates anterior cingulate gyrus activations during the cold pressor test. *Neuroimage* 2001; 14:827–836.

Frost JJ, Mayberg HS, Sadzot B, et al. Comparison of [¹¹C]diprenorphine and [¹¹C]carfentanil binding to opiate receptors in humans by positron emission tomography. *J Cereb Blood Flow Metab* 1990; 10:484–492.

Fukumoto M, Ushida T, Zinchuk VS, Yamamoto H, Yoshida S. Contralateral thalamic perfusion in patients with reflex sympathetic dystrophy syndrome. *Lancet* 1999; 354:1790–1791.

Gracely RH, Petzke F, Wolf JM, Clauw DJ. Functional magnetic resonance imaging evidence of augmented pain processing in fibromyalgia. *Arthritis Rheum* 2002; 46:1333–1343.

Grachev ID, Fredrickson BE, Apkarian AV. Abnormal brain chemistry in chronic back pain: an in vivo proton magnetic resonance spectroscopy study. *Pain* 2000; 89:7–18.

Hagelberg N, Martikainen IK, Mansikka H, et al. Dopamine D2 receptor binding in the human brain is associated with the response to painful stimulation and pain modulatory capacity. *Pain* 2002; 99:273–279.

Hagelberg N, Forssell H, Rinne JO, et al. Striatal dopamine D1 and D2 receptors in burning mouth syndrome. *Pain* 2003; 101:149–154.

Hofbauer RK, Rainville P, Duncan GH, Bushnell MC. Cortical representation of the sensory dimension of pain. *J Neurophysiol* 2001; 86:402–411.

Hsieh JC, Belfrage M, Stone-Elander S, Hansson P, Ingvar M. Central representation of chronic ongoing neuropathic pain studied positron emission tomography. *Pain* 1995; 63:225–236.

Hsieh JC, Meyerson BA, Ingvar M. PET study on central processing of pain in trigeminal neuropathy. *Eur J Pain* 1999a; 3:51–65.

Hsieh JC, Stone-Elander S, Ingvar M. Anticipatory coping of pain expressed in the human anterior cingulate cortex: a positron emission tomography study. *Neurosci Lett* 1999b; 262:61–64.

Hume SP, Opacka-Juffry J, Myers R, et al. Effect of L-dopa and 6-hydroxydopamine lesioning on [^{11}C]raclopride binding in rat striatum, quantified using PET. *Synapse* 1995; 21:45–53.

Hyder F, Behar KL, Martin MA, Blamire AM, Shulman RG. Dynamic magnetic resonance imaging of the rat brain during forepaw stimulation. *J Cereb Blood Flow Metab* 1994; 14:649–655.

Iadarola MJ, Max MB, Berman KF, et al. Unilateral decrease in thalamic activity observed with positron emission tomography in patients with chronic neuropathic pain. *Pain* 1995; 63:55–64.

Jaaskelainen SK, Rinne JO, Forssell H, et al. Role of the dopaminergic system in chronic pain—a fluorodopa-PET study. *Pain* 2001; 90:257–260.

Jochimsen TH, Norris DG, Moller HE. Is there a change in water proton density associated with functional magnetic resonance imaging? *Magn Reson Med* 2005; 53:470–473.

Kim SG, Ugurbil K. High-resolution functional magnetic resonance imaging of the animal brain. *Methods* 2003; 30:28–41.

Kornelsen J, Stroman PW. fMRI of the lumbar spinal cord during a lower limb motor task. *Magn Reson Med* 2004; 52:411–414.

Koyama T, McHaffie JG, Laurienti PJ, Coghill RC. The single-epoch fMRI design: validation of a simplified paradigm for the collection of subjective ratings. *Neuroimage* 2003; 19:976–987.

Lassen NA, Ingvar DH, Skinhoj E. Brain function and blood flow: changes in the amount of blood flowing in areas of the human cerebral cortex, reflecting changes in the activity of those areas, are graphically revealed with the aid of a radioactive isotope. *Sci Am* 1978; 139:62–71.

Lawrence J, Stroman PW, Bascaramurty S, Jordan LM, Malisza KL. Correlation of functional activation in the rat spinal cord with neuronal activation detected by immunohistochemistry. *Neuroimage* 2004; 22:1802–1807.

Longe SE, Wise R, Bantick S, et al. Counter-stimulatory effects on pain perception and processing are significantly altered by attention: an fMRI study. *Neuroreport* 2001; 12:2021–2025.

Lorenz J, Cross DJ, Minoshima S, et al. A unique representation of heat allodynia in the human brain. *Neuron* 2002; 35:383–393.

Lorenz J, Minoshima S, Casey KL. Keeping pain out of mind: the role of the dorsolateral prefrontal cortex in pain modulation. *Brain* 2003; 126:1079–1091.

Lyoo IK, Kim MJ, Stoll AL, et al. Frontal lobe gray matter density decreases in bipolar I disorder. *Biol Psychiatry* 2004; 55:648–651.

Malisza KL, Stroman PW. Functional imaging of the rat cervical spinal cord. *Magn Reson Imaging* 2002; 16:553–558.

Malisza KL, Gregorash L, Turner A, et al. Functional MRI involving painful stimulation of the ankle and the effect of physiotherapy joint mobilization. *Magn Reson Imaging* 2003a; 21:489–496.

Malisza KL, Stroman PW, Turner A, et al. Functional MRI of the rat lumbar spinal cord involving painful stimulation and the effect of peripheral joint mobilization. *Magn Reson Imaging* 2003b; 18:152–159.

Mandeville JB, Marota JJ, Kosofsky BE, et al. Dynamic functional imaging of relative cerebral blood volume during rat forepaw stimulation. *Magn Reson Med* 1998; 39:615–624.

Marota JJ, Ayata C, Moskowitz MA, et al. Investigation of the early response to rat forepaw stimulation. *Magn Reson Med* 1999; 41:247–252.

Mertz H, Morgan V, Tanner G, et al. Regional cerebral activation in irritable bowel syndrome and control subjects with painful and nonpainful rectal distention. *Gastroenterology* 2000; 118:842–848.

Moorhead TW, Job DE, Whalley HC, et al. Voxel-based morphometry of comorbid schizophrenia and learning disability: analyses in normalized and native spaces using parametric and nonparametric statistical methods. *Neuroimage* 2004; 22:188–202.

Naliboff BD, Derbyshire SW, Munakata J, et al. Cerebral activation in patients with irritable bowel syndrome and control subjects during rectosigmoid stimulation. *Psychosom Med* 2001; 63:365–375.

Olausson H, Marchand S, Bittar RG, et al. Central pain in a hemispherectomized patient. *Eur J Pain* 2001; 5:209–218.

Petrovic P, Ingvar M, Stone-Elander S, Petersson KM, Hansson PA. PET activation study of dynamic mechanical allodynia in patients with mononeuropathy. *Pain* 1999; 83:459–470.

Petrovic P, Petersson KM, Ghatan PH, Stone-Elander S, Ingvar M. Pain-related cerebral activation is altered by a distracting cognitive task. *Pain* 2000; 85:19–30.

Petrovic P, Kalso E, Petersson KM, Ingvar M. Placebo and opioid analgesia—imaging a shared neuronal network. *Science* 2002; 295:1737–1740.

Peyron R, Garcia-Larrea L, Gregoire MC, et al. Allodynia after lateral-medullary (Wallenberg) infarct. A PET study. *Brain* 1998; 121 (Pt 2):345–356.

Peyron R, Larrea L, Gregoire MC, et al. Parietal and cingulate processes in central pain. A combined positron emission tomography (PET) and functional magnetic resonance imaging (fMRI) study of an unusual case. *Pain* 2000; 84:77–87.

Ploghaus A, Tracey I, Gati JS, et al. Dissociating pain from its anticipation in the human brain. *Science* 1999; 284:1979–1981.

Porro CA, Baraldi P, Pagnoni G, et al. Does anticipation of pain affect cortical nociceptive systems? *J Neurosci* 2002; 22:3206–3214.

Pukall CF, Strigo I, Binik YM, et al. Neural correlates of painful genital touch in women with vulvar vestibulitis syndrome. *Pain* 2005; 115:118–127.

Rainville P, Duncan GH, Price DD, Carrier B, Bushnell MC. Pain affect encoded in human anterior cingulate but not somatosensory cortex. *Science* 1997; 277:968–971.

Rainville P, Hofbauer RK, Paus T, et al. Cerebral mechanisms of hypnotic induction and suggestion. *J Cogn Neurosci* 1999; 11:110–125.

Sawamoto N, Honda M, Okada T, et al. Expectation of pain enhances responses to nonpainful somatosensory stimulation in the anterior cingulate cortex and parietal operculum/posterior insula: an event-related functional magnetic resonance imaging study. *J Neurosci* 2000; 20:7438–7445.

Shyu BC, Lin CY, Sun JJ, Chen SL, Chang C. BOLD response to direct thalamic stimulation reveals a functional connection between the medial thalamus and the anterior cingulate cortex in the rat. *Magn Reson Med* 2004; 52:47–55.

Silverman DH, Munakata JA, Ennes H, et al. Regional cerebral activity in normal and pathological perception of visceral pain. *Gastroenterology* 1997; 112:64–72.

Stroman PW, Ryner LN. Functional MRI of motor and sensory activation in the human spinal cord. *Magn Reson Imaging* 2001; 19:27–32.

Stroman PW, Nance PW, Ryner LN. BOLD MRI of the human cervical spinal cord at 3 tesla. *Magn Reson Med* 1999; 42:571–576.

Stroman PW, Krause V, Malisza KL, Frankenstein UN, Tomanek B. Functional magnetic resonance imaging of the human cervical spinal cord with stimulation of different sensory dermatomes. *Magn Reson Imaging* 2002; 20:1–6.

Stroman PW, Kornelsen J, Bergman A, et al. Noninvasive assessment of the injured human spinal cord by means of functional magnetic resonance imaging. *Spinal Cord* 2004; 42:59–66.

Talbot JD, Marrett S, Evans AC, et al. Multiple representations of pain in human cerebral cortex. *Science* 1991; 251:1355–1358.

Tölle TR, Kaufmann T, Siessmeier T, et al. Region-specific encoding of sensory and affective components of pain in the human brain: a positron emission tomography correlation analysis. *Ann Neurol* 1999; 45:40–47.

Tracey I, Ploghaus A, Gati JS, et al. Imaging attentional modulation of pain in the periaqueductal gray in humans. *J Neurosci* 2002, 22:2748–2752.

Valet M, Sprenger T, Boecker H, et al. Distraction modulates connectivity of the cingulo-frontal cortex and the midbrain during pain—an fMRI analysis. *Pain* 2004; 109:399–408.

Villemagne VL, Frost JJ, Dannals RF, et al. Comparison of [^{11}C]diprenorphine and [^{11}C]carfentanil in vivo binding to opiate receptors in man using a dual detector system. *Eur J Pharmacol* 1994; 257:195–197.

Wager TD, Rilling JK, Smith EE, et al. Placebo-induced changes in FMRI in the anticipation and experience of pain. *Science* 2004; 303:1162–1167.

Wik G, Fischer H, Bragee B, Finer B, Fredrikson M. Functional anatomy of hypnotic analgesia: a PET study of patients with fibromyalgia. *Eur J Pain* 1999; 3:7–12.

Wilke M, Kowatch RA, DelBello MP, Mills NP, Holland SK. Voxel-based morphometry in adolescents with bipolar disorder: first results. *Psychiatry Res* 2004; 131:57–69.

Willoch F, Rosen G, Tölle TR, et al. Phantom limb pain in the human brain: unraveling neural circuitries of phantom limb sensations using positron emission tomography. *Ann Neurol* 2000; 48:842–849.

Wise RG, Williams P, Tracey I. Using fMRI to quantify the time dependence of remifentanil analgesia in the human brain. *Neuropsychopharmacology* 2004; 29:626–635.

Yoshizawa T, Nose T, Moore GJ, Sillerud LO. Functional magnetic resonance imaging of motor activation in the human cervical spinal cord. *Neuroimage* 1996; 4:174–182.

Zubieta JK, Dannals RF, Frost JJ. Gender and age influences on human brain mu-opioid receptor binding measured by PET. *Am J Psychiatry* 1999; 156:842–848.

Zubieta JK, Smith YR, Bueller JA, et al. Regional mu opioid receptor regulation of sensory and affective dimensions of pain. *Science* 2001; 293:311–315.

Zubieta JK, Heitzeg MM, Smith YR, et al. COMT val158met genotype affects mu-opioid neurotransmitter responses to a pain stressor. *Science* 2003; 299:1240–1243.

Correspondence to: M. Catherine Bushnell, PhD, McGill Centre for Research on Pain, 3640 University Street, Room M19, Montreal, Quebec, Canada H3A 2B2. Tel: 514 398-3493; Fax: 514 398-7464; email: catherine.bushnell@mcgill.ca.

Emerging Strategies for the Treatment of Neuropathic Pain, edited by James N. Campbell, Allan I. Basbaum, André Dray, Ronald Dubner, Robert H. Dworkin, and Christine N. Sang, IASP Press, Seattle, © 2006.

19

Microarray Studies and Pain

Fredrik Kamme and Sandra R. Chaplan

Johnson & Johnson Pharmaceutical Research & Development, LLC, San Diego, California, USA

Microarrays are powerful tools for the molecular analysis of tissues. The ability to assay the expression of (in principle) every gene offers a comprehensive view of a biological sample. This chapter will give an overview of microarray studies with relevance to pain in the literature.

Pain is a crossroads field, overlapping with inflammation, neurodegeneration, learning and memory, and regeneration, among other areas of investigation. We have attempted to bring together studies from disparate fields that are noteworthy in a discussion of where microarray studies on pain have been, and could yet go. The techniques and methods of microarray hybridization will not be covered in this chapter, and are well described in sources such as the following Web sites: www.bio.davidson.edu/courses/genomics/chip/chip.html, www.deathstarinc.com/science/biology/chips.html, and industry.ebi.ac.uk/~alan/MicroArray/IntroMicroArrayTalk/.

A review of the progress using microarrays in this field highlights many of the benefits and caveats of microarray technology. Several good reviews on this subject have recently compared microarray studies to other molecular techniques for pain-related mechanistic studies (Mogil and McCarson 2000; Reilly et al. 2004). The final part of this chapter will describe possible additional applications of microarrays to the field of pain that have not yet been fully realized.

From an application point of view, three major types of microarray experiments have been performed in the pain field: anatomy/cell type classification, description of disease processes/target identification, and studies of drug effects. Although they share much in terms of technical approach, they differ, particularly in how they are analyzed.

ANATOMY/CELL TYPE CLASSIFICATION

Much interest centers on the differential roles of identifiably different neuronal subtypes in the transduction and maintenance of pain states. Subpopulations of primary afferent neurons have been mainly studied, due to their accessibility. Small-diameter peripheral nerve fibers (myelinated and unmyelinated) are classically regarded as nociceptive; however, large-diameter myelinated fibers, while traditionally held to be responsible only for the transduction of the non-noxious sensations of touch, vibration, and proprioception, have more recently been implicated in the sensation of allodynia and may include a subpopulation of nociceptors (Djouhri and Lawson 2004).

Shortly after the introduction of microarray technology, Luo et al. (1999a) combined laser capture microdissection and cDNA microarrays to explore expression differences between groups of normal rat dorsal root ganglion (DRG) neurons distinguished by simple morphological criteria, with the goal of identifying potentially useful pain targets expressed in specific neuronal populations. A comparison of 1,000 pooled small neurons (diameter < 25 microns) with a matching number of large neurons (diameter > 40 microns) yielded the major conclusions that differentially expressed gene populations could be reliably detected, as evidenced by reproducibility of array studies and by verification using in situ hybridization. Fourteen mRNAs were preferentially expressed in large neurons, including those encoding the proinflammatory cytokine osteopontin, the sodium channel β_1 subunit, neuromedin B, and all three neurofilament proteins—heavy, medium, and light. Twenty-six mRNAs were preferentially expressed in small neurons, including those encoding sodium channel $Na_V1.9$ (NaN), the purinergic $P2X_3$ receptor, the proteasome activator receptor PA28 subunit α, calcitonin gene-related peptide, and the serotonin $5HT_3$ receptor. While this study was the first of its kind, classification of DRG neurons merely into small versus large leaves much to be desired.

A preliminary microarray study has been reported in abstract form comparing the trigeminal and dorsal root ganglia (Ahn and Basbaum 2001); a few transcripts were found to be overrepresented in the trigeminal ganglion, and a larger number in the DRG; however, details of this work have not been published. A recent comparison was performed of cranial sensory ganglia only: the trigeminal or Gasserian ganglion, giving rise to the trigeminal nerve; the petrosal ganglion, giving rise to the glossopharyngeal nerve; the geniculate ganglion, one of the two ganglia of the facial nerve, and the nodose ganglion of the vagus nerve (Matsumoto et al. 2003). These four ganglia have mixed sensory functions. This study correlated gene expression patterns with the differential overlap in sensory functions of these ganglia with respect to general visceral sensations (petrosal and nodose ganglia), general somatic sensations (trigeminal, glossopharyngeal, and geniculate ganglia), and gustatory sensations (geniculate, petrosal, and nodose).

Sun and colleagues (2002) chose a regional approach to the dorsal spinal cord, separating the entire cord into dorsal and ventral halves and hybridizing these separately. Genes expressed preferentially (twofold or more) in the dorsal half included those encoding somatostatin, proenkephalin, neuropeptide Y, protachykinin, the cannabinoid CB1 receptor, nociceptin, the NR1 subunit of the *N*-methyl-D-aspartate (NMDA) receptor, as well as the gene for potassium channel 3.1 (*Kv3.1*), the sodium channel gene *Scn6a* (*Na$_V$2.1*), and a transcript resembling a voltage-gated ion channel of uncertain identity (Lee et al. 1999).

DESCRIPTION OF DISEASE PROCESSES AND TARGET IDENTIFICATION

Perhaps the application in which expectations from microarrays have been the greatest involves the description of disease processes and identification of therapeutic targets. Great expectations are understandable, since a comprehensive scan of genes that change in a disease state provides us with an unbiased view and the opportunity to discover the unexpected.

NERVE INJURY MODELS

Nerve injury results in degenerative and reparative processes, and may result in neuropathic pain. A number of microarray studies, including the earliest studies in the field, have been directed at identifying gene regulation involved in the regeneration process after peripheral nerve or spinal cord injury in the mouse or rat. Many of these studies include efforts to examine the limitations to regeneration evident after spinal cord injury, compared with peripheral nerve injury (Fan et al. 2001; Bonilla et al. 2002; Tachibana et al. 2002; Gris et al. 2003; Di Giovanni et al. 2004; Resnick et al. 2004; Zhang et al. 2004). Despite a lack of emphasis on pain, these studies provide a useful background toward the task of distinguishing changes that are more likely to contribute to sensory abnormalities.

The first published pain-related peripheral nerve injury study is surprisingly recent, and was done by Xiao et al. (2002), who studied axotomized sciatic nerve rat DRG using custom-generated cDNA arrays. Among numerous changes, they described significant upregulation of genes encoding the α_5 subunit of the γ-aminobutyric acid A (GABA$_A$) receptor, the peripheral benzodiazepine receptor, the nicotinic α_7 subunit, the P2Y1 purinoceptor, the β_2 sodium channel subunit, and the $\alpha_2\delta_1$ calcium channel subunit. Costigan et al. (2002) also published a study of axotomy-induced changes. In this study, a mid-thigh sciatic nerve transection was performed 3 days prior to L5/L6 DRG harvest for microarray analysis. Among the most notable changes reported was the identification of 240 genes that showed both a >1.5-fold change and statistical significance using an uncorrected two-tailed t-test. Previously uncharacterized changes reported included downregulation of the CB1 and $5HT_{3A}$ receptors and upregulation of the endothelin-1 receptor. This study noted that sensitivity problems exist with the Affymetrix oligonucleotide array (U34A) that was used. Specifically, many G-protein-coupled receptors, including the μ-opioid receptor, are expressed at low levels, and fell below the sensitivity of this methodology.

The sciatic nerve transection preparation is technically straightforward. Due to the earlier branching of the femoral, sural, and saphenous nerves from the lumbar plexus, sciatic transection does not uniformly injure all neurons in the DRG from which it is derived. Furthermore, since sciatic transection results in profound distal motor deficits to the limb, assessment of a resulting pain state is difficult. Withdrawal behaviors cannot be performed, and the incidence of other behaviors thought to be related to pain, such as autotomy, is variable (Zeltser et al. 2000). Wang et al. (2002) performed tight ligation of the L5/L6 spinal nerves and carefully documented pain behavior prior to collection of DRG 2 weeks later. They reported profound changes in L5/L6 DRG, with some parallel but lesser changes in the spared L4 DRG. Upregulated DRG genes included those encoding neuropeptide Y (*M15880*), galanin (*J03624*), vasoactive intestinal peptide (*X02341*), pituitary adenylate cyclase-activating peptide (*A1228407*), NADH dehydrogenase (*AA874803*), calcium channel $\alpha_2\delta$ (*M86621*), activating transcription factor 3 (ATF3) (*M63282*), early growth response 1 (*M18416*), and cysteine-rich protein 3 (*X81193*). Markedly downregulated genes included those encoding somatostatin (*K02248*), amylin (*X52820*), tachykinin 1 (*X56306*), the $5HT_3$ receptor (*D49395*), and $Na_V1.9$ (*AF059030*), $Na_V1.8$ (*X92184*), and $Na_V1.1$ (*M22253*). This study went on to examine spinal cord changes ipsilateral to the nerve lesion relative to the uninjured side in the same preparation, although the exact anatomy of the spinal cord dissection is not clearly specified. Fewer changes were seen; notable examples include upregulation of genes encoding the chemokine receptor CCR5 (*Y12009*), ATF3 (*M63282*), and the peripheral benzodiazepine receptor (*J05122*).

The inclusion of extraneous tissue clearly influences the sensitivity of a microarray study. Analysis of the whole hemisected spinal cord may have diluted regional changes of interest in the Wang et al. study. Members of the Shanghai team (Yang et al. 2004) performed a similar study to examine changes in the spinal cord after nerve injury, with perhaps a key difference that they refined the area of study to the dissected L4/L5 dorsal hemisection. Again, this team studied changes 14 days after sciatic transection, as opposed to selective spinal nerve ligation. The most heavily upregulated channels included calcium channel α_{1E} (*NM_019291*), $\alpha_2\delta$ subunit 1 (*NM_012919*), and Scn6a ($Na_V2.1$) (*NM_031686*), and the most heavily upregulated receptors included $5HT_{5B}$ (*L10073*), nicotinic cholinergic α_5 (*NM_017078*) and β_2 (*NM_019297*) subunits, $AMPA_3$ (*NM_032990*), and vasopressin V_2 (*Z11932*). Among strongly upregulated signal transduction molecules, protein kinase C-α stood out, with a more than 14-fold change.

With so many changes in gene expression, a systematic approach is needed to assess which genes may contribute to sensory abnormalities, and which may be involved other processes that are in the "background" from the standpoint of pain investigations. Valder ct al. (2003) performed an intriguing study of injured DRG using Affymetrix oligonucleotide microarrays to compare outcomes of L5/L6 nerve ligation in two strains of Sprague-Dawley rat: the Holtzman strain, previously documented to sustain minimal behavioral change after nerve injury (Okuse et al. 1997), and the Harlan strain, known to develop robust and persisting allodynia. This study noted a number of genes differentially expressed at baseline in the two strains. Interestingly, this genetic background did not clearly affect subsequent findings, as these genes did not display regulation. Using a threshold of at least twofold change, the investigators identified 35 genes as differentially upregulated between the two strains (upregulated in one but not the other), whereas 37 genes were differentially downregulated. A total of 63 similarly upregulated and 76 downregulated genes were also identified. Similar upregulation was found in neuropeptides galanin, neuropeptide Y, and vasoactive intestinal peptide, as well as the calcium channel $\alpha_2\delta$ subunit and the peripheral benzodiazepine receptor. Profound downregulation was seen in parallel in preprosomatostatin and the $5HT_3$ receptor. Changes are suggestive of both alterations in membrane neurotransmission apparatus and intracellular signaling pathways. Tyrosine phosphatase was unchanged in Harlan rats but increased 2–4-fold in Holtzman rats. $Na_V1.1$ decreased 23–26-fold in Harlan rats but was unchanged in Holtzmans, and diacylglycerol kinase decreased 2–3 fold in Harlans but not in Holtzmans, as did mitogen-activated protein kinase (MAPK)-upstream protein kinase (MUK) and putative protein kinase C regulatory protein. This study did not suggest specific hypotheses to explain the difference in behavior between the two strains, but it did demonstrate the feasibility of interstrain comparisons using microarrays. A logical extension of this effort would be the use of microarrays to examine inbred mouse strains in which careful studies have shown specific differences in pain behaviors under different conditions (Kest et al. 2002; Smith et al. 2004).

INFLAMMATORY STATES WITH RELEVANCE TO PAIN

Early to join those using microarray studies were multiple sclerosis investigators. Several studies have looked at the gene profiles of human lesions (Whitney et al. 1999; Chabas et al. 2001) or murine models such as experimental autoimmune encephalitis (Chabas et al. 2001; Carmody et al. 2002; Matejuk et al. 2003; Paintlia et al. 2004; Spach et al. 2004). In a postmortem study of lesions from a single multiple sclerosis patient, Whitney et al. (1999) identified several upregulated genes associated with acute plaques. These included leukotriene A-4 hydrolase, tumor necrosis factor (TNF)-α receptor 2, the Duffy chemokine receptor, and retinoic acid receptor α_1. Microarray studies of both murine experimental autoimmune encephalitis and plaques from multiple sclerosis patients have also identified upregulation of the cytokine osteopontin (*X13694*) (Chabas et al. 2001), leading to the identification of elevated plasma osteopontin levels in multiple sclerosis patients (Comabella et al. 2005). Of interest, osteopontin has been identified in other microarray studies as being upregulated in the axotomized sympathetic ganglion, in addition to several malignancies, including pancreatic adenocarcinoma, squamous cell carcinoma of the head and neck, and ovarian carcinoma (Kim et al. 2002; Le et al. 2003; Boeshore et al. 2004; Koopmann et al. 2004).

STUDIES OF PATHWAYS AND MECHANISMS

A few studies have examined the effect of inflammatory mediator provocation on gene expression profiles. In perhaps the only study mentioned in this chapter performed on a non-neuronal tissue, Saban et al. (2002) found that while there were histological profiles of bladder inflammation produced by the instillation of lipopolysaccharide, substance P, or antigen in previously albumen-sensitized mice, and many genes were up or downregulated in common, 82 genes were upregulated in response to antigen alone, six genes were upregulated by substance P alone, and 39 genes were upregulated specifically by lipopolysaccharide. This kind of study is potentially very useful in that it not only holds the promise of diagnostic utility, but it also has the power to illuminate previously unsuspected pathway participants in inflammatory cascades. In addition, since other studies have demonstrated the sufficiency of antagonists such as naloxone to block the gene regulation effects of morphine, this type of study could provide additional confirmation of the specificity of eventual agonist or antagonist drugs to be countered by their respective counterpart.

In another mechanistic study, Linnarsson et al. (2001) used glial-derived neurotrophic factor (GDNF) to probe regulated pathways in mouse DRG in culture. This study identified GDNF-related downregulation of a set of genes resulting in neurite growth and branching inhibition. Given the important roles of several neurotrophic factors in pain states due to nerve injury and inflammation, this kind of study helps to shed further light on pathways that may not previously have been known to be implicated.

The pain field has historically looked to the learning and memory field for inspiration. Small but significant changes in transcriptional profiles were found by Irwin and colleagues after a brief swimming task, and maze-learning led to changes in hippocampal profiles (Irwin 2001; Luo et al. 2001). Using electrical pathway stimulation and pharmacological intervention, Thompson et al. (2003) have examined NMDA-receptor-independent long-term potentiation in the hippocampus. Upregulated genes included those encoding NMDA-receptor 2D, neuropeptide Y, proenkephalin, brain-derived neurotrophic factor, and nerve growth factor receptor. Thus, pathway facilitation can be detected by microarray, and much probably remains to be gleaned from comparative studies.

DRUG OR COMPOUND EFFECTS

Loguinov et al. (2001) have investigated the effects of acute morphine administration on gene expression in mice in the absence of a pain state. Thirty or 120 minutes after intraperitoneal administration of 10 mg/kg morphine sulfate, the medial striatum and lumbar spinal cord were harvested and hybridized to a cDNA microarray. Changes of note (many confirmed by RNAse protection) included upregulation of P/Q calcium channel α_{1A} (*AB025352*), c-src tyrosine kinase (*NM_007783*), and cyclin D1 (*NM_00763*), and downregulation of fatty acid binding protein (*X70100*), enzymes involved in glycolysis and oxidation, and the sodium channel β_1 subunit (*U85786*), as well as several proteins involved in cellular secretion. Importantly, these changes were prevented by the concomitant intraperitoneal administration of 15 mg/kg naloxone. Thus, acute effects of drug administration are detectable by microarray. The impact of morphine on energy and secretory pathways is speculated to have to do with the role of opioids in thermoregulation and metabolism.

An interesting study was performed by Nesic et al. (2002) using a T8 spinal cord contusion model. Noting that an increase in extracellular glutamate to neurotoxic levels is one of the earliest events after spinal cord injury (Liu et al. 1999) and that administration of an NMDA antagonist in proximity to the injury is neuroprotective (Faden and Simon 1988; Kochhar et al. 1988; Gomez-Pinilla et al. 1989), they studied three experimental groups: animals with sham injury, with injury alone, and with injury plus lumbar intrathecal administration of MK-801. Notwithstanding the lack of a sham injury plus MK-801 group, the findings are interesting. Fifty percent of genes upregulated by contusion alone were not upregulated in the presence of MK-801, suggesting a role for the activation of the NMDA receptor in their regulation. An additional 168 genes not upregulated by spinal cord injury alone were altered in the MK-801 group, suggestive of a drug effect.

Another quite different use of microarrays is as a tool in reverse pharmacological investigations. More than a few clinically reproducible drug effects are not yet attributable to a known mechanism, with the result that—from a subsequent drug discovery point of view—optimization of the desired effect is difficult, hit-or-miss, or impossible. Cited here are a few studies that have attempted to shed light on marketed drug mechanisms in disease states relevant to pain. Therapeutic effects of statins, or 3-hydroxy-3 methylglutaryl coenzyme A (HMG-CoA) reductase inhibitors, have been documented in multiple sclerosis and appear to be independent of their cholesterol-modulating effects. Effects on TNF-α and inducible nitric oxide synthase have been shown (Pahan 1997), and results of a clinical trial (Vollmer et al. 2004) are encouraging in terms of reduction of central lesions. A microarray study recently has been performed in search of a mechanistic explanation for the effects of lovastatin in the experimental autoimmune encephalomyelitis model in mice (Paintlia et al. 2004). In addition to improving the clinical score in the treated mice, lovastatin exposure resulted in decreased inflammatory cell infiltrate and demyelination in the central nervous system. Differential gene expression profiles included modulation of 114 genes including inflammatory transcription factors. Support for a role in regulating the infiltration of B cells and other lymphocytes through the blood-brain barrier was identified. Upregulation of peroxisome proliferator-activated receptors γ and δ as well as 12-lipoxygenase was seen.

No doubt similar studies have been performed in search of the mechanism for the mechanism of action of drugs such as gabapentin in pain and epilepsy. It is to be hoped that the results will be shared with the pain research community in the near future.

A more workhorse application of the reverse pharmacological technique appears to be gaining favor in the toxicological literature. Since many of the reasons why promising compounds fail early in the drug discovery process relate to toxicological findings, microarrays have become an increasingly common reverse pharmacological application in drug discovery. Clustering of microarray data generated from incubation of dissociated hepatocytes with novel compounds and compounds with identified toxic potential makes it possible to identify the toxic liability of a new compound (Hamadeh et al. 2002a,b). This approach exploits the power of microarrays. While the large number of genes assayed by a microarray complicates gene-by-gene analysis, it makes pattern matching, as is done in clustering of toxic compounds, very powerful.

COLLECTION OF CELLS FOR MICROARRAY ANALYSIS

Pain is a pathway phenomenon involving peripheral, spinal, and supraspinal components. Many of the regions involved in pain processing are highly heterogeneous in cell composition, with the DRG serving as a prime example. On top of the neuronal component, immune cells play an important role in disease. Predictably, data generated at the gross sample level may yield different conclusions than data generated within a defined cellular context. Strongly expressed transcripts in a minority of cells in a homogenized sample are likely to be diluted to the point of eluding detection or attracting minimal attention. In "before" and "after" studies, important neural plasticity may be missed altogether if it is highly cell-specific. A classic example is the case of substance P, where investigators analyzing homogenized DRG reported a large decrease in net protachykinin transcripts after axotomy. However, in subpopulations of neurons, protachykinin transcripts are known to be considerably induced by axotomy (Henken et al. 1990; Noguchi et al. 1994). Thus, conclusions based on microarray data must take into account the limitation that complex gene induction effects may occur in the tissue in question, and that observations based on whole tissues may obscure significant changes in specific cell types.

Considerable effort was thus made early on to collect specific cell populations for microarray analysis. Indeed, the combination of laser capture microdissection and microarrays was first applied to the DRG. Laser microdissection allows for the collection of individual cells from tissue sections. This technique is not without some drawbacks. As dendrites and axons cannot be collected, a certain population of mRNAs is missed. Cells are collected from thin frozen sections and may be more or less readily identified under these conditions. Other techniques for collecting "identified neurons" have been used to pick neurons of interest for other molecular biological studies, usually polymerase chain reaction (PCR). While these selection techniques hold exciting possibilities, their extension to microarray studies has not yet been published. For example, cells from dissociated DRG have been characterized by calcium imaging and then collected individually and analyzed by quantitative reverse transcription (RT)-PCR (Martin et al. 2002; Nealen et al. 2003; Spehr et al. 2004). This method adds functional description to the gene expression data. Liss and Roeper (Liss et al. 2001; Liss 2002) have performed electrophysiological characterization of individual neurons in brain slice preparations, followed by aspiration of cytoplasmic contents and examination using quantitative PCR for specified targets. Again, this technique has not yet been extended to microarray studies, but it is highly promising.

SOME CHALLENGES OF MICROARRAY STUDIES

The studies described above have produced a wealth of valuable data; however, it is questionable whether or not any drug targets have emerged. The reasons may be manifold, but interpretation of microarray data has emerged as the largest hurdle in its application to disease process characterization and drug target identification. Interpretation is complicated by several factors. For example, the sheer number of differences that may be identified in a microarray experiment simply makes it humanly impossible to cover the literature on the genes involved. The interpretation therefore becomes heavily biased toward the investigator's favorite genes. If analysis is done on a gene-by-gene basis, the effect of a gene induction is usually considered as the effect of its corresponding protein. This is a perilous extrapolation. For example, we have found that although microarray, quantitative RT-PCR and immunohistochemical studies demonstrated a decrease in the two major forms of hyperpolarization-activated, cyclic nucleotide-modulated channels, expressed in the DRG after nerve ligation, the corresponding Ih current was in fact dramatically upregulated. Evidently, despite a reduced amount of membrane channel protein, a mechanism exists whereby there is a gain of function of the remaining protein (Chaplan et al. 2003). Perhaps the gravest caveat in the gene-by-gene approach in data analysis is that we are attempting to explain the emergent property of a complex system, such as a cell or a pathway, basically as the sum of the functions of the genes that change. Due to the often extensive interactions between gene products, the functional link between a change in expression of a particular gene and its role in a disease state may be tortuous indeed, rendering it difficult to interpret. For example, a study by Luo et al. (1999b) found a massive upregulation of neuronal nitric oxide synthase (nNOS) in the DRG in neuropathic pain models, without a corresponding pharmacological implication of this enzyme in allodynia. The role of nNOS upregulation has not been clarified.

It should be acknowledged that even before microarray data are analyzed for biological importance, mathematical preprocessing of the raw array data is an art in itself. Normalization between samples and between experiments, for example, is not always straightforward. Going further back, to the arrays themselves, it is important to appreciate that array platforms have different sensitivities and show a selected part of the genes present. It is quite possible that depending on the complexity of the sample, there might be 20–40% false negatives. Consequently, great care should be exercised when comparing data across platforms.

FUTURE APPLICATIONS

The pain field adopted microarrays early on, but it is probably safe to claim that the real gains of this technology have not yet been actualized. What developments do we see in tools, technologies, and software that will improve the utility of expression profiling in pain research?

INTERPRETATION OF DATA

A move away from the gene-by-gene analysis approach is needed to better exploit the value of microarray data. Pathway tools, such as KEGG (www.genome.jp/kegg/pathway.html), Jubilant (jubilantbiosys.com), and Ingenuity (www.ingenuity.com), allow microarray data to be mapped on top of wiring diagrams of metabolic and signaling networks, facilitating their detection of modulation. However, detection of signal *flow* through such signaling transduction chains may require a different approach. One possibility is the utilization of known stimuli to generate a reference dataset. An expression pattern generated in an experiment is then compared to the reference dataset, and by similarity in gene expression, the stimulus is identified. Examples to date include a stress reference dataset generated by Murray et al. (2004) and a yeast knockout reference dataset by Hughes et al. (2000). To our knowledge, this approach has not yet been attempted in the pain field.

DEFINITION OF CELL TYPES

Attempts to generate data in a defined cell population have made it clear that our appreciation of the taxonomy of neurons in the DRG, spinal cord, and brain is far from complete. The DRG is a good case in point.

While Lawson and Harper's studies of the heterogeneity of DRG neurons related conduction velocity and cell diameter in three categories of neurons, C, Aδ, and Aα/β, these categories are clearly neither internally homogeneous nor crisply delineated distinctions (Harper and Lawson 1985). Within small neurons, it is well known that within the diameter range accepted as "small," subpopulations exist with respect to expression of many molecules, one obvious example being the ligand for the plant lectin IB4.

It is not known how many kinds of DRG neurons there are, however. Investigators have used electrophysiological techniques to attempt to further catalogue the variety of neuronal subtypes in the DRG. In an extension of an approach first used by Scroggs and Cardenas (Cardenas et al. 1995), Petruska et al. (2000) performed an analysis of acutely dissociated adult rat DRG neurons, classifying them by "signature" electrophysiological profiles into nine clusters of small and medium neurons based on responsiveness to capsaicin, adenosine triphosphate, and protons, and on histochemical properties. Four of the nine profiles were associated with small diameters, and five with medium diameters. Petruska's group observed that unique neural signatures provided by DRG neurons could predict more than 25 functionally diverse afferent populations.

We have previously demonstrated the feasibility of segregating cell types based on clustering of single-cell array data (Kamme et al. 2003). We are applying this technology to molecularly define cell types in the DRG by single-cell profiling of a large number of neurons (Fig. 1). The output of the data analysis is a dendrogram, or phylogeny tree, where cells are grouped based on their similarity to each other in gene expression (Fig. 2). The groups defined are expected to represent cell types, or perhaps subtypes of cells. The mathematical processing to build these dendrograms based on expression data can be done in several ways, each producing slightly different groupings. We lack the knowledge to define a priori which algorithms are suitable for defining cell types. Fortunately, much is already known about gene expression in the DRG, allowing us to judge if a particular clustering algorithm produces groupings consistent with known markers. The data from 103 single DRG neurons produced a dendrogram with 12 groups, corresponding to what we believe to be 12 cell types. Markers for the individual cell types isolated in this experiment will provide a foundation to address transcriptome changes in a cell type-specific fashion in disease states.

In the spinal cord, cell type definition is also a pressing matter (Zhang and Craig 1997; Yu et al. 1999). The spinal cord may equal the DRG in terms of cellular heterogeneity, but it has a more complex topography, which complicates molecular analysis. We have used single-cell profiling to characterize spinothalamic tract neurons in lamina I, identified by retrograde tracing (technique described in Kamme et al. 2004). Cluster analysis showed

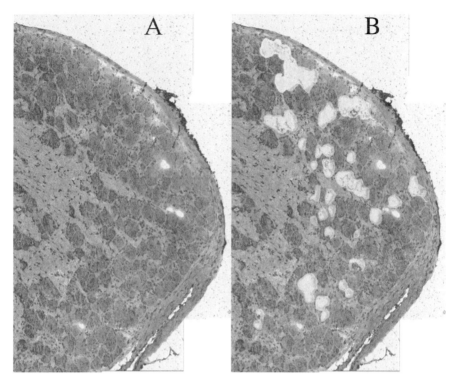

Fig. 1. Laser microdissection of single cells in the dorsal root ganglion. Fifty-two cells were individually collected using the PALM instrument (A) before capture and (B) after capture. The "After" picture is a montage of individual capture images superimposed on the "Before" image using Photoshop.

molecularly distinct classes, supporting the cellular heterogeneity of this population.

It can be readily appreciated that is surprisingly hard to select any group of neurons or cells with any confidence that they are homogeneous, whether in a sensory ganglion, the spinal cord, or the brain. We need cell type markers that can be used to immunohistochemically define cells so that when control and disease state data are collected, we can be certain we are studying the same population of cells. This is a fundamental problem that requires more than just an effort to collect massive amounts of cell-type-specific expression data. How do we molecularly define a cell type? This question has ramifications into the very heart of cell biology. What is a cell type? How different can cells within a given cell type be? What is a subtype of a cell? While it might be argued that cell types can be defined differently using different techniques such as gene expression, morphology, and electrophysiology, we believe that gene expression most reliably detects cell

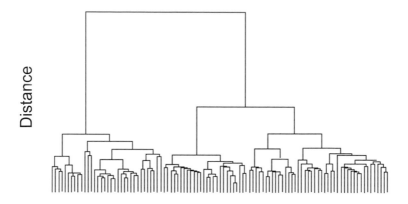

Fig. 2. Cluster dendrogram of array data from 103 individual dorsal root ganglion neurons. The vertical distance between nodes indicates the degree of difference between samples or groups of samples. The samples were grouped based on hierarchical clustering of the array data. Based on this dendrogram and consecutive subclustering (not shown), we found 12 stable clusters, which we suggest corresponds to 12 cell types.

type. Thus, two cells that have the same gene expression pattern are the same cell type, and two cells that are of different types cannot have the same expression pattern. A key point is that we do not know *how* different two expression patterns need be for the cells to be of different types. We already know that cells belonging to the same type based on morphological and functional criteria are not transcriptionally identical in vivo (Kamme et al. 2003).

DRUG EFFECTS

Using expression profiles as snapshots of cellular physiology, Gunther et al. (2003) were able to accurately predict the clinical effects of drugs by microarray experiments in vitro. Gonzalez-Maeso et al. (2003) took this approach one step further and demonstrated that by using the expression levels of a small number of genes they could differentiate between hallucinogenic and non-hallucinogenic $5HT_{2A}$-receptor agonists in vivo. Expression profiles were used in these experiments as a representation of physiology in that they were analyzed and grouped based on similarity to other expression patterns, much like the classification of cell types described previously. Therefore, this approach does not require an interpretation of the meaning of the expression profiles, which is an inherent strength. The use of expression profiling as a surrogate for physiology in vitro and in vivo has potentially vast implications. If implemented in screening, it would allow for compound search based on similarity to model compounds without knowledge of the underlying mechanism of action. Implemented in vivo, it will allow us to characterize the physiological effects of drug action in a very efficient way. Importantly, using a physiological surrogate as an endpoint in an assay or an experiment allows us to find compounds that act via multiple targets. Applying microarrays and expression profiling as a physiological surrogate in pain research, particularly in vivo, will depend on a new generation of high-throughput arrays, high-throughput target preparation methods, and most likely high-throughput laser microdissection, at a per sample cost that is a fraction of what it is today. Cost may well be the limiting factor. At a current cost of U.S.$300 or more per sample for target

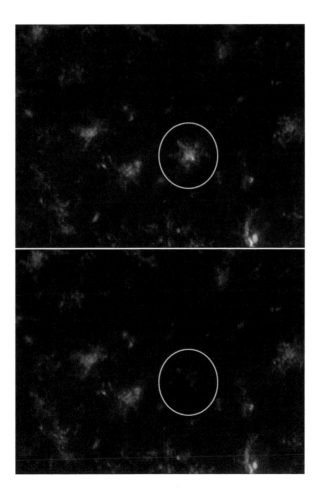

Fig. 3. Laser capture of immunostained microglia from the rat forebrain. Microglia were stained with OX-42 antibody and a Qdot-labeled secondary antibody. Nuclei were counterstained green. The labeled cell inside the yellow circle was captured using an Arcturus Pixcell 2 instrument.

preparation and array analysis, these studies are prohibitively expensive. Consider a hypothetical experiment looking at drug effects on responses in the DRG following axotomy: Not knowing which cell type is the target of our drug, we need to sample each of the 10–20 cell types present and do this in each of our experimental animals, perhaps including different time points. We may want to compare our drug with a series of known drugs. It is easy to see that the number of samples can reach several hundreds. Affymetrix, Illumina, and Quantum Dot Corporation offer high-throughput arrays based on different platforms. A major determinant for the suitability of these arrays to drug effect studies will simply be the cost per array.

IMMUNE CELLS

Immune cells, microglia in particular, have been implicated in the induction phase of neuropathic pain after peripheral nerve injury (Raghavendra et al. 2003). Studying immune cells in situ using microarrays is difficult because these cells require positive histochemical staining to be detected, which has compromised RNA integrity in the past. Once techniques for maintaining RNA during immunohistochemistry are established, we should see more studies on the transcriptonomics of immune cells in pain. Fig. 3 illustrates laser capture of immunostained microglia in the rat central nervous system.

CONCLUSION

Pain researchers were participants at the forefront of microarray technology. For example, the anatomical complexity of pain pathways fueled efforts to combine laser capture with microarrays. Studies of pain-related structures, disease processes, and the effects of drugs have certainly added large amounts of information to the pain field, and at the same time have exposed some of the challenges of using microarrays in tissues. Clearly we are at the early stages of transcriptonomics and have yet to fully exploit the potential of such massively parallel data. To help us meet these challenges, a series of new technical and analytical developments are emerging. If these efforts are successful, the contribution of expression profiling to pain drug discovery will increase.

REFERENCES

Ahn AH, Basbaum AI. Dorsal root and trigeminal ganglion neurons have overlapping but distinct gene expression. *Soc Neurosci Abstracts* 2001; 162.20. Available at: http://sfn.scholarone.com/itin2001/.

Boeshore KL, Schreiber RC, Vaccariello SA, et al. Novel changes in gene expression following axotomy of a sympathetic ganglion: a microarray analysis. *J Neurobiol* 2004; 59:216–235.

Bonilla IE, Tanabe K, Strittmatter SM. Small proline-rich repeat protein 1A is expressed by axotomized neurons and promotes axonal outgrowth. *J Neurosci* 2002; 22:1303–1315.

Cardenas CG, Del Mar LP, Scroggs RS. Variation in serotonergic inhibition of calcium channel currents in four types of rat sensory neurons differentiated by membrane properties. *J Neurophysiol* 1995; 74:1870–1879.

Carmody RJ, Hilliard B, Maguschak K, Chodosh LA, Chen YH. Genomic scale profiling of autoimmune inflammation in the central nervous system: the nervous response to inflammation. *J Neuroimmunol* 2002; 133:95–107.

Chabas D, Baranzini SE, Mitchell D, et al. The influence of the proinflammatory cytokine, osteopontin, on autoimmune demyelinating disease. *Science* 2001; 294:1731–1735.

Chaplan SR, Guo HQ, Lee DH, et al. Neuronal hyperpolarization-activated pacemaker channels drive neuropathic pain. *J Neurosci* 2003; 23:1169–1178.

Comabella M, Pericot I, Goertsches R, et al. Plasma osteopontin levels in multiple sclerosis. *J Neuroimmunol* 2005; 158:231–239.

Costigan M, Befort K, Karchewski L, et al. Replicate high-density rat genome oligonucleotide microarrays reveal hundreds of regulated genes in the dorsal root ganglion after peripheral nerve injury. *BMC Neurosci* 2002; 3:16.

Di Giovanni S, Faden AI, Yakovlev A, et al. Neuronal plasticity after spinal cord injury: identification of a gene cluster driving neurite outgrowth. *FASEB J* 2005;19:153–154.

Djouhri L, Lawson SN. A-beta-fiber nociceptive primary afferent neurons: a review of incidence and properties in relation to other afferent A-fiber neurons in mammals. *Brain Res Brain Res Rev* 2004; 46:131–145.

Faden AI, Simon RP. A potential role for excitotoxins in the pathophysiology of spinal cord injury. *Ann Neurol* 1988; 23:623–626.

Fan M, Mi R, Yew DT, Chan WY. Analysis of gene expression following sciatic nerve crush and spinal cord hemisection in the mouse by microarray expression profiling. *Cell Mol Neurobiol* 2001; 21:497–508.

Gomez-Pinilla F, Tram H, Cotman CW, Nieto-Sampedro M. Neuroprotective effect of MK-801 and U-50488H after contusive spinal cord injury. *Exp Neurol* 1989; 104:118–124.

Gonzalez-Maeso J, Yuen T, Ebersole BJ, et al. Transcriptome fingerprints distinguish hallucinogenic and nonhallucinogenic 5-hydroxytryptamine 2A receptor agonist effects in mouse somatosensory cortex. *J Neurosci* 2003; 23:8836–8843.

Gris P, Murphy S, Jacob JE, Atkinson I, Brown A. Differential gene expression profiles in embryonic, adult-injured and adult-uninjured rat spinal cords. *Mol Cell Neurosci* 2003; 24:555–567.

Gunther EC, Stone DJ, Gerwien RW, Bento P, Heyes MP. Prediction of clinical drug efficacy by classification of drug-induced genomic expression profiles in vitro. *Proc Natl Acad Sci USA* 2003; 100:9608–9613.

Hamadeh HK, Bushel PR, Jayadev S, et al. Prediction of compound signature using high density gene expression profiling. *Toxicol Sci* 2002a; 67:232–240.

Hamadeh HK, Bushel PR, Jayadev S, et al. Gene expression analysis reveals chemical-specific profiles. *Toxicol Sci* 2002b; 67:219–231.

Harper AA, Lawson SN. Conduction velocity is related to morphological cell type in rat dorsal root ganglion neurones. *J Physiol* 1985; 359:31–46.

Henken DB, Battisti WP, Chesselet MF, Murray M, Tessler A. Expression of beta-preprotachykinin mRNA and tachykinins in rat dorsal root ganglion cells following peripheral or central axotomy. *Neuroscience* 1990; 39:733–742.

Hughes TR, Marton MJ, Jones AR, et al. Functional discovery via a compendium of expression profiles. *Cell* 2000; 102:109–126.

Irwin LN. Gene expression in the hippocampus of behaviorally stimulated rats: analysis by DNA microarray. *Brain Res Mol Brain Res* 2001; 96:163–169.

Kamme F, Salunga R, Yu J, et al. Single-cell microarray analysis in hippocampus CA1: demonstration and validation of cellular heterogeneity. *J Neurosci* 2003; 23:3607–3615.

Kamme F, Zhu J, Luo L, et al. Single-cell laser-capture microdissection and RNA amplification. *Methods Mol Med* 2004; 99:215–223.

Kest B, Hopkins E, Palmese CA, Adler M, Mogil JS. Genetic variation in morphine analgesic tolerance: a survey of 11 inbred mouse strains. *Pharmacol Biochem Behav* 2002; 73:821–828.

Kim JH, Skates SJ, Uede T, et al. Osteopontin as a potential diagnostic biomarker for ovarian cancer. *JAMA* 2002; 287:1671–1679.

Kochhar A, Zivin JA, Lyden PD, Mazzarella V. Glutamate antagonist therapy reduces neurologic deficits produced by focal central nervous system ischemia. *Arch Neurol* 1988; 45:148–153.

Koopmann J, Fedarko NS, Jain A, et al. Evaluation of osteopontin as biomarker for pancreatic adenocarcinoma. *Cancer Epidemiol Biomarkers Prev* 2004; 13:487–491.

Le QT, Sutphin PD, Raychaudhuri S, et al. Identification of osteopontin as a prognostic plasma marker for head and neck squamous cell carcinomas. *Clin Cancer Res* 2003; 9:59–67.

Lee JH, Cribbs LL, Perez-Reyes E. Cloning of a novel four repeat protein related to voltage-gated sodium and calcium channels, *FEBS Lett* 1999; 445:231–236.

Linnarsson S, Mikaels A, Baudet C, Ernfors P. Activation by GDNF of a transcriptional program repressing neurite growth in dorsal root ganglia. *Proc Natl Acad Sci USA* 2001; 98:14681–14686.

Liss B. Improved quantitative real-time RT-PCR for expression profiling of individual cells. *Nucleic Acids Res* 2002; 30:e89.

Liss B, Franz O, Sewing S, et al. Tuning pacemaker frequency of individual dopaminergic neurons by Kv4.3L and KChip3.1 transcription. *Embo J* 2001; 20:5715–5724.

Liu D, Xu GY, Pan E, McAdoo DJ. Neurotoxicity of glutamate at the concentration released upon spinal cord injury. *Neuroscience* 1999; 93:1383–1389.

Loguinov AV, Anderson LM, Crosby GJ, Yukhananov RY. Gene expression following acute morphine administration. *Physiol Genomics* 2001; 6:169–181.

Luo L, Salunga RC, Guo H, et al. Gene expression profiles of laser-captured adjacent neuronal subtypes. *Nat Med* 1999a; 5:117–122.

Luo ZD, Chaplan SR, Scott BP, et al. Neuronal nitric oxide synthase mRNA upregulation in rat sensory neurons after spinal nerve ligation: lack of a role in allodynia development. *J Neurosci* 1999b; 19:9201–9208.

Luo Y, Long JM, Spangler EL, et al. Identification of maze learning-associated genes in rat hippocampus by cDNA microarray. *J Mol Neurosci* 2001; 17:397–404.

Martin DJ, McClelland D, Herd MB, et al. Gabapentin-mediated inhibition of voltage-activated Ca^{2+} channel currents in cultured sensory neurones is dependent on culture conditions and channel subunit expression. *Neuropharmacology* 2002; 42:353–366.

Matejuk A, Hopke C, Dwyer J, et al. CNS gene expression pattern associated with spontaneous experimental autoimmune encephalomyelitis. *J Neurosci Res* 2003; 73:667–678.

Matsumoto I, Emori Y, Nakamura S, et al. DNA microarray cluster analysis reveals tissue similarity and potential neuron-specific genes expressed in cranial sensory ganglia. *J Neurosci Res* 2003; 74:818–828.

Mogil JS, McCarson KE. Identifying pain genes: bottom-up and top-down approaches. *J Pain* 2000; 1:66–80.

Murray JI, Whitfield ML, Trinklein ND, et al. Diverse and specific gene expression responses to stresses in cultured human cells. *Mol Biol Cell* 2004;15:2361–2374.

Nealen ML, Gold MS, Thut PD, Caterina MJ. TRPM8 mRNA is expressed in a subset of cold-responsive trigeminal neurons from rat. *J Neurophysiol* 2003; 90:515–520.

Nesic O, Svrakic NM, Xu GY, et al. DNA microarray analysis of the contused spinal cord: effect of NMDA receptor inhibition. *J Neurosci Res* 2002; 68:406–423.

Noguchi K, Dubner R, De Leon M, Senba E, Ruda MA. Axotomy induces preprotachykinin gene expression in a subpopulation of dorsal root ganglion neurons. *J Neurosci Res* 1994; 37:596–603.

Okuse K, Chaplan SR, McMahon SB, et al. Regulation of expression of the sensory neuron-specific sodium channel SNS in inflammatory and neuropathic pain. *Mol Cell Neurosci* 1997; 10:196–207.

Paintlia AS, Paintlia MK, Singh AK, et al. Regulation of gene expression associated with acute experimental autoimmune encephalomyelitis by Lovastatin. *J Neurosci Res* 2004; 77:63–81.

Petruska JC, Napaporn J, Johnson RD, Gu JG, Cooper BY. Subclassified acutely dissociated cells of rat DRG: histochemistry and patterns of capsaicin-, proton-, and ATP-activated currents. *J Neurophysiol* 2000; 84:2365–2379.

Raghavendra V, Tanga F, DeLeo JA. Inhibition of microglial activation attenuates the development but not existing hypersensitivity in a rat model of neuropathy. *J Pharmacol Exp Ther* 2003; 306:624–630.

Reilly SC, Cossins AR, Quinn JP, Sneddon LU. Discovering genes: the use of microarrays and laser capture microdissection in pain research. *Brain Res Brain Res Rev* 2004; 46:225–233.

Resnick DK, Schmitt C, Miranpuri GS, et al. Molecular evidence of repair and plasticity following spinal cord injury. *Neuroreport* 2004; 15:837–839.

Saban MR, Nguyen NB, Hammond TG, Saban R. Gene expression profiling of mouse bladder inflammatory responses to LPS, substance P, and antigen-stimulation. *Am J Pathol* 2002; 160:2095–2110.

Smith SB, Crager SE, Mogil JS. Paclitaxel-induced neuropathic hypersensitivity in mice: responses in 10 inbred mouse strains. *Life Sci* 2004; 74:2593–2604.

Spach KM, Pedersen LB, Nashold FE, et al. Gene expression analysis suggests that 1,25-dihydroxyvitamin D3 reverses experimental autoimmune encephalomyelitis by stimulating inflammatory cell apoptosis. *Physiol Genomics* 2004; 18:141–151.

Spehr J, Spehr M, Hatt H, Wetzel CH. Subunit-specific P2X-receptor expression defines chemosensory properties of trigeminal neurons. *Eur J Neurosci* 2004; 19:2497–510.

Sun H, Xu J, Della Penna KB, et al. Dorsal horn-enriched genes identified by DNA microarray, in situ hybridization and immunohistochemistry. *BMC Neurosci* 2002; 3:11.

Tachibana T, Noguchi K, Ruda MA. Analysis of gene expression following spinal cord injury in rat using complementary DNA microarray. *Neurosci Lett* 2002; 327:133–137.

Thompson KJ, Orfila JE, Achanta P, Martinez JL Jr. Gene expression associated with in vivo induction of early phase-long-term potentiation (LTP) in the hippocampal mossy fiber-Cornus Ammonis (CA)3 pathway. *Cell Mol Biol* 2003; 49:1281–1287.

Valder CR, Liu JJ, Song YH, Luo ZD. Coupling gene chip analyses and rat genetic variances in identifying potential target genes that may contribute to neuropathic allodynia development. *J Neurochem* 2003; 87:560–573.

Vollmer T, Key L, Durkalski V, et al. Oral simvastatin treatment in relapsing-remitting multiple sclerosis. *Lancet* 2004; 363:1607–1608.

Wang H, Sun H, Della Penna K, et al. Chronic neuropathic pain is accompanied by global changes in gene expression and shares pathobiology with neurodegenerative diseases. *Neuroscience* 2002; 114:529–546.

Whitney LW, Becker KG, Tresser NJ, et al. Analysis of gene expression in multiple sclerosis lesions using cDNA microarrays. *Ann Neurol* 1999; 46:425–428.

Xiao HS, Huang QH, Zhang FX. et al. Identification of gene expression profile of dorsal root ganglion in the rat peripheral axotomy model of neuropathic pain. *Proc Natl Acad Sci USA* 2002; 99:8360–8365.

Yang L, Zhang FX, Huang F, et al. Peripheral nerve injury induces trans-synaptic modification of channels, receptors and signal pathways in rat dorsal spinal cord. *Eur J Neurosci* 2004; 19:871–883.

Yu XH, Zhang ET, Craig AD, et al. NK-1 receptor immunoreactivity in distinct morphological types of lamina I neurons of the primate spinal cord. *J Neurosci* 1999; 19:3545–3555.

Zeltser R, Beilin B, Zaslansky R, Seltzer Z. Comparison of autotomy behavior induced in rats by various clinically-used neurectomy methods. *Pain* 2000; 89:19–24.

Zhang ET, Craig AD. Morphology and distribution of spinothalamic lamina I neurons in the monkey. *J Neurosci* 17 1997; 3274–3284.

Zhang KH, Xiao HS, Lu PH, et al. Differential gene expression after complete spinal cord transection in adult rats: an analysis focused on a subchronic post-injury stage. *Neuroscience* 2004; 128:375–388.

Correspondence to: Sandra R. Chaplan, MD, Johnson & Johnson Pharmaceutical Research & Development, LLC, 3210 Merryfield Row, San Diego, CA 92107, USA. Tel: 858-784-3280; Fax: 858-450-2040; email: schaplan@prdus.jnj.com.

Emerging Strategies for the Treatment of Neuropathic Pain, edited by James N. Campbell, Allan I. Basbaum, André Dray, Ronald Dubner, Robert H. Dworkin, and Christine N. Sang, IASP Press, Seattle, © 2006.

20

Psychophysical Models for Neuropathic Pain

Rolf-Detlef Treede

Institute of Physiology and Pathophysiology,
Johannes Gutenberg University, Mainz, Germany

Neuropathic pain is defined as pain initiated or caused by a primary lesion or dysfunction in the nervous system (Merskey and Bogduk 1994). Current efforts to refine this definition focus on the terms "dysfunction" and "nervous system" with the intention to clarify that there must be an identifiable disease process and that this process has to affect the somatosensory system. Experimental models of neuropathic pain according to either of these definitions are expected to imitate mechanisms of nerve damage within the peripheral or central parts of the somatosensory system and the ensuing processes of degeneration or regeneration. Whereas this strategy of reproducing the etiology and pathophysiology of the underlying disease process is the focus of various animal models of neuropathic pain, for obvious ethical reasons this approach cannot be used in healthy human subjects.

Human surrogate models of neuropathic pain focus on sensory symptoms and not on mechanisms of nerve damage, degeneration, or regeneration (Klein et al. 2005). On the one hand, this can be considered a limitation of such models, but on the other hand, the investigation of sensory symptoms exploits the human capacity for verbal communication, which is not possible in animal studies. Verbal communication allows the direct assessment of ongoing symptoms (pain and paresthesias) and evoked signs (evoked pain and sensory loss) without relying on reflexes. In addition, laboratory studies have been conducted in human surrogate models using electrophysiological and imaging techniques. Although the array of available methods in humans is limited when compared with animal models, such research has the advantage of being immediately transferable to patient populations. This chapter outlines the potential of human surrogate models of neuropathic pain, regardless of whether or not this potential has already been exploited in experimental studies, and explores the role of such models in translational research on mechanism-based treatments for neuropathic pain.

HUMAN SURROGATE MODELS OF ONGOING PAIN AND PARESTHESIAS

Neuropathic pain is considered to be characterized by several sensory qualities (Bouhassira et al. 2004). Some neuropathic pains are reported as continuous and burning and others as paroxysmal and shooting. Although little is known about the mechanisms by which these different pain qualities are encoded in the nociceptive system, qualitatively similar sensations can be elicited experimentally in healthy human subjects. Thus, some experimental models that use evoked pain may be conceived as surrogate models of ongoing neuropathic pain (Table I).

A burning pain quality is a feature of experimental first- and second-degree burn injuries (Raja et al. 1984; Moiniche et al. 1993). Similar pain qualities are induced by topical application of capsaicin or mustard oil to the skin (Koltzenburg et al. 1994; Petersen and Rowbotham 1999). Whereas the tonic burning pain quality might serve as a model for certain aspects of ongoing, constant neuropathic pain, activation of the nociceptive system occurs via adequate stimulation of its peripheral nerve terminals in these models. Strictly speaking, these models actually simulate nociceptive pain, hence the concern that they may mimic inflammatory pain conditions better than neuropathic pain.

The unnatural dysesthetic sensations that may be representative of certain paroxysmal neuropathic pain qualities are often described as being "shooting" or "electric," analogous to electrical stimulation. Hence, electrical stimulation of nerve trunks might serve as a surrogate model of this type of neuropathic pain. Many clinical trials on analgesic efficacy have used electrical stimulation, but those trials were not designed to model neuropathic pain (Dowman 1991; Scharein and Bromm 1998). According to the differential electrical excitability of large and small nerve fibers, electrical stimuli to the nerve trunk primarily activate large myelinated A fibers. It is questionable whether conventional electrical nerve stimulation at clinical intensities activates any C fibers. Given the evidence that some neuropathic pains are mediated by large myelinated A fibers (Wallin et al. 1976; Campbell et al. 1988; Gracely et al. 1992; Torebjörk et al. 1992), standard electrical nerve stimulation may be a good model for these clinical entities. Several strategies have been developed to favor C-fiber recruitment by electrical stimuli, including intracutaneous electrodes (Koppert et al. 2001), punctate epicutaneous electrodes (Klein et al. 2004), ramp-shaped stimuli (Zimmermann 1968), and slow sine waves (Wallace et al. 1996).

Another ongoing symptom of neuropathic pain is paresthesia. This sensation can be safely induced in humans by reperfusion following nerve compression or ischemia (Ochoa and Torebjörk 1980; Reinert et al. 2000). Studies using this technique have also been conducted in rats (Sher et al. 1992). Microneurographic recordings in humans have shown that paresthesias are accompanied by ectopic spontaneous activity in large myelinated A fibers (Ochoa and Torebjörk 1980; Campero et al. 1998). Sometimes these sensations are described as being painful (Reinert et al. 2000).

HUMAN SURROGATE MODELS OF EVOKED PAIN

Dynamic mechanical allodynia, wherein gentle tactile stimuli elicit a pain sensation, was described as a puzzling clinical phenomenon in many early studies on neuropathic pain (Lindblom and Verillo 1979; Merskey 1982). Later studies recognized that this sensation is elicited best when tactile stimuli are moved across the skin in a stroking movement (Koltzenburg et al. 1992; Ochoa and Yarnitsky 1993). Allodynia is also one of the sensory characteristics in the area of secondary hyperalgesia surrounding an injury site and in the area of referred hyperalgesia that occurs with referred visceral or muscle pain (Treede et al. 1992). Secondary hyperalgesia can be induced without injury by intradermal injection of small amounts of capsaicin (LaMotte et al. 1991). Many pharmacological studies have used this human surrogate model of one of the sensory signs of neuropathic pain (Liu et al. 1998).

Punctate mechanical hyperalgesia occurs in similar conditions as dynamic mechanical allodynia, but in contrast to allodynia it is assessed by static contact with small probes such as von Frey probes (LaMotte et al. 1991; Koltzenburg et al. 1992; Ziegler et al. 1999). Whereas dynamic mechanical allodynia appears to be maintained by a tonic sensitizing input from the periphery, static mechanical hyperalgesia does not depend on a maintaining sensitizing input, and hence it may reflect a more chronic mechanism than allodynia in experimental models (LaMotte et al. 1991; Koltzenburg et al. 1994). There is some evidence that punctate mechanical hyperalgesia is a more frequent symptom than allodynia (Liu et al. 1998; Petersen and Rowbotham 1999; Baumgärtner et al. 2002). This human surrogate model of another one of the sensory signs of neuropathic pain has also been used in many pharmacological studies (Liu et al. 1998).

Hyperalgesia to cooling stimuli has also been listed as a cardinal symptom of neuropathic pain (Frost et al. 1988). This sign has not been reproduced

Table I

Pattern of representation of clinical characteristics of neuropathic pain in human surrogate models

Human Surrogate Models	Ongoing Pain/Paresthesia[a]				Sensory Loss				
	Continuous Burning	Continuous Squeezing/ Pressure	Paroxysmal Shooting	Nonpainful Paresthesia	Tactile Hypo-esthesia	Cold Hypo-esthesia	Hypo-algesia to Pinprick	Warm Hypo-esthesia	Heat Hypo-algesia
Burn injury	++	–	–	–	–	–	–	(+)	(+)[c]
Freeze lesion	+	–	–	–	?	?	–	?	–
UVB	–	–	–	–	–	–	–	–	–
Intradermal capsaicin	++	–	–	–	+	?	–	?	(+)[b]
Topical capsaicin (acute)	++	–	–	–	?	?	–	?	–
Topical mustard oil	++	–	–	–	?	?	–	?	–
Topical menthol	(+)	–	–	–	–	–	–	–	–
Burn injury/ capsaicin/heat	+	–	–	–	?	?	?	?	–
Painful electrical stim. (skin)	+	–	+	–	–	–	–	–	–
Painful electrical stim. (nerve)	–	–	+	+	?	?	?	?	?
Reperfusion	–	–	(+)	++	–	–	–	–	–
Ischemia/compression	–	+	–	–	++	++	++	(–)	?
Topical capsaicin (chronic)	(+)	–	–	–	–	–	(+)	(+)	++
Local anesthetic	–	–	–	–	++	++	++	++	++

Evoked Pain

Human Surrogate Models	Mechanical Allodynia	Punctate Hyper-algesia	Static Hyper-algesia	Heat Hyper-algesia	Cold Hyper-algesia/ Allodynia	Paradoxical Heat Sensation	After-sensation	Radiation	Referred Pain
Burn injury	+	++	+[b]	++[b]	–	(+)	?	?	–
Freeze lesion	(+)	+	++[b]	++[b]	?	?	?	?	–
UVB	++	++	+[b]	++[b]	+[b]	–	?	?	–
Intradermal capsaicin	+	++	–	(+)[b]	–	–	?	?	–
Topical capsaicin (acute)	(+)	+	+[b]	++[b]	?	?	?	?	–
Topical mustard oil	+	++	+[b]	++[b]	?	?	?	?	–
Topical menthol	–	+	–	–	+[b]	–	?	?	–
Burn injury/ capsaicin/heat (skin)	+	++	?	++[b]	?	?	?	?	–
Painful electrical stim. (skin)	+	++	+[b]	–	–	–	?	?	–
Painful electrical stim. (nerve)	–	–	–	–	–	–	?	+	+
Reperfusion	–	–	–	–	–	–	+	+	+
Ischemia/compression	–	–	–	–	+	++	?	?	?
Topical capsaicin (chronic)	–	–	–	–	–	–	–	–	–
Local anesthetic	–	–	–	–	–	–	–	–	?

Source: Modified from Klein et al. (2005).

Symbols: ++: pronounced; +: present; (+): weak, may not be exploitable; –: absent; ?: not (sufficiently) tested.
[a] In surrogate models only experienced during conditioning stimulation. [b] Zone of primary hyperalgesia. [c] Zone of secondary hyperalgesia.

successfully in any of the models of secondary hyperalgesia. Recently, experimental cold hyperalgesia was induced by topical application of high concentrations of menthol (Wasner et al. 2004). This model may be useful for future study of the mechanisms and treatment of cold hyperalgesia in neuropathic pain.

Paradoxical heat sensation is a phenomenon in which gentle cooling is erroneously perceived as a hot or burning feeling. It might be a sign of central disinhibition of a polymodal nociceptive pathway that is supposed to be under tonic inhibitory control by a thermoreceptive pathway (Yarnitsky and Ochoa 1990; Craig and Bushnell 1994). Paradoxical heat sensation occurs with both peripheral and central neuropathic pain (Yosipovitch et al. 1995; Hansen et al. 1996). It is easily induced in healthy subjects by preferential A-fiber block by nerve compression (Fruhstorfer 1984; Susser et al. 1999; Ziegler et al. 1999; Fruhstorfer et al. 2003).

HUMAN SURROGATE MODELS OF SENSORY LOSS

A selective sensory loss of functions mediated by Aβ and Aδ fibers can be induced by a transient ischemic nerve block. For this purpose, either the whole limb is rendered ischemic by inflating a blood pressure cuff above systolic blood pressure, or pressure is exerted directly onto a nerve overlying a bone (the superficial radial nerve at the wrist, the ulnar at the elbow, or the peroneal below the knee). The transient sensory loss includes loss of tactile and cold detection, and with a longer latency it also includes loss of the ability to detect punctate mechanical stimuli (Gasser and Erlanger 1929; Fruhstorfer 1984; Ziegler et al. 1999). This pattern of partial sensory loss is similar to that in certain patients with neuropathic pain (Baumgärtner et al. 2002).

A selective sensory loss of functions mediated by primary nociceptive afferents that express the TRPV1 receptor ("capsaicin-sensitive afferents") can be induced by long-term epicutaneous application of capsaicin (Nolano et al. 1999; Magerl et al. 2001). Skin biopsies have shown that TRPV1-expressing nerve fibers withdraw from the epidermis and dermis when exposed to this treatment and regrow after cessation of treatment. This selective nerve block is a model of partial nociceptive denervation lasting for days to a few weeks and affects mostly C fibers. The sensory loss includes heat pain perception and only minor effects on mechanical pain perception. It is unclear which aspects of neuropathic pain are mimicked by this model.

Total nerve block with local anesthetic mimics regional deafferentation. Several studies have investigated the effects of this model on cortical reorganization and sensory capacities, reproducing certain aspects of phantom limb sensations and phantom limb pain (Flor et al. 1995; Knecht et al. 1996; Gandevia and Phegan 1999; Paqueron et al. 2003; Waberski et al. 2003).

OBJECTIVE MEASURES IN HUMAN SURROGATE MODELS

There is no laboratory measure for ongoing pain that would bypass subjective report, but development of such a measure remains a hopeful aim for the future (Cruccu et al. 2004). Direct recordings from nociceptive neurons in humans would be the ideal technique by which to assess neural processing in patients with neuropathic pain and in human surrogate models of neuropathic pain. Microneurography of primary nociceptive afferents has been applied both in healthy subjects and in patients with neuropathic pain (Ochoa and Torebjörk 1980; Ørstavik et al. 2003). However, it is a difficult technique that is only available in a few centers, and since it yields only a small amount of data per individual, it is unlikely that it will become much more widely available. A few direct recordings from the human spinal cord have been performed in the course of neurodestructive procedures such as percutaneous anterolateral cordotomy and dorsal root entry zone lesion, but no single-unit recordings have been made (Campbell and Lipton 1983). At the thalamic level, single-unit recordings are regularly performed in some centers in the course of stereotactic placement of stimulating electrodes for neuroaugmentative procedures to treat movement disorders and chronic pain (Lenz et al. 1989; Lenz and Dougherty 1997; Dostrovsky 2000). This technique has yielded valuable insights into thalamic neural processing in patients with neuropathic pain. Since for evident ethical reasons these recordings cannot be performed in healthy subjects, it is difficult to define an adequate control group (usually patients with movement disorders serve as controls), and there are no recordings in human surrogate models of neuropathic pain.

There are several objective clinical neurophysiological methods by which to demonstrate a correlate of sensory loss, including assessment of peripheral nerve conduction velocity, somatosensory evoked potentials, laser-evoked potentials, and electromyography (Cruccu et al. 2004). These methods can be applied equally well in patients with neuropathic pain and in healthy human subjects. Of these neurophysiological techniques, only laser-evoked potentials and the R-III component of the withdrawal reflex assess the function of the nociceptive system. The other, more widely used, tests assess the function of the tactile system. Both nociceptive and tactile functions can be assessed by quantitative sensory testing. This psychophysical method involves precisely controlled and reproducible stimuli, but the response is still subjective (Hansson 2002). Functional magnetic resonance imaging (fMRI) and positron emission tomography (PET) provide indirect but objective measures of brain activation. The signal-to-noise ratio in PET, and in particular in fMRI, is relatively low, and neither method is sensitive enough to demonstrate the normal function of the somatosensory system in all healthy subjects; hence, these neuroimaging methods cannot be used to prove sensory loss.

Laser-evoked potentials can detect sensory loss in a broad variety of neurological diseases, but this technique is insensitive to gains in sensitivity such as in allodynia and hyperalgesia (Garcia-Larrea et al. 2002; Treede et al. 2003). The R-III component of the withdrawal reflex may be useful to demonstrate central sensitization, since it was found to be enhanced in secondary hyperalgesia (Grönroos and Pertovaara 1993). Functional imaging studies have shown enhanced processing of sensory input in such conditions, but only on a group level (Iadarola et al. 1998; Baron et al. 1999).

CORRELATION OF PAIN PSYCHOPHYSICS
WITH PAIN MECHANISMS

As illustrated in Fig. 1, pain mechanisms can conveniently be divided into three phases (Cervero and Laird 1991; Woolf and Salter 2000). Phase 1 represents the transient *activation* of the nociceptive system by adequate stimuli and the processing of this information in the central nervous system. Phase 2 mechanisms represent the acute plasticity of the nociceptive system that is invoked with each persistent pain state and comprises reversible *modulation* of the nociceptive system. Phase 3 mechanisms represent chronic abnormal pain sensations due to *modification* of the nociceptive system.

It is important to recognize that these three sets of mechanisms are activated in different sequences in nociceptive and neuropathic pain (Table II). The initiating event in nociceptive pain is actual or impending tissue damage, which leads to the activation of peripheral nociceptive nerve terminals by an adequate stimulus. This signal is conducted toward the central nervous system, where it is processed according to the current balance of excitatory and inhibitory influences (phase 1). When nociceptive discharges reach the cerebral cortex, they are eventually perceived as a pain sensation. Whenever tissue damage has occurred, phase 2 mechanisms are also activated, including peripheral and central sensitization, as well as modulation of descending inhibition and facilitation. These mechanisms are part of the

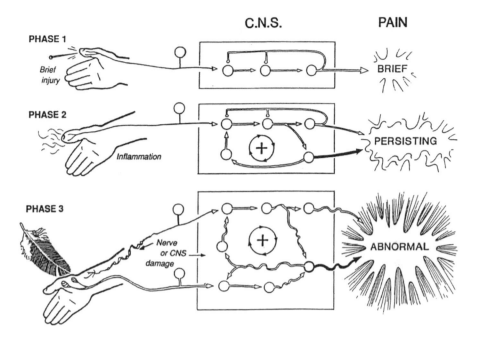

Fig. 1. Models of nociceptive signal processing for three phases of pain. It had long been recognized that phase 1 mechanisms (the processing of brief noxious stimuli) are insufficient to explain the abnormal pain of neuropathic states, where response properties of the nociceptive system may be modified to a large extent (phase 3). It is important to keep in mind, however, that the nociceptive system can also modulate its response properties as a normal component of the reactions to tissue damage (phase 2). Chronic persistence of phase 2 mechanisms contributes to chronic pain, but by definition these mechanisms are spontaneously reversible upon removal of the driving force for their maintenance. From Cervero and Laird (1991), with permission.

normal response of the nociceptive system, and they are usually fully reversible within a few hours or days. Phase 2 mechanisms are typical in postoperative pain and other types of acute pain. In chronic inflammatory diseases, some modification of the nociceptive system may occur (e.g., altered gene expression in primary nociceptive neurons) that may lead to long-lasting changes in its responsiveness. These phase 3 mechanisms contribute to chronic inflammatory pain.

The initiating event in neuropathic pain is damage to the nervous system, or more precisely the somatosensory system, which leads to a loss of function (negative sensory signs). If this damage also leads to ongoing pain, there must be an activation somewhere along the nociceptive system, for example in a peripheral neuroma, the dorsal root ganglion, dorsal horn neurons, or thalamic neurons. The generation of this ectopic activity is a consequence of modification of the nociceptive system, such as altered expression of

Table II
Mechanistic comparison of nociceptive and neuropathic pain

Nociceptive Pain	Neuropathic Pain
Tissue damage	Damage to the nervous system

Phase 1 (activation):
   Peripheral nociceptive nerve terminals
   Impulse conduction
   Synaptic transmission in the CNS
	Phase 3 (modification):
	   Ectopic activity
	   Loss of inhibition

Phase 2 (modulation):
   Peripheral and central sensitization
	Phase 1 (activation):
	   Impulse conduction
	   Synaptic transmission in the CNS

Phase 3 (modification):
   Phenotype changes, etc.
	Phase 2 (modulation):
	   Central sensitization
	   Disinhibition
	   Descending facilitation

Source: Modified from Klein et al. (2005).

sodium, potassium, or calcium channels. Thus, neuropathic pain begins with phase 3 mechanisms. Once neural discharges are generated at one level of the nociceptive system, normal synaptic transmission (phase 1) and normal modulation of the nociceptive system (phase 2) occur at all higher levels of the system. Apart from the fact that ongoing neuropathic pain does not involve transduction at the peripheral nerve terminals, nociceptive and neuropathic pain share many of the phase 1 and 2 mechanisms. Positive sensory symptoms and signs of neuropathic pain thus may be conceived as manifestations of either chronically persisting phase 2 modulation or phase 3 modification. The rapid reversibility of hyperalgesia following nerve blocks in some patients suffering from chronic neuropathic pain suggests that in these cases a persisting phase 2 mechanism was still operating (Gracely et al. 1992).

Table II lists fewer mechanisms than have been described in animal experiments, as it includes only those that can be grouped according to the symptoms that they are likely to generate. This grouping is illustrated in Table III, where neural mechanisms are compared with clinically observable manifestations. Clinical manifestations basically consist of sensory loss, ongoing pain, and evoked pain. Sensory loss plays a prominent role in the assessment of neuropathic pain, because it gives evidence of damage to the nervous system, or more precisely damage to the nociceptive system. The pattern of affected modalities allows us to distinguish which afferent fiber classes (Aβ, Aδ, C) and which central pathways (dorsal column, spinothalamic tract) are involved in the nervous system damage. The spatial pattern of sensory loss allows us to make inferences about the site of damage.

Ongoing pain and paresthesias give evidence of spontaneous activity generated within the nociceptive system in the absence of an adequate peripheral stimulus. In the peripheral nervous system, this activity may take the form of ectopic impulses generated at a neuroma site or in the dorsal root ganglion. Various changes in ion channel expression (subtypes of sodium, potassium, and calcium channels) may be responsible for ectopic impulse generation. Given that central neurons are spontaneously active under normal conditions, a reduction in inhibitory input is sufficient to generate enhanced spontaneous activity, leading to ongoing pain. Again, reduced efficacy of several inhibitory transmitter systems might be responsible.

The positive sensory signs of hyperalgesia and allodynia may be due to central sensitization, for example in the spinal cord. Currently there is no way to distinguish whether this sensitization is mediated by glutamate, substance P, or some other change in excitatory neurotransmission. In addition, reduced descending inhibition or enhanced descending facilitation should also lead to positive sensory signs. The lack of a validated strategy makes it impossible to distinguish between these possibilities with certainty. Central sensitization can cross the boundaries of the innervation territory of a peripheral nerve (Sang et al. 1996); nevertheless, its effects are limited to the immediate vicinity of the affected peripheral nerve or segment. In contrast, descending inhibition typically has remote effects (Millan 2002), so that a deficit in descending inhibition would be expected to affect larger areas or even the whole body. Peripheral and central sensitization may be distinguished according to the modality that is affected: peripheral sensitization leads to heat hyperalgesia, whereas central sensitization leads to mechanical hyperalgesia (Treede et al. 1992). Some evidence indicates that paradoxical heat sensations and cold hyperalgesia may stem from the loss of central inhibition from a thermoreceptive pathway (Craig and Bushnell 1994; Fruhstorfer et al. 2003). We can tentatively interpret localized mechanical hyperalgesia as evidence for central sensitization, generalized hyperalgesia

Table III
Clinical manifestations and mechanisms of neuropathic pain

Clinical Manifestation	Probable Mechanisms
Sensory loss	Damage to the nociceptive system (peripheral or central)
Ongoing pain	Ectopic activity Loss of inhibition
Mechanical or cold hyperalgesia, allodynia	Central sensitization Disinhibition Descending facilitation

as evidence for disinhibition, cold hyperalgesia as evidence for disinhibition, and heat hyperalgesia as evidence for peripheral sensitization.

Clearly there are gaps in our knowledge about the relationship between neurobiological mechanisms and the resulting pattern of sensory symptoms and signs. These gaps can be narrowed by studies that evaluate a standardized set of variables such as quantitative sensory tests (Rolke et al. 2006) or pain questionnaires (Bouhassira et al. 2004) in a broad variety of human surrogate models with known mechanisms of symptom generation. For this purpose, human models are superior to animal models because they can assess both ongoing and evoked symptoms and signs, whereas current animal models are restricted to the study of evoked signs. Pharmacological treatment strategies can also be grouped according to the mechanisms of symptom generation that they are designed to address (Table IV). This grouping allows us to formulate testable hypotheses about mechanism-based treatment of neuropathic pain that can be checked in both human surrogate models and selected patient populations.

These hypotheses appear to be formulated less precisely than those used in many previous studies. For example, instead of asking "Do NK1 receptors mediate neuropathic pain?" or "Do NMDA receptors mediate neuropathic pain?" we might ask "Which manifestations of neuropathic pain are due to central sensitization?" There is a good reason for this lack of precision, because testable hypotheses should be based on observable clinical manifestations, which do not allow the same level of sophistication as neuropharmacology. The proposed grouping, however, represents an increase in sophistication over the common practice in large clinical trials that use daily

Table IV
Rational treatment of neuropathic pain

Target Mechanism	Current Treatment Options
Neural damage	Disease-modifying treatment (if available)
Ectopic activity	Anticonvulsants, sodium channel blockers Potassium channel openers? Calcium channel modulators?
Loss of inhibition	Opiate receptor agonists, antidepressants Alpha-2 adrenoreceptor agonists GABA- or glycine receptor agonists?
Central sensitization	Glutamate receptor antagonists Calcium channel modulators (e.g., NK1, COX-2, NOS)?

Abbreviations: COX-2 = cyclooxygenase 2; GABA = gamma-aminobutyric acid; NK1 = neurokinin 1; NOS = nitric oxide synthase.

pain ratings as the end point, because it allows the formulation of rational inclusion criteria. If the pharmacological mechanism of action of a drug addresses aspects of central sensitization, the drug should primarily be assessed in patients who exhibit evidence of central sensitization. If its pharmacological mechanism is directed toward ectopic impulse generation, patients with evidence of ectopic activity should be recruited.

SUMMARY AND CONCLUSIONS

Disease mechanisms and molecular and cellular mechanisms of neuropathic pain are studied in animal models. Human surrogate models of neuropathic pain focus on the investigation of mechanisms of symptom generation. As listed above, a vast array of human surrogate models is available for ongoing symptoms, for positive sensory symptoms, and for sensory loss. By design, human surrogate models of neuropathic pain involve a reversible modulation of the properties of the nociceptive system, i.e., its acute plasticity (phase 2 mechanisms). They usually do not create a long-lasting and potentially irreversible modification (phase 3 mechanisms). The denervation and ectopic activity of phase 3 can be modeled to a certain extent by transient nerve compression and ischemia or by topical capsaicin. By invoking phase 2 mechanisms, however, most human models mimic sensory signs that may occur in both neuropathic and nociceptive pain (e.g., central sensitization). Thus, the findings from such models are relevant for, but not restricted to, neuropathic pain.

Each sensory finding is basically compatible with multiple neurobiological and neuropharmacological mechanisms, because many molecular and cellular mechanisms converge in the generation of a relatively small number of observable clinical manifestations. By using clinical manifestations as a guide for the classification of neuropathic pain and its models (both human and animal), an intermediate level of sophistication can be created to bridge the gap between highly complex pharmacological mechanisms of action and a simple clinical assessment of daily pain intensity. This intermediate level of sophistication should prove useful for translational research. A more thorough characterization of human surrogate models, such as the identification of the differential clinical manifestations of descending facilitation and spinal sensitization, would allow us to refine the proposed grouping scheme. At the present stage, however, human surrogate models of neuropathic pain are already very useful for the investigation of pharmacological mechanisms of action and therapeutic efficacy because they are based on the same assessment techniques used in clinical studies.

ACKNOWLEDGMENTS

The author's work has been supported by the Deutsche Forschungsgemeinschaft (Tr 236/13-3, Tr 236/16-1) and by the Bundesministerium für Bildung und Forschung (01EM0107).

REFERENCES

Baron R, Baron Y, Disbrow E, Roberts TPL. Brain processing of capsaicin-induced secondary hyperalgesia. A functional MRI study. *Neurology* 1999; 53:548–557.

Baumgärtner U, Magerl W, Klein T, Hopf HC, Treede R-D. Neurogenic hyperalgesia versus painful hypoalgesia: two distinct mechanisms of neuropathic pain. *Pain* 2002; 96:141–151.

Bouhassira D, Attal N, Fermanian J, et al. Development and validation of the neuropathic pain symptom inventory. *Pain* 2004; 108:248–257.

Campbell JA, Lipton S. Somatosensory evoked potentials recorded from within the anterolateral quadrant of the human spinal cord. In: Bonica JJ, Lindblom U, Iggo A (Eds). *Proceedings of the Third World Congress on Pain,* Advances in Pain Research and Therapy, Vol. 5. New York: Raven Press, 1983, pp 193–196.

Campbell JN, Raja SN, Meyer RA, Mackinnon SE. Myelinated afferents signal the hyperalgesia associated with nerve injury. *Pain* 1988; 32:89–94.

Campero M, Serra J, Marchettini P, Ochoa JL. Ectopic impulse generation and auto excitation in single myelinated afferent fibers in patients with peripheral neuropathy and positive sensory symptoms. *Muscle Nerve* 1998; 21:1661–1667.

Cervero F, Laird JMA. One pain or many pains? A new look at pain mechanisms. *News Physiol Sci* 1991; 6:268–273.

Craig AD, Bushnell MC. The thermal grill illusion: Unmasking the burn of cold pain. *Science* 1994; 265:252–255.

Cruccu G, Anand P, Attal N, et al. EFNS guidelines on neuropathic pain assessment. *Eur J Neurol* 2004; 11:153–162.

Dostrovsky JO. Role of thalamus in pain. In: Sandkühler J, Bromm B, Gebhart GF (Eds). *Nervous System Plasticity and Chronic Pain,* Progress in Brain Research. Vol. 129. Amsterdam: Elsevier, 2000, pp 245–257.

Dowman R. Spinal and supraspinal correlates of nociception in man. *Pain* 1991; 45:269–281.

Flor H, Elbert T, Knecht S, et al. Phantom-limb pain as a perceptual correlate of cortical reorganization following arm amputation. *Nature* 1995; 375:482–484.

Frost SA, Raja SN, Campbell JN, Meyer RA, Khan AA. Does hyperalgesia to cooling stimuli characterize patients with sympathetically maintained pain (reflex sympathetic dystrophy)? In: Dubner R, Gebhart GF, Bond MR (Eds). *Proceedings of the Vth World Congress on Pain.* Amsterdam: Elsevier, 1988, pp 151–156.

Fruhstorfer H. Thermal sensibility changes during ischemic nerve block. *Pain* 1984; 20:355–361.

Fruhstorfer H, Harju E-L, Lindblom UF. The significance of A-delta and C fibres for the perception of synthetic heat. *Eur J Pain* 2003; 7:63–71.

Gandevia SC, Phegan CML. Perceptual distortions of the human body image produced by local anaesthesia, pain and cutaneous stimulation. *J Physiol* 1999; 514:609–616.

García-Larrea L, Convers P, Magnin M, et al. Laser-evoked potential abnormalities in central pain patients: the influence of spontaneous and provoked pain. *Brain* 2002; 125:2766–2781.

Gasser HS, Erlanger J. The role of fiber size in the establishment of a nerve block by pressure or cocaine. *Am J Physiol* 1929; 88:581–591.

Gracely RH, Lynch SA, Bennett GJ. Painful neuropathy: altered central processing, maintained dynamically by peripheral input. *Pain* 1992; 51:175–194.

Grönroos M, Pertovaara A. Capsaicin-induced central facilitation of a nociceptive flexion reflex in humans. *Neurosci Lett* 1993; 159:215–218.

Hansen C, Hopf HC, Treede R-D. Paradoxical heat sensation in patients with multiple sclerosis. Evidence for a supraspinal integration of temperature sensation. *Brain* 1996; 119:1729–1736.

Hansson P. Neuropathic pain: clinical characteristics and diagnostic workup. *Eur J Pain* 2002; 6(Suppl A):47–50.

Iadarola MJ, Berman KF, Zeffiro TA, et al. Neural activation during acute capsaicin-evoked pain and allodynia assessed with PET. *Brain* 1998; 121:931–947.

Klein T, Magerl W, Hopf HC, Sandkühler J, Treede RD. Perceptual correlates of nociceptive long-term potentiation and long-term depression in humans. *J Neurosci* 2004; 24:964–971.

Klein T, Magerl W, Rolke R, Treede RD. Human surrogate models of neuropathic pain. *Pain* 2005; 115:227–233.

Knecht S, Henningsen H, Elbert T, et al. Reorganizational and perceptional changes after amputation. *Brain* 1996; 119:1213–1219.

Koltzenburg M, Lundberg LER, Torebjörk HE. Dynamic and static components of mechanical hyperalgesia in human hairy skin. *Pain* 1992; 51:207–219.

Koltzenburg M, Torebjörk HE, Wahren LK. Nociceptor modulated central sensitization causes mechanical hyperalgesia in acute chemogenic and chronic neuropathic pain. *Brain* 1994; 117:579–591.

Koppert W, Dern SK, Sittl R, et al. A new model of electrically evoked pain and hyperalgesia in human skin: the effects of intravenous alfentanil, S^+-ketamine, and lidocaine. *Anesthesiology* 2001; 95:395–402.

LaMotte RH, Shain CN, Simone DA, Tsai E-FP. Neurogenic hyperalgesia: psychophysical studies of underlying mechanisms. *J Neurophysiol* 1991; 66:190–211.

Lenz FA, Dougherty PM. Pain processing in the human thalamus. In: Steriade M, Jones EG, McCormick DA (Eds). *Thalamus. Experimental/Clinical Aspects*, Vol. II. Oxford: Elsevier Press, 1997, pp 617–651.

Lenz FA, Kwan HC, Dostrovsky JO, Tasker RR. Characteristics of the bursting pattern of action potentials that occurs in the thalamus of patients with central pain. *Brain Res* 1989; 496:357–360.

Lindblom U, Verrillo RT. Sensory functions in chronic neuralgia. *J Neurol Neurosurg Psychiatry* 1979; 42:422–435.

Liu MW, Max MB, Robinovitz E, Gracely RH, Bennett GJ. The human capsaicin model of allodynia and hyperalgesia: sources of variability and methods for reduction. *J Pain Symptom Manage* 1998; 16:10–20.

Magerl W, Fuchs PN, Meyer RA, Treede R-D. Roles of capsaicin-insensitive nociceptors in pain and secondary hyperalgesia. *Brain* 2001; 124:1754–1764.

Merskey H. Pain terms: a supplementary note. *Pain* 1982; 14:205–206.

Merskey H, Bogduk N. *Classification of Chronic Pain: Descriptions of Chronic Pain Syndromes and Definitions of Pain Terms*, 2nd ed. Seattle: IASP Press, 1994.

Millan MJ. Descending control of pain. *Prog Neurobiol* 2002; 66:355–474.

Moiniche S, Dahl JB, Kehlet H. Time course of primary and secondary hyperalgesia after heat injury to the skin. *Br J Anaesth* 1993; 71:201–205.

Nolano M, Simone DA, Wendelschafer-Crabb G, et al. Topical capsaicin in humans: parallel loss of epidermal nerve fibers and pain sensation. *Pain* 1999; 81:135–145.

Ochoa JL, Torebjörk HE. Paraesthesiae from ectopic impulse generation in human sensory nerves. *Brain* 1980; 103:835–853.

Ochoa JL, Yarnitsky D. Mechanical hyperalgesias in neuropathic pain patients: dynamic and static subtypes. *Ann Neurol* 1993; 33:465–472.

Ørstavik K, Weidner C, Schmidt R, et al. Pathological C-fibres in patients with a chronic painful condition. *Brain* 2003; 126:567–578.

Paqueron X, Leguen M, Rosenthal D, et al. The phenomenology of body image distortions induced by regional anaesthesia. *Brain* 2003; 126:702–712.

Petersen KL, Rowbotham MC. A new human experimental pain model: the heat/capsaicin sensitization model. *Neuroreport* 1999; 10:1511–1516.

Raja SN, Campbell JN, Meyer RA. Evidence for different mechanisms of primary and secondary hyperalgesia following heat injury to the glabrous skin. *Brain* 1984; 107:1179–1188.

Reinert A, Treede R-D, Bromm B. The pain inhibiting pain effect: an electrophysiological study in humans. *Brain Res* 2000; 862:103–110.

Rolke R, Magerl W, Andrews-Campbell K, et al. Quantitative sensory testing: a comprehensive protocol for clinical trials. *Eur J Pain* 2006; 10:77–88.

Sang CN, Gracely RH, Max MB, Bennett GJ. Capsaicin-evoked mechanical allodynia and hyperalgesia cross nerve territories: evidence for a central mechanism. *Anesthesiology* 1996; 85:491–496.

Scharein E, Bromm B. The intracutaneous pain model in the assessment of analgesic efficacy. *Pain Rev* 1998; 5:216–246.

Sher GD, Cartmell SM, Gelgor L, Mitchell D. Role of N-methyl-D-aspartate and opiate receptors in nociception during and after ischaemia in rats. *Pain* 1992; 49:241–248.

Susser E, Sprecher E, Yarnitsky D. Paradoxical heat sensation in healthy subjects: peripherally conducted by A delta or C fibres? *Brain* 1999; 122:239–246.

Torebjörk HE, Lundberg LER, LaMotte RH. Central changes in processing of mechanoreceptive input in capsaicin-induced secondary hyperalgesia. *J Physiol* 1992; 448:765–780.

Treede R-D, Meyer RA, Raja SN, Campbell JN. Peripheral and central mechanisms of cutaneous hyperalgesia. *Prog Neurobiol* 1992; 38:397–421.

Treede R-D, Lorenz J, Baumgärtner U. Clinical usefulness of laser-evoked potentials. *Neurophysiol Clin* 2003; 33:303–314.

Waberski TD, Gobbelé R, Kawohl W, Cordes C, Buchner H. Immediate cortical reorganization after local anesthetic block of the thumb: source localization of somatosensory evoked potentials in human subjects. *Neurosci Lett* 2003; 347:151–154.

Wallace MS, Dyck JB, Rossi SS, Yaksh TL. Computer-controlled lidocaine infusion for the evaluation of neuropathic pain after peripheral nerve injury. *Pain* 1996; 66:69–77.

Wallin G, Torebjörk E, Hallin R. Preliminary observations on the pathophysiology of hyperalgesia in the causalgic pain syndrome. In: Zotterman Y (Ed). *Sensory Functions of the Skin in Primates.* Oxford: Pergamon Press, 1976, pp 489–502.

Wasner G, Schattschneider J, Binder A, Baron R. Topical menthol—a human model for cold pain by activation and sensitization of C nociceptors. *Brain* 2004; 127:1159–1171.

Woolf CJ, Salter MW. Neuronal plasticity: increasing the gain in pain. *Science* 2000; 288:1765–1769.

Yarnitsky D, Ochoa JL. Release of cold-induced burning pain by block of cold-specific afferent input. *Brain* 1990; 113:893–902.

Yosipovitch G, Yarnitsky D, Mermelstein V, et al. Paradoxical heat sensation in uremic polyneuropathy. *Muscle Nerve* 1995; 18:768–771.

Ziegler EA, Magerl W, Meyer RA, Treede R-D. Secondary hyperalgesia to punctate mechanical stimuli: central sensitization to A-fibre nociceptor input. *Brain* 1999; 122:2245–2257.

Zimmermann M. Selective activation of C-fibers. *Pflügers Arch* 1968; 301:329–333.

Correspondence to: Prof. Dr. Rolf-Detlef Treede, Institute of Physiology and Pathophysiology, Johannes Gutenberg University, Saarstr. 21, D-55099 Mainz, Germany. Tel: 49-6131-392-5715; Fax: 49-6131-392-5902; e-mail: treede@uni-mainz.de.

21

Psychophysical Tests that Characterize Pathological Mechanisms of Pain in Humans

Donald D. Price,[a] Charles J. Vierck,[b]
and Roland Staud[c]

[a]Departments of Oral and Maxillofacial Surgery, College of Dentistry,
and Departments of [b]Neuroscience and [c]Medicine, College of Medicine,
University of Florida, Gainesville, Florida, USA

Psychophysics has an important role in elucidating the neurophysiological basis for pain. In addition, it provides a scientific basis for modern noninvasive methods of pain measurement and assessment (Marks 1974; Gracely and Dubner 1981; Price 1999). Psychophysical methods of sensory testing also play a pivotal role in understanding pathophysiological mechanisms of pain, including neuropathic pain. The main objective of this chapter is to explain how the combination of direct scaling methods and sensory testing can be used to identify some of the mechanisms of neuropathic pain. Psychophysical methods of direct scaling, in combination with tests of elicited pain sensations that reflect abnormal or enhanced pain mechanisms, are useful in characterizing different types of persistent pain conditions, including neuropathies. We consider this objective to be useful in aiding diagnoses and ultimately in matching treatments to pain syndromes.

APPLICATION OF DIRECT SCALING METHODS TO CHARACTERIZE PATHOLOGICAL PAIN

All methods of pain measurement share a common goal of accurately representing the human pain experience. Threshold measures of pain sensitivity are limited in that they do not assess changes in pain sensitivity that may occur over a wide range of nociceptive stimulus intensities. Although multiple methods of sensory testing are useful, including threshold and discriminability measures, this chapter will focus on direct scaling methods because they have the capacity to assess a wide range of responses to threshold and suprathreshold intensities, a characteristic that is most relevant to clinical pain assessment.

Direct scales include numerical rating scales (NRS), verbal rating scales (VRS), verbal descriptor scales (VDS), cross-modality matching, magnitude estimation, and visual analogue scales (VAS). VAS have emerged as having psychometric properties that are superior to the other pain-scaling methods just mentioned because they fulfill multiple criteria for ideal pain measurement and assessment (Gracely and Dubner 1981; Price et al. 2002). These criteria include ratio scale properties (Price et al. 1983, 1994a; Myles et al. 1999), high test-retest reliability and repeatability (Rosier et al. 2002), internally consistent measures of clinical and experimental pain (Price et al. 1983, 1994a; Price and Harkins 1987), sensitivity to variables that increase or decrease pain (Price et al. 1985, 2001), capacity to measure multiple dimensions of pain (Price et al. 1983, 1987, 1994a; Price and Harkins 1987), strong correlation with measures of pain-related activity in the human brain (Coghill et al. 2003), and in the case of mechanical or electronic VAS, simplicity and ease of use (Gracely and Dubner 1981; Price et al. 1994a). Probably as a consequence of these characteristics, VAS is the most commonly used single scale in human research studies of pain. For example, among 121 human studies using single pain scales that were published in *PAIN* in 2004, 49% used VAS, 36% used numerical rating scales, 8% used verbal rating scales, and 6.6% used another type of rating scale. The latter category included three studies that used faces scales for children. Proportions are similar in other years and other pain journals.

It is not widely recognized that VAS have measurement properties that are superior to other commonly used scales, such as the NRS. Unlike VAS, the 11-point NRS clearly does not have ratio scale properties and has no distinct zero point (see Fig. 4 and associated data in Price et al. 1994a). Compared to VAS ratings, NRS ratings have been shown to be artificially higher for both clinical and experimental pain (Price et al. 1994a). The notion that NRS ratings can easily substitute for VAS ratings because they are highly correlated with each other is very misguided. For example, both are monotonic functions of heat stimulus intensity and are likely to be highly correlated, yet the 11-point NRS stimulus-response curve is displaced above the VAS curve. This displacement has two consequences. The first is that, unlike the VAS, the NRS does not accurately predict subjects' separate judgments of ratios of pain intensity. Thus, 49.6°C is judged on average as twice as painful as 47°C, a judgment that is consistent with the stimulus-VAS response curve but *not* with the stimulus-NRS response curve. The consistency between independent judgments of ratios and VAS rating curves provides a critical line of evidence for ratio scale properties. The second consequence is that ratings of pain, especially near pain threshold, are artificially high in the case of NRS. For example, subjects' average NRS rating of 45°C, a stimulus that is on average at or very near pain threshold, is 2.2 on a scale of 0–10 and is significantly above zero. Thus, it is highly questionable as to whether NRS have a true zero point for pain. In contrast, VAS ratings of 45°C are much lower and not significantly different from zero (the mean is slightly above zero because a few individuals have pain thresholds below 45°C). These issues apply to both clinical and experimental pain for two reasons. First, it has been repeatedly demonstrated that patients give higher NRS ratings than VAS ratings to both clinical and experimental pain (Wallenstein et al. 1980; Price et al. 1983, 1994a). Second, similar to the ratio scale test of experimental pain (Price et al. 1983, 1994a), Myles et al. (1999) showed that VAS ratings of clinical pain accurately predict patients' separate judgments of ratios of clinical pain.

Given the superior psychometric characteristics of VAS, it is astonishing that NRS have been recommended over other pain scales, including VAS, in clinical research and practice (Jensen and Karoly 2001; Dworkin et al. 2005). Because of their measurement advantages, studies that use VAS to conduct sensory tests on patients with pathological pain are emphasized in this chapter.

PSYCHOPHYSICAL CHARACTERIZATION OF PATHOLOGICAL PAIN

The psychophysical attributes of pain that relate to pathological pain have been characterized using several measurement methods, including direct scaling methods. These include thresholds for pain, adaptation of pain intensity, nociceptive stimulus intensity-pain intensity relationships, discriminability between pain intensities, and temporal and spatial summation of suprathreshold pain. Here we focus on a few tests that we consider to be the most useful in characterizing hyperalgesia and allodynia in patients with complex regional pain syndrome (CRPS) and other types of pain, including fibromyalgia. These tests mainly rely on VAS ratings of graded painful stimuli or, in combination with brief repeated stimuli, test temporal summation mechanisms. Responses to these sensory tests have been useful in characterizing the variability and severity of pain conditions and their central pathophysiological mechanisms.

DIRECT RATINGS OF RAMP-AND-HOLD
NOCICEPTIVE TEMPERATURES

A reliable and valid test of heat allodynia and hyperalgesia consists of having subjects rate pain intensity on a VAS in response to ramp-and-hold contact heat stimuli delivered to skin of body areas that are proximate to the source of ongoing pain (e.g., the hand and forearm of a CRPS patient whose pain includes these areas). An example of heat-induced hyperalgesia is shown in Fig. 1 for one CRPS patient taken from a series of 31 patients (Price et al. 1992). Exaggerated perceptions of pain occurred throughout a wide range of 5-second stimulus intensities (43°–49°C) presented in random order. However, the differences between normal responses to pain, obtained from stimuli delivered to a homologous contralateral nonpathological zone, and abnormal responses to pain, obtained from stimuli delivered to a pathological zone, were greatest toward the lower end of the stimulus range, 43°–45°C (Fig. 1). This pattern of increased responsiveness is remarkably similar to that obtained for C-polymodal nociceptive afferents and for human ratings of heat-induced pain after heat-induced injury of the skin (Meyer and Campbell 1981; Campbell et al. 1988). Both in the case of CRPS and skin injury, the hyperalgesia is likely to be dynamically maintained by tonic input from primary nociceptive afferents, particularly C-nociceptive afferents (Gracely et al. 1992). However, in some cases of CRPS, especially CRPS-II (i.e., CRPS with evidence of a nerve lesion), tonic input is more likely to be related to ectopic foci within peripheral nerve axons because the skin is not injured. Based on the curves presented in Fig. 1, it is also likely that the

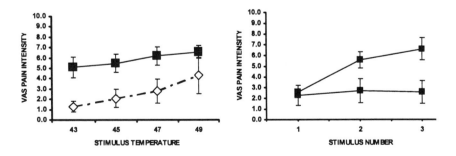

Fig. 1. Left panel: Pain intensity ratings of a CRPS patient who had heat-induced hyperalgesia. Five-second skin temperature stimuli applied to the pathological right foot (upper black squares) resulted in much higher VAS ratings than those applied to the normal left foot (lower open squares). Each data point is based on five trials; vertical error bars are standard deviations. Right panel: Pain ratings of the same patient in response to trains of gentle mechanical stimuli (15 g/mm, 1-second duration) applied to the pathological right foot. Note that temporal summation of mechanical allodynia occurred with stimuli delivered at 1/3 seconds but not at 1/5 seconds. Each data point is based on four trials.

thermal thresholds for pain were lowered, so that heat *allodynia* was also likely to be present in this patient. Cold and mechanical allodynia have been shown to be more common characteristics of CRPS patients (Campbell et al. 1988).

Fibromyalgia patients also have heat allodynia/hyperalgesia when tested with ramp-and-hold skin temperatures, as shown in Fig. 2 (Price et al. 2002). However, unlike CRPS, fibromyalgia patients are more likely to have pain referred to many body areas. Consequently, their heat hyperalgesia has been established by comparing their pain ratings to those of age- and sex-matched control subjects (Fig. 2). Rates of ramp-and-hold heat stimuli can be adapted to predominantly stimulate Aδ-fiber (2°–10°C/sec) or C-fiber (<2°C/sec) heat-sensitive nociceptors (Yeomans and Proudfit 1996; Yeomans et al. 1996a,b). C-fiber testing is more directly relevant for persistent clinical pain. These stimuli can be applied to both humans and animals.

TEMPORAL SUMMATION OF SECOND PAIN

A brief nociceptive stimulus, such as a heat tap at 51°C or percutaneous electrical stimulation of A- and C-fiber axons, can evoke two distinct pain

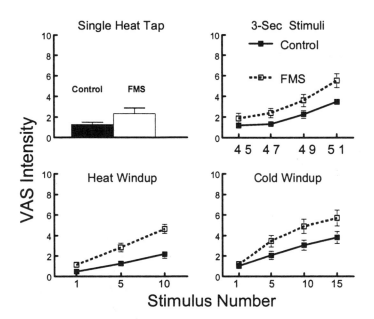

Fig. 2. Mean VAS ratings of fibromyalgia syndrome (FMS) and normal control (NC) subjects to single heat taps (top left), graded 3-second heat stimuli (top right), repeated thenar heat taps (bottom left), and repeated cold taps (bottom right). (From Price et al. 2002.)

sensations called "first" and "second" pain (Price 1972; Price et al. 1977; Vierck et al. 1997; Staud et al. 2001, 2004). First pain is usually an immediate sharp sensation, whereas second pain occurs about a second later and can be a dull, throbbing, or burning sensation depending on the type of stimulus used to evoke it. Second pain often lingers well beyond this brief stimulus. Cross-modality matching and VAS scaling methods have been used to analyze the temporal summation found in second pain (Price et al. 1977; Vierck et al. 1997). Examples of temporal summation of second pain in normal subjects and fibromyalgia patients are shown in Fig. 2. Among normal pain-free subjects, C-fiber-evoked second pain increases in intensity whenever the interstimulus interval is 3 seconds or less but does not change when the interstimulus interval is 5 seconds or greater. This slow temporal summation occurs even when the stimulus moves from spot to spot during the train of heat pulses, and even after total blockade of the peripheral impulses in the A-fiber axons necessary for first pain (Price 1972; Price et al. 1977). Temporal summation of second pain usually results in a continuous burning pain after several stimuli, and this burning pain often continues for several seconds after termination of the stimuli. This aftersensation has long been noted to be a common feature of pain evoked by stimulation of C-fiber nociceptive afferent neurons (Staud et al. 2001, 2004). Temporal summation of second pain reflects early mechanisms that lead to central sensitization, secondary hyperalgesia, and persistent pain states. For example, dorsal horn neurons show temporal summation or "wind-up" in response to repeated C-fiber stimulation (Mendell and Wall 1965; Li et al. 1999).

Given the parallels between wind-up and temporal summation of second pain, enhanced second pain most likely reflects activation of N-methyl-D-aspartate (NMDA) and/or substance P receptors as well as intracellular mechanisms of sensitization in the spinal dorsal horn (Price et al. 1994b, 1994c). The neurotransmitters involved in wind-up include excitatory amino acids, tachykinins, substance P, and neurokinin A, which lead to progressive removal of the Mg block and activation of NMDA receptors in dorsal horn neurons. Both wind-up and temporal summation of second pain reflect an early stage of central sensitization in which activated receptors allow increased calcium influx and initiate cascades of intracellular biochemical events (reviewed in Staud et al. 2004). The latter are associated with long-term neuroplastic changes that lead to increased excitability of pain-related neurons.

Experiments on both normal volunteers and patients provide support for NMDA mechanisms of both normal and abnormal slow temporal summation. Temporal summation of heat-induced second pain can be attenuated by dextromethorphan, an uncompetitive NMDA-receptor antagonist (Price et al. 1994b; Vierck et al. 1997; Staud et al. 2005). Another NMDA-receptor antagonist, ketamine, reduces both mechanical allodynia and spontaneous pain associated with intradermal capsaicin injection and various types of nerve injury (Park et al. 1994; Byas-Smith et al. 1993). Intravenous ketamine (0.15 mg/kg) was effective in simultaneously reducing ongoing pain, mechanical allodynia, and temporal summation of mechanical allodynia in postherpetic neuralgia patients, reflecting clinically relevant demonstration of NMDA-receptor antagonism of temporal summation of mechanical allodynia (Eide et al. 1994).

It is also important to recognize that the characteristics of temporal summation of second pain just described have been observed in several different laboratories using different methods. Temporal summation of second pain occurs in response to repeated cutaneous electric shocks before and after blockade of myelinated axons (Price 1972). It occurs in response to repeated brief heat pulses of 51°C (Price 1977; Price et al. 1989, 1994b; Maixner et al. 1998) or to repeated 53°C heat taps to the skin (Vierck et al. 1997). Slow temporal summation occurs with repetitive stimulation of muscle nociceptive afferents (Staud et al. 2003, 2005) and with repetitive stimulation of visceral nociceptive afferents (Arendt-Nielsen et al. 1997).

We have previously reported that in comparison to normal control subjects, fibromyalgia patients respond to repeated heat taps with enhanced slow temporal summation and more prolonged aftersensations (Staud et al. 2001, 2004; Vierck et al. 2001; Price et al. 2002) (Fig. 2). Summation also occurs at a lower frequency (i.e., 0.2 Hz) in fibromyalgia patients, similar to patients with temporomandibular joint disease (Maixner et al. 1998). Furthermore, once it occurs, enhanced second pain can be maintained by very low frequencies of stimulation in fibromyalgia patients but not in normal controls (Staud et al. 2004). This characteristic is parallel to that of responses of dorsal horn nociceptive neurons to repetitive stimulation of C fibers (Li et al. 1999). Once wind-up reaches a plateau, only very low frequencies (e.g., one C-fiber volley every 10 seconds) are required to maintain enhanced responsiveness. The enhanced responsiveness is accompanied by expanded receptive fields (Li et al. 1999). All of these changes are likely to be integral to early mechanisms of central sensitization, allodynia, and secondary hyperalgesia. Enhanced aftersensations, measured just after second pain summation, are also salient predictors of fibromyalgia patients' ratings of clinical pain, accounting for 27% of the variance in ratings (Staud et al. 2003). Tender point count and pain-related emotions accounted for about 22% of the remaining variance. A similar approach of using psychophysical tests to characterize neuropathic pain states could be used, as discussed below.

TESTS OF MECHANICAL ALLODYNIA

Studies of neuropathic pain patients have shown pathological conditions characterized by zones of skin in which heat hyperalgesia is present in some patients and by larger zones in which mechanical hyperalgesia and/or allodynia is present in all or most patients (Price et al. 1989, 1992; Gracely et al. 1992). Two distinct types of mechanical allodynia have been characterized in neuropathic pain patients. The first is termed low-threshold Aβ allodynia (Price et al. 1989, 1992). Its presence is based on several lines of evidence. First, it occurs in response to electrical stimulation of the lowest threshold axons in nerves supplying the pathological zone. Second, it occurs in response to very gentle mechanical stimuli. Third, it is abolished by blockade of the largest, fastest conducting axons within nerves (Gracely et al. 1992). Finally, it has a reaction time consistent with conduction in myelinated afferents (Gracely et al. 1992). It is also commonly characterized by the fact that moving stimuli or stimulus onset or offset are more painful than static mechanical stimuli (Price et al. 1989, 1992). The other type of mechanical allodynia is characterized by evidence that Aβ afferents do *not* seem to be involved (see above) and that more intense but normally painless stimuli are required to evoke pain. For example, 15–600-g von Frey filament stimuli, which are well above threshold for Aβ primary mechanoreceptive afferents but are rarely painful under normal circumstances, evoke pain when applied to the pathological zones of these patients. This type of mechanical allodynia is termed high-threshold and may well be mediated by activation of nociceptive afferents under conditions that normally do not produce pain.

High threshold allodynia is likely to be triggered by A-fiber nociceptors under at least some circumstances. For example, high-threshold allodynia corresponds to phenomena that have been referred to as static hyperalgesia and punctate hyperalgesia. Punctate hyperalgesia can survive capsaicin desensitization (all epidermal C fibers are gone), and it disappears with an A-fiber block (Fuchs et al. 2000; Magerl et al. 2001). Central sensitization to input from these Aδ nociceptors could be a mechanism that accounts for enhanced pain in response to punctate mechanical stimuli within zones of secondary hyperalgesia (Magerl et al. 2001). Therefore, capsaicin-insensitive A-fiber nociceptors may be at least one of the mediators of hyperalgesia in neuropathic pain.

ABNORMAL TRIGGERING OF TEMPORAL SUMMATION BY PRIMARY MECHANORECEPTIVE AFFERENT NEURONS

Regardless of whether the mechanical allodynia is Aβ or high threshold, it often has characteristics similar to pains evoked by unmyelinated C-nociceptive afferents described above for normal pain (Price et al. 1994b). Thus, repeated brief mechanical stimulation of allodynic patients often evokes slow temporal summation of burning pain, as shown in Fig. 1 (right panel). For some CRPS patients, slow temporal summation of burning pain occurs when gentle mechanical stimuli or electrical stimulation of Aβ afferents are applied at rates of once per 3 seconds. For other patients, slow temporal summation occurs only with more intense but normally nonpainful mechanical stimuli. Still other patients do not exhibit slow temporal summation with these types of repetitive mechanical stimuli. Both mechanical allodynia and slow temporal summation of allodynia are completely or nearly completely reversed by anesthetic blockade of sympathetic ganglia in some CRPS patients, indicating that these sensory abnormalities can sometimes be dynamically maintained by sympathetic efferent activity, presumably activity that induces continuous input over nociceptive afferents. Slow temporal summation of mechanical allodynia, particularly that induced by stimulation of Aβ afferents, is abnormal since such types of stimuli evoke pain neither in pain-free subjects nor when delivered to homologous contralateral pain-free zones in CRPS patients. In fact, Aβ-afferent stimulation, even at extremely high frequencies, does not evoke pain in normal human subjects (Collins et al. 1960). Therefore, Aβ mechanical allodynia and abnormal slow temporal summation of mechanical allodynia may represent an exaggeration or abnormal triggering of physiological mechanisms that already exist in normal pain-free individuals. Such mechanisms can be demonstrated in the latter by temporal summation of experimentally induced second pain, as described earlier. Thus, under some pathological conditions after nerve injury or nerve dysfunction, Aβ input may somehow gain access to and trigger the same temporal summation mechanisms normally activated by C-afferent stimulation. In other pathological conditions, sensitized nociceptors themselves are likely to be the direct proximal cause of the slow temporal summation of mechanical allodynia.

Regardless of the exact mechanisms by which temporal summation of allodynia is generated, the phenomenon is likely to be at least part of the basis for CRPS patients' ongoing "spontaneous" pain. It has been suggested that temporal summation of Aβ allodynia provides at least part of the basis for ongoing background pain in neuropathic pain patients (Price et al. 1992). This relationship could occur if continuous input from Aβ low-threshold afferents (evoked in the normal course of mechanical stimulation from walking, sitting, or even contact with clothes) activated slow temporal summation of a type of burning, aching, or throbbing pain that built up slowly and dissipated slowly over time. This possibility was explicitly tested in a group of 31 CRPS patients by recording the intensity of ongoing pain in 10 patients who demonstrated slow temporal summation compared with 17 patients who did not (Price et al. 1992). The former had significantly higher intensities of ongoing pain (mean = 7.02 on VAS) than the latter (mean = 4.04 on VAS; P < 0.001). Therefore, exaggerated or abnormally triggered mechanisms of slow temporal summation are likely to form at least part of the basis of persistent pain that usually occurs in CRPS patients. Abnormally triggered temporal summation of mechanical allodynia also appears to be related to paroxysmal pains in some cases of trigeminal neuralgia, and this summation can be reduced by anticonvulsants such as carbamazepine (Dubner et al. 1987).

Studies of both fibromyalgia and neuropathic pain patients indicate that "spontaneous" or ongoing clinical pain may be co-determined by two major factors: (1) tonic impulse input from nociceptive afferents in damaged or otherwise dysfunctional nerves and (2) central sensitization mechanisms mediated by NMDA-receptor mechanisms, including sensitization of postsynaptic membrane glutamate receptors and excitotoxic loss of inhibitory mechanisms. The interrelationship between these two general factors is evident in other ways as well. For example, zones of hyperalgesia and allodynia that extend well beyond the cutaneous territory innervated by the injured nerve indicate that altered central processing is dynamically maintained by ongoing nociceptor input. Evidence for this conclusion comes from experiments on patients who had one or more foci of unusually high sensitivity and areas of allodynic and hyperalgesic skin that were spatially remote from these small foci (Gracely et al. 1992). Local anesthesia of these small foci eliminated the ongoing pain and abolished the allodynia and hyperalgesia in areas of skin spatially remote from the local injections of anesthetics. A similar reversal occurs with sympathetic blocks in some CRPS patients (Price et al. 1989, 1998). This principle applies to other pain conditions as well. For example, rectal administration of lidocaine gel not only normalizes rectal hyperalgesia in patients with irritable bowel syndrome but also resolves cutaneous heat hyperalgesia in their lower extremities (Verne et al. 2003).

USING SENSORY TESTS TO MATCH
TREATMENTS TO MECHANISMS

Sensory tests may offer a strategy of matching treatments to mechanisms. For example, temporal summation of Aβ allodynia may be mediated by NMDA-receptor mechanisms. If this is the case, and if this type of allodynia is present in some but not all CRPS patients (37% in the study described above), then a clinical trial of a NMDA-receptor blocker might detect a clinical benefit only if patients have been carefully examined for the presence of this particular sensory abnormality. In another example, evoked pains that radiate (i.e., shooting pain) may be particularly responsive to treatment with anticonvulsants. Sensory tests may also be used in combination with local anesthetic blocks to identify peripheral sources of tonic impulse input that sustain neuropathic and other types of pain conditions. An obvious example is that of using lidocaine patches to treat postherpetic neuralgia. This same principle may be used to treat irritable bowel syndrome (Verne et al. 2003).

APPLICATION OF PSYCHOPHYSICAL METHODS IN ANIMAL MODELS OF PATHOLOGICAL PAIN

Studies of neuropathic pain patients provide an understanding of the general physiological factors involved in various persistent pain conditions, such as temporal summation and the role of tonic afferent input. However, knowledge of detailed peripheral and central neural mechanisms of persistent pain conditions also requires physiological and neurochemical approaches that can only be used in animal models of persistent pain conditions. An optimum approach is to combine physiological measurements or manipulations with psychophysical tests in animals that evaluate the same mechanisms elaborated above for human subjects. Many of the same stimulus paradigms and features described above can be utilized in laboratory animal experiments, and psychophysical ratings of humans can help evaluate the clinical relevance of results from animal experiments. Although simple withdrawal tests (e.g., the tail-flick test or the Hargreaves test) have dominated the field of animal studies of pain, including pathological pain, we think there are good reasons for a shift in emphasis to operant-escape paradigms, as discussed in the chapter on animal studies of pain by Vierck in this volume. For example, operant escape paradigms permit evaluation of responses to a greater spectrum of nociceptive stimulus conditions than do reflex tests, and stimulus-response functions from escape are more commensurate with those obtained from humans, using the same stimulus conditions (Vierck et al. 2004).

CONCLUSIONS

Psychophysical tests that are of considerable relevance to pathophysiological mechanisms of pain include direct ratings of threshold and suprathreshold controlled stimuli, particularly those that exaggerate or abnormally trigger the same mechanisms observed for normal pain processing.

Relevant examples include tests of pain from low or slowly rising nociceptive temperatures that preferentially produce tonic activity in C nociceptors, tests of temporal summation of pain from phasic stimuli that activate C-nociceptive afferent neurons, and tests of mechanical allodynia. Pathological expressions of pain mechanisms can be identified in individual patients through the use of these standardized sensory tests. The test results have important implications for treating various types of pathological pain. The same tests can be modeled to some extent in animal operant-escape paradigms, thereby increasing their relevance to human pain conditions. Psychophysical characterization of pathological pain mechanisms is useful in aiding diagnoses, in understanding mechanisms of pain diseases or syndromes, and ultimately in matching treatments to mechanisms.

REFERENCES

Arendt-Nielson L, Graven-Nielsen T, Svennson P, Jensen TS. Temporal summation in muscles and referred pain areas: an experimental human study. *Muscle Nerve* 1997; 10:1311–1313.

Byas-Smith MG, Max MB, Gracely RH, Bennett GJ. Intravenous ketamine and alfentanil in patients with chronic causalgic pain and allodynia. *Abstracts: 7th World Congress on Pain.* Seattle: IASP Press, 1993, p 454.

Campbell JN, Raja SN, Meyer RA. Painful sequelae of nerve injury. In: Dubner R, Gebhart GF, Bond MR (Eds). *Proceedings of The Vth World Congress on Pain,* Pain Research and Clinical Management, Vol. 3. New York: Elsevier, 1988, pp 135–143.

Coghill RC, McHaffie JG, Yen YF. Neural correlates of interindividual differences in the subjective experience of pain. *Proc Natl Acad Sci USA* 2003; 100:8538–8542.

Collins WF, Nulsen FE, Randt CT. Relation of peripheral nerve fiber size and sensation in man. *Arch Neurol (Chic)* 1960; 3:381–385.

Dubner R, Sharav Y, Gracely RH, Price DD. Idiopathic trigeminal neuralgia: sensory features and pain mechanisms. *Pain* 1987; 31:23–33.

Dworkin RH, Turk DC, Farrar JT, et al. Core outcome measures for chronic pain clinical trials: IMMPACT recommendations. *Pain* 2005; 113:1–2.

Eide PK, Jorum E, Stubhaug A, Bremnes J, Breivik H. Relief of post-herpetic neuralgia with the *N*-methyl-D-aspartate acid receptor antagonist ketamine: a double blind, crossover comparison with morphine and placebo. *Pain* 1994; 58:347–355.

Fuchs PN, Campbell JN, Meyer RA. Secondary hyperalgesia persists in capsaicin desensitized skin. *Pain* 2000; 84:141–149.

Gracely RH, Dubner R. Pain assessment in humans: a reply to Hall. *Pain* 1981; 11:109–120.

Gracely RH, Lynch SA, Bennett GJ. Painful neuropathy: altered central processing maintained dynamically by peripheral input. *Pain* 1992; 51:175–194.

Jensen MP, Karoly P. Self-report scales and procedures for assessing pain in adults. In: Turk DC, Melzack R (Eds). *Handbook of Pain Assessment.* New York: Guilford Press, 2001, pp 135–151.

Li J, Simone DA, Larson AA. Windup leads to characteristics of central sensitization. *Pain* 1999; 79(1):75–82.

Maixner W, Fillingim R, Sigurdsson A, Kincais S, Silva S. Sensitivity of patients with painful temporomandibular disorders to experimentally evoked pain: evidence for altered temporal summation of pain. *Pain* 1998; 76(1–2):71–81.

Magerl W, Fuchs PN, Meyer RA, Treede RD. Roles of capsaicin-insensitive nociceptors in cutaneous pain and secondary hyperalgesia. *Brain* 2001; 124(pt 9):1754–1764.

Marks LW. *Sensory Processes: The New Psychophysics.* New York: Academic Press, 1974.

Mendell LM, Wall PD. Responses of single dorsal cord cells to peripheral cutaneous unmyelinated fibres. *Nature* 1965; 206:97–99.

Meyer RA, Campbell JN. Myelinated nociceptive afferents account for the hyperalgesia that follows a burn to the hand. *Science* 1981; 213:1527–1529.

Myles PS, Troedel S, Boquest M, Reeves M. The pain visual analog scale: is it linear or nonlinear? *Anesth Analg* 1999; 89(6):1517–1520.

Park KM, Max MB, Robinovitz E, Gracely RH, Bennett G J. Effects of intravenous ketamine and alfentanil on hyperalgesia induced by intradermal capsaicin, In: Gebhart GF, Hammond DL, Jensen TS (Eds.) *Proceedings of the 7th World Congress on Pain,* Progress in Pain Research and Management, Vol. 2. Seattle: IASP Press, 1994, pp 647–656.

Price DD. Characteristics of second pain and flexion reflexes indicative of prolonged central summation. *Exp Neurol* 1972; 37:371–391.

Price DD. *Psychological Mechanisms of Pain and Analgesia,* Progress in Pain Research and Management, Vol. 15. Seattle: IASP Press, 1999.

Price DD, Harkins SW. Combined use of experimental pain and visual analogue scales in providing standardized measurement of clinical pain. *Clin J Pain* 1987; 3:3–11.

Price DD, Hu JW, Dubner R, Gracely R. Peripheral suppression of first pain and central summation of second pain evoked by noxious heat pulses. *Pain* 1977; 3:57–68.

Price DD, McGrath PA, Rafii A, Buckingham B. The validation of visual analogue scales as ratio scale measures for chronic and experimental pain. *Pain* 1983; 17:45–56.

Price DD, Von der Gruen A, Miller J, Rafii A, Price C. A psychophysical analysis of morphine analgesia. *Pain* 1985; 22:261–269.

Price DD, Harkins SW, Baker C. Sensory affective relationships among different types of clinical and experimental pain. *Pain* 1987; 28(3):291–299.

Price DD, Bennett GJ, Rafii A. Psychophysical observations on patients with neuropathic pain relieved by a sympathetic block. *Pain* 1989; 36:209–218.

Price DD, Long S, Huitt C. Sensory testing of pathophysiological mechanisms of pain in patients with reflex sympathetic dystrophy. *Pain* 1992; 49:163–173.

Price DD, Bush FM, Long S, Harkins SW. A comparison of pain measurement characteristics of mechanical visual analogue and simple numerical rating scales. *Pain* 1994a; 56:217–226.

Price DD, Mao J, Frenk H, Mayer DJ. The *N*-methyl-D-aspartate receptor antagonist dextromethorphan selectively reduces temporal summation of second pain in man. *Pain* 1994b; 59:165–174.

Price DD, Mao J, Mayer DJ. Central neural mechanisms of normal and abnormal pain states. In: Fields HL, Liebeskind JC (Eds). *Pharmacological Approaches to the Treatment of Chronic Pain: New Concepts and Critical Issues,* Progress in Pain Research and Management, Vol. 1. Seattle: IASP Press, 1994c, pp 61–84.

Price DD, Long S, Wilsey B, Rafii A. Analysis of peak magnitude and duration of analgesia produced by local anesthetics injected into sympathetic ganglia of complex regional pain syndrome patients. *Clin J Pain* 1998; 14(3):216–226.

Price DD, Staud R, Robinson ME, et al. Enhanced temporal summation of second pain and its central modulation in fibromyalgia patients. *Pain* 2002; 99(1–2):49–60.

Rosier EM, Iadarola MJ, Coghill RC. Reproducibility of pain measurement and pain perception. *Pain* 2002; 98(1–2):205–216.

Staud R, Vierck CJ, Cannon RL, Mauderli AP, Price DD. Abnormal sensitization and temporal summation of second pain (wind-up) in patients with fibromyalgia syndrome. *Pain* 2001; 91:165–175.

Staud R, Robinson ME, Vierck CJ Jr, et al. Ratings of experimental pain and pain-related negative affect predict clinical pain in patients with fibromyalgia syndrome. *Pain* 2003; 105(1–2):215–222.

Staud R, Price DD, Robinson ME, Mauderli AP, Vierck CJ. Maintenance of windup of second pain requires less frequent stimulation in fibromyalgia patients compared to normal controls. *Pain* 2004; 110(3):689–696.

Staud RM, Robinson ME, Vierck CJ, Price DD. The N-methyl-d-aspartate receptor antagonist dextromethorphan attenuates second pain summation in fibromyalgia patients and normal control subjects. *J Pain* 2005; 6(5):323–332.

Verne GN, Robinson ME, Vase L, Price DD. Reversal of visceral and cutaneous hyperalgesia by local rectal anesthesia in irritable bowel syndrome patients. *Pain* 2003; 105(1–2):223–230.

Vierck CJ, Cannon RL, Fry G, Maixner W, Whitsel BL. Characteristics of temporal summation of second pain sensations elicited by brief contact of glabrous skin by a pre-heated thermode. *J Neurophysiol* 1997; 78(2):992–1002.

Vierck CJ, Staud R, Price DD, et al. The effect of maximal exercise on temporal summation of second pain (wind-up) in patients with fibromyalgia syndrome. *J Pain* 2001; 2(6):334–344.

Vierck CJ Jr, Kline RL III, Wiley RG. Comparison of operant escape and innate reflex responses to nociceptive skin temperatures produced by heat and cold stimulation of rats. *Behav Neurosci* 2004; 118:627–635.

Wallenstein SL, Heidrich G III, Kaiko R, Houde RW. Clinical evaluation of mild analgesics: the measurement of clinical pain. *Br J Clin Pharm* 1980; 10:319S–327S.

Yeomans DC, Proudfit HK. Nociceptive responses to high and low rates of noxious cutaneous heating are mediated by different nociceptors in the rat: electrophysiological evidence. *Pain* 1996; 68:141–150.

Yeomans DC, Cooper BY, Vierck CJ Jr. Effects of systemic morphine on responses of primates to first or second pain sensation. *Pain* 1996a; 66:253–263.

Yeomans DC, Pirec V, Proudfit HK. Nociceptive responses to high and low rates of noxious cutaneous heating are mediated by different nociceptors in the rat: behavioral evidence. *Pain* 1996b; 86:141–150.

Correspondence to: Donald D. Price, PhD, Departments of Oral and Maxillofacial Surgery, University of Florida College of Dentistry, PO Box 100416, Gainesville, FL 326510, USA. Tel: 352-846-2718; Fax: 352-846-0588.

Emerging Strategies for the Treatment of Neuropathic Pain, edited by James N. Campbell, Allan I. Basbaum, André Dray, Ronald Dubner, Robert H. Dworkin, and Christine N. Sang, IASP Press, Seattle, © 2006.

22

Biomarkers in Pain

Laszlo Urban,[a] Istvan Nagy,[b,c] Katalin Lukacs,[c] and Peter Santha[d]

[a]Preclinical Compound Profiling, Lead Discovery Center, Discovery Technologies, Novartis Institutes for BioMedical Research, Inc., Cambridge, Massachusetts, USA; [b]Department of Anaesthesiology and Intensive Care, Imperial College London, London, United Kingdom; [c]School of Medicine, Chelsea and Westminster Hospital, London, United Kingdom; [d]Department of Physiology, University of Szeged, Szeged, Hungary

Biomarkers are specific biochemicals in the body with a well-defined molecular feature that makes them useful for diagnosing a disease, measuring the progress of a disease, or determining the effects of a treatment. They have revolutionized the diagnosis of cancer and have become essential in the development of new medications, particularly in the area of cardiovascular, metabolic, and hormonal diseases. The correct use of biomarkers basically depends on a single principle—close association of a molecule, or a pattern of expression of several molecules, with a disease. This association can relate simply to the presence of a disease or to its pathophysiological mechanism, severity, or time course, and sometimes to the progress and outcome of treatment.

Approaches to using biomarkers vary from the definition of protein expression patterns by using chip technology to the detection and behavior of single disease-associated molecules, obtained by either invasive or non-invasive technologies. The chosen molecule can be any biologically active molecule that acts as a diagnostic or prognostic indicator through its alteration in abundance, structure, or function as linked with defined pathology. Most biomarkers are obtained from blood and urine samples, smears, and cerebrospinal fluid (CSF) samples, but advanced technologies require only a tiny amount of almost any tissue from a biopsy.

Novel detection and information technologies applied in biomarker research are providing unprecedented insight into disease mechanisms and hold the promise of revolutionizing medical diagnosis and treatment. The biomarker field is expanding rapidly from experimental status into medical applications. Patterns of protein expression used for diagnostic purposes can reveal subclasses of pathophysiological mechanisms, highlight gene polymorphisms, and bring greater precision to therapeutic decision making. Clinical trials can benefit from the use of biomarkers because analysis of molecular patterns in large-scale trials can help to define the disease under investigation, identify subpopulations of patients, and determine the best use of novel medications.

PROTEOMIC PATTERNS AND THEIR POTENTIAL FOR DISEASE DIAGNOSIS, PROGNOSIS, AND THERAPY

Combined advances in separation technologies and in biomolecular mass spectrometry have opened new avenues for the use of biomarkers. Surface-enhanced laser desorption ionization associated with time-of-flight mass spectrometry (SELDI-TOF-MS) is a novel, state-of-the-art technology that is increasingly being used to diagnose disease and to assess the effectiveness of therapies (for a detailed review, see Merchant and Weinberger 2000). This approach can detect differentially captured proteins from clinical samples and thus provide fine patterns of protein expression (for review, see Bischoff and Luider 2004; Xiao et al. 2004). In addition to the increased sensitivity of new mass spectrometry technologies, another essential advance has been the parallel development of sample preparation and purification steps, the revolutionary use of protein chip arrays, and the application of a variety of statistical methods and bioinformatics software (Fung and Enderwick 2002; Reddy and Dalmasso 2003). The SELDI protein chip platform incorporates a complex technology that can identify and characterize proteins associated with diseases (see Li et al. 2002). In essence, it provides high-throughput analysis of the fine pattern of protein expression in biological samples (Fig. 1).

The main advantage of this technology is that it automates the tedious job of purification and separation of proteins, and more importantly, it does not require prior knowledge of the specific protein (or for that matter any specific molecule). The use of various chips also allows investigators to profile protein expression as modified by disease or therapy. SELDI-TOF-MS, which requires an extremely small quantity of virtually any tissue, can identify and compare hundreds of thousands of proteins in just a microliter sample of blood, urine, cell lysates, cellular secretion products, tissue biopsy,

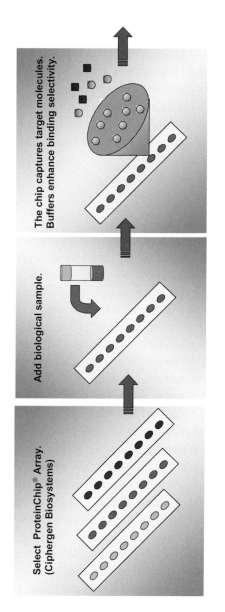

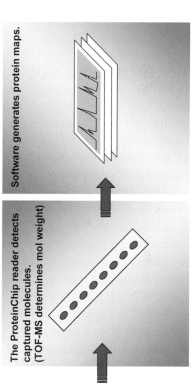

Select ProteinChip® Array.
(Ciphergen Biosystems)

Add biological sample.

The chip captures target molecules.
Buffers enhance binding selectivity.

The ProteinChip reader detects
captured molecules.
(TOF-MS determines mol weight)

Software generates protein maps.

Fig. 1. Simple diagram of the SELDI-TOF-MS protocol using chip technology.

CSF, or lymph. Although it has rarely been used for the diagnosis of pain syndromes, it has found widespread use in the diagnosis of ovarian, prostate, and breast cancer (Adam et al. 2002; for reviews, see Wulfkuhle et al. 2003; Conrads et al. 2004).

However, the broad use of this technology is limited by its high sensitivity for detection of any change in protein expression associated with pathophysiological mechanisms unrelated to the disease of interest—for example, a combination of a common cold, local inflammation, and bacterial infections can significantly modify the expression pattern of the targeted disease. Also, commonly used biomarkers might be relevant to several different diseases, thus diminishing their diagnostic value.

USE OF BIOMARKERS FOR PAIN STUDIES

Although the literature is extensive on the use of biomarkers in the clinic, relatively little information has been published on their use in association with pain diagnosis and medication. Pain is usually treated as a symptom associated with major disease groups such as osteoarthritis, rheumatoid arthritis, diabetes, or cancer. In the case of arthritis, although biomarkers are available that can fairly successfully predict the state and prognosis of the disease, pain is not necessarily closely associated with the progress of the disease. The level of available biomarkers that relate to the progress of tissue damage may not measure the extent of pain.

Neuropathies associated with damage to peripheral nerves, such as some types of low back pain, constitute another area in which biomarkers have been identified, largely in animal models. The application of these biomarkers has been limited because CSF samples are required. Neuropathic low back pain and other peripheral neuropathies are mostly diagnosed based on anamnesis and physical examination, without the use of biomarkers. Diagnosis and prescription of analgesic medications are based, to great extent, on subjective feedback from the patient, with a strong influence from environmental, social, and psychological factors. Assessments may include testing of stimulus-evoked pain and verbal or visual analogue scales designed to measure spontaneus or movement-related pain. Quality-of-life assessment is also influenced by the level of pain and the effectiveness of pain therapy. However, these assessment methods are generally less precise than biomarker techniques. Because of the considerable subjectivity involved, most pain trials must deal with a sizeable placebo effect. In multicenter, international trials, the social, cultural, and linguistic diversity among patients and staff contribute further to the subjective component of pain studies.

However, some promising clinical efforts have begun to investigate the use of biomarkers in chronic diseases associated with a prominent pain component, such as malignant bone pain, osteoarthritis, rheumatoid arthritis, diabetic neuropathy, and postherpetic neuralgia. Good progress has been made in the field of chest pain associated with acute myocardial infarction and in gynecological pain associated with extrauterine pregnancy. In these two latter cases, the presence of pain triggered studies to find biomarkers to define the prognosis or differential diagnosis of the disease and ultimately define the treatment regimen. The need to make a rapid and reliable diagnosis in these life-threatening conditions stimulated clinicians to demand effective biomarkers for use in emergency situations.

Efforts to introduce well-defined biomarkers for the objective measurement of pain will be greatly welcomed. Several preclinical mechanistic studies using animal models and clinical trials testing novel methodologies offer hope that specific biological markers exist for pain. Such biomarkers could revolutionize the study, diagnosis, and treatment of pain. They could also serve as a measure of stimulus-independent pain in animal models and could therefore be used to foster drug development.

BIOMARKERS IN EXPERIMENTAL PAIN RESEARCH

Several efforts have been made to validate the SELDI-TOF-MS method in animal models of inflammatory and neuropathic pain. Data obtained from models of inflammatory pain induced by complete Freund's adjuvant (CFA) and from models of neuropathic pain induced by chronic nerve constriction suggest that this method can differentiate between the two types of pain and provide information on the analgesic actions of anti-inflammatory agents such as cyclooxygenase-2 (COX-2) inhibitors (Gineste 2003). The protein expression profile in the CSF revealed that levels of two metal-binding proteins and three anionic proteins were selectively increased in the rat CFA model. The expression of the proteins matched the time course of the development of pain. Nimesulide, a selective COX-2 inhibitor, prevented the increase of protein expression in this model, and this finding correlated well with the antinociceptive effect of the drug.

In another study, Cornefjord and colleagues (2004) used CSF samples to determine whether protein expression was altered after experimental disk injury. Several biomarker candidates such as neurofilaments, the neuropeptide nociceptin, glial fibrillary acidic protein, neuron-specific enolase, S-100 protein, the cytokine interleukin-8 (IL-8), and substance P endopeptidase levels were examined in a pig model that mimics clinical disk herniation with associated pain behavior. The study found increases in neurofilament and nociceptin levels, but reported no changes for the other molecules.

The above efforts show that both inflammatory and neuropathic pain can be characterized with different biomarkers. Some of these markers, such as IL-8, have also been tested in human clinical pain conditions, but few comprehensive protein expression studies have been reported in the clinical setting.

BIOMARKERS IN RHEUMATOID ARTHRITIS

An array of biomarkers can be used to differentiate between rheumatoid arthritis and other inflammatory joint disorders. These molecules can predict the subtype and progression of the disease and may be used to monitor the effectiveness of therapies. Although our understanding of its pathophysiological mechanisms is far from complete, rheumatoid arthritis is considered to be an autoimmune inflammatory disease of the synovial membrane, which results in the degradation of the cartilage matrix and destruction of the arthritic bone. Thus, rheumatoid arthritis has various biomarkers that can be measured in the synovial fluid, plasma, mononuclear blood cells, and urine. These molecules include a series of antibodies, inflammatory mediators, enzymes, activating factors, and structural proteins (Visser et al. 2002; Marvin et al. 2003; Dotzlaw et al. 2004; Kantor et al. 2004; Liao et al. 2004). Although pain is a major symptom in rheumatoid arthritis, few studies have investigated the correlation between pain and levels of biomarkers.

A large proportion of patients with rheumatoid arthritis show elevated serum levels of immune complexes, such as rheumatoid factor and antibodies that recognize various filaggrin-related proteins. The anti-filaggrin-related antibodies include antiperinuclear factor and anticyclic citrullinated peptide, a molecule that binds to the synthetic human filaggrin derivative, cyclic citrullinated peptide (Ward 2003).

While no evidence exists for a correlation between rheumatoid factor levels and pain, an association has been found between pain and serum concentrations of perinuclear factor, an autoantibody detected in more than 50% of patients with rheumatoid arthritis (Munoz-Fernandez et al. 1999). A recent report indicates that the level of antibodies recognizing cyclic citrullinated peptide is also positively correlated with pain in the erosive, persistent form of rheumatoid arthritis (Visser at al. 2002). Since the expression of anticyclic citrullinated peptide antibodies is highly selective and specific in rheumatoid arthritis, its measurement is worth considering as a biomarker for the severity of pain.

In addition to selective biomarkers, nonselective ones are also often used to assess rheumatoid arthritis. For example, the level of C-reactive protein (CRP) increases in a variety of inflammatory diseases, including rheumatoid arthritis. This important acute-phase protein is commonly used as a serological marker in confirming the diagnosis and the effectiveness of treatments. Sarzi-Puttini et al. (2002) have recently found a correlation between pain and serum CRP levels in patients with rheumatoid arthritis. In addition, CRP proved to be a valuable marker in assessing the efficacy and safety of treatment with anakinra, a recombinant form of the naturally occurring IL-1 receptor antagonist, in combination with methotrexate, in reducing the signs and symptoms of rheumatoid arthritis. Clinically meaningful and statistically significant responses were seen with both CRP and pain (Cohen et al. 2004). However, other investigators have failed to reproduce such a correlation (Arvidson et al. 2002).

Vitamin B6 is also used as a nonspecific biomarker in various disorders, and its levels have been found to correlate with pain in rheumatoid arthritis. Chiang et al. (2003) reported that pyridoxal 5'-phosphate levels, which are indicative of vitamin B6 status, were inversely correlated with the degree of pain. Interestingly, low plasma levels of vitamin B6 seem to be associated with increased CRP levels (Friso et al. 2001). While CRP and vitamin B6 might be good biomarkers in rheumatoid arthritis, one should not forget their non-specificity. Thus, any concomitant infectious disease can influence results obtained with these biomarkers.

Another potential biomarker for rheumatoid arthritis may be CD57-positive T cells. Several lines of evidence suggest that in addition to killer cells, a subset of non-killer T lymphocytes also express the CD57 antigen, and that the number of these cells is higher than normal in the peripheral blood, knee joint fluid, knee synovial membrane, and bone marrow of rheumatoid arthritis patients (Loughran 1993; Arai et al. 1998). Maeda et al. (2002) have reported recently a positive correlation between the number of CD57-positive T cells in the peripheral blood and visual analogue pain scores in rheumatoid arthritis sufferers. However, CD57 is not a selective marker for rheumatoid arthritis because the number of CD57-positive cells also increases in other disorders (Rose and Berliner 2004).

Inflammatory markers, such as the cytokine interleukin-6 (IL-6), tumor necrosis factor alpha (TNF-α), and CRP are also used as biomarkers, particularly in rheumatoid arthritis, but their specificity is highly debated because other inflammatory diseases can mask the diagnostic or prognostic value of the data obtained. In addition, there is no evidence that levels of these markers correlate well with pain scores.

BIOMARKERS IN OSTEOARTHRITIS

Because the etiology of osteoarthritis is far from clear and the progress of the disease is difficult to predict (it is often episodic and erratic), many teams are attempting to determine biomarkers that would shed light on the pathophysiological mechanisms of this disease, provide a reliable prognosis, and be useful in monitoring the effects of treatment. The major changes are associated with the cartilage, the synovium, and the subarthritic bone, and so successful markers would be likely to reflect changes in bone or cartilage tissue (Garnero and Delmas 2003).

Although all clinical trials of osteoarthritis measure pain among other symptoms, a correlation between pain and serum or urine biomarkers has not been satisfactorily studied. Thus, biomarkers described in this chapter are more closely linked to cartilage, synovial, and bone pathology and only correlate to a certain extent with associated pain.

Bruyere et al. (2003) describe these correlations in a well-designed 3-year study in patients with knee osteoarthritis. The investigators compared data from an extensive list of biomarkers to the pain, stiffness, and physical function subscales of the Western Ontario and McMaster Universities Osteoarthritis (WOMAC) index at baseline and after 1 year. In addition, mean and minimal joint space width of the femorotibial joint was measured after 3 years. The aim was to investigate the relationship between the biomarkers and bone and cartilage remodeling and progression of the disease. Biomarkers under investigation were serum keratan sulfate, serum hyaluronic acid, urine

Table I
Biomarkers for osteoarthritis degradation products

Bone	Cartilage	Synovium
Pyridinoline	Pyridinoline	Pyridinoline, CTX-I, NTX-I
Deoxypyridinoline, collagen telopeptides (CTX-I, NTX-I, ICTP)	CTX-II, collagen α-chain fragments: COL2-3/4 (long) and COL2-3/4C (short)	Glucosyl galactosyl pyridinoline
Bone sialoprotein	Core protein fragments, keratan sulfate (epitopes 5D4, ANP9[1])	
Tartrate-resistant acid phosphatase (5b isoenzyme)	Cartilage oligomeric matrix protein	

Source: Modified from Garnero et al. (2003).
Abbreviations: CTX-I = carboxy-terminal crosslinking telopeptide of type I collagen; CTX-II = carboxy-terminal cross-linking telopeptide of type II collagen; ICTP = pyridinoline cross-linking carboxy-terminal telopeptide of type I collagen; NTX-I = N-terminal cross-linking telopeptide of type I collagen.

pyridinoline, urine deoxypyridinoline, serum osteocalcin, and cartilage oligomeric matrix protein. At baseline, no correlation was observed between any of the measured parameters. However, the 3-year radiological progression of knee osteoarthritis was correlated with a 1-year increase in osteocalcin and a 1-year decrease in hyaluronic acid levels. Unfortunately, although the study found a correlation between biomarker scores and physical measurement of disease progression (narrowing of joint space, ankylotic processes), it did not find a correlation with pain scores.

In an other large-scale study involving 1235 subjects over 6 years, Reijman et al. (2004) found a strong association between concentrations of C-terminal crosslinking telopeptide of type II collagen (CTX-II, a marker of collagen degradation) and the prevalence and progression of radiographic osteoarthritis of the knee and hip. This study clearly showed that the observed association was stronger in patients with joint pain.

Some studies question the predictive value of broadly used biomarkers. Schmidt-Rohlfing et al. (2002) used pyridinoline, deoxypyridinoline, N-telopeptide, carboxyterminal propeptide of type I collagen, matrix metalloproteinases 1 and 3, and a tissue inhibitor of matrix metalloproteinases to detect and monitor the progression of osteoarthritis. For the majority of markers, the study found a very low correlation with different phases of the disease.

Based on the outcome of numerous clinical studies, biomarkers yield the best predictive value for diagnosis and progression of osteoarthritis when used in cohorts and compared with complex clinical scores. When single markers such as cartilage oligomeric matrix protein are used, the substantial between-subjects variation could strongly influence the correlation (Sharif et al. 2004). The episodic and erratic nature of the disease further complicates matters.

BIOMARKERS IN NEUROPATHIC PAIN SYNDROMES

Neuropathic pain is associated with various major diseases such as diabetes, herpes zoster, and peripheral nerve injury. Thus, it is difficult to find a unifying platform of biomarkers that relate to neuropathic pain. In fact, studies of biomarkers associated with diabetic neuropathic pain and low back pain are rare.

A human study (Brisby et al. 2002) examined the concentration of IL-1β, IL-6, IL-8, interferon-gamma (IFN-γ), and TNF-α in the CSF and plasma of patients with diagnosed herniated intervertebral disks. This study is particularly informative from the point of view as to whether pain can be objectively monitored by biomarkers, because the biochemical laboratory results were directly matched with pain measurements. Only the concentration of IL-8 was increased, in about one-third of the patients, and this increase correlated with a brief duration of pain and more pronounced herniation. However, there was no correlation between pain intensity and IL-6 concentration. Unfortunately, there are no data on the effects of any analgesic treatment on the level of IL-8 in disk herniation.

Some studies were based on the observation that serum levels of keratan sulfate are strongly associated with massive and rapid degradation of intervertebral disks (Kuiper et al. 1998). Analysis of several human studies suggests that keratan sulfate could be used as a biomarker for disk hernia, at least at the acute phase.

Postherpetic neuralgia (PHN) is the most severe consequence of shingles. At present, we do not know how and in which patients PHN develops. Two recent studies addressed this question. The first study examined serum levels of T-helper (Th) 1 and 2 cytokines, IFN-γ, IL-6, and IL-8 in 30 zoster patients (Zak-Prelich et al. 2003). No significant change was found for any of these markers in comparison to controls. Antibody titers to varicella zoster virus were high in the patient group, but did not differ between patients who developed PHN and those who did not. Thus, the conventional use of several molecules associated with inflammation did not prove to be a good biomarker. However, a second study (Kotani et al. 2004) examined whether increased levels of IL-8 in the CSF during the full crusting of herpetic rash can identify patients who are likely to develop PHN. The study, which took age and acute pain into account, concluded that IL-8 content in the CSF, when measured at the right time, is a good predictor of the development of PHN.

Comparison of the two studies above suggests that the suitability of a given substance as a biomarker depends, at least in this case, on the timing of measurement. The importance of the right timing further highlights the difficulties of biomarker use in pain syndromes.

BIOMARKERS AND CHEST PAIN

The significant overlap of symptoms, including chest pain, in acute coronary syndromes and pulmonary embolism hampers accurate diagnosis in this "mixed" patient population. As in many other diseases, one of the patients' major complaints is pain, which presents as the earliest symptom. As chest pain signals potentially life-threatening conditions, it is imperative to make fast decisions as to appropriate treatment. Thus, pain is used for initial diagnosis. Subsequent identification of biomarkers could accelerate or optimize differential diagnosis (see reviews, see Gibler et al. 2003; Jesse et al. 2004).

Imaging technologies such as ventilation/perfusion scan, echocardiography, pulmonary arteriography, magnetic resonance imaging, and coronary arteriography constitute differential diagnostic tools. In addition, recently identified biomarkers such as d-dimers, troponins, and natriuretic peptides can further refine the diagnosis or can be used in the absence of expensive diagnostic equipment (Rahimtoola and Bergin 2005).

The existing literature on various biomarkers is extensive, with information on well-established methods, but many of the recommendations are based on only a few studies or on a single study and need validation with larger patient populations before they can be broadly accepted as diagnostic tools. Below, we discuss the use of established biomarkers in the emergency room and highlight a couple of studies with promising results.

Creatine kinase myocardial band, cardiac troponin T, troponin I, myoglobin, and β-type natriuretic peptide (for congestive heart failure) are established biomarkers for the rapid diagnosis of acute myocardial infarction in patients with chest pain (Gibler et al. 2003; Jesse et al. 2004; Wu et al. 2004). Troponin is the gold standard biomarker for the diagnosis and prognosis of acute myocardial infarction. The value of these markers often depends on the turnaround time of the assay. Accuracy thus depend on logistics and on the rapidity of the laboratory test. These markers do not correlate well with pain sensation, but rather they relate to myocardial damage and identify cases of acute myocardial infarction among patients with acute chest pain.

In addition to the above-mentioned biomarkers, ischemia-modified albumin may be a reliable biomarker for the identification of acute coronary syndrome in patients with typical acute chest pain (Roy et al. 2004). Interestingly, CRP was also considered to be a good biomarker for acute coronary syndrome; however, this marker is present in many diseases that have an inflammatory component (see the sections above on osteoarthritis and rheumatoid arthritis). Thus, it is questionable whether CRP is really a marker for acute coronary syndrome or simply a risk factor.

BIOMARKERS AND BONE CANCER PAIN

Biomarkers that take advantage of serum proteomics methods are being successfully used in cancer research, particularly for diagnosis. However, some shortcomings of the SELDI-TOF-MS technology were highlighted in some recent reviews (Rocken et al. 2004; Rosenblatt et al. 2004). The sensitivity of the proteomic approach, comorbidities such as influenza, dietary changes, or episodic drug use (e.g., a single dose of analgesic) can complicate the interpretation of study results (Rocken et al. 2004; Rosenblatt et al. 2004).

This section focuses on metastasis of cancer to bone. One of the major symptoms of bone metastasis is pain, which is different in its characteristics from neuropathic or inflammatory pain. This pain is very difficult to manage, and evidence from animal models suggests that the underlying mechanisms differ from those of other types of chronic pain (Mantyh 2004).

Bone metastases are a common cause of morbidity in patients with prostate, ovarian, or breast cancer. Palliative treatments such as bisphosphonates, particularly zoledronic acid, have been developed to alleviate pain and reduce the number of metastases. A randomized, placebo-controlled clinical trial of zoledronic acid for hormone-refractory prostate cancer assessed pain scores, skeletal-related events, and drug safety (Saad et al. 2002). Levels of prostate-specific antigen (PSA), serum bone alkaline phosphatase, and testosterone and parathyroid hormones were monitored from blood samples, while N-telopeptide, pyridinoline, deoxypyridinoline, and creatinine were measured from urine samples to monitor bone resorption activity. A bone survey was made with various imaging approaches. Quality-of-life parameters were also measured, of which pain was the primary efficacy variable. Analgesic scores were taken during the course of treatment. The pain score, as assessed on the Brief Pain Inventory, was a composite of four items (worst pain, least pain, average pain during the last 7 days, and present pain). This trial involved 634 patients. Zoledronic acid did not have any effect on the secretion, clearance, and measurement of PSA, nor on overall tumor progression or survival. This outcome was expected because treatment addressed metastatic bone disease, rather than the prostate cancer itself. However, further studies evaluating the effects of treatment with an earlier starting point are needed to reveal any disease-modifying effect. However, the significantly increased median time to skeletal-related events and significant changes in serum and urine markers of bone metabolism indicated a positive effect on bone conditions in the 4-mg treatment group in comparison to the placebo group. In parallel, a "modest but consistent" effect on pain was measured, which reached significance by the end of the trial. Although earlier trials for bisphosphonates measured pain scores, this is the first time that analgesic effect was reported in a randomized, controlled trial.

Based on the success of the original trial for prostate cancer, further trials were conducted with a similar regimen expanded to breast cancer and multiple myeloma (Vogel et al. 2004). The main aim of this trial was to prove the safety of zoledronic acid and address nephrotoxicity concerns. The therapeutic regimen was the same as for the study described above. Again, in addition to blood and urine samples for biochemical measurements, pain and quality-of-life assessments were used. Pain scores decreased within the range of acceptable serum creatinine levels. Although these trials used biomarkers extensively, no direct correlation between pain scores and other descriptors were established in clinical cases. However, other evidence shows a close correlation between skeletal remodeling and pain during bisphosphonate treatment (Walker et al. 2002; Sevcik et al. 2004). Unfortunately, while alendronate treatment had positive effects on bone remodeling and pain scores, it did not diminish the tumor burden; in fact, both tumor growth and tumor necrosis increased (Sevcik et al. 2004).

Interestingly, Tiffany et al. (2004) used a combination of imatinib and zoledronic acid for the treatment of androgen-independent prostate cancer, but the results were negative. The Present Pain Intensity Scale was used to measure pain. Prostate-specific antigen response and decrease of bone turnover were monitored in parallel. This study was not able to detect any palliative effect, and PSA responses were unchanged. Urine N-telopeptides were reduced, and there was a trend toward reduction of serum osteocalcin. No change was measured in bone-specific alkaline phosphatase. However, the trial was abandoned early because of lack of clinical activity.

The above examples demonstrate that the complex nature of metastatic cancer pain complicates trial design and sometimes makes the interpretation of the outcome controversial. However, increasing evidence from clinical case studies and from more focused trials indicates that bisphosphonates, in addition to their effects on biomarkers associated with bone metabolism, do produce pain relief. So far, no proteomics approaches have been applied to this disease. As knowledge is limited about the mechanisms of bone cancer pain, the use of SELDI-TOF might reveal more relevant biomarkers that could provide a tighter correlation with pain.

BIOMARKERS AND GYNECOLOGICAL PAIN

Pain and bleeding during the first trimester of pregnancy are the major symptoms of ectopic pregnancy. The rapid growth of the fetus can lead to life-threatening consequences for the mother. Early detection of ectopic pregnancy is not reliable using imaging technologies, and no serum test can provide an early warning. Symptoms such as bleeding and pain associated with the condition could, in fact, be a late warning. A new approach using

SELDI-TOF-MS is currently being applied to this problem (Gerton et al. 2004). The trial is based on the assumption that women presenting with pain or bleeding during the first trimester of pregnancy may have an ectopic pregnancy. Serum markers from patients indicate that a reliable test can be produced to enable the clinical differentiation between women in need of immediate intervention for ectopic pregnancy, women with normal pregnancy, and women who require further monitoring.

Although the data are controversial, it is worth mentioning that cystatin C, a secreted cysteine protease inhibitor that is induced in the spinal dorsal horn by inflammation, might be a good biomarker for labor pain (Mannes et al. 2003). CSF samples from 10 patients with or without pain were examined by immunoassay and SELDI-TOF-MS. The study found that cystatin C levels were elevated in the CSF of patients with pain in comparison to those without pain. However, a subsequent extended trial in 131 subjects involving labor pain and chronic neuropathic pain could not confirm the results of the earlier study (Eisenach et al. 2004). Cystatin C was increased in pregnant women with or without pain in comparison to normal volunteers. No increase was measured in the neuropathic pain group. Furthermore, an independent study identified cystatin C as a biomarker of Creutzfeldt-Jakob disease (Sanchez et al. 2004). Thus, cystatin C seems to be an unreliable diagnostic marker for pain in humans.

CONCLUDING REMARKS

Although the use of biomarkers is expanding rapidly, and novel technologies such as SELDI-TOF-MS are proving useful to clinicians and research scientists, applications in the field of pain are still rare. Pain is typically considered a symptom; it is very common and thus extremely nonspecific. The underlying mechanisms can vary greatly, and even within the context of the same disease, pain can have many mediators and substrates. These factors all help to explain why so many nonspecific biomarkers are used in diseases associated with severe pain (i.e., osteoarthritis and rheumatoid arthritis). Recent studies indicate that a set of biomarkers is more useful in most cases than a single one.

Because pain is often the most common symptom of a disease, many trials include it as a diagnostic marker to measure disease progress or the effect of therapies. In this context, although pain might not correlate well with changes in biomarker content, its measurement is a very important element of clinical evaluations.

The introduction of proteomics has established that patterns of biomarker expression are emerging during clinical trials (e.g., for cancer therapies). These patterns can be highly characteristic and have great diagnostic and prognostic potential. This approach has proven very successful in oncology. In pain studies, definitive biomarker patterns could provide a more objective measure of the "nociceptive" component of pain, as opposed to psychosocial contributions. Some of the studies discussed above have already introduced proteomics to create biomarkers. It is too early to judge the results of these pilot studies, but based on experience from other fields, we can be confident that clinical pain studies will increasingly turn to this powerful technology, produce novel and exciting insights into pain mechanisms, and promote better pain management.

REFERENCES

Adam BL, Qu Y, Davies JV, et al. Serum protein fingerprinting coupled with pattern-matching algorithm distinguishes prostate cancer from benign prostate hyperplasia and healthy men. *Cancer Res* 2002; 62:3609–3614.

Arai K, Yamamura S, Seki S, et al. Increase of CD57+ T cells in knee joints and adjacent bone marrow of rheumatoid arthritis (RA) patients: implication for an anti-inflammatory role. *Clin Exp Immunol* 1998; 111:345–352.

Arvidson NG, Larsson A, Larsen A. Simple function tests, but not the modified HAQ, correlate with radiological joint damage in rheumatoid arthritis. *Scand J Rheumatol* 2002; 31:146–150.

Bischoff R, Luider TM. Methodological advances in the discovery of protein and peptide disease markers. *J Chromatogr* 2004; 803:27–44.

Brisby H, Tao H, Ma DD, Diwan AD. Cell therapy for disc degeneration—potentials and pitfalls. *Orthop Clin* 2004; 35:85–93.

Bruyere O, Collette JH, Ethgen O, et al. Biochemical markers of bone and cartilage remodeling in prediction of long-term progression of knee osteoarthritis. *J Rheumatol* 2003; 30:1043–1050.

Chiang EP, Bagley PJ, Selhub J, Nadeau M, Roubenoff R. Abnormal vitamin B(6) status is associated with severity of symptoms in patients with rheumatoid arthritis. *Am J Med* 2003; 114:283–287.

Cohen SB, Moreland LW, Cush JJ, et al. A multicentre, double blind, randomised, placebo controlled trial of anakinra (Kineret), a recombinant interleukin 1 receptor antagonist, in patients with rheumatoid arthritis treated with background methotrexate. *Ann Rheum Dis* 2004; 63:1062–1068.

Conrads TP, Hood BL, Issaq HJ, Veenstra TD. Proteomic patterns as a diagnostic tool for early-stage cancer: a review of its progress to a clinically relevant tool. *Mol Diagn* 2004; 8:77–85.

Cornefjord M, Nyberg F, Rosengren L, Brisby H. Cerebrospinal fluid biomarkers in experimental spinal nerve root injury. *Spine* 2004; 29:1862–1868.

Dotzlaw H, Schulz M, Eggert M, Neeck G. A pattern of protein expression in peripheral blood mononuclear cells distinguishes rheumatoid arthritis patients from healthy individuals. *Biochim Biophys Acta* 2004; 1696:121–129.

Eisenach JC, Thomas JA, Rauck RL, Curry R, Li X. Cystatin C in cerebrospinal fluid is not a diagnostic test for pain in humans. *Pain* 2004; 107:207–212.

Friso S, Jacques PF, Wilson PW, Rosenberg IH, Selhub J. Low circulating vitamin B(6) is associated with elevation of the inflammation marker C-reactive protein independently of plasma homocysteine levels. *Circulation* 2001; 103:2788–2791.

Fung ET, Enderwick C. ProteinChip® clinical proteomics: computational challenges and solutions. *Biotechniques* 2002; 32(Suppl):34–41.

Garnero P, Delmas PD. Biomarkers in osteoarthritis. *Curr Opin Rheumatol* 2003; 15:641–646.

Gerton GL, Fan XJ, Chittams J, et al. A serum proteomics approach to the diagnosis of ectopic pregnancy. *Ann NY Acad Sci* 2004; 1022:306–316.

Gibler WB, Blomkalns AL, Collins SP. Evaluation of chest pain and heart failure in the emergency department: impact of multimarker strategies and B-type natriuretic peptide. *Rev Cardiovasc Med* 2003; (Suppl 4):S47–55.

Gineste C, Ho L, Pompl P, Bianchi M, Pasinetti GM. High-throughput proteomics and protein biomarker discovery in an experimental model of inflammatory hyperalgesia: effects of nimesulide. *Drugs* 2003; 63(Suppl 1):23–29.

Jesse RL, Kontos MC, Roberts CS. Diagnostic strategies for the evaluation of the patient presenting with chest pain. *Prog Cardiovasc Dis* 2004; 46:417–437.

Kantor AB, Wang W, Lin H, Govindarajan H, et al. Biomarker discovery by comprehensive phenotyping for autoimmune diseases. *Clin Immunol* 2004; 111:186–195.

Kotani N, Kudo R, Sakurai Y, et al. Cerebrospinal fluid interleukin 8 concentrations and the subsequent development of postherpetic neuralgia. *Am J Med* 2004; 116:318–324.

Kuiper JI, Verbeek JHAM, Frings-Dresen MHW, Ikkink AJK. Keratan sulfate as a potential biomarker of loading of the intervertebral disc. *Spine* 1998; 23:657–663.

Li J, Zhang Z, Rosenzweig J, Wang YY, Chan DW. Proteomics and bioinformatics approaches for identification of serum biomarkers to detect breast cancer. *Clin Chem* 2002; 1296–1304.

Liao H, Wu J, Kuhn E, et al. Use of mass spectrometry to identify protein biomarkers of disease severity in the synovial fluid and serum of patients with rheumatoid arthritis. *Arthritis Rheum* 2004; 50:3792–3803.

Loughran TP Jr. Clonal diseases of large granular lymphocytes. *Blood* 1993; 82:1–14.

Maeda T, Yamada H, Nagamine R, et al. Involvement of CD4+, CD57+ T cells in the disease activity of rheumatoid arthritis. *Arthritis Rheum* 2002; 46:379–384.

Mannes AJ, Martin BM, Yang HYT, et al. Cystatin C as a cerebrospinal fluid biomarker for pain in humans. *Pain* 2003; 102:251–256.

Mantyh PW. A mechanism-based understanding of bone cancer pain. *Novartis Found Symp* 2004; 261:194–214.

Marvin LF, Roberts MA, Fay LB. Matrix-assisted laser desorption/ionization time-of-flight mass spectrometry in clinical chemistry. *Clin Chim Acta* 2003; 337:11–21.

Merchant M, Weinberger SC. Recent advancements in surface-enhanced laser desorption/ ionization time of flight mass spectrometry. *Electrophoresis* 2000; 21:1164–1167.

Munoz-Fernandez S, Alvarez-Doforno R, Gonzalez-Tarrio JM, et al. Antiperinuclear factor as a prognostic marker in rheumatoid arthritis. *J Rheumatol* 1999; 26:2572–2577.

Rahimtoola A, Bergin JD. Acute pulmonary embolism: an update on diagnosis and management. *Curr Probl Cardiol* 2005; 30:61–114.

Reddy G, Dalmasso EA. SELDI ProteinChip® Array Technology: protein-base predictive medicine and drug discovery applications. *J Biomed Biotechnol* 2003; 4:237–241.

Reijman M, Hazes JM, Bierma-Zeinstra SM, et al. A new marker for osteoarthritis: cross-sectional and longitudinal approach. *Arthritis Rheum* 2004; 50:2471–2478.

Rocken C, Ebert MPA, Roessner A. Proteomics in pathology, research and practice. *Pathol Res Practice* 2004; 200: 69–82.

Rose MG, Berliner N. T-cell large granular lymphocyte leukemia and related disorders. *Oncologist* 2004; 9:247–258.

Rosenblatt KP, Bryant-Greenwood P, Killian JK, et al. Serum proteomics in cancer diagnosis and management. *Ann Rev Med* 2004; 55:97–112.

Roy D, Quiles J, Aldama G, et al. Ischemia modified albumin for the assessment of patients presenting to the emergency department with acute chest pain but normal or non-diagnostic 12-lead electrocardiograms and negative cardiac troponin T. *Int J Cardiol* 2004; 97:297–301.

Saad F, Gleason DM, Murray R, et al. A randomized, placebo-controlled trial of zoledronic acid in patients with hormone-refractory metastatic prostate carcinoma. *Natl Cancer Inst* 2002; 94:1458–1468.

Sanchez JC, Guillaume E, Lescuyer P, et al. Cystatin C as a potential cerebrospinal fluid marker for the diagnosis of Creutzfeldt-Jakob disease. *Proteomics* 2004; 4:2229–2233.

Sarzi-Puttini P, Fiorini T, Panni B, et al. Correlation of the score for subjective pain with physical disability, clinical and radiographic scores in recent onset rheumatoid arthritis. *BMC Musculoskelet Disord* 2002; 19:18.

Schmidt-Rohlfing B, Thomsen M, Niedhart C, Wirtz DC, Schneider U. Correlation of bone and cartilage markers in the synovial fluid with the degree of osteoarthritis. *Rheumatol Int* 2002; 21:193–199.

Sevcik MA, Luger NM, Mach DB, et al. Bone cancer pain: the effects of the bisphosphonate alendronate on pain, skeletal remodeling, tumor growth and tumor necrosis. *Pain* 2004; 111:169–180.

Sharif M, Kirwan JR, Elson CJ, Granell R, Clarke S. Suggestion of nonlinear or phasic progression of knee osteoarthritis based on measurements of serum cartilage oligomeric matrix protein levels over five years. *Arthritis Rheum* 2004; 50:2479–2488.

Tiffany NM, Wersinger EM, Garzotto M, Beer TM. Imatinib mesylate and zoledronic acid in androgen-independent prostate cancer. *Urology* 2004; 63:934–939.

Visser H, le Cessie S, Vos K, Breedveld FC, Hazes JM. How to diagnose rheumatoid arthritis early: a prediction model for persistent (erosive) arthritis. *Arthritis Rheum* 2002; 46:357–365.

Vogel CL, Yanagihara RH, Wood AJ, et al. Safety and pain palliation of zoledronic acid in patients with breast cancer, prostate cancer, or multiple myeloma who previously received bisphosphonate therapy. *Oncologist* 2004; 9:687–695.

Walker K, Medhurst S, Kidd BL, et al. Disease modifying and antinociceptive effects of the bisphosphonate, zoledronic acid in a novel rat model of bone cancer pain. *Pain* 2002; 304:219–229.

Ward MM. Clinical epidemiology: diagnostic and prognostic tests. *Rheumatol* 2003; 15:105–109.

Wu AH, Smith A, Christenson RH, Murakami MM, Apple FS. Evaluation of a point-of-care assay for cardiac markers for patients suspected of acute myocardial infarction. *Clin Chim Acta* 2004; 346:211–219.

Wulfkuhle JD, Paweletz CP, Steeg PS, Petricoin EF, Liotta L. Proteomic approaches to the diagnosis, treatment, and monitoring of cancer. *Adv Exp Med Biol* 2003; 532:59–68.

Xiao Z, Prieto D, Conrads TP, Veenstra TD, Issaq HJ. Proteomic patterns: their potential for disease diagnosis. *Mol Cell Endocrinol* 2005; 230:95–106.

Zak-Prelich M, McKenzie RC, Sysa-Jedrzejowska A, Norval M. Local immune responses and systemic cytokine responses in zoster: relationship to the development of postherpetic neuralgia. *Clin Exp Immunol* 2003; 131:318–323.

Correspondence to: Laszlo Urban, MD, PhD, Preclinical Compound Profiling, Lead Discovery Center, Discovery Technologies, NIBRI, Cambridge, MA 01932, USA. Email: laszlo.urban@novartis.com.

Emerging Strategies for the Treatment of Neuropathic Pain, edited by James N. Campbell, Allan I. Basbaum, André Dray, Ronald Dubner, Robert H. Dworkin, and Christine N. Sang, IASP Press, Seattle, © 2006.

23

Animal Studies of Pain: Lessons for Drug Development

Charles J. Vierck

Department of Neuroscience and McKnight Brain Institute, University of Florida College of Medicine, Gainesville, Florida, USA

METHODOLOGICAL CONSIDERATIONS FOR PAIN TESTING IN LABORATORY ANIMALS

For 34 years, my collaborators and I have proposed and documented the need for, even the necessity of using, operant testing methods for modeling pain sensitivity in laboratory animals. In the meantime, pain researchers have almost exclusively employed reflex measures of nociceptive sensitivity, providing a massive experimental evaluation of reflex modulation involving spinal and brainstem circuits. Some discussion at the conference that inspired this volume focused on whether reflex tests used for laboratory animal screening have optimally provided new agents that effectively control clinical pain. However, the answer is unknown, because there has been so little use of behavioral endpoints that appropriately assess pain perception. The thesis of this chapter is that nociceptive stimulation should continue to be used to validate ratings of clinical pain and that operant escape from similar forms of exteroceptive stimulations should constitute the dependent variable for associated laboratory animal models. Advantages of exteroceptive stimulation for relating laboratory animal experiments to human experiments are described, and methods of operant escape testing are outlined. The chapter aims to encourage investigators to employ operant behavioral procedures that reflect processing of nociception throughout the neuraxis. Emphasis on exteroceptive stimulation is not meant to discount methods of intentional interoceptive stimulation that are not covered here but have been used to characterize visceral pain conditions.

Limitations inherent to reflex tests can be appreciated logically, without extensive experimental verification. For example, there has been widespread recognition for some time that recordings from spinal neurons represent mechanisms of first-order coding of pain only if the neurons can be back-fired from the thalamus (Willis and Coggeshall 1978). The implication of this procedural requirement, which substantially increases the difficulty of neurophysiological experiments, is clear. It is necessary to know that the recorded output of spinal neurons reaches the cerebrum and is not limited to spinal or brainstem levels of processing. However, afferent driving of moto-neurons, without the necessity of cerebral processing, evokes limb and tail withdrawal, which are the predominant reflexes utilized for behavioral evalu-ation of nociceptive sensitivity in laboratory animals (Hargreaves et al. 1988). Withdrawal and flexion reflex circuits are classically described as disynaptic, involving afferent input to interneurons and motoneurons in the ventral horn, and it cannot be presumed that motoneuronal output to muscles is identical to the discharge of spinothalamocortical projection neurons in response to nociceptive stimulation.

Motoneurons provide the output for all behavioral responses, so a ques-tion analogous to backfiring for spinal recordings concerns the origin of input to motoneurons involved in a behavioral response. If we require that nociceptive spinal neurons encoding pain constitute a link in a spinothalamocortical projection system, then pain behaviors should neces-sarily depend on input to the cerebral cortex and on subsequent output from the cortex and associated cerebral structures that ultimately reaches moto-neurons. Because there are long-loop spinal-cortical-spinal reflexes (Bard 1933), additional criteria must be applied for a behavior that reveals levels of pain sensitivity. Briefly, these criteria involve evidence that the behavior is motivated, intentional, complex, and learned. These characteristics de-pend on cerebral processing and exemplify pain behaviors of humans that we particularly care about. For example, when I get a sinus headache (or anticipate one), I am motivated to do something about it; consequently, I decide to take whatever remembered route leads me to the medicine cabinet (or drive to the pharmacist if required), and I take medication that I have learned is effective. These actions are comparable to operant escape, which requires laboratory animals to perform a learned response in order to termi-nate a nociceptive stimulus. In contrast, a variety of less complex, unlearned responses to nociceptive stimulation are not necessarily associated with pain sensations, although they can appear to be motivationally derived, even intentional.

Examples of unlearned behaviors that are more complex than simple flexion are struggling, jumping, and orienting to and attacking a stimulus or the site of stimulation. These responses depend on supraspinal projections and are not present in spinalized animals. However, these and other complex responses to nociceptive stimulation (e.g., licking, biting, guarding, and vocalizing) are retained after high decerebration (Woolf 1984; Berridge 1989; Matthies and Franklin 1992). Particularly in mammals less encephalized than primates, a number of unlearned defensive behaviors are organized within and can be elicited by direct stimulation of the brainstem (Morgan and Whitney 2000). Because the brainstem coordinates motor and autonomic responses to stimuli that threaten homeostasis, behavioral consequences of brainstem activation by nociceptive stimulation can appear to include the emotional tone we associate with pain. However, there are a number of reasons for not relying on these responses to model pain sensitivity.

If our goal is to simulate human pain reactions in laboratory animal experiments, it is necessary to come as close as possible to monitoring responses that depend upon neural connections required for conscious appreciation of pain in humans. The closest we can come to justifying the inference that sensory perception has occurred is to ensure that an animal has learned complex relationships between (1) the duration, intensity, and quality of nociceptive sensations; (2) environmental contingencies such as stimulus location and the availability of escape; and (3) response strategies that optimally attenuate or eliminate pain. Learned responses to nociceptive stimulation require sensory perception and subsequent cerebral processing that occurs outside the realm of spinal and brainstem circuits that mediate unlearned reactions. Therefore, pharmacological agents and other experimental manipulations can be expected to have different effects on the neural circuits integral to learned (operant) and unlearned (reflex) responses to nociceptive stimulation.

THE IMPORTANCE OF EXTEROCEPTIVE STIMULATION
FOR EVALUATION OF PAIN CONDITIONS

To this point, my comments have been restricted to behavioral models involving nociceptive stimulation, but the sources of (or stimuli for) clinical pain in humans often are unknown or are not adaptable to experimental simulation. In some cases, there are sources of neuronal hyperactivity within pain transmission systems (Weng et al. 2000) that result from a prior injury and produce "spontaneous" sensations that can include pain. Consequently, animal models involving observation of spontaneous behaviors such as overgrooming or autotomy have frequently been used for behavioral evaluation after peripheral and central lesions (Coderre et al. 1986). These models are problematic in a number of respects (as discussed below); they have arisen in part from a misconception that chronic pain and elicited pain are so fundamentally different that humans with chronic pain do not respond uniquely to exteroceptive stimulation (Mogil and Crager 2004; Vierck et al. 2005b).

Exteroceptive stimulation has been used effectively to evaluate many forms of chronic clinical pain, including neurogenic pain. Patterns of activity at projection targets within pain transmission systems should be modifiable by any stimuli that access neurons at these sites. In order for chronic pain to be unresponsive to any form of stimulation, neurons from the source of abnormal activity through all subsequent "relays" in nociceptive pathways would have to be completely isolated—an impossible condition for a sensate individual. Thus, studies of chronic pain patients should be able to identify methods of stimulation that reveal characteristics of the offending neuronal systems. Once methods of stimulation that can reveal or modify abnormal sensations are identified for a specific condition, then these techniques can be used in animal models for that form of clinical pain. For example, injury to a peripheral nerve can produce chronic pain, and when this occurs, allodynia is pronounced for certain forms of cutaneous stimulation in the region of referred clinical pain (see Price et al., this volume) and within and adjacent to the receptive field of an injured nerve in an animal model (Vierck et al. 2005a).

Spinal cord injury (SCI), like peripheral nerve injury, produces chronic pain in a subset of patients with apparently similar injuries. Below-level SCI pain is referred to dermatomes well caudal to the spinal level of injury and is particularly refractory to treatment. Below-level pain can progress gradually after apparently complete spinal transection, and rostral deafferentation of pain transmission systems must be a contributing factor. When there is a complete loss of somatosensory input to the cerebrum from segments caudal to a spinal transection, exteroceptive stimulation of dermatomes below the lesion is not useful, except to document that the lesion is complete. However, recent studies have revealed abnormal sensitivity to stimulation of dermatomes above a spinal lesion in humans (Cohen et al. 1996; Vierck et al. 2002b). Heightened activity among spinal neurons in the vicinity of the lesion and by deafferented cells rostral to the lesion has produced a widespread alteration of neuronal excitability.

Similar phenomena occur after incomplete spinal lesions involving the spinothalamic tract. Spinothalamic tractotomy for severe chronic pain, such as pain produced by a cancerous growth affecting an extremity, substantially reduces sensitivity to nociceptive stimulation caudal and contralateral to the lesion. However, chronic pain referred to the affected extremity returns for a subset of patients, and sensitivity to nociceptive stimulation of this limb recovers (Vierck et al. 1986). In addition, stimulation within dermatomes ipsilateral and caudal to the lesion reveals hypersensitivity (Bowsher 1988). These results have been confirmed by operant escape testing before and after unilateral spinothalamic tractotomy of monkeys and rats (Vierck and Luck 1979; Vierck et al. 1990; Vierck and Light 1999). With time after surgery, contralateral nociceptive sensitivity recovers for a subset of animals, and ipsilateral sensitivity becomes abnormally increased. The animal models of spinothalamic tractotomy have additionally shown that excitotoxic influences at the lesion site contribute to the bilateral increase in nociceptive sensitivity over time. Thus, gray matter damage in the region of a spinal white matter lesion can be sufficient to produce an excitatory central generator with widespread influences on pain sensitivity. These effects have been revealed by exteroceptive stimulation of humans and laboratory animals after SCI. The resulting departure from the classical assumption that chronic pain from central lesions results entirely from white matter damage has been confirmed in studies of humans (Finnerup and Jensen 2004), and it has important therapeutic implications. Regeneration of damaged axons to their normal targets is unrealistic, but attenuation of excitotoxicity is feasible.

Another advantage of exteroceptive stimulation for investigation of mechanisms and treatments is revealed by fibromyalgia—a puzzling condition involving widespread pain referred to deep tissues. Because it has been difficult to detect overt pathology within the peripheral or central nervous system, fibromyalgia pain often has been regarded as psychogenic, implying that sensation intensity would be exaggerated in a psychophysical experiment. How do we know that fibromyalgia patients' ratings of clinical pain intensity are comparable to those of control subjects experiencing the same pain intensity? One solution to this problem is to present a variety of stimulus conditions in a manner that precludes knowledge about the parameters presented so that subjects cannot know the relationships between stimulus intensities and experimental manipulations. Studies of this type have revealed a hypersensitivity for thermal and mechanical stimuli among fibromyalgia patients (Price et al. 2002; Staud et al. 2003). A consistent feature of the thermal hypersensitivity is a substantially enhanced duration of elicited pain (Staud et al. 2004), suggesting afterdischarge among central cells in pain projection systems that receive convergent input from deep and superficial nociceptive afferents. Thus, it is useful to verify ratings of human clinical pain with studies of elicited pain. Similar forms of verification are needed for laboratory animal models of clinical pain.

OBSERVATION OF BEHAVIORS THAT ARE NOT ELICITED BY EXTEROCEPTIVE STIMULATION

Attempts to detect the presence of chronic pain in laboratory animals have often involved observation of spontaneous behaviors that are protective of a limb or have the appearance of ongoing aversive reactions. However, it is risky to interpret these behaviors as "pain-related." First, it is not clear whether they are reflexive sensory-motor adaptations or represent intentional protection of a limb. For example, guarding of a limb has been regarded as an intentional response to tonic pain when flexion of a limb is prolonged, i.e., longer in duration than a flexion or withdrawal response to phasic stimulation. However, prolonged flexion of a limb can occur in spinalized rats (Price 1972), and other spontaneous behaviors that imply intent occur in decerebrate rats (Woolf 1984). Therefore, observations of spontaneous behaviors are subject to concerns that apply to reflex measures of nociception.

An example of difficulties interpreting spontaneous behaviors is provided by a prominent model of peripheral neuropathy—chronic constriction injury (CCI). Following unilateral CCI of the sciatic nerve, spontaneous behaviors of the affected limb occur over approximately 40 days (e.g., Kupers et al. 1992), and reflex testing has repeatedly revealed lowered thresholds or latencies for mechanical and thermal (hot and cold) stimulation over a comparable duration (e.g., Kingery et al. 1994). Consistent with cautions that motor deficits of the affected limb predispose it to flex during weight bearing (Kauppila et al. 1998), the spontaneous behaviors and reflex effects can be ascribed to a time-limited postural asymmetry resulting from unilateral injury to peripheral afferent and efferent nerves. Spontaneous behaviors such as guarding are not seen after bilateral CCI of the sciatic nerves, and operant testing reveals no allodynia or hyperalgesia for heat (Vierck et al. 2005a) (Fig. 1). The latter result is supported by recordings from the dorsal horn of rats that have revealed no increase in neuronal sensitivity to heat after unilateral CCI (Palecek et al. 1992; Laird and Bennett 1993; Takaishi et al. 1996). However, operant escape from cold is enhanced for more than 100 days (Fig. 1), in contrast to the temporary appearance of spontaneous behaviors and enhancement of segmental reflex responses to cold or heat after unilateral CCI. The longevity of enhanced escape from cold after CCI is consistent with an extended duration of chronic pain when it results from nerve injury in humans, but recovery of asymmetric postures and reflex effects after CCI is not. Thus, CCI differentially affects sensory projection neurons and spinal circuits involved in reciprocal motor innervation.

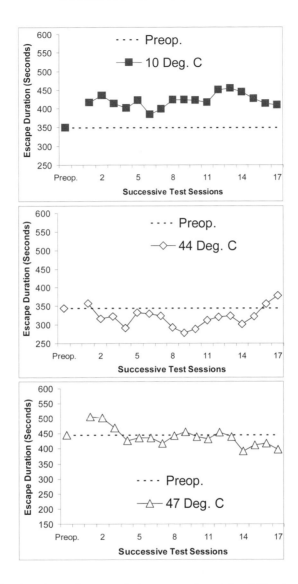

Fig. 1. Cascaded durations of escape during successive trials of 10 minutes (600 s) are shown for a group of nine female rats tested before (preop.) and after bilateral ligation of the sciatic nerves (chronic constriction injury; CCI). The top panel shows that escape from 10°C was consistently (and significantly) enhanced over 17 testing sessions after CCI (approximately 100 days). In contrast, escape from 44°C (middle panel) or 47°C (bottom panel) was not increased over the same period after CCI, compared to preoperative means (dashed lines). The lowest ordinate value for each graph approximates the preoperative mean of time spent on the thermally regulated plate (600 s minus the cumulative escape duration). Note that 44°C and 10°C are equally matched in aversiveness (preop. escape duration), but responses to these temperatures were affected differentially by CCI. Also note the presence of a stimulus-response function (more escape from 47°C than from 44°C). Data are from Vierck et al. (2005a).

IS SELF-INJURIOUS BEHAVIOR NECESSARILY
INDICATIVE OF CHRONIC PAIN?

Special considerations apply to spontaneous behaviors that are self-injurious, such as autotomy or overgrooming. Rather than appearing to protect a
limb affected by neuronal injury, laboratory animals can engage in self-
injurious behavior directed at a peripheral region affected by injury to a
nerve or the spinal cord. When nociceptive afferents or central nociceptive
pathways are damaged, self-injurious behavior directed at the affected peripheral region will be less punishing than similar treatment of a normally
innervated limb, or it may not be painful at all, depending upon the injury.
Experimental reduction of this behavior by local anesthesia and other manipulations indicates that these animals are experiencing an abnormal sensation (Seltzer et al. 1991). A recent case report of self-injurious scratching by
a patient with an excitotoxic spinal lesion (a cavernous hemangioma) docu-
ments referral of both pain and itching to the affected region and makes a
case for itch as the stimulus that elicits self-injurious behavior (Dey et al.
2005). From the perspective of research concerning control over abnormal
central activity in pain transmission systems, it makes little difference whether
it is itch or pain that elicits self-injurious behavior. It is likely that both pain
and itch derive from tonic ongoing activity among neurons with axons in the
spinothalamic tract (Craig 2001), and both sensations are aversive. However, sensations of itch are rare, relative to pain, and nonaversive paresthesias
are reported considerably more often than itch or pain after nerve or spinal
cord injury in humans. Therefore, it cannot be concluded that autotomy is
elicited by either pain or itch in an animal model.

Not only is it impossible to identify an eliciting sensation for self-
injurious behavior in a laboratory animal, but autotomy often is highly variable in time and between animals with peripheral or central injuries. The
reasons for this variability are unclear. Autotomy has not been associated
with hyperalgesia in our primate and rodent studies of spinothalamic tractotomy (Vierck et al. 1990; Vierck and Light 1999), a procedure that produces
abnormal activity in pain transmission pathways (Weng et al. 2000). In other
animal models that can produce autotomy reliably (e.g., peripheral nerve
section or rhizotomy), it is unlikely that the behavior is driven by tonic pain
in all animals, based on comparisons with the incidence of tonic pain in
humans with similar injuries. Abnormal activity among dorsal root ganglion
cells and central cells may well elicit reflexive chewing or scratching with
or without referral of tonic sensations of pain or itch to the anesthetic receptive field of the nerve.

AVAILABLE OPERANT METHODS FOR EVALUATING NOCICEPTIVE RESPONSES OF LABORATORY ANIMALS

An overriding consideration for animal models of pain is to mimic, as nearly as possible, methods that are used for pain testing of humans. It is desirable that such methods reveal unique characteristics of disordered pain sensitivity in humans with different forms of chronic pain. As outlined by Noordenbos (1959), nociceptive sensitivity in the presence of clinical pain can exist in at least three basic forms: (1) a lowering of pain threshold, ordinarily with increased sensitivity throughout the range of stimuli that normally produce tolerable levels of pain (allodynia and hyperalgesia); (2) a normal pain threshold but an increased slope of pain intensities relative to ratings of control subjects for suprathreshold pain (hyperalgesia); and (3) an elevated pain threshold but a dramatically increased slope of pain intensities over the higher range of normally tolerable nociceptive stimuli (hyperpathia). It is clear that detection of each of these types of abnormal nociceptive sensitivity cannot rely solely upon threshold testing, which is typically attempted with reflex measures. Plotting of a stimulus-response function across a wide range of stimulus intensities is needed to fully describe the nociceptive sensitivity of a laboratory animal or human subject. For example, in a study involving interruption of descending spinal pathways in the dorsolateral column of monkeys—a lesion expected to increase sensitivity to nociceptive input to segments below the lesion—thresholds for operant escape were not affected, but the slope of the function relating escape to stimulus intensity was considerably enhanced (Vierck et al. 1971), indicating hyperalgesia. In contrast, flexion reflex amplitudes of the ipsilateral limb are reduced by this lesion (Vierck et al. 2002b).

Early studies of nociceptive sensitivity of human and nonhuman primates in my laboratory utilized electrical stimulation of the lateral calf. Parenthetical comments about electrical stimulation are presented here, because of a bias among some that it is an "unnatural" stimulus. Electrical stimulation of a nerve trunk, often used by neurophysiologists, produces discharge in an unphysiologically large population of afferents, and psychophysical characterization of sensations elicited by a wide range of intensities delivered directly to a nerve is virtually nonexistent. In contrast, parameters of electrical stimulation of the skin (away from a nerve trunk) can be adjusted to produce quite natural sensations of pain with many discriminable intensities, from those below pain detection threshold to levels approaching the pain tolerance threshold (Vierck et al. 1983a, 1995; Vierck and Cooper 1984). Intensities subthreshold for pain have a tingling (sometimes an itching) quality that gives way to an increasingly intense sensation of heat pain as the current is increased.

In studies with monkeys, we started with a paradigm having features that are adaptable to many laboratory animal species and methods of stimulation. The monkeys were gently restrained in a testing chair for short daily sessions of 15 to 30 minutes. Electrical stimulation was applied to either lateral calf and could be terminated (escaped) by pressing a panel (Lineberry and Vierck 1975) or by pulling on a manipulandum (Vierck et al. 1990) with either hand. We chose electrical stimulation for several reasons: it is easy to present different intensities from trial to trial; sensation intensity is immediately proportional to stimulus intensity (rather than increasing gradually within a trial); the stimulus terminates abruptly, providing the animals with immediate reinforcement for responding; and there is no tissue injury.

An important feature of this or any operant escape task is that the stimulus intensity presented in an individual trial should not be contingent upon whether or not an animal responded on the previous trial. For example, in a typical operant titration paradigm, stimulus intensity is increased from trial to trial until the animal escapes. The transition from no response to termination of a trial provides an estimate of threshold. Because stimulation intensity is decreased for trials immediately (or soon) after a response occurs in titration paradigms, the animals learn to avoid high levels of stimulation by responding to low levels. Titration thresholds for electrical stimulation correspond to detection thresholds for a non-nociceptive sensation (Greenspan et al. 1986); typically they are an order of magnitude lower than escape thresholds obtained when stimulus intensity is not contingent upon responding (Vierck and Cooper 1984). Thus, titration thresholds result from avoidance learning, not from escape learning.

Similar problems have plagued reflex tests—particularly methods such as the Hargreaves test (Hargreaves et al. 1988), which is the most prevalent method for evaluating reflexes. On the first few exposures to radiant heat or mechanical stimulation of a foot, a pure reflex response probably occurs. However, with repeated trials, an animal can learn to withdraw the foot as soon as the radiant thermal stimulus is applied or a low level of heat is felt, or the animal can learn to withdraw from any detectable level of mechanical stimulation. There is no deterrent to avoidance learning in this paradigm, and reflex withdrawal responses cannot be discriminated subjectively from avoidance responses. In addition, because delivery of the stimulus and judgment of a criterion response depend upon a number of experimenter-related factors, this procedure is susceptible to experimenter bias. In an extensive study of reflex thresholds using the Hargreaves procedure, the most potent determinant of variability was the experimenter (Chesler et al. 2002).

   Avoidance learning can be prevented and evaluated by parametric design of an operant test. First, it is important to present stimuli that are below pain threshold but clearly detectable by the animals. Also, the duration of the target stimulus intensity on each trial must be long enough for the animals to evaluate sensation intensity. If most or all of the stimuli are high in intensity, above the pain threshold, animals learn to respond quickly and often. When many of the stimuli are below pain threshold or mildly painful, animals typically restrict reliable and fast responding to high intensities. A stimulus-response function with significant slope demonstrates that avoidance learning has not been a factor on a paradigm intended to evaluate escape. Avoidance responding will occur similarly in response to different intensities, producing a flat stimulus-response function. Stimulus-response functions for escape should reveal few or no responses to intensities below pain threshold and progressively faster, more vigorous, and more reliable responding to high intensities. A plateau region of maximal responding will depend upon the response variable. For example, the percentage of trials escaped at each intensity determines escape threshold (e.g., 50% escape) and provides an estimate of sensitivity to the low end of painful stimuli (from 50% to 100% escape). Response latency extends the stimulus-response function up to moderate to high levels of tolerable pain. Animals typically terminate the stimulus at shorter and shorter latencies for stimulus intensities at which escape first occurs, through intensities above the level that elicits escape on 100% of the trials. Understandably, the variability of response latencies decreases as stimulus intensity increases, and at high intensities the animals have short latency responses on a high percentage of trials. Similarly, we have used response force as a dependent variable, because responses become reliably more imperative as stimulus intensity increases for both humans and laboratory animals (Vierck et al. 1971, 1983a,b).

   To ensure that learned escape responses do not have a reflexive component, precautions should be taken so that reflex responses cannot operate a manipulandum used to trigger escape. For example, bar or panel presses that terminate stimulation should be made with a limb other than the one stimulated. Additionally, because reflex responses to electrical stimulation occur at latencies shorter than the minimal reaction time for an operant response, we have utilized an interval of 200 ms after stimulus onset in which reactions such as the startle reflex are not measured and do not terminate the nociceptive stimulus. Unfortunately, nearly all reflex assays involve observation of the stimulated limb, which is the limb (or tail) affected by an experimental manipulation, and there is no objective way of separating reflex and operant responses using these methods.

For any stimulus continuum utilized to generate stimulus-response functions for escape, it is important to be aware of the receptor populations activated across the intensities delivered. Electrocutaneous stimulation has advantages and limitations such as the following: (1) It bypasses receptor transduction and can be compared to methods that selectively activate a subpopulation of nociceptors. (2) It activates afferents in sequence according to size and myelination, so that non-nociceptive Aβ axons are activated at low intensities, then nociceptive Aδ axons, and then C nociceptors as the stimulus intensity increases. Generally, stimulus-response functions will plateau before intensities are reached that activate C nociceptors. Therefore, electrical stimulation delivered in brief trains provides a model of Aδ-fiber nociception. (3) Stimulus parameters can be monitored with precision and adjusted so that the skin is not traumatized by the range of intensities needed. (4) Responses to non-nociceptive stimulation can be observed readily, to determine whether allodynia has been produced by a manipulation.

Operant escape paradigms using electrical stimulation have revealed stimulus-response functions for escape that are compatible with expectations from human studies but different from the functions for flexion reflex thresholds or amplitudes. For example, the threshold for flexion is below that for escape (Cooper and Vierck 1986), demonstrating that limb flexion is not necessarily a nociceptive reflex, as is often assumed and stated. A surprising finding in these studies was that neither escape nor flexion reflexes of monkeys in response to Aδ-fiber nociceptive input were sensitive to low doses of morphine. This finding prompted us to evaluate the effects of morphine on psychophysical ratings of pain by human subjects. For electrical, mechanical, and thermal stimulation, second pain from activation of C nociceptors is attenuated substantially by a therapeutic dose of morphine for opioid-naive human subjects (less than 0.25 mg/kg), but first pain from activation of Aδ nociceptors is not significantly affected (Vierck et al. 1984; Cooper et al. 1986). For primates, there is a hierarchy of sensitivity to systemic morphine: C nociception >> Aδ nociception > Aδ flexion reflex. These findings prompted us to develop an operant paradigm that would be sensitive to input from C nociceptors. The clinical effectiveness of systemic morphine, together with suspicions that numerous forms of chronic pain result from abnormal input from C nociceptors, makes this an important priority for translational research. Also, the need to evaluate responses to C nociception constitutes another important rationale for operant methodology, because protective reflex behaviors such as limb withdrawal or flexion are elicited by input from myelinated afferents.

Repetitive stimulation of C nociceptors produces temporal summation of second pain (Price et al. 1977), and tests of temporal summation can reveal central mechanisms relevant to chronic pain (Staud et al. 2001). There-fore, our first operant procedure for evaluation of C nociception used a paradigm modeled after procedures that "wind up" neuronal activity (Yeomans et al. 1996). Monkeys were trained to terminate series of thermal stimuli by pulling a manipulandum after the fourth, fifth, sixth, or last of seven pulses of thermal stimulation when a tone was presented (signaled escape). Brief (700-ms) pulses of stimulation were applied by tapping the skin with a preheated thermode. The force of escape responses was related to stimulus intensity, an important indication that escape responding was dictated by sensation magnitude. A low dose of morphine (0.25 mg/kg) significantly reduced escape responding. Although this paradigm successfully evaluated responsivity to C nociception, the training time was prolonged. Subsequently, a simpler paradigm was utilized with rats, using thermal stimulation of the hindpaws (C. Vierck and A. Light, unpublished data), but the rats were unable to learn that lever presses terminated the train of stimuli. Because second pain responses are delayed, it is not obvious to an animal that a response has terminated stimulation. Therefore, our attempts to selectively stimulate C nociceptors of laboratory animals have not continued to use pulsatile stimulation paradigms that are effective for human psychophysical evaluation of second pain and temporal summation (see Price et al., this volume).

Fortunately, maintained stimulation that is just suprathreshold for pain can be used to preferentially stimulate C nociceptors, as demonstrated by Yeomans and Proudfit (1996). Based on these findings, we developed an operant escape paradigm for rodents that tests sensitivity to thermal stimulation (Mauderli et al. 2000) (Fig. 2). Because pain from heat stimulation develops gradually, there is a potential for avoidance responding. One solution for this problem is to set up a conflict paradigm. Rats or mice are placed in an enclosure with the floor temperature set to an aversive level of heat or cold. Escape to another compartment with a thermally neutral platform is always available, but the escape compartment is brightly lit, which is aversive for rodents. The animals cycle back and forth between compartments, and time on the escape platform is determined by the level of thermal stimulation. Stimulus-response functions for heat and cold are consistent with expectations from human psychophysics (Vierck et al. 2004) (Fig. 2).

Additional validation of this paradigm by injection of systemic morphine has shown that escape from 44°C is decreased by a low dose (0.5 mg/kg) that has the opposite effect on (i.e., increases) reflex lick/guard responding to the same temperature (Vierck et al. 2002a). This finding is an important demonstration that central inhibitory modulation of reflex circuits differs critically from that of pain pathways. Other disparate effects on lick/

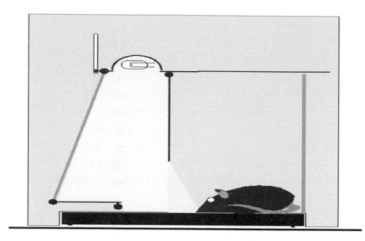

Fig. 2. A thermal escape apparatus, adaptable to operant testing of rats or mice. The animal is shown on a plate that is thermally regulated by circulation of water through internal channels. A hanging septum separates the relatively dark compartment for thermal stimulation from a brightly lit compartment with a thermally neutral escape platform. Occupancy of the escape platform is detected by switches triggered by the animal's weight. Custom-designed software keeps track of the onset and duration of each period of time on the plate and the platform during trials of 10 to 15 minutes. It also is used to calibrate and set the light intensity level. Redrawn from Mauderli et al. (2000).

guard reflexes and operant escape have been obtained in studies using the thermal/light conflict paradigm. Excitotoxic injury to the thoracic spinal gray matter produces a below-level enhancement of escape but not of lick/guard responses (Acosta-Rua 2003). Prior restraint stress enhances escape but attenuates lick/guard responses (King et al. 2003). Intrathecal injection of substance P-saporin over lumbosacral spinal segments reduces escape but not lick/guard responses (Vierck et al. 2003). Spinothalamic tractotomy selectively attenuates contralateral escape responses but reduces flexion reflexes bilaterally (Vierck et al. 1990; Vierck and Light 2000). These direct comparisons of escape and reflex responses to identical stimuli are required to determine whether unlearned responses can be used for screening of antinociceptive treatments. In order to conclude that reflex assays can suffice, it is necessary to show that they *always* produce results comparable to those obtained with measures sensitive to cerebral processing of nociception, and this is not the case.

Reflex assays appear to have flourished because they are perceived to be time-efficient and because of investigators' interest in spinal processing of nociception. However, without the training required for operant testing, animals are not fully acclimated to handling and nociceptive stimulation during reflex testing, and stress effects become a concern. In general, acute stress depresses reflexes and activates systems that promote immobility (Morgan and Whitney 2000). Furthermore, reflex testing requires observation of the animal and subjective interpretation of responsivity. Data collection during operant testing can be automated, and stimulus delivery and response interpretation are objectively independent of the investigator. For reflex testing, high stimulus intensities of thermal stimulation have been employed consistently in order to minimize variability between animals and trials. Again, this method is efficient, but it has a number of undesirable consequences. Responses to high intensities of heat practically preclude demonstrations of hypersensitivity, because of a floor effect—the primary reflex measure, latency, is already minimal in the absence of an experimental manipulation. Moreover, the initial response latency was the least reliable measure in our studies of lick/guard and escape responding (Vierck et al. 2004). The first response latency is influenced by the strong exploratory tendencies of rodents. Additional measures of responsivity, such as the duration or frequency of licking or guarding, are limited by the necessity of short trial durations at high stimulus intensities, to prevent trauma to the skin. This factor does not apply to operant testing over a wide range of intensities, because the animals can escape the thermal stimulus and prevent skin temperatures from reaching traumatic levels.

Not only have investigators using reflex assays made parametric choices designed to limit variability, but the standard animal for these experiments is an inbred albino male rat with poor vision and strong tendencies toward immobility. Females are avoided because of potential variability associated with the estrous cycle. Our experiments with rodents have primarily utilized Long-Evans hooded females for a number of reasons. They are active and inquisitive animals that are well suited to behavioral experiments. A number of chronic pain conditions primarily affect females, and hormonal variations related to estrus may be a contributing factor that can be evaluated. In our operant and reflex studies of untreated males and females, we have not encountered substantial differences in variability that increase the number of females needed for statistical comparisons. For our long-term studies of recovery from neuronal injury, females are advantageous because they remain docile and do not gain as much weight with age. Furthermore, they are more suitable than male rats for thermal stimulation paradigms because thermal stimulation of the scrotum substantially increases the influences of temperature regulation on responses that are intended to reflect nociceptive sensitivity of the paws (Gordon and Heath 1986; Hole and Tjolsen 1993).

CONTROL PROCEDURES AND PARAMETRIC VARIATIONS FOR EVALUATION OF NOCICEPTION

Regardless of the behavioral assay utilized, controls for confounding effects must be incorporated. For reflexes, motoneuronal excitability is the principal concern, in contrast to operant tests involving behaviors that can be sufficient to execute an escape response over a wide range of excitability states for motoneurons. Testing the effects of experimental manipulations on non-nociceptive reflexes would provide useful controls to determine whether an effect on a nociceptive reflex results from sensory or motor modulation (Kiernan et al. 1995; Schomburg 1997), but this additional testing is almost never done. For operant responses, a variety of motor controls are available. For example, some manipulations have produced a selective effect on escape responses from heat but not cold (e.g., morphine; Vierck et al. 2002a) or from cold but not heat (CCI; Vierck et al. 2005b). Similarly, escape from a lighted compartment to a dark compartment has been used to control for motor effects of a treatment (Mauderli et al. 2000). Escape responses that are unaffected provide the most stringent control for possible motor and motivational effects of a manipulation on escape responses to another stimulus. For example, unaffected responses to light indicate that aversion has not changed independently of the stimulus and show that neither activity levels nor motor capacities have been altered to a degree that thermal escape is modified independently of sensory modulation. In addition, we present two trials each day and vary the temperatures. For example, depending on the experimental goals, two or more temperatures can be sequenced according to a preselected schedule (e.g., 36°–44°C, 44°–36°C, 36°–10°C, 10°–36°C, 10°–44°C, 44°–10°C). With sequences like this example, the animals learn to sample the stimulus during each trial and adjust escape according to relative sensation intensity. Responsivity to the neutral stimulus (36°C) should be less than that for nociceptive stimulation, demonstrating that the animals have not developed avoidance tendencies. An additional goal of presenting two trials per day is to stabilize and manipulate skin and body temperature on the first trial, prior to a critical test on the second trial.

Final methodological considerations concern behavioral training and the variety of behavioral paradigms that can be used to evaluate cerebrally mediated nociceptive responses. Learning of an escape response can occur quickly with structuring to encourage responding. For example, we acclimate animals to the test apparatus without light over the escape platform and gradually increase heat or decrease cold plate temperatures over days. Once the animals have learned to escape, the light is turned on over the platform, and the sequence of temperatures is repeated. After training, some testing sessions are required to stabilize performance. A useful variation for training can be to provide food or liquid reinforcement in the escape compartment to establish responding, and then change the paradigm so that the same response terminates nociceptive stimulation. Innumerable responses can be required for escape. For example, bar pressing on a fixed ratio schedule requiring a certain number of responses per escape is effective when the nociceptive stimulus can be turned on and off during a trial.

A variation of conflict paradigms has been used to manipulate the stimulus-response function into moderate to high levels of pain. For some experiments, there may be reasons to evaluate pain tolerance rather than to measure responsivity to low and intermediate levels of nociceptive stimulation (Manning and Vierck 1973). For example, when access to food or liquid reinforcement is contingent on receipt of nociceptive stimulation, interruption of ingestion provides a measure of aversion associated with different temperatures (Casey and Morrow 1989; Neubert et al. 2005).

Another variation of conflict paradigms provides important confirmation that a manipulation selectively affects either cold or heat pain (e.g., Vierck et al. 2002a, 2005a). We have tested animals in a two-compartment preference test, with one floor hot and the other cold (Vierck et al. 2002a). The animals learn quickly to alternate occupancy of the two compartments, and they consistently apportion time in the compartments according to the relative aversiveness of the two temperatures. This test has revealed substantial sex differences for Long-Evans rats that are not apparent for lick/guard testing (Acosta-Rua 2003). Temperatures that resulted in 50% exposures for cold and heat for females were determined to be 10°C and 45°C. Males were then tested at these parameters, and they strongly preferred the cold side. Temperatures that stabilized the males at 50% occupancy of each side were 0.3°C and 43°C. Thus, heat is more aversive for males, and cold is more aversive for females. These differences in stimulus preference cannot be accounted for in terms of motivational, emotional, or motor (activity) differences.

SUMMARY

Arguments against the use of reflex assays of nociception are particularly relevant for screening of systemic pharmacological agents that might attenuate clinical pain. Implicit in the use of reflex measures is an assumption that pain modulation is best achieved at early stages of nociceptive processing. For example, morphine acts in part at spinal levels, presynaptically, inhibiting input from C nociceptors (Taddese et al. 1995). This mechanism is ideal for clinical pain control—attenuation of tonic pain at the entry level and preservation of input from Aδ nociceptors that elicits protective reflexes and warns against damaging exposure to external sources of pain. However, reflexes that are observable behaviorally are highly insensitive to morphine and presumably to new and improved opioid agonists. Furthermore, opioid receptors are located throughout the nervous system, as are receptors for most transmitters and modulators. It is crucial that actions all along the neuraxis should be accounted for in a drug screening. Routine use of algesic assays that depend upon cerebral processing would provide the potential for identifying pharmacological agents that are effective *because* they act preferentially at high levels of nociceptive processing. For example, systemic morphine may attenuate the affective dimension of pain (Beecher 1957), and operant escape is sensitive to such a reduction of aversion that normally accompanies nociceptive sensations.

From the perspective of basic science, it is reasonable and logical to seek an understanding of early nociceptive processing in order to appreciate upstream elaborations. The goal of reflex assessments for procedures such as intrathecal pharmacological administration has been to reflect actions on sensory transduction in the dorsal horn. However, receptors for nearly all neurotransmitters and peptide modulators that have been studied extensively using nociceptive reflex assays are located on motoneurons and/or on ventral horn interneurons that modulate motoneurons. Reflex measures are highly susceptible to motoneuronal modulation. This applies to intrathecal pharmacological application and to descending modulation initiated by pharmacological influences on the brainstem (Morgan and Whitney 2000; Jankowska et al. 2003). Thus, reflex assessment without an appropriate control for effects on motoneurons cannot be relied upon to reflect alterations of sensory transduction at spinal levels, and it is not capable of revealing supraspinal effects on sensory intensity. It is inappropriate and misleading to refer to altered excitability of a reflex circuit as analgesia, allodynia, or hyperalgesia. If the sensitivity of a reflex response is altered, this effect should be referred to as hyper- or hyporeflexia.

As an alternative to reflex testing, this chapter has presented some examples and principles behind operant testing paradigms, based on my experience with techniques using exteroceptive stimulation that can be terminated (escaped from) by animal subjects or rated by human subjects. A simple escape response is impoverished relative to verbal or visual analogue scale ratings by humans, but with variation of stimulus parameters, a high degree of correspondence can be shown for effects of pharmacological agents and other manipulations on different forms of human pain and on animal models of these conditions. These laboratory animal studies can then form an appropriate basis for clinical trials.

REFERENCES

Acosta-Rua A. Effects of midthoracic gray matter damage on below-level pain sensitivities. Dissertation. University of Florida, 2003.

Bard P. Studies on the cerebral cortex. I. Localized control of placing and hopping reaction in the cat and their normal management by small cortical remnants. *Arch Neurol Psychiatry* 1933; 30:40–74.

Beecher HK. Measurement of pain: prototype for the quantitative study of subjective sensations. *Pharmacol Rev* 1957; 9:59–209.

Berridge KC. Progressive degradation of serial grooming chains by descending decerebration. *Behav Brain Res* 1989; 33:241–253.

Bowsher D. Contralateral mirror-image pain following anterolateral chordotomy. *Pain* 1988; 18:63–65.

Casey KL, Morrow TJ. Effect of medial bulboreticular and raphe nuclear lesions on the excitation and modulation of supraspinal nocifensive behaviors in the cat. *Brain Res* 1989; 501:150–161.

Chesler E, Wilson S, Lariviere W, Rodriguez-Zas S, Mogil J. Influences of laboratory environment on behavior. *Nature Neurosci* 2002; 5:1101–1102.

Coderre T, Grines R, Melzack R. Deafferentation and chronic pain in animals: an evaluation of evidence suggesting autotomy is related to pain. *Pain* 1986; 26:61–84.

Cohen M, Song Z, Schandler S, Ho W, Vulpe M. Sensory detection and pain thresholds in spinal cord injury patients with and without dysesthetic pain, and in chronic low back pain patients. *Somatosens Mot Res* 1996; 13:29–37.

Cooper BY, Vierck CJ Jr. Measurement of pain and morphine hyperalgesia in monkeys. *Pain* 1986; 26:361–392.

Cooper BY, Vierck CJ Jr, Yeomans DC. Selective reduction of second pain sensations by systemic morphine in humans. *Pain* 1986; 24:93–116.

Craig A. Spinothalamic lamina I neurons selectively sensitive to histamine: a central neural pathway for itch. *Nat Neurosci* 2001; 4:9–10.

Dey D, Oandrum O, Oaklander A. Central neuropathic itch from spinal-cord cavernous hemangioma: a human case, a possible animal model, and hypotheses about pathogenesis. *Pain* 2005; 13:233–237.

Finnerup N, Jensen T. Spinal cord injury pain: mechanisms and treatment. *Eur J Neurol* 2004; 11:73–82.

Gordon C, Heath J. Integration and central processing in temperature regulation. *Ann Rev Physiol* 1986; 48:595–612.

Greenspan JD, Vierck CJ Jr, Ritz LA. Sensitivity to painful and non-painful electrocutaneous stimuli in monkeys: effects of anterolateral chordotomy. *J Neurosci* 1986; 6:380–390.

Hargreaves K, Dubner R, Brown F, Flores C, Joris J. A new and sensitive method for measuring thermal nociception in cutaneous hyperalgesia. *Pain* 1988; 32:77–88.

Hole K, Tjolsen A. The tail-flick and formalin tests in rodents: changes in skin temperature as a confounding factor. *Pain* 1993; 53:247–254.

Jankowska E, Hammar I, Slawinska U, Maleszak K, Edgley S. Neuronal basis of crossed actions from the reticular formation on feline hindlimb motoneurons. *J Neurosci* 2003; 23:1867–1878.

Kauppila T, Kontinen VK, Pertovaara A. Weight bearing of the limb as a confounding factor in assessment of mechanical allodynia in the rat. *Pain* 1998; 74:55–59.

Kiernan B, Phillips J, Price D. Hypnotic analgesia reduces R-III nociceptive reflex: further evidence concerning the multifactorial nature of hypnotic analgesia. *Pain* 1995; 63:391–392.

King C, Rodgers J, Devine D, Vierck CJ, Yezierski R. Differential effects of stress on escape versus reflex responses to nociceptive thermal stimuli in the rat. *Brain Res* 2003; 987:214–222.

Kingery WS, John JDL, Roffers A, Kell DR. The resolution of neuropathic hyperalgesia following motor and sensory functional recovery in sciatic axonotmetic mononeuropathies. *Pain* 1994; 58:157–168.

Kupers RC, Nuytten D, De Castro-Costa M, Gybels JM. A time course analysis of the changes in spontaneous and evoked behaviour in a rat model of neuropathic pain. *Pain* 1992; 50:101–111.

Laird JMA, Bennett GJ. An electrophysiological study of dorsal horn neurons in the spinal cord of rats with an experimental peripheral neuropathy. *J Neurophysiol* 1993; 69:2072–2085.

Lineberry CG, Vierck CJ Jr. Attenuation of pain reactivity by caudate nucleus stimulation in monkeys. *Brain Res* 1975; 98:119–134.

Manning AA, Vierck CJ Jr. Behavioral assessment of pain detection and tolerance in monkeys. *J Exp Anal Behav* 1973; 19:125–132.

Matthies BK, Franklin KBJ. Formalin pain is expressed in decerebrate rats but not attenuated by morphine. *Pain* 1992; 51:199–206.

Mauderli A, Acosta-Rua A, Vierck CJ. An operant assay of thermal pain in conscious, unrestrained rats. *J Neurosci Methods* 2000; 97:19–29.

Mogil J, Crager S. What should we be measuring in behavioral studies of chronic pain in animals? *Pain* 2004; 112:12–15.

Morgan MM, Whitney PK. Immobility accompanies the antinociception mediated by the rostral ventromedial medulla of the rat. *Brain Res* 2000; 872:276–281.

Neubert JK, Widmer C, Malphurs W, et al. Use of a novel thermal operant behavioral assay for characterization of orofacial pain sensitivity. *Pain* 2005; 116:386–395.

Noordenbos W. *Pain.* New York: Elsevier, 1959.

Palecek J, Paleckova V, Dougherty PM, Carlton SM, Willis WD. Responses of spinothalamic tract cells to mechanical and thermal stimulation of skin in rats with experimental peripheral neuropathy. *J Neurophysiol* 1992; 67:1562–1573.

Price DD. Characteristics of second pain and flexion reflexes indicative of prolonged central summation. *Exp Neurol* 1972; 37:371–387.

Price DD, Hu JW, Dubner R, Gracely RH. Peripheral suppression of first pain and central summation of second pain evoked by noxious heat pulses. *Pain* 1977; 3:57–68.

Price DD, Staud R, Robinson ME, et al. Enhanced temporal summation second pain and its central modulation in fibromyalgia patients. *Pain* 2002; 99:49–59.

Schomburg ED. Restrictions on the interpretation of spinal reflex modulation in pain and analgesia research. *Pain Forum* 1997; 6:101–109.

Seltzer Z, Beilin B, Ginzburg R, Paran Y, Shimko T. The role of injury discharge in the induction of neuropathic pain behavior in rats. *Pain* 1991; 46:327–336.

Staud R, Vierck CJ, Cannon RL, Mauderli AP, Price DD. Abnormal sensitization and temporal summation of second pain (wind-up) in patients with fibromyalgia syndrome. *Pain* 2001; 91:165–175.

Staud R, Cannon RC, Mauderli AP, et al. Temporal summation of pain from mechanical stimulation of muscle tissue in normal controls and subjects with fibromyalgia syndrome. *Pain* 2003; 102:87–95.

Staud R, Price D, Robinson M, Mauderli A, Vierck C. Maintenance of windup of second pain requires less frequent stimulation in fibromyalgia patients compared to normal controls. *Pain* 2004; 110:689–696.

Taddese A, Nah S-Y, McCleskey EW. Selective opioid inhibition of small nociceptive neurons. *Science* 1995; 270:1366–1369.

Takaishi K, Eisele JH, Carstens E. Behavioral and electrophysiological assessment of hyperalgesia and changes in dorsal horn responses following partial sciatic nerve ligation in rats. *Pain* 1996; 66:297–306.

Vierck CJ Jr, Cooper BY. Guidelines for assessing pain reactions and pain modulation in laboratory animal subjects. In: Kruger L, Liebeskind J (Eds). *Neural Mechanisms of Pain.* New York: Raven Press, 1984, pp 305–322.

Vierck C Jr, Light A. Effects of combined hemotoxic and anterolateral spinal lesions on nociceptive sensitivity. *Pain* 1999; 83:447–457.

Vierck CJ Jr, Light AR. Allodynia and hyperalgesia within dermatomes caudal to a spinal cord injury in primates and rodents. *Prog Brain Res* 2000; 129:411–428.

Vierck CJ Jr, Luck MM. Loss and recovery of reactivity to noxious stimuli in monkeys with primary spinothalamic chordotomies, followed by secondary and tertiary lesions of other cord sectors. *Brain* 1979; 102:233–248.

Vierck CJ Jr, Hamilton DM, Thornby JI. Pain reactivity of monkeys after lesions to the dorsal and lateral columns of the spinal cord. *Exp Brain Res* 1971; 13:140–158.

Vierck CJ Jr, Cooper BY, Cohen RH. Human and non-human primate reactions to painful electrocutaneous stimuli and to morphine. In: Kitchell R, Erickson H (Eds). Animal pain perception and alleviation. *Am Physiol Soc* 1983a, pp 117–132.

Vierck CJ Jr, Cooper BY, Franzen O, Ritz LA, Greenspan JD. Behavioral analysis of CNS pathways and transmitter systems involved in conduction and inhibition of pain sensations and reactions in primates. In: Sprague J, Epstein A (Eds). *Progress in Psychobiology and Physiological Psychology*. New York: Academic Press, 1983b, pp 113–165.

Vierck CJ Jr, Cooper BY, Cohen RH, Yeomans DC, Franzen O. Effects of systemic morphine on monkeys and man: generalized suppression of behavior and preferential inhibition of pain elicited by unmyelinated nociceptors. In: von Euler C, Franzen O, Lindblom U, Ottoson D (Eds). *Somatosensory Mechanisms*, Wenner-Gren International Symposium Series, Vol. 41. London: MacMillan Press, 1984, pp 309–323.

Vierck CJ Jr, Greenspan JD, Ritz LA, Yeomans DC. The spinal pathways contributing to the ascending conduction and the descending modulation of pain sensations and reactions. In: Yaksh T (Ed). *Spinal Systems of Afferent Processing*. Plenum Press, 1986, pp 275–329.

Vierck CJ Jr, Greenspan JD, Ritz LA. Long term changes in purposive and reflexive responses to nociceptive stimulation in monkeys following anterolateral chordotomy. *J Neurosci* 1990; 10:2077–2095.

Vierck CJ Jr, Lee CL, Willcockson HH, et al. Effects of anterolateral spinal lesions on escape responses of rats to hindpaw stimulation. *Somatosens Mot Res* 1995; 12:163–174.

Vierck CJ, Acosta-Rua A, Nelligan R, Tester N, Mauderli A. Low dose systemic morphine attenuates operant escape but facilitates innate reflex responses to thermal stimulation. *J Pain* 2002a; 3:309–319.

Vierck C, Cannon R, Stevens K, Acosta-Rua A, Wirth E. Mechanisms of increased pain sensitivity within dermatomes remote from an injured segment of the spinal cord. In: Yezierski RP, Burchiel KJ (Eds). *Spinal Cord Injury Pain: Assessment, Mechanisms, Management*, Progress in Pain Research and Management, Vol. 23. Seattle: IASP Press, 2002b, pp 155–173.

Vierck CJ, Kline R, Wiley R. Intrathecal substance P-saporin attenuates operant escape from nociceptive thermal stimuli. *Neurosci* 2003; 119:223–232.

Vierck C, Kline R IV, Wiley R. Comparison of operant escape and innate reflex responses to nociceptive skin temperatures produced by heat and cold stimulation of rats. *Behav Neurosci* 2004; 118:627–635.

Vierck CJ, Acosta-Rua A, Johnson RD. Bilateral chronic constriction of the sciatic nerve: a model of long-term cold hyperalgesia. *J Pain* 2005a; 6:507–517.

Vierck CJ, Mauderli AP, Wiley RG. Assessment of pain in laboratory animals: a comment on Mogil and Crager. *Pain* 2005b; 114:520–523.

Weng H-R, Lee J, Lenz F, et al. Functional plasticity in primate somatosensory thalamus following chronic lesion of the ventral lateral spinal cord. *Neuroscience* 2000; 101:393–401.

Willis WD, Coggeshall RE. *Sensory Mechanisms of the Spinal Cord*. New York: Plenum Press, 1978.

Woolf CJ. Long term alterations in the excitability of the flexion reflex produced by peripheral tissue injury in the chronic decerebrate rat. *Pain* 1984; 18:325–343.

Yeomans DC, Proudfit HK. Nociceptive responses to high and low rates of noxious cutaneous heating are mediated by different nociceptors in the rat: electrophysiological evidence. *Pain* 1996; 68:141–150.

Yeomans DC, Cooper BY, Vierck CJ Jr. Effects of systemic morphine on responses of primates to first or second pain sensation. *Pain* 1996; 66:253–263.

Correspondence to: Charles J. Vierck, PhD, Department of Neuroscience and McKnight Brain Institute, University of Florida College of Medicine, P.O. Box 100244, Gainesville, FL 32610-0244, USA. Tel: 352-371-2378; Fax: 352-392-8513; email: vierck@mbi-ufl.edu.

Index